Chronic Obstructive Pulmonary Disease

Editor

PETER J. BARNES

CLINICS IN CHEST MEDICINE

www.chestmed.theclinics.com

March 2014 • Volume 35 • Number 1

ELSEVIER

1600 John F. Kennedy Boulevard • Suite 1800 • Philadelphia, Pennsylvania, 19103-2899

http://www.theclinics.com

CLINICS IN CHEST MEDICINE Volume 35, Number 1
March 2014 ISSN 0272-5231, ISBN-13: 978-0-323-26090-9

Editor: Patrick Manley
Developmental Editor: Casey Jackson

Clinics in Chest Medicine (ISSN 0272-5231) is published quarterly by Elsevier Inc., 360 Park Avenue South, New York, NY 10010-1710. Months of issue are March, June, September, and December. Periodicals postage paid at New York, NY and additional mailing offices. Subscription prices are $345.00 per year (domestic individuals), $556.00 per year (domestic institutions), $165.00 per year (domestic students/residents), $380.00 per year (Canadian individuals), $690.00 per year (Canadian institutions), $470.00 per year (international individuals), $690.00 per year (international institutions), and $230.00 per year (international and Canadian students/residents). International air speed delivery is included in all Clinics subscription prices. All prices are subject to change without notice. **POSTMASTER:** Send address changes to Clinics in Chest Medicine, Elsevier Health Sciences Division, Subscription Customer Service, 3251 Riverport Lane, Maryland Heights, MO 63043. **Customer Service: Telephone: 1-800-654-2452** (U.S. and Canada); **1-314-447-8871** (outside U.S. and Canada). **Fax: 1-314-447-8029. E-mail: journalscustomerservice-usa@elsevier.com** (for print support); **journalsonlinesupport-usa@elsevier.com** (for online support).

Reprints. For copies of 100 or more of articles in this publication, please contact the Commercial Reprints Department, Elsevier Inc., 360 Park Avenue South, New York, NY 10010-1710. Tel.: 212-633-3874; Fax: 212-633-3820; E-mail: reprints@elsevier.com.

Clinics in Chest Medicine is covered in *MEDLINE/PubMed (Index Medicus), Current Contents/Clinical Medicine, EMBASE/ Excerpta Medica, Science Citation Index,* and *ISI/BIOMED.*

Printed and bound by CPI Group (UK) Ltd, Croydon, CR0 4YY

Contributors

EDITOR

PETER J. BARNES, FRS, FMedSci
Head of Respiratory Medicine, National Heart and Lung Institute, Imperial College, London, United Kingdom

AUTHORS

ALVAR AGUSTI, MD, PhD
Professor, Thorax Institute, Hospital Clinic, IDIBAPS, Universitat de Barcelona and CIBER Enfermedades Respiratorias (CIBERES), Mallorca, Spain

PETER J. BARNES, FRS, FMedSci
Head of Respiratory Medicine, National Heart and Lung Institute, Imperial College, London, United Kingdom

PETER CALVERLEY, DSc, FMedSc
Professor, Respiratory Research, Clinical Sciences Department, Professor of Respiratory Medicine, Institute of Ageing & Chronic Diseases, University Hospital Aintree, Liverpool, United Kingdom

CARLOS AUGUSTO CAMILLO, PT, MSc
Respiratory Rehabilitation and Respiratory Division, University Hospital Leuven; Faculty of Kinesiology and Rehabilitation Sciences, Department of Rehabilitation Sciences, Katholieke Universiteit Leuven, Leuven, Belgium

MARIO CAZZOLA, MD
Professor of Respiratory Medicine, University of Rome Tor Vergata, Rome, Italy

GOURAB CHOUDHURY, MBBS, MRCP(UK)
ELEGI and COLT Laboratories, Queens Medical Research Institute, Edinburgh, United Kingdom

DAVID M. DAUGHTON, MS
University of Nebraska Medical Center, Division of Pulmonary, Critical Care, Sleep and Allergy, 985910 Nebraska Medical Center, Omaha, Nebraska

HELEEN DEMEYER, PT, MSc
Respiratory Rehabilitation and Respiratory Division, University Hospital Leuven; Faculty of Kinesiology and Rehabilitation Sciences, Department of Rehabilitation Sciences, Katholieke Universiteit Leuven, Leuven, Belgium

ENRIQUE DIAZ-GUZMAN, MD
Division of Pulmonary, Critical Care, and Sleep Medicine, University of Alabama at Birmingham, Birmingham, Alabama

MARK A. GIEMBYCZ, BSc, PhD
Professor, Tier 1 Canada Research Chair in Pulmonary Pharmacology, Department of Physiology & Pharmacology, Airways Inflammation Research Group, Snyder Institute for Chronic Diseases, University of Calgary, Calgary, Alberta, Canada

TREVOR T. HANSEL, FRCPath, PhD
Imperial Clinical Respiratory Research Unit (ICRRU), Biomedical Research Centre (BMRC), Centre for Respiratory Infection (CRI), National Heart and Lung Institute (NHLI), St Mary's Hospital, Imperial College, Paddington, London, United Kingdom

MIEK HORNIKX, PT, MSc
Respiratory Rehabilitation and Respiratory
Division, University Hospital Leuven;
Faculty of Kinesiology and Rehabilitation
Sciences, Department of Rehabilitation
Sciences, Katholieke Universiteit Leuven,
Leuven, Belgium

WIM JANSSENS, MD, PhD
Respiratory Rehabilitation and Respiratory
Division, University Hospital Leuven;
Faculty of Kinesiology and Rehabilitation
Sciences, Department of Rehabilitation
Sciences, Katholieke Universiteit Leuven,
Leuven, Belgium

PIERANTONIO LAVENEZIANA, MD, PhD
Laboratoire de Physio-Pathologie Respiratoire,
Faculté de Médecine Pierre et Marie Curie
(site Pitié-Salpêtrière), Université Pierre et
Marie Curie (Paris VI), Paris, France

**DAVID A. LOMAS, PhD, ScD, FRCP,
FMedSci**
Professor, University College London, London,
United Kingdom

ALEX J. MACKAY, BSc(Hons), MRCP
Clinical Fellow in Respiratory Medicine, Centre
for Respiratory Medicine, Royal Free Campus,
University College London, London, United
Kingdom

**WILLIAM MACNEE, MBChB, MD, FRCP(G),
FRCP(E)**
ELEGI and COLT Laboratories, Queens Medical
Research Institute, Edinburgh, United Kingdom

DAVID M. MANNINO, MD
Division of Pulmonary, Critical Care, and Sleep
Medicine, University of Alabama at
Birmingham, Birmingham, Alabama;
Department of Preventive Medicine and
Environmental Health, University of Kentucky
College of Public Health, Lexington, Kentucky

STEFAN J. MARCINIAK, PhD, FRCP
Doctor, Division of Respiratory Medicine,
Department of Medicine, Addenbrooke's
Hospital; Cambridge Institute for Medical
Research (CIMR), University of Cambridge,
Cambridge, United Kingdom

MARIA GABRIELLA MATERA, MD, PhD
Professor of Pharmacology, Second University
of Naples, Naples, Italy

PATRICK BRIAN MURPHY, MRCP, PhD
Lane Fox Clinical Respiratory Physiology
Group, Guy's & St Thomas' NHS Foundation
Trust, London, United Kingdom

J. ALBERTO NEDER, MD, DSc
Division of Respiratory and Critical Care
Medicine, Department of Medicine, Kingston
General Hospital, Queen's University,
Kingston, Ontario, Canada

ROBERT NEWTON, BSc, PhD
Professor, Alberta Innovates-Health Solutions
Senior Scholar, Department of Cell Biology &
Anatomy, Airways Inflammation Research
Group, Snyder Institute for Chronic Diseases,
University of Calgary, Calgary, Alberta, Canada

**DENIS E. O'DONNELL, MD, FRCP(I),
FRCP(C)**
Division of Respiratory and Critical Care
Medicine, Department of Medicine, Kingston
General Hospital, Queen's University,
Kingston, Ontario, Canada

MICHAEL IAIN POLKEY, PhD, FRCP
NIHR Respiratory Biomedical Research Unit,
Royal Brompton and Harefield NHS
Foundation Trust, Imperial College London,
London, United Kingdom

DIRKJE S. POSTMA, MD, PhD
Department of Pulmonology, GRIAC
Research Institute, University Medical Center
Groningen, University of Groningen,
Groningen, The Netherlands

ROBERTO RABINOVICH, MBBS, MD, PhD
ELEGI and COLT Laboratories, Queens
Medical Research Institute, Edinburgh,
United Kingdom

KAMEN RANGELOV, MD
Fellow, Pulmonary and Critical Care Medicine,
University at Buffalo, SUNY, Buffalo, New York

HELEN K. REDDEL, MD, PhD
Woolcock Institute of Medical Research,
University of Sydney, Sydney, New South
Wales, Australia

STEPHEN I. RENNARD, MD
University of Nebraska Medical Center, Larson
Professor of Medicine, Division of Pulmonary,
Critical Care, Sleep and Allergy, 985910
Nebraska Medical Center, Omaha, Nebraska

CLARE L. ROSS, MRCP
Imperial Clinical Respiratory Research Unit (ICRRU), Biomedical Research Centre (BMRC), Centre for Respiratory Infection (CRI), National Heart and Lung Institute (NHLI), St Mary's Hospital, Imperial College, Paddington, London, United Kingdom

SUNDEEP SALVI, MD, DNB, PhD, FCCP
Director, Chest Research Foundation, Pune, India

SANJAY SETHI, MD
Professor of Medicine, Division Chief, Pulmonary, Critical Care, and Sleep Medicine, Staff Physician, VA Western New York Healthcare System, University at Buffalo, The State University of New York, Buffalo, New York

DON D. SIN, MD, PhD
Professor, Division of Respirology, Department of Medicine, The Institute for Heart and Lung Health, James Hogg Research Center, St. Paul's Hospital, University of British Columbia, Vancouver, British Columbia, Canada

RICHA SINGH, BSc(Hons), MRCP
Clinical Fellow in Respiratory Medicine, Centre for Respiratory Medicine, Royal Free Campus, University College London, London, United Kingdom

ROBERT A. STOCKLEY, MD, DSc, FRCP
Professor of Medicine, ADAPT Project, Lung Function & Sleep Department, Queen Elizabeth Hospital Birmingham, Birmingham, United Kingdom

NICK H.T. TEN HACKEN, MD, PhD
Department of Pulmonology, Groningen Research Institute of Asthma and COPD, University Medical Center Groningen, University of Groningen, Groningen, The Netherlands

THIERRY TROOSTERS, PT, PhD
Respiratory Rehabilitation and Respiratory Division, University Hospital Leuven; Faculty of Kinesiology and Rehabilitation Sciences, Department of Rehabilitation Sciences, Katholieke Universiteit Leuven, Leuven, Belgium

MAARTEN VAN DEN BERGE, MD, PhD
Department of Pulmonology, Groningen Research Institute of Asthma and COPD, University Medical Center Groningen, University of Groningen, Groningen, The Netherlands

JØRGEN VESTBO, DMSc, FRCP
Professor of Respiratory Medicine, Department of Respiratory Medicine J, Odense University Hospital, Clinical Institute, University of Southern Denmark, Odense, Denmark; Respiratory Research Group, Manchester Academic Sciences Centre, University Hospital South Manchester NHS Foundation Trust, Manchester, United Kingdom

KATHERINE WEBB, MSc
Division of Respiratory and Critical Care Medicine, Department of Medicine, Kingston General Hospital, Queen's University, Kingston, Ontario, Canada

JADWIGA A. WEDZICHA, MD, FRCP
Professor of Respiratory Medicine, Centre for Respiratory Medicine, Royal Free Campus, University College London, London, United Kingdom

ZAID ZOUMOT, MBBS, MRCP, MSc
NIHR Respiratory Biomedical Research Unit, Royal Brompton and Harefield NHS Foundation Trust, Imperial College London, London, United Kingdom

Contents

Preface: Chronic Obstructive Pulmonary Disease   xiii

Peter J. Barnes

COPD: Definition and Phenotypes   1

Jørgen Vestbo

> Chronic obstructive pulmonary disease (COPD) is currently defined as a common preventable and treatable disease that is characterized by persistent airflow limitation that is usually progressive and associated with an enhanced chronic inflammatory response in the airways and the lung to noxious particles or gases. Exacerbations and comorbidities contribute to the overall severity in individual patients. The evolution of this definition and the diagnostic criteria currently in use are discussed. COPD is increasingly divided in subgroups or phenotypes based on specific features and association with prognosis or response to therapy, the most notable being the feature of frequent exacerbations.

Epidemiology and Prevalence of Chronic Obstructive Pulmonary Disease   7

Enrique Diaz-Guzman and David M. Mannino

> Chronic obstructive pulmonary disease (COPD) represents one of the main causes of morbidity and mortality worldwide. According to the World Health Organization, approximately 3 million people in the world die as a consequence of COPD every year. Tobacco use remains the main factor associated with development of disease in the industrialized world, but other risk factors are important and preventable causes of COPD, particularly in the developing world. The purpose of this review is to summarize the literature on the subject and to provide an update of the most recent advances in the field.

Tobacco Smoking and Environmental Risk Factors for Chronic Obstructive Pulmonary Disease   17

Sundeep Salvi

> The development of chronic obstructive pulmonary disease (COPD) is multifactorial, and the risk factors include both genetic and environmental factors. Although tobacco smoking is an established risk factor for COPD, many other associated factors remain underappreciated or neglected. Up to 50% of cases of COPD can be attributed to nonsmoking risk factors. This article describes the role of tobacco smoking and the various environmental risk factors associated with the development of COPD.

Genetic Susceptibility   29

Stefan J. Marciniak and David A. Lomas

> Why only 20% of smokers develop clinically relevant chronic obstructive pulmonary disease (COPD) was a puzzle for many years. Now, epidemiologic studies point clearly toward a large heritable component. The combination of genome-wide association studies and candidate gene analysis is helping to identify those genetic variants responsible for an individual's susceptibility to developing COPD. In this

review, the current data implicating specific loci and genes in the pathogenesis of COPD are examined.

Alpha1-antitrypsin Review   39

Robert A. Stockley

> Alpha1-antitrypsin (AAT) deficiency was first described in 1963 together with its associations with severe early-onset basal panacinar emphysema. The genetic defects leading to deficiency have been elucidated and the pathophysiologic processes, clinical variation in phenotype, and the role of genetic modifiers have been recognized. Strategies to increase plasma (and hence tissue) concentrations of AAT have been developed. The only recognized specific therapeutic strategy is regular infusions of the purified plasma protein, and evidence confirms its efficacy in protecting the lung (at least partially). Early detection and modification of lifestyle remains crucial to the management of AAT deficiency.

Chronic Obstructive Pulmonary Disease: Clinical Integrative Physiology   51

Denis E. O'Donnell, Pierantonio Laveneziana, Katherine Webb, and J. Alberto Neder

> Peripheral airway dysfunction, inhomogeneous ventilation distribution, gas trapping, and impaired pulmonary gas exchange are variably present in all stages of chronic obstructive pulmonary disease (COPD). This article provides a cogent physiologic explanation for the relentless progression of activity-related dyspnea and exercise intolerance that all too commonly characterizes COPD. The spectrum of physiologic derangements that exist in smokers with mild airway obstruction and a history compatible with COPD is examined. Also explored are the perceptual and physiologic consequences of progressive erosion of the resting inspiratory capacity. Finally, emerging information on the role of cardiocirculatory impairment in contributing to exercise intolerance in patients with varying degrees of airway obstruction is reviewed.

Cellular and Molecular Mechanisms of Chronic Obstructive Pulmonary Disease   71

Peter J. Barnes

> Chronic obstructive pulmonary disease is associated with chronic inflammation affecting predominantly lung parenchyma and peripheral airways and results in largely irreversible and progressive airflow limitation. This inflammation is characterized by increased numbers of alveolar macrophages, neutrophils, and T lymphocytes, which are recruited from the circulation. Oxidative stress plays a key role in driving this inflammation. The pulmonary inflammation may enhance the development and growth of lung cancer. The peripheral inflammation extends into the circulation, resulting in systemic inflammation with the same inflammatory proteins. Systemic inflammation may worsen comorbidities. Treatment of pulmonary inflammation may therefore have beneficial effects.

Role of Infections   87

Kamen Rangelov and Sanjay Sethi

> This article represents a review of the current literature on the role of infection in the pathogenesis of chronic obstructive pulmonary disease (COPD), in stable disease, exacerbations, and pneumonia. It outlines the complex interactions between respiratory pathogens and host immune defenses that underlie the clinical manifestations of infection in COPD.

Comorbidities and Systemic Effects of Chronic Obstructive Pulmonary Disease   101

Gourab Choudhury, Roberto Rabinovich, and William MacNee

Although primarily a lung disease, chronic obstructive pulmonary disease (COPD) is now recognized to have extrapulmonary effects on distal organs, the so-called systemic effects and comorbidities of COPD. Skeletal muscle dysfunction, nutritional abnormalities including weight loss, cardiovascular complications, metabolic complications, and osteoporosis, among others, are all well-recognized associations in COPD. These extrapulmonary effects add to the burden of mortality and morbidity in COPD and therefore should be actively looked for, assessed, and treated.

Biomarkers in COPD   131

Alvar Agusti and Don D. Sin

Chronic obstructive pulmonary disease (COPD) is a heterogeneous disease that cannot be described by the severity of airflow limitation (forced expiratory volume in the first second of expiration) only. Other measures are needed in clinical practice to assess patients, predict their risk, guide their treatment, and assess their response to it. Over the past few years, there has been a great deal of interest in the identification and validation of biomarkers of potential clinical use in COPD. Here, the authors review some general concepts in the field, discuss currently validated biomarkers in COPD, and speculate on potential future developments.

Asthma and Chronic Obstructive Pulmonary Disease: Similarities and Differences   143

Dirkje S. Postma, Helen K. Reddel, Nick H.T. ten Hacken, and Maarten van den Berge

Asthma and COPD are both heterogeneous lung diseases including many different phenotypes. The classical asthma and COPD phenotypes are easy to discern because they reflect extremes of a phenotypical spectrum. Thus asthma in childhood and COPD in smokers have their own phenotypic expression with underlying pathophysiological mechanisms that differ importantly. In older adults, asthma and COPD are more difficult to differentiate and there exists a bronchodilator response in most but not all patients with asthma and persistent airway obstruction in most but not all patients with COPD where even up to 50% have been reported to have some bronchodilator response as assessed with FEV_1. Airway obstruction is generated in the large and small airways both in asthma and COPD, and this small airway obstruction is located more proximally in asthma, yet is found more distally in severe and older individuals with asthma, comparable to COPD. Though the underlying inflammation and remodelling processes in asthma and COPD are different in their extreme phenotypes, there are overlap phenotypes with eosinophilic inflammation even in stable COPD and neutrophilic inflammation in longstanding and severe asthma.

Acute COPD Exacerbations   157

Jadwiga A. Wedzicha, Richa Singh, and Alex J. Mackay

Exacerbations are important events for patients with chronic obstructive pulmonary disease (COPD) and key outcomes in COPD studies and trials. Exacerbations have an impact on health status and contribute to disease progression, and exacerbation prevention is a key goal of therapy in COPD. A majority of COPD exacerbations are triggered by respiratory viral infections and/or bacterial infections. Several pharmacologic therapies can prevent COPD exacerbations and reduce hospital admissions. Nonpharmacologic interventions for exacerbation prevention include pulmonary rehabilitation, long-term oxygen therapy, and home noninvasive ventilator support.

Improved management of acute exacerbations also prolongs the time to the next exacerbation event.

Smoking Cessation

165

Stephen I. Rennard and David M. Daughton

Cigarette smoking is a major preventable cause of morbidity and mortality. It is the major risk factor for chronic obstructive pulmonary disease in the developed world. Smoking is a chronic relapsing disease. Optimal treatment includes nonpharmacologic support, together with pharmacotherapy. All clinicians should be comfortable with the use of nicotine replacement therapy, bupropion, and varenicline. Second-line therapies can be used by those familiar with their use. Effective use of these medications requires their integration into an effective management plan, which is likely to be a long-term undertaking, involving several cycles of remission and relapse.

Current Drug Treatment, Chronic and Acute

177

Peter Calverley

The appropriate management of chronic obstructive pulmonary disease (COPD) involves more than taking prescription medicines. The key components have been set out in detail in many treatment guidelines, both national and international. They include the avoidance of identified risk factors, especially tobacco smoking, and the optimization of daily physical activity. This article reviews the key components of the pharmacologic treatment of COPD, both acute and chronic, with an emphasis on those recent studies, which are likely to change practice in the next few years.

Bronchodilators: Current and Future

191

Mario Cazzola and Maria Gabriella Matera

Bronchodilators are central in the symptomatic treatment of chronic obstructive pulmonary disease (COPD), although there is often limited reversibility of airflow obstruction. Three classes of bronchodilators (β_2-agonists, antimuscarinic agents, methylxanthines) are currently available, which can be used individually, or in combination with each other or inhaled corticosteroids. Novel classes of bronchodilators have proved difficult to develop. The muscarinic β_2-agonist molecules approach likely provides the best opportunity to develop combinations that combine corticosteroids with dual-bronchodilator activities, and thus potentially achieve better efficacy than is apparent with the current combination products that dominate the treatment of COPD.

How Phosphodiesterase 4 Inhibitors Work in Patients with Chronic Obstructive Pulmonary Disease of the Severe, Bronchitic, Frequent Exacerbator Phenotype

203

Mark A. Giembycz and Robert Newton

Current international guidelines recommend that roflumilast be added on to an inhaled corticosteroid/long-acting β_2-adrenoceptor agonist (LABA) combination therapy in high-risk patients with severe, bronchitic chronic obstructive pulmonary disease who have frequent acute exacerbations. This article presents evidence that a glucocorticoid, LABA, and phosphodiesterase (PDE) 4 inhibitor in combination can interact in a complex manner to induce a panel of genes that could act collectively to suppress inflammation and improve lung function. The possibility that multivalent ligands may deliver superior efficacy is also being explored. Single molecules that inhibit PDE4 and activate β_2-adrenoceptors at similar concentrations have been described.

New Drug Therapies for COPD   219

Clare L. Ross and Trevor T. Hansel

Clinical trials with new drugs for chronic obstructive pulmonary disease (COPD) have been performed. Viruses exacerbate COPD and bacteria may play a part in severe COPD; therefore, antibiotic and antiviral approaches have a sound rationale. Antiinflammatory approaches have been studied. Advances in understanding the molecular basis of other processes have resulted in novel drugs to target reactive oxidant species, mucus, proteases, fibrosis, cachexia, and muscle wasting, and accelerated aging. Studies with monoclonal antibodies have been disappointing, highlighting the tendency for infections and malignancies during treatment. Promising future directions are lung regeneration with retinoids and stem cells.

Pulmonary Rehabilitation   241

Thierry Troosters, Heleen Demeyer, Miek Hornikx, Carlos Augusto Camillo, and Wim Janssens

Pulmonary rehabilitation is a therapy that offers benefits to patients with chronic obstructive pulmonary disease that are complementary to those obtained by pharmacotherapy. The main objective of pulmonary rehabilitation is to restore muscle function and exercise tolerance, reverse other nonrespiratory consequences of the disease, and help patients to self-manage chronic obstructive pulmonary disease and its exacerbations and symptoms. To do so, a multidisciplinary program tailored to the patient in terms of program content, exercise prescription, and setting must be offered. Several settings and programs have shown to spin off in significant immediate results. The challenge lies in maintaining the benefits outside the program.

Noninvasive Ventilation and Lung Volume Reduction   251

Patrick Brian Murphy, Zaid Zoumot, and Michael Iain Polkey

As parenchymal lung disease in chronic obstructive pulmonary disease becomes increasingly severe there is a diminishing prospect of drug therapies conferring clinically useful benefit. Lung volume reduction surgery is effective in patients with heterogenous upper zone emphysema and reduced exercise tolerance, and is probably underused. Rapid progress is being made in nonsurgical approaches to lung volume reduction, but use outside specialized centers cannot be recommended presently. Noninvasive ventilation given to patients with acute hypercapnic exacerbation of chronic obstructive pulmonary disease reduces mortality and morbidity, but the place of chronic non-invasive ventilatory support remains more controversial.

Index   271

CLINICS IN CHEST MEDICINE

FORTHCOMING ISSUES

June 2014
Pulmonary Rehabilitation
Linda Nici, MD and Richard ZuWallack, MD,
Editors

September 2014
Sleep and Breathing Beyond Obstructive Sleep Apnea
Carolyn D'Ambrosio, *Editor*

December 2014
ARDS
Lorraine Ware, *Editor*

RECENT ISSUES

December 2013
Pulmonary Arterial Hypertension
Terence K. Trow, *Editor*

September 2013
Interventional Pulmonology
Ali I. Musani, *Editor*

June 2013
HIV and Respiratory Disease
Kristina Crothers, MD, Laurence Huang, MD,
and Alison Morris, MD, MS, *Editors*

RELATED INTEREST

Clinics in Chest Medicine, Vol. 33, No. 4 (December 2012)
Occupational Pulmonology
Carrie A. Redlich, Paul D. Blanc, Mridu Gulati, and Ware G. Kuschner, *Editors*

DOWNLOAD
Free App!

Review Articles
THE CLINICS

NOW AVAILABLE FOR YOUR iPhone and iPad

Preface
Chronic Obstructive Pulmonary Disease

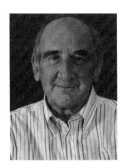

Peter J. Barnes, FRS, FMedSci
Editor

Chronic obstructive pulmonary disease (COPD) is a major global health problem that is increasing throughout the world, especially in developing countries. This increase reflects continuing cigarette smoking, which remains the commonest cause, but also relates to aging populations since COPD is a disease of the elderly and may be regarded as accelerated aging of the lung. In addition to cigarette smoking, other causal mechanisms, such as exposure to biomass fuels, air pollution, and poor nutrition, as well as poverty, are also recognized as contributory risk factors. COPD is now the third most prevalent cause of death in Western countries and its mortality is rising in developing countries. It has now become one of the most frequent causes of hospitalization. Although it is one of the most common chronic diseases, it is still poorly recognized among the general public and among doctors, with over half of the patients undiagnosed and many of the diagnosed cases mistreated. There is a major need to better understand this complex disease, which appears to include many poorly understood phenotypes. It is increasingly recognized that COPD occurs with several comorbidities, including cardiovascular and metabolic diseases and lung cancer, which have a major effect on clinical outcomes and management. This volume brings together current knowledge of COPD, written by international experts, and explores every aspect of the disease from epidemiology, through clinical presentation, to underlying mechanisms and clinical management.

Although major progress has been made in understanding COPD, many questions about COPD remain unanswered. We do not understand why only a minority of smokers develop airway obstruction, nor the complex interplay between different risk factors in addition to smoking and biomass smoke exposure. We do not understand how the underlying inflammatory process is linked to pathophysiology and disease progression and the reason inflammation and disease progression persist even after smoking cessation is not understood. The different phenotypes may respond differently to different treatments, but this is poorly understood. Although long-acting bronchodilators have proved to be the most effective therapies so far available, we still do not have treatments that suppress the underlying inflammatory process to prevent disease progression and exacerbations. This suggests that much more research is needed in the future.

This issue brings together our current understanding of COPD and provides a sound up-to-date synopsis of the disease that will provide a valuable basis for future research into this devastating disease. I wish to thank all of the authors for their excellent articles and to keeping to the deadlines, and the publishers for putting together this volume.

Peter J. Barnes, FRS, FMedSci
National Heart and Lung Institute
Imperial College, Dovehouse Street
London, SW3 6LY, UK

E-mail address:
p.j.barnes@imperial.ac.uk

Clin Chest Med 35 (2014) xiii
http://dx.doi.org/10.1016/j.ccm.2013.11.003
0272-5231/14/$ – see front matter © 2014 Published by Elsevier Inc.

COPD: Definition and Phenotypes

Jørgen Vestbo, DMSc, FRCP[a,b,*]

KEYWORDS

- COPD • Definition • Diagnosis • Lung function • Chronic inflammation

KEY POINTS

- The definition of chronic obstructive pulmonary disease (COPD) is pragmatic and highlights the chronicity, the enhanced inflammation, and the importance of exacerbations and comorbidities.
- For the clinical diagnosis of COPD, exposures, symptoms, and airflow limitation are all required.
- Phenotypes are distinct COPD subgroups that deserve attention because they have either specific outcomes or require specific management.
- The frequent exacerbator is an important phenotype with higher future risks and a requirement for preventive treatments.

The definition and phenotypes in chronic obstructive pulmonary disease (COPD) are important topics. Not only should the definition clearly outline the disease but it is also, to a large extent, the conceptual framework on which we build the diagnostic criteria for the disease. *Phenotype* is a more recent term in COPD; however, the notion of COPD consisting of several subgroups is not new at all. In fact, it is often stated that COPD is a syndrome rather than a disease. Snider[1] has dealt with this COPD nosology quite extensively, and this article only deals briefly with these concepts. More space is devoted to the operationalization of the definition, diagnostic criteria, and phenotypes.

DEFINITION

Several definitions of COPD exist, and it would be wrong to say that one is clearly superior to another. The first definitions arising from working groups of the major respiratory societies came in 1995 from the American Thoracic Society (ATS)[2] and the European Respiratory Society (ERS).[3] Significant national guidelines have subsequently adopted and modified these definitions. The ATS and ERS definitions are shown in **Box 1**.

Neither of these definitions is particularly precise and can easily include disease entities that are not usually regarded as COPD, such as cystic fibrosis, sarcoidosis, and bronchiectasis. Importantly, neither of these definitions differentiates COPD from chronic asthma with airway remodeling. There are reasons for this; there is a significant overlap, and as acknowledged by the ATS mentioning airway hyperreactivity, one of the hallmarks of asthma, some patients with COPD do have features that make it difficult to separate them from patients with chronic ongoing asthma.

In 2001, the Global Initiative for Chronic Obstructive Lung Diseases (GOLD) was launched; in their seminal document from 2001,[4] COPD is

Disclosure of Interests: J. Vestbo has received honoraria for advising Bioxydyn, Chiesi, GlaxoSmithKline, Novartis, Syntaxin, and Takeda. J. Vestbo has received honoraria for presenting from AstraZeneca, Boehringer-Ingelheim, Chiesi, GlaxoSmithKline, Novartis, and Takeda. J. Vestbo is a member (vice-chair) of the Board of Directors of the Global Initiative for Obstructive Lung Diseases (GOLD), and he is the chair of the GOLD Scientific Committee.
[a] Department of Respiratory Medicine J, Odense University Hospital, Clinical Institute, University of Southern Denmark, Odense, Denmark; [b] Respiratory Research Group, Manchester Academic Sciences Centre, University Hospital South Manchester NHS Foundation Trust, Southmoor Road, M23 9LT Manchester, UK
* Department of Respiratory Medicine J, Odense University Hospital, Sdr Boulevard 29, 5000 Odense C, Denmark.
E-mail address: Jorgen.vestbo@manchester.ac.uk

Clin Chest Med 35 (2014) 1–6
http://dx.doi.org/10.1016/j.ccm.2013.10.010

defined as "a disease state characterized by airflow limitation that is not fully reversible. The airflow obstruction is usually both progressive and associated with an abnormal response of the lungs to noxious particles or gases."[4]

This definition differs fundamentally from those of the ATS and ERS in its inclusion of inflammation as well as the disease being a consequence of external stimuli (ie, noxious particles and gases). The GOLD document has been revised twice, in 2006 and 2011. On both occasions, the definition has been changed. In 2006[5] it was changed as follows:

Chronic obstructive pulmonary disease (COPD) is a preventable and treatable disease with some significant extrapulmonary effects that may contribute to the severity in individual patients. Its pulmonary component is characterized by airflow limitation that is not fully reversible. The airflow limitation is usually progressive and associated with an abnormal inflammatory response of the lung to noxious particles or gases.[5]

The phrase *preventable and treatable* was also included in the definition proposed by the joint ATS/ERS document from 2004 and reflects an attempt to leave previous therapeutic nihilism regarding COPD behind. Importantly, this definition includes extrapulmonary effects as a contributor to severity in individual patients. These extrapulmonary effects were, however, not clearly

defined; subsequently, many of these effects were seen as comorbidities. This point is reflected in the most recent GOLD definition[6] and is shown in **Box 2**.

The most recent changes reflect the increased knowledge of the disease that had accumulated since 2006. It has become clear that calling airflow limitation reversible in asthma and irreversible in COPD is too simplistic because patients with COPD can show significant reversibility with bronchodilators. However, airflow is never normalized; the airflow limitation was, thus, described as persistent. Similarly, we have seen that the chronic inflammation in airways and lung parenchyma does not have any specific abnormal characteristics. Rather, it seems that patients with COPD are unable to switch off inflammation; it was, therefore, thought that the phrase *enhanced inflammation* was a better descriptor. Extrapulmonary effects were replaced by comorbidities, and it was thought that the importance of exacerbations for individual patients was sufficient to warrant the inclusion of the term *exacerbations* in the definition.

DIAGNOSTIC CRITERIA

Is the current definition as proposed by GOLD ideal? The many different suggestions for a definition probably illustrates that this is not the case. The most important limitation is probably that it seems difficult to directly translate the definition into diagnostic criteria. In particular, we have no means of easily measuring the enhanced inflammation that we think is the basis for COPD. For this reason, our diagnostic criteria have heavily relied on the physiologic ascertainment of airflow limitation in patients with relevant exposure presenting to a physician.

In the GOLD 2011 revision,[6] the main section on diagnosis states that

A clinical diagnosis of COPD should be considered in any patient who has dyspnea, chronic cough or sputum production, and/or a history of exposure to risk factors for the

disease. *Spirometry is required to make the diagnosis in this clinical context; the presence of a post-bronchodilator [forced expiratory volume in the first second of expiration/forced vital capacity] FEV_1/FVC <0.70 confirms the presence of persistent airflow limitation and thus of COPD.*[6]

It is important to note that the aforementioned definition relates to a clinical diagnosis (ie, a doctor making a diagnosis in a patient). Although this is clearly the most important aspect of a diagnosis, the epidemiology of COPD has for decades relied on field measurements of lung function using spirometry and simple questions excluding asthma and sometimes other respiratory disease. It may seem trivial, but this distinction has significant implications, not the least of which is for the discussion on the spirometric criteria for airflow limitation. In epidemiology, there is no proxy for patients going to a doctor; diagnostic criteria in epidemiology, therefore, resemble the criteria that would be used for screening, a tool not advocated by any major respiratory society or body.

However, the devil is often in the details. Importantly, in the 2013 update,[7] the terms *and/or* in the second line have been substituted by the term *and* as shown in **Box 3**.

In simple words, this means that in patients with relevant exposure and respiratory symptoms, a spirometry should be obtained; if airflow limitation (here defined as a postbronchodilator FEV_1/FVC <0.70) is found, this constitutes a diagnosis of COPD unless patients have other respiratory conditions, such as asthma, bronchiectasis, stenosing bronchial tumor, and so forth. Using the aforementioned strategy for COPD case finding will often result in a favorable yield; in Denmark, programs using this approach have resulted in diagnoses in 20% to 30% of those fulfilling the criteria for spirometry.[8]

Unfortunately, most of the debate on diagnostic criteria has focused on the choice of an FEV_1/FVC

Box 3
COPD diagnostic criteria according to GOLD 2013

"A clinical diagnosis of COPD should be considered in any patient who has dyspnea, chronic cough or sputum production, and a history of exposure to risk factors for the disease. Spirometry is required to make the diagnosis in this clinical context; the presence of a post-bronchodilator FEV_1/FVC <0.70 confirms the presence of persistent airflow limitation and thus of COPD."[7]

---

of less than 0.70 as the defining cutoff for airflow limitation. This cutoff is somewhat arbitrary, and opponents often argue that it has no scientific validity; instead, the lower limit of normal (LLN) is proposed.[9] There is little doubt that in most populations, the fixed 0.70 cutoff will result in more abnormal FEV_1/FVC ratios in the elderly and fewer in patients younger than 50 years.[10] This has led to a heated debate that seems futile because no gold standard exists; therefore, little real evidence exists in this area. In the epidemiologic setting, LLN should be preferred,[11] although great care should be taken when selecting reference values. In the clinical setting, no comparative studies exist. The virtue of the fixed 0.70 cutoff is simplicity and familiarity, and this is the reason why GOLD[7] and the UK National Center for Clinical Excellence have kept this criterion. The LLN is the physiologists' choice because it is anchored in our usual scientific definition of normality. However, this author really does not think it matters in clinical practice, and it seems that far too much energy has been spent on this issue considering the underrecognition, underdiagnosis, and undertreatment of COPD globally.

The probably most critical issue with the current diagnostic criteria is that they do not capture patients with pure emphysema until relatively late in the course of the disease. With an increasing focus on early diagnosis, the lack of sensitivity to a major COPD component – such as emphysema – reliance on simple spirometry for diagnosis may no longer be sufficient.

CONSIDERATIONS FOR FUTURE DIAGNOSTIC CRITERIA

So, because the current diagnostic criteria are far from ideal and the spirometric criteria are frequently the topic of futile debates, it may be worth considering if it is time to rethink diagnosis. When comparing with another chronic illness that in many ways resembles COPD, heart failure, it is clear that others have avoided debate on very specific cutoff values.[12] If we were to transfer similar thinking to COPD as that of the cardiologists when diagnosing heart failure, future COPD diagnostic criteria could take the shape of 'Symptoms and clinical features compatible with COPD in an individual with relevant exposures, where either physiologic measures or imaging support the presence of functional or structural abnormalities supporting a diagnosis of COPD.'

With the very general definition of COPD and the debated diagnostic criteria, those favoring the use of diagnoses such as emphysema and chronic bronchitis (the splitters) instead of COPD (the lumpers) may wish to go back to the time before the umbrella term *COPD* was launched. But there is little doubt that COPD has come to stay. However, the splitters can comfort themselves in the fact that most COPD researchers and many clinicians find increasing value in splitting COPD into subgroups, into *phenotypes*.

COPD PHENOTYPES

A phenotype is usually considered the physical appearance or biochemical characteristic resulting from an interaction between its genotype and the environment. In COPD, whereby the underlying genes are mainly unknown or poorly characterized, *phenotype* has become almost synonymous with *clinical subgroup*. Several researchers have come up with a consensus definition of phenotypes[13] as shown in **Box 4**. This definition emphasizes that a phenotype has to be a subgroup that impacts on the outcome, that is, that having a particular phenotype means a different prognosis, a higher risk of exacerbation, a better response to a particular therapy, and so forth.

There are a few important issues regarding the concept of phenotypes. One phenotype is unlikely to be unique to one patient. In Snider's[14] original nonproportional Venn diagram, several overlapping subgroups were presented; subsequent studies trying to implement Snider's diagram to patients and populations showed that the overlap was indeed substantial. In addition to belonging to several phenotypes, patients can also have phenotypical traits. Considering emphysema as a phenotype, a patient could have mild emphysema and quite significant airflow limitation; one could speculate if emphysema had any importance in this particular patient. Also, specific combinations of phenotypes could be more important than others. Finally, in asthma, there is a move away from phenotypes toward endotypes,[15] whereby an endotype is basically a phenotype defined by a distinct pathophysiologic mechanism.

SPECIFIC COPD PHENOTYPES

The classic phenotypes of Snider's[14] diagram are asthma, emphysema, and chronic bronchitis.

Box 4
Phenotype definition

"A COPD phenotype is a single or combination of disease attributes that describe differences between individuals with COPD as they relate to clinically meaningful outcomes (symptoms, exacerbations, response to therapy, rate of disease progression, or death)."[13]

Asthma is likely to be considered a disease entity of its own, or a separate syndrome, despite the significant clinical overlap and the fact that asthma can be regarded as a risk factor for persistent airflow limitation. Features of asthma, such as airway hyperresponsiveness and reversibility, have been associated with a worse prognosis in some studies[16,17]; but particularly reversibility seems to be a very instable phenotype in COPD.[17]

Emphysema is a significant component of COPD and the extent of emphysema increases with increasing severity of airflow limitation. Emphysema is associated with a significantly increased decline in FEV_1, the hallmark of COPD.[18] Emphysema is a stable phenotype. The same can be said for chronic bronchitis, which in some studies has been associated with excess FEV_1 decline, particularly in younger adults,[19] with hospital admission as well as mortality.

Many other phenotypes are likely to exist as suggested in **Box 5**.

Having frequent exacerbations is a feature that has attracted considerable attention in recent years. Several studies have shown that only some patients with COPD experience exacerbations. But with the analyses of the Evaluation of COPD Longitudinally to Identify Predictive Surrogate Endpoints (ECLIPSE) study,[20] it became evident that having 2 or more exacerbations per year seemed a stable phenotype. This has significant implications. First, exacerbations are associated with a poor prognosis[21] and an excess FEV_1 decline[18,22]; secondly, several treatments are aimed at reducing exacerbations.[7] It can be argued whether 2 annual exacerbations is the right threshold for defining the frequent exacerbator, but at least the current literature seems to support this cutoff.

Another characteristic that has attracted attention lately is the presence of systemic inflammation. Early studies saw systemic inflammation as

---

Box 5
Features of suggested phenotypes in COPD

Asthma

Bronchial hyperresponsiveness

Bronchodilator reversibility

Emphysema

Hyperinflation

Cachexia

Chronic bronchitis

Frequent exacerbations

Systemic inflammation

a feature of COPD; but with larger patient cohorts studied, we have learned more. First, not all patients with COPD have elevated markers of systemic inflammation. The markers most frequently measured have been C-reactive protein (CRP) and fibrinogen, and both are associated with subsequent hospital admission and death.[23] Recent analyses from the ECLIPSE study showed that multiple markers were likely to provide more relevant information than single markers,[24] and an epidemiologic study has shown that the use of 3 biomarkers (CRP, fibrinogen, and white blood cell count) seemed to provide prognostic value regarding incident comorbidities.[25] However, we currently have no treatment aimed at systemic inflammation in COPD.

Several other phenotypes exist and could be discussed. They are all based on our understanding of the disease, and most of them rely on single observational characteristics. Several groups have made an attempt at developing phenotypes based on an unbiased approach, including machine learning. They have been applied in both stable COPD and exacerbations; but, to date, the value of these approaches is difficult to evaluate.

Thus, the whole concept of COPD as a syndrome with specific entities is constantly evolving. The current definition has changed only a little over the last decade. It is likely to change within the coming decade. Whether the concept of phenotypes will evolve and be included in future standards for diagnosis and management remains to be seen.

REFERENCES

1. Snider GL. Definition of chronic obstructive pulmonary disease. In: Calverley PM, MacNee W, Pride NB, et al, editors. Chronic obstructive pulmonary disease. 2nd edition. London: Arnold; 2003. p. 1–10.

2. American Thoracic Society. Standards for the diagnosis and care of patients with chronic obstructive pulmonary disease. Am J Respir Crit Care Med 1995;152:S77–121.

3. Siafakas NM, Vermeire P, Pride NB, et al. Optimal assessment and management of chronic obstructive pulmonary disease (COPD). The European Respiratory Society Task Force. Eur Respir J 1995;8:1398–420.

4. Pauwels RA, Buist AS, Calverley PM, et al. Global strategy for the diagnosis, management, and prevention of chronic obstructive pulmonary disease. NHLBI/WHO Global Initiative for Chronic Obstructive Lung Disease (GOLD) workshop summary. Am J Respir Crit Care Med 2001;163:1256–76.

5. Rabe KF, Hurd S, Anzueto A, et al. Global strategy for the diagnosis, management and prevention of chronic obstructive pulmonary disease, GOLD executive summary. Am J Respir Crit Care Med 2007;176(6):532–55.

6. Vestbo J, Hurd SS, Agusti AG, et al. Global strategy for the diagnosis, management and prevention of chronic obstructive pulmonary disease, GOLD executive summary. Am J Respir Crit Care Med 2013;187:347–65.

7. Available at: http://www.goldcopd.org/uploads/users/files/GOLD_Report_2013_Feb20.pdf. Accessed May 2, 2013.

8. Ulrik CS, Løkke A, Dahl R, et al. Early detection of COPD in general practice. Int J Chron Obstruct Pulmon Dis 2011;6:123–7.

9. Pellegrino R, Brusasco V, Viegi G, et al. Definition of COPD: based on evidence or opinion? Eur Respir J 2008;31:681–2.

10. Vollmer WM, Gislason T, Burney P, et al. Comparison of spirometry criteria for the diagnosis of COPD: results from the BOLD study. Eur Respir J 2009;34:588–97.

11. Bakke PS, Rönmark E, Eagan T, et al. Recommendations for epidemiological studies on COPD. ERS Task Force Report. Eur Respir J 2011;38:1261–77.

12. McMurray JJ, Adamopoulos S, Anker SD, et al. The Task Force for the Diagnosis and Treatment of Acute and Chronic Heart Failure 2012 of the European Society of Cardiology. ESC guidelines for the diagnosis and treatment of acute and chronic heart failure 2012. Eur Heart J 2012;33:1787–847.

13. Han MK, Agusti A, Calverley PM, et al. COPD phenotypes: the future of COPD. Am J Respir Crit Care Med 2010;182:598–604.

14. Snider G. Chronic obstructive pulmonary disease: a definition and implications of structural determinants of airflow obstruction for epidemiology. Am Rev Respir Dis 1989;140(3 Pt 2):S3–8.

15. Lötvall J, Akdis CA, Bacharier LB, et al. Asthma endotypes: a new approach to classification of disease entities within the asthma syndrome. J Allergy Clin Immunol 2011;127:355–60.

16. Scott TW, Sparrow D, editors. Airways responsiveness and atopy in the development of chronic lung disease. New York: Raven Press; 1989.

17. Albert PS, Agusti A, Edwards LD, et al. Bronchodilator responsiveness is not a consistent phenotypic characteristic of COPD. Thorax 2012;67:701–8.

18. Vestbo J, Edwards LD, Scanlon PD, et al, for the ECLIPSE Investigators. Change in forced expiratory volume in 1 second over time in COPD. N Engl J Med 2011;365:1184–92.

19. Guerra S, Sherrill DL, Venker C, et al. Chronic bronchitis before age 50 years predicts incident airflow limitation and mortality risk. Thorax 2009;64:894–900.

20. Hurst JR, Vestbo J, Anzueto A, et al, for the Evaluation of COPD Longitudinally to Identify Predictive

Surrogate Endpoints (ECLIPSE) investigators. Susceptibility to exacerbation in chronic obstructive pulmonary disease. N Engl J Med 2010;363:1128–38.

21. Soler-Cataluña JJ, Martínez-García MA, Román Sánchez P, et al. Severe acute exacerbations and mortality in patients with chronic obstructive pulmonary disease. Thorax 2005;60:925–31.

22. Celli BR, Thomas NE, Anderson JA, et al. Effect of pharmacotherapy on rate of decline of lung function in COPD: results from the TORCH study. Am J Respir Crit Care Med 2008;178:332–8.

23. Celli BR, Locantore N, Yates J, et al, for the ECLIPSE investigators. Inflammatory biomarkers improve clinical prediction of mortality in chronic obstructive pulmonary disease. Am J Respir Crit Care Med 2012;185:1065–72.

24. Agusti A, Edwards LD, Rennard SI, et al, for the Evaluation of COPD Longitudinally to Identify Predictive Surrogate Endpoints (ECLIPSE) investigators. Persistent systemic inflammation is associated with poor clinical outcomes in COPD: a novel phenotype. PLoS One 2012;7:e37483.

25. Thomsen M, Dahl M, Lange P, et al. Inflammatory biomarkers and comorbidities in chronic obstructive pulmonary disease. Am J Respir Crit Care Med 2012;186:982–8.

Epidemiology and Prevalence of Chronic Obstructive Pulmonary Disease

Enrique Diaz-Guzman, MD[a], David M. Mannino, MD[a,b],*

KEYWORDS

- Chronic obstructive pulmonary disease • Prevalence • Trends • Epidemiology

KEY POINTS

- In most studied countries, about 8% to 10% of the adult population has chronic obstructive pulmonary disease, with cigarette smoking as the main risk factor.
- Occupational and environmental exposures are important in the development and progression of chronic obstructive pulmonary disease, particularly in the developing world.
- Recent data suggest that rates of chronic obstructive pulmonary disease morbidity and mortality are starting to decrease in some parts of the world.

INTRODUCTION

Chronic obstructive pulmonary disease (COPD) is a preventable and treatable disease characterized by progressive airflow limitation and represents one of the most prevalent human health disorders in the world.[1] Although mortality associated with cardiovascular disease has been significantly reduced during the last 2 decades, the number of deaths associated with COPD has almost doubled, and COPD is now the fourth leading cause of death globally. More than 15 million people have the disease in the United States[2] and more than 210 million globally.[3] Despite significant public health efforts aimed to better understand and prevent the burden of this disease, the World Health Organization (WHO) has predicted that COPD will become the third most common cause of death in the world by 2030.[4] Moreover, prevalence estimates suggest that up to a quarter of

adults 40 years or older have evidence of airflow obstruction.[5] Because of the increase in prevalence, many efforts have been made to measure the epidemiology of COPD at national and international levels. Studies such as the Global Burden of Disease (GBD) and the Global Initiative for Chronic Obstructive Lung Disease (GOLD), have affected our understanding of the burden and impact of chronic respiratory disease.[6,7] This review provides a summary of the most important recent reports addressing the epidemiology of COPD and a description of new COPD guidelines.

DEFINITION OF COPD

The most recent GOLD guidelines define COPD as "a common preventable and treatable disease characterized by persistent airflow limitation that is usually progressive and associated with an enhanced chronic inflammatory response in the

Conflict of Interest Statement: E. Diaz-Guzman reports no conflicts of interest. D.M. Mannino has served as a consultant for Boehringer Ingelheim, GlaxoSmithKline, Astra-Zeneca, Novartis, Merck and Forest and has received research grants from GlaxoSmithKline, Novartis, Boehringer-Ingelheim, Forest and Pfizer.
[a] Division of Pulmonary, Critical Care, and Sleep Medicine, University of Alabama at Birmingham, 625 19th Street, Birmingham, AL 35249, USA; [b] Department of Preventive Medicine and Environmental Health, University of Kentucky College of Public Health, 111 Washington Avenue, Lexington, KY 40536, USA
* Corresponding author.
E-mail address: dmannino@uky.edu

Clin Chest Med 35 (2014) 7–16
http://dx.doi.org/10.1016/j.ccm.2013.10.002
0272-5231/14/$ – see front matter © 2014 Elsevier Inc. All rights reserved.

chestmed.theclinics.com

airways and the lungs to noxious particles or gases. Exacerbations and comorbidities contribute to the overall severity in individual patients."[7] Although this definition includes the major components of the disease, in practice, COPD consists of different clinical syndromes whose definitions vary according to the presence or absence of symptoms and measures of airflow limitation and reversibility. The following components are frequently considered when defining COPD.

Measures of Airflow Limitation and Reversibility

Airflow limitation, defined as a reduction in velocity of expiratory airflow, consists of a low forced expiratory volume in 1 second (FEV_1) and a low FEV_1 to forced vital capacity (FVC) ratio despite bronchodilator therapy. An FEV_1/FVC ratio of less than 70% continues to be used to identify airflow limitation in patients with COPD.[7,8] The use of lower limit of normal (LLN) values (based on the normal distribution of the population) has been proposed as a more specific tool to diagnose airflow limitation, but current GOLD and American Thoracic Society/European Respiratory Society guidelines continue to recommend the use of a fixed ratio instead of an LLN. Some studies have found that the use of a fixed FEV_1/FVC ratio will result in underestimation of COPD in patients less than 45 years of age (particularly those with mild disease), may overestimate the prevalence of COPD in older adults, and can result in misclassification in some patients.[9] Other studies, however, suggest that the use of a fixed ratio of 0.70 functions reasonably well in classifying most patients.[10]

In addition to airflow limitation, reversibility of airflow obstruction in response to an inhaled bronchodilator or to oral or inhaled corticosteroid is frequently used to identify patients who benefit from bronchodilator therapy.[7,11] Airflow reversibility, defined as an increase in FEV_1 of 200 mL and 12% improvement greater than baseline FEV_1, has been traditionally used to further characterize patients with airflow obstruction. Nevertheless, the degree of reversibility has not been found to increase sensitivity or specificity to diagnose COPD,[12] and current GOLD guidelines do not recommend the use of airflow reversibility as a criterion for the definition of COPD.[7]

Clinical Features and Overlap Syndromes

The characterization of COPD has included the terms *chronic bronchitis* (CB) and *emphysema*. CB is defined as the presence of a chronic productive cough for 3 months in each of 2 consecutive years provided that other medical causes have

been excluded.[13] Emphysema is defined as the destruction of alveolar walls and permanent enlargement of the airspaces distal to the terminal bronchioles.[14] Although significant improvements in imaging technologies currently allow of the accurate detection of emphysema in most patients, significant variability in physician diagnosis of emphysema and CB exist, and current GOLD guidelines do not include the use of these terms in the definition of COPD.[7]

Asthma is defined as a "chronic inflammatory disorder of the airways in which many cells and cellular elements play a role. The chronic inflammation causes an associated increase in airway hyper-responsiveness that leads to recurrent episodes of wheezing, breathlessness, chest tightness and coughing, particularly at night or in the early morning. These episodes are usually associated with widespread but variable airflow obstruction that is often reversible either spontaneously or with treatment."[15] Asthma and COPD represent 2 distinct entities with different pathogeneses and risk factors; nevertheless, clinical features of both diseases may overlap, and large population studies have found that a high proportion of patients with respiratory problems are classified with more than one diagnosis (ie, asthma and chronic bronchitis or emphysema).[16,17] Moreover, overlapping diagnoses of asthma and COPD occur more commonly in patients older than 50 years, and its frequency increases with age.[16,18]

RISK FACTORS

The pathophysiology of COPD is complex, and the disease is related to genetic and environmental factors. In addition to smoking tobacco, additional important risk factors have been recognized as important and preventable causes of COPD in industrialized and developing countries. The list of risk factors associated with this condition is extensive and has been previously well described in the literature. Following is a brief description of the most commonly known risk factors in COPD.

Active and Passive Cigarette Smoking

There is overwhelming epidemiologic evidence that confirms that smoking tobacco remains the main risk factor for COPD. Several studies have found increased risk of airway obstruction measured by spirometry[19,20] and increased risk of COPD and hospitalizations for COPD exacerbations.[21] A 25-year follow-up study of the general population in Denmark that included 8045 men and women age 30 to 65 years, found that the risk of COPD for continuous smokers was at least 25%.[22] The BOLD (Burden of Obstructive Lung

Disease) project analyzed data from 14 different populations older than 40 years and found that pack-years of smoking were associated with increased risk of COPD, including passive cigarette smoke exposure (odds ratio [OR], 1.24, 95% confidence interval [CI], 1.05–1.47 for each 10 pack-year increase).[23] In addition to the risk for COPD, results of a recent study involving 26,851 participants from Sweden found that current smoking is a strong risk factor for any wheeze (including asthmatic wheezing), particularly among young women.[24] Tobacco use remains a major cause of morbidity and mortality, particularly in patients with COPD. A recent study using pooled data from 7 different cohort studies in the United States, analyzed 50-year trends in smoking-related mortality and found that the overall risks associated with smoking plateau compared with the levels seen 2 decades ago, except for a continuing increase in mortality from COPD.[25]

Occupational Risk Factors

Several occupational exposures may increase the risk for COPD. Activities such as farming (exposure to high levels of organic particles such as vegetable dust and bacterial or fungal toxins), textile industry work (exposure to cotton dust), and industrial work (mining, smelting, wood work, building) have been associated with an increased risk for obstructive lung disease.[26] The overall work-related burden of COPD at a population level has been well-characterized. Blanc[27] performed a review of several studies and found a median PAR% (population-attributable risk) for occupationally related COPD of 15% (range 0%–37%) and 15% for occupationally related CB (range 0%–35%). A more recent prospective cohort study by Mehta and colleagues[28] evaluated the incidence of COPD in 4267 Swiss workers exposed to biologic dusts, mineral dusts, gases/fumes, and vapors and found an increased risk (2- to 5-fold) of COPD (stage 2 according to GOLD). The PAR of stage 2 COPD was between 31% and 32% for biologic dusts among smokers and ranged between 43% and 56% for nonsmokers depending on type and level of exposure.

Air Pollution

Environmental exposure to air pollution or inside of the home (particularly among habitants of under-developed countries) represents an important risk factor for COPD and other obstructive lung diseases. A multinational study from 3 metropolitan areas in Latin America (ESCALA), recently described that levels of particulate matter are significantly associated with increased mortality

from respiratory and cardiovascular causes, including COPD.[29] A more recent population cohort study assessed the risk of COPD associated with residential exposures to traffic-related air pollutants (black carbon, particulate matter <2.5 μm in aerodynamic diameter, nitrogen dioxide, and nitric oxide) and wood smoke. The study found a 7% increased risk of mortality and 15% increased risk of hospitalizations associated with COPD.[30]

Genetic Factors

Genetic factors determining the lung responses to environmental exposures are key for the development of COPD. Nevertheless, the specific genes responsible for this enhanced risk and increase in susceptibility remains poorly understood. The best described genetic factor in COPD is a deficiency in α_1-antitrypsin (PIZZ phenotype), but this abnormality accounts for only 1% to 3% of patients with COPD.[31] Numerous other genes have been studied and implicated in COPD susceptibility, based on different pathogenetic pathways: inflammatory (interleukin-4, -6, -13), tumor necrosis factor, transforming growth factor-β, protease/antiprotease (MMP9, TIMP2, SERPINA3), oxidative stress (glutathione transferase, superoxide dismutase) and others (ACE, ADRB2). A recent review of the literature summarizing possible genetic associations is shown in **Fig. 1**.[32]

PREVALENCE OF COPD

Even though COPD represents one of the most significant health care problems in the world, ascertainment of true prevalence among different countries has been difficult. Estimates of the prevalence of COPD depend on the criteria used. Significant differences in prevalence estimates from well-designed epidemiologic studies have been reported, particularly among studies completed before standardization of an epidemiologic definition of COPD. Furthermore, until recently, few studies were able to provide an estimate of disease prevalence using a standard spirometry-based definition.

Criteria and Impact on Disease Prevalence

In 1997, GOLD recommended spirometry as the gold standard diagnostic test for COPD. Estimations of COPD prevalence before GOLD guidelines were published were plagued with methodologic issues because of lack of quality assurance measures, frequent use of prebronchodilator values (which may result in overestimation of COPD), and inconsistencies in the definition of obstruction

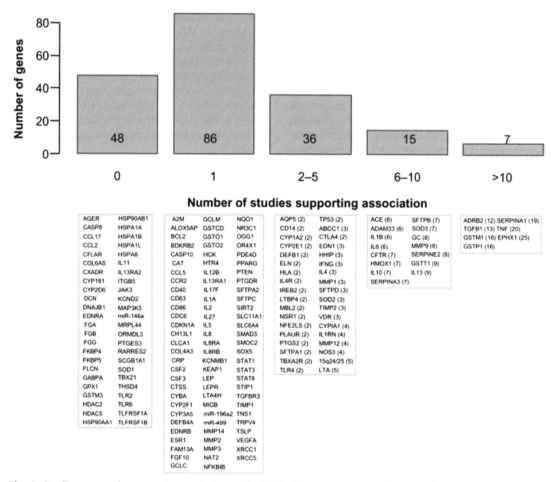

Fig. 1. Studies supporting genetic association with COPD. (*From* Bosse Y. Updates on the COPD gene list. Int J Chron Obstruct Pulmon Dis 2012;7:613.)

being used.[33] In 2002, the Burden of Obstructive Lung Disease (BOLD) project set standards for definition of COPD in epidemiologic studies and recommended the use of a postbronchodilator FEV_1/FVC ratio of less than 0.7 to define the presence of the disease. The 2013 GOLD guidelines continue to use an FEV_1/FVC ratio of less than 0.7 to define the presence of COPD, and studies have found that the observed prevalence of COPD using the GOLD definition is higher than when using the lower limit of normal criteria.[33,34]

Prevalence Estimates

In the United States, several national surveys have been conducted to establish the prevalence of COPD. Two main limitations must be taken into account when considering COPD prevalence based on survey estimates: (1) they rely on both study participants and health care providers in proper recognition and diagnosis of COPD and

(2) they lack objective spirometry data to corroborate the presence of airflow limitation.

The National Health Interview Survey, a national representative survey that included more than 40,000 households in the United States, reported in 2011 that between 2007 and 2009 approximately 5.1% (11.8 million) of adults 18 years and older had COPD. The survey also reported that the prevalence of COPD was higher in older age groups, and women had higher rates than men throughout most of the lifespan (6.1% of women [7.4 million] had COPD compared with 4.1% of men [4.4 million]). The prevalence rate of COPD is reported to be stable from 1998 through 2009.[35]

Data from the Third National Health and Nutrition Examination Survey (NHANES III), a national survey that included a representative sample of the civilian noninstitutionalized US population from 1988 and 1994 and that included data from questionnaires in the household, physical examination, and pulmonary function testing, estimated that 23.6 million adults (13.9%) met GOLD definition of COPD (stage 1 or higher) in 2000.[36] This study concluded that most subjects classified as having COPD by GOLD criteria had mild to moderate disease and that approximately 1.4% of the population (2.4 million adults) had an FEV_1 less than 50% of the predicted value.[36]

In 2011, a national telephone survey performed by the Centers for Disease Control in the United States Behavioral Risk Factor Surveillance System (BRFSS), estimated that approximately 15 million adults in the United States have COPD (age-adjusted prevalence of 6.0%). In addition, the survey reported that the prevalence increased from 3.2% among those less than 44 years of age, to 11.6% among those ≥65 years. The prevalence varied significantly across different states (**Fig. 2**).[2]

A previous meta-analysis of 62 studies published between 1990 and 2004 that included prevalence estimates from 28 different countries, reported a pooled prevalence of COPD of 7.6%. The prevalence estimate increased to 8.9% from studies that included spirometry data.[37] A recent review of the literature that included articles in English published between 2000 and 2010, reported that most estimates in the adult population varied widely across countries and populations, with a range from 0.2% in Japan to 37% in the United States. Consistent with previous observations, COPD prevalence was higher among studies using GOLD criteria to define COPD compared with other classification methods.[38] **Table 1** includes a summary of recent studies that have included spirometry data to estimate prevalence of COPD.

The table highlights how different definitions and exclusion criteria can result in different estimates of disease prevalence, even when using data from the same study.

Prevalence of COPD and Gender Differences

COPD historically has been considered a disease of male predominance; nevertheless, a significant shift in gender prevalence has been observed over the last few decades. In the United States, data from NHANES studies showed that the prevalence of moderate COPD increased during the last 2 decades in women (50.8–58.2 per 1000), whereas the prevalence decreased in men during the same period (108.1–74.3 per 1000).[39,40] Similarly, the National Health Interview Survey study reported that although the prevalence of COPD has been stable from 1998 through 2009, it has remained higher in women than in men (**Fig. 3**).[35] A similar trend has been observed in other developed countries,[41,42] whereas in developing countries, prevalence of COPD is still higher in men compared with women.[43]

BURDEN OF COPD AND MORTALITY

The GBD study has provided estimates of worldwide global and regional mortality. In 2006, GBD reported that COPD caused the death of at least 3.1 million people, representing the fourth leading cause of mortality in the world.[44] A subsequent report of the GBD that included mortality between 1990 and 2010 shows that COPD is now the third leading cause of mortality in the world, although

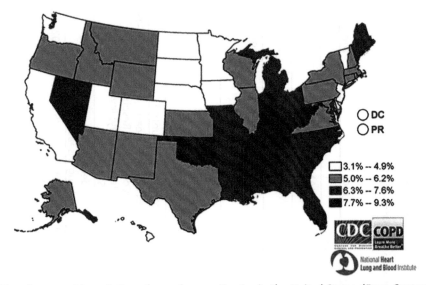

Fig. 2. BRFSS and geographic variation of prevalence estimates in the United States. (*From* Centers for Disease Control and Prevention. Chronic pulmonary obstructive disease among adults - United States 2011. MMWR Morb Mortal Wkly Rep 2012;61(46):938–42.)

Table 1
Prevalence estimates of COPD

Reference	Study	Dates	Sample	Diagnosis of COPD	Prevalence (%)	Comments
United States						
Celli et al[9]	NHANES III	1988–1994	9838 adults (30–80 y)	GOLD Stage ≥I (2001 criteria)	16.8	Smokers had 21.9% vs never smokers 9.1%
Hnizdo et al[50]	NHANES III	1988–1994	13,824 adults (20–80 y)	GOLD Stage >I (2001 criteria)	14.2	Prevalence by LLN criteria (ATS 1991) of 12.3%
Mannino et al[40]	NHANES III	1991–1994	6600 adults (>25 y) with spirometry data	GOLD Stage >II (2001 criteria)	7.4	Prevalence rates age adjusted to 2000 US population
Vaz Fragoso et al[51]	NHANES III	1988–1994 (followed up until 12/2000)	3502 adults (40–80 y)	GOLD Stage >I (2006 criteria)	27	Mean age 60.7 y. LLN (2008 criteria) prevalence of 13.8%
Multicentric, International (>1 country)						
Cerveri et al[52]	ECRHS (European Community Respiratory Health Survey) involving 25 countries	1991–1993	17,966 adults (20–44 y)	Stage >I (2004 criteria)	3.6	Prevalence for GOLD stage 0 was 11.8%
Buist et al[53]	Burden of Obstructive Lung Disease (BOLD)	—	9425 adults (40 y of age and older)	GOLD Stage >II (2006 criteria)	10.1	11.8% for men and 8.5% for women
Menezes et al[54]	PLATINO Study (5 Latin American countries)	2002–2005	5315 adults (>40 y)	GOLD Stage >0 (2004 criteria)	7.8–19.7	Rates varied significantly across Latin American countries

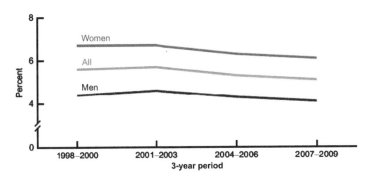

Fig. 3. Prevalence of COPD among adults aged 18 and older: United States, 1998 to 2009. (*From* Akinbami LJ, Liu X. Chronic obstructive pulmonary disease among adults aged 18 and over in the United States, 1998–2009. NCHS Data Brief 2011;(63):1–8.)

the number of deaths attributed to COPD decreased from 3.1 million to 2.9 million annually.[45]

In contrast to these optimistic estimates in developed countries, the problem of COPD continues to increase in the rest of the world. Studies estimate that up to 50% of all households in developing countries use coal and biomass as primary sources of energy and therefore are exposed to smoke produced during heating and cooking.[46] The WHO has estimated that approximately 700,000 annual deaths from COPD are caused by solid fuel smoke exposure, although these numbers may severely underestimate the real burden of COPD in underdeveloped countries.[47] Studies calculate that in Latin America, between 30% and 75% of people living in rural areas use biomass fuels for cooking[48] and in India, China, and sub-Saharan Africa, as much as 80%.[49] In 2000, the WHO estimated that approximately 1.6 million deaths in the world were attributed to indoor air pollution. Ten years later, the WHO raised the estimate to 2.0 million deaths annually.

A recent review of the literature that included 58 studies between 2000 and 2010 describes significant variations in mortality rates in the world, with overall mortality rate of 3 to 9 deaths per 100,000 people in Japan to 7 to 111 deaths per 100,000 in the United States. This review found that studies reported an overall increase in COPD mortality rates within the last 30 to 40 years, with a much greater increase in mortality in women compared with men, with some studies suggesting a slight decrease in COPD mortality among men.[38]

In the United States, studies have reported that the age-adjusted mortality rate for COPD doubled from 1970 to 2000.[41] Nevertheless, a recent report by Ford and colleagues[10] that included an analysis from data in the NHANES I and NHANES III studies, found that compared with NHANES I, the mortality rate among participates in the NHANES III decreased by 15.8% for participants with moderate or severe COPD and 25.2% for those with mild COPD, suggesting that overall mortality attributed to COPD may be decreasing,

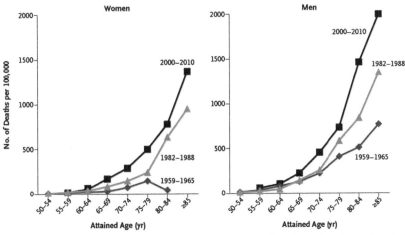

Fig. 4. Changes in rates of death from COPD over time among current female and male smokers in 3 time periods. (*From* Thun MJ, Carter BD, Feskanich D, et al. 50-year trends in smoking-related mortality in the United States. N Engl J Med 2013;368(4):360; with permission.)

but there was a lesser decrease in mortality rate in women with moderate or severe COPD compared with men (3% vs 17.8%).

A recent assessment of smoking-related mortality in the United States evaluated temporal trends in sex-specific, smoking-related mortality across 3 time periods (1959–1965, 1982–1988, and 2000–2010) in 7 large cohorts. In the contemporary cohort that encompassed the years 2000 to 2010, male and female current smokers had similar relative risks for mortality from COPD (26.61 for men, 22.35 for women), with these relative risks representing almost a doubling of risk when compared with the 1982 to 1988 period (**Fig. 4**).[25]

SUMMARY

Estimating the true prevalence of COPD in the world is a difficult task. Nevertheless, during the last couple of decades, there has been significant progress made in identification and classifications of populations with COPD that currently allow us to determine the impact of this deadly disease in the world. In developed countries, current information estimates a prevalence of 8% to 10% among adults 40 years of age and older, whereas in developing countries, prevalence varies significantly among countries and is difficult to estimate. Recent reports also suggest that prevalence of COPD might have plateaued or even decreased in developed countries, whereas there is overwhelming evidence to suggest that most of the world population is still exposed to biomass fuels and likely will see an increase in prevalence of COPD. Overall, the mortality associated with COPD appears to be improving, except for a trend increase in mortality in women. Further studies will help us better understand these geographic and mortality differences.

REFERENCES

1. Decramer M, Janssens W, Miravitlles M. Chronic obstructive pulmonary disease. Lancet 2012; 379(9823):1341–51.
2. Centers for Disease Control and Prevention. Chronic pulmonary obstructive disease among adults - United States 2011. MMWR Morb Mortal Wkly Rep 2012;61(46):938–42.
3. Bousquet J, Kiley J, Bateman ED, et al. Prioritised research agenda for prevention and control of chronic respiratory diseases. Eur Respir J 2010; 36(5):995–1001.
4. WHO. World health statistics. 2008. Available at: http://www.whoint/whosis/whostat/EN_WHS08_Full. pdf. Accessed February 15, 2012.
5. Mannino DM, Buist AS. Global burden of COPD: risk factors, prevalence, and future trends. Lancet 2007;370(9589):765–73.
6. Murray CJ, Lopez AD. Alternative projections of mortality and disability by cause 1990-2020: Global Burden of Disease Study. Lancet 1997; 349(9064):1498–504.
7. Global strategy for the diagnosis, management, and prevention of chronic obstructive pulmonary disease. NHLBI/WHO Global Initiative for Chronic Obstructive Lung Disease (GOLD) Workshop summary (Revised 2013). Available at: http://www. goldcopd.org. Accessed February 15, 2013.
8. Celli BR, MacNee W. Standards for the diagnosis and treatment of patients with COPD: a summary of the ATS/ERS position paper. Eur Respir J 2004; 23(6):932–46.
9. Celli BR, Halbert RJ, Isonaka S, et al. Population impact of different definitions of airway obstruction. Eur Respir J 2003;22(2):268–73.
10. Ford ES, Mannino DM, Zhao G, et al. Changes in mortality among US adults with COPD in two national cohorts recruited from 1971-1975 and 1988-1994. Chest 2012;141(1):101–10.
11. Dirksen A, Christensen H, Evald T, et al. Bronchodilator and corticosteroid reversibility in ambulatory patients with airways obstruction. Dan Med Bull 1991;38(6):486–9.
12. Albert P, Agusti A, Edwards L, et al. Bronchodilator responsiveness as a phenotypic characteristic of established chronic obstructive pulmonary disease. Thorax 2012;67(8):701–8.
13. Standards for the diagnosis and care of patients with chronic obstructive pulmonary disease. American Thoracic Society. Am J Respir Crit Care Med 1995;152(5 Pt 2):S77–121.
14. Snider GL. Chronic obstructive pulmonary disease: a definition and implications of structural determinants of airflow obstruction for epidemiology. Am Rev Respir Dis 1989;140(3 Pt 2):S3–8.
15. Masoli M, Fabian D, Holt S, et al. The global burden of asthma: executive summary of the GINA Dissemination Committee report. Allergy 2004; 59(5):469–78.
16. Soriano JB, Davis KJ, Coleman B, et al. The proportional Venn diagram of obstructive lung disease: two approximations from the United States and the United Kingdom. Chest 2003;124(2):474–81.
17. Shaya FT, Dongyi D, Akazawa MO, et al. Burden of concomitant asthma and COPD in a Medicaid population. Chest 2008;134(1):14–9.
18. Gibson PG, Simpson JL. The overlap syndrome of asthma and COPD: what are its features and how important is it? Thorax 2009;64(8):728–35.
19. Gold DR, Wang X, Wypij D, et al. Effects of cigarette smoking on lung function in adolescent boys and girls. N Engl J Med 1996;335(13):931–7.

20. Langhammer A, Johnsen R, Gulsvik A, et al. Sex differences in lung vulnerability to tobacco smoking. Eur Respir J 2003;21(6):1017–23.

21. Prescott E, Bjerg AM, Andersen PK, et al. Gender difference in smoking effects on lung function and risk of hospitalization for COPD: results from a Danish longitudinal population study. Eur Respir J 1997;10(4):822–7.

22. Lokke A, Lange P, Scharling H, et al. Developing COPD: a 25 year follow up study of the general population. Thorax 2006;61(11):935–9.

23. Hooper R, Burney P, Vollmer WM, et al. Risk factors for COPD spirometrically defined from the lower limit of normal in the BOLD project. Eur Respir J 2012;39(6):1343–53.

24. Bjerg A, Ekerljung L, Eriksson J, et al. Higher Risk of wheeze in female than male smokers. Results from the Swedish GA(2)LEN Study. PLoS One 2013;8(1):e54137.

25. Thun MJ, Carter BD, Feskanich D, et al. 50-year trends in smoking-related mortality in the United States. N Engl J Med 2013;368(4):351–64.

26. Diaz-Guzman E, Aryal S, Mannino DM. Occupational chronic obstructive pulmonary disease: an update. Clin Chest Med 2012;33(4):625–36.

27. Blanc PD. Occupation and COPD: a brief review. J Asthma 2012;49(1):2–4.

28. Mehta AJ, Miedinger D, Keidel D, et al. Occupational exposure to dusts, gases and fumes and incidence of COPD in SAPALDIA. Am J Respir Crit Care Med 2012;185:1292–300.

29. Romieu I, Gouveia N, Cifuentes LA, et al. Multicity study of air pollution and mortality in Latin America (the ESCALA study). Res Rep Health Eff Inst 2012;(171):5–86.

30. Gan WQ, Fitzgerald JM, Carlsten C, et al. Associations of ambient air pollution with chronic obstructive pulmonary disease hospitalization and mortality. Am J Respir Crit Care Med 2013;187:721–7.

31. Stoller JK, Aboussouan LS. Alpha1-antitrypsin deficiency. Lancet 2005;365(9478):2225–36.

32. Bosse Y. Updates on the COPD gene list. Int J Chron Obstruct Pulmon Dis 2012;7:607–31.

33. Shirtcliffe P, Weatherall M, Marsh S, et al. COPD prevalence in a random population survey: a matter of definition. Eur Respir J 2007;30(2):232–9.

34. Colak Y, Lokke A, Marott JL, et al. Impact of diagnostic criteria on the prevalence of COPD. Clin Respir J 2013;7:297–303.

35. Akinbami LJ, Liu X. Chronic obstructive pulmonary disease among adults aged 18 and over in the United States, 1998-2009. NCHS Data Brief 2011;(63):1–8.

36. Mannino DM, Gagnon RC, Petty TL, et al. Obstructive lung disease and low lung function in adults in the United States: data from the National Health and Nutrition Examination Survey, 1988–1994. Arch Intern Med 2000;160(11):1683–9.

37. Halbert RJ, Natoli JL, Gano A, et al. Global burden of COPD: systematic review and meta-analysis. Eur Respir J 2006;28(3):523–32.

38. Rycroft CE, Heyes A, Lanza L, et al. Epidemiology of chronic obstructive pulmonary disease: a literature review. Int J Chron Obstruct Pulmon Dis 2012;7:457–94.

39. Camp PG, Goring SM. Gender and the diagnosis, management, and surveillance of chronic obstructive pulmonary disease. Proc Am Thorac Soc 2007; 4(8):686–91.

40. Mannino DM, Homa DM, Akinbami LJ, et al. Chronic obstructive pulmonary disease surveillance–United States, 1971-2000. MMWR Surveill Summ 2002;51(6):1–16.

41. Gershon AS, Wang C, Wilton AS, et al. Trends in chronic obstructive pulmonary disease prevalence, incidence, and mortality in ontario, Canada, 1996 to 2007: a population-based study. Arch Intern Med 2010;170(6):560–5.

42. Bischoff EW, Schermer TR, Bor H, et al. Trends in COPD prevalence and exacerbation rates in Dutch primary care. Br J Gen Pract 2009;59(569):927–33.

43. Menezes AM, Perez-Padilla R, Jardim JR, et al. Chronic obstructive pulmonary disease in five Latin American cities (the PLATINO study): a prevalence study. Lancet 2005;366(9500):1875–81.

44. Lopez AD, Shibuya K, Rao C, et al. Chronic obstructive pulmonary disease: current burden and future projections. Eur Respir J 2006;27(2): 397–412.

45. Lozano R, Naghavi M, Foreman K, et al. Global and regional mortality from 235 causes of death for 20 age groups in 1990 and 2010: a systematic analysis for the Global Burden of Disease Study 2010. Lancet 2012;380(9859):2095–128.

46. Perez-Padilla R, Schilmann A, Riojas-Rodriguez H. Respiratory health effects of indoor air pollution. Int J Tuberc Lung Dis 2010;14(9):1079–86.

47. Zhang J, Smith KR. Indoor air pollution: a global health concern. Br Med Bull 2003;68:209–25.

48. Romieu I, Riojas-Rodriguez H, Marron-Mares AT, et al. Improved biomass stove intervention in rural Mexico: impact on the respiratory health of women. Am J Respir Crit Care Med 2009;180(7):649–56.

49. Desai M, Mehta S, Smith K. Indoor smoke from solid fuels: assessing the environmental burden of disease at national and local levels. Geneva (Switzerland): World Health Organization; 2004.

50. Hnizdo E, Sullivan PA, Bang KM, et al. Association between chronic obstructive pulmonary disease and employment by industry and occupation in the US population: a study of data from the Third National Health and Nutrition Examination Survey. Am J Epidemiol 2002;156(8):738–46.

51. Vaz Fragoso CA, Concato J, McAvay G, et al. The ratio of FEV1 to FVC as a basis for establishing chronic obstructive pulmonary disease. Am J Respir Crit Care Med 2010;181(5): 446–51.

52. Cerveri I, Accordini S, Verlato G, et al. Variations in the prevalence across countries of chronic bronchitis and smoking habits in young adults. Eur Respir J 2001;18(1):85–92.

53. Buist AS, McBurnie MA, Vollmer WM, et al. International variation in the prevalence of COPD (the BOLD Study): a population-based prevalence study. Lancet 2007;370(9589):741–50.

54. Menezes AM, Perez-Padilla R, Hallal PC, et al. Worldwide burden of COPD in high- and low-income countries. Part II. Burden of chronic obstructive lung disease in Latin America: the PLATINO study. Int J Tuberc Lung Dis 2008;12(7):709–12.

Tobacco Smoking and Environmental Risk Factors for Chronic Obstructive Pulmonary Disease

Sundeep Salvi, MD, DNB, PhD

KEYWORDS

- Chronic obstructive pulmonary disease • Risk factors • Environmental • Tobacco smoking
- Biomass smoke

KEY POINTS

- A better understanding of the risk factors associated with chronic obstructive pulmonary disease (COPD) is important to help prevent the development and progression of COPD.
- Tobacco smoking is an established risk factor for COPD. Tobacco can be smoked in different forms apart from cigarettes, many of which are more harmful. Exposure to second-hand smoke is also a risk factor for COPD.
- However, many other risk factors associated with COPD remain underappreciated or neglected. More than 50% of cases of COPD can be attributed to nonsmoking risk factors.
- Exposure to indoor air pollution resulting from the burning of biomass fuels is a major risk factor for COPD, especially in developing countries.
- Other indoor air pollutants and outdoor air pollutants also contribute to the risk of COPD.
- Occupational causes contribute to up to 30% of COPD cases, but very little is known about this risk factor. Farming is a neglected risk factor for COPD.

INTRODUCTION

Chronic obstructive pulmonary disease (COPD) is a chronic progressive disease of the airways and lung parenchyma that is associated with exposure to tobacco smoke and other environmental insults in genetically susceptible individuals. The damaged lungs in COPD are difficult to revert back to normal. Current management is therefore aimed at reducing the symptoms and rapid decline in lung function, and preventing acute exacerbations. The economic burden associated with COPD is huge. Preventing the development of COPD, therefore, seems to be the only cost-effective public health intervention strategy that can reduce the global burden. Understanding the risk factors associated with the development of COPD is important so that primary, secondary, and even tertiary preventive strategies can be developed.

The development of COPD is multifactorial, and the risk factors include both genetic and environmental factors. The association between tobacco smoking and chronic bronchitis was first highlighted in 1955 by Oswald and Medvei.[1] However, the landmark study that established the association between tobacco smoking and COPD was the 8-year prospective study of 792 British men by Feltcher and Peto,[2] which observed that susceptible smokers showed a sharp and progressive decline in lung function that was the hallmark of this disease. The larger and longer Framingham study from the United States has confirmed these earlier reports.[3] For the last 5 decades, tobacco smoking has remained the most important risk

Chest Research Foundation, Marigold Complex, Kalyaninagar, Pune 411014, India
E-mail address: ssalvi@crfindia.com

Clin Chest Med 35 (2014) 17–27
http://dx.doi.org/10.1016/j.ccm.2013.09.011

chestmed.theclinics.com

factor associated with COPD across the world. In fact, the term COPD is used synonymously with smoking-induced lung disease.

As early as 1958, Fairbairn and Reid[4] reported that outdoor air pollution was an important risk factor for COPD, and in 1963 Phillips[5] reported that risk factors other than tobacco smoking were associated with COPD. However, the overwhelming interest in smoking as the main risk factor for COPD overshadowed these nonsmoking causes. In 2003, Lundbäck and colleagues[6] from Sweden and Mannino and colleagues[7] from the United States reported that the population-attributable risk of tobacco smoking for COPD was 45% and 44%, respectively, indicating that more than half of the cases of COPD were due to nonsmoking causes. In the same year, Ezatti and Lopez[8] published global mortality rates attributable to smoking from all causes in *The Lancet*, and reported that 47% of COPD deaths in men and 78% of COPD deaths in women were not attributable to tobacco smoking (**Fig. 1**). In 2009, Salvi and Barnes[9] reviewed the global literature on the prevalence of COPD among never-smokers, and reported that between 25% and 45% of patients with COPD across the globe had never smoked; highlighting the fact that COPD in never-smokers is much more common than was previously believed. A recent study on COPD prevalence from 14 countries, defined by postbronchodilator spirometry values, reported that 23.3% of the COPD subjects were never-smokers.[10]

This article describes the role of tobacco smoking and the various environmental risk factors associated with the development of COPD. Other risk factors for COPD such as poorly treated chronic severe asthma, status post pulmonary tuberculosis, poor socioeconomic status, and nutritional factors are not covered herein, and for a discussion of these factors the reader is referred to the review by Salvi and Barnes.[9]

TOBACCO SMOKING

The cigarette looks deceptively simple, but it is one of the most effectively engineered inhaler devices that delivers a steady dose of nicotine to the human body. Nicotine is present in the tobacco leaf, and its concentration varies depending on the variety of tobacco leaf. For example, the bright variety, which was originally grown in Virginia, United States, contains 2.5% to 3% nicotine, whereas the burley type of tobacco contains 3.5% to 4% nicotine and the oriental tobacco type contains less than 2% nicotine.

Nicotine is an alkaloid that is an extremely powerful drug. It stimulates the central nervous system and also increases the heart rate and blood pressure. Nicotine causes addiction similar to that of heroin and cocaine,[11] and is contained in the moisture of the tobacco leaf. When the cigarette is lit it evaporates, attaching itself to minute droplets in the tobacco smoke inhaled by the smoker. After being deposited in the lung, nicotine is absorbed very quickly and reaches the brain within 10 to 19 seconds. The damage that occurs in the lungs of tobacco smokers is mainly mediated by the tar present in the smoke, whereas the nicotine is relatively harmless.

Tar is the sticky brown substance that stains smokers' fingers and teeth yellow-brown. All cigarettes produce tar, but different brands produce different amounts. Earlier cigarettes (1950s) contained 30 mg tar per cigarette, but because of strict legislation modern cigarettes have tar levels lower than 11 mg per cigarette. According to the European Union directives, upper limits of tar, nicotine, and carbon monoxide have been set at

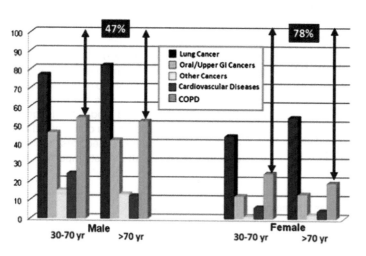

Fig. 1. Global mortality attributable to smoking: 47% of male COPD deaths and 78% of female COPD deaths are not attributable to tobacco smoking. (*Data from* Ezatti M, Lopez AD. Estimates of global mortality attributable to smoking in 2000. Lancet 2003;362(9387):847–52.)

10 mg, 1 mg, and 10 mg, respectively. The type of paper used in the cigarette determines the amount of tar and nicotine that will be delivered into the lungs. Using more porous paper will let more air into the cigarette, diluting the smoke and reducing the amount of tar and nicotine entering into the lungs. Filters are made of cellulose acetate, and trap some of the tar and smoke particles from the inhaled smoke. Filters also cool the smoke slightly, making it easier to breathe.

Apart from the dried tobacco leaf, the cigarette also contains fillers made from the stems and other bits of tobacco, which are otherwise waste products. These fillers are mixed with water and various flavorings and additives. Additives are used to make the tobacco products more acceptable to the smoker, and include humectants (moisturizers) to prolong shelf life, and sugars to make the smoke milder and easier to inhale. A total of 600 such additives have been permitted by the Department of Health in the United States. Although many of these additives may seem quite harmless on their own, they may be toxic in their combination with other substances. Tobacco smoke contains 4000 chemicals, at least 20 of which are known to be carcinogenic.

Tobacco is inhaled in various other forms also. In India and other Asian countries, tobacco is rolled in dried tendu leaves (*Diospyros melanoxylon*), called bidi, and smoked (**Fig. 2**). Seventy percent of people in India smoke bidis mainly because they are cheap and easily available. Compared with cigarettes, bidis contain lesser amounts of nicotine (one-fourth of that in a cigarette) but produce 3 to 5 times the amount of tar, making it more harmful than cigarettes. Moreover, bidi smoking requires the person to smoke continuously and deeper to keep the bidi lit, which further increases the tar deposition in the lungs. Other forms of tobacco smoking include the hookah or water-pipe and the chillum, which also contain other additives apart from tobacco leaf. These forms of smoking have been shown to be more harmful than cigarette smoke.[12] Water-pipe smoking, which is common in the Middle East and Asia (**Fig. 3**), is perceived to be safer than cigarettes because the smoke passes through water, but studies have shown that this smoke is as harmful as cigarette smoke.[13]

Associations between tobacco smoking and COPD have been shown in a large number of studies.[14] It was earlier reported that 15% of smokers develop COPD, indicating a strong genetic basis, because a significant proportion of smokers do not develop COPD. However, Lundbäck and colleagues[6] have reported that up to 50% of smokers can develop COPD, indicating that tobacco smoking poses a substantial risk for COPD in the general population.

SECOND-HAND SMOKE OR ENVIRONMENTAL TOBACCO SMOKE

The sidestream smoke from the burning of cigarettes is called second-hand smoke or

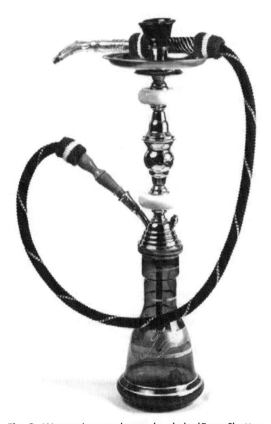

Fig. 3. Water-pipe smoker or hookah. (*From* Shutterstock, with permission. Available at: www.shutterstock.com.)

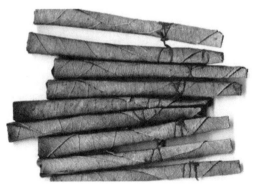

Fig. 2. Bidi: Tobacco wrapped in dried tendu leaf. (*From* Shutterstock, with permission. Available at: www.shutterstock.com.)

environmental tobacco smoke, which mainly comes from the burning tip of the cigarette. Many toxins are present in higher concentrations in the sidestream smoke than in the mainstream smoke.[15] Typically, 85% of smoke in a room is due to sidestream smoke. Woodruff and colleagues[16] and, more recently, Goldklang and colleagues[17] studied the mechanisms by which second-hand smoke causes emphysema in animal experiments. Apart from cellular and mediator inflammation triggered by second-hand smoke, they report evidence of recruitment and activation of alveolar macrophages along with generation of reactive oxygen species, which together trigger the development of alveolar wall destruction. Exposure to second-hand smoke in human subjects has been shown to cause degradation of body elastin and possible injury to lung structure, thereby indicating a mechanism by which second-hand smoke can lead to the development of emphysema.[18]

Earlier observational studies reported an association between exposure to second-hand tobacco smoke and the risk of COPD.[19–21] A case-control study conducted by Kalandidi and colleagues[19] reported that women married to smokers and exposed to 1 pack per day or less were at a 2.5-times greater risk of having COPD than those married to nonsmokers. Sandler and colleagues[20] followed 14,783 healthy subjects exposed to second-hand smoke for 12 years and reported that the estimated relative risk of death from COPD was 5.65. Female spouses of smokers from Italy were reported to be at a 2.24-fold greater risk of developing obstructive lung disease than those married to nonsmokers.[21]

A cross-sectional study from China reported an association between self-reported exposure to passive smoking at home and work and the risk of COPD.[22] An average exposure of 40 hours per week for more than 5 years was associated with a 48% increased odds of contracting COPD. A similar cross-sectional study from the United States involving 2113 adults between the ages of 55 and 75 years reported that exposure to second-hand smoke was associated with a 36% greater odds of contracting COPD.[23] More recently, a study from Taiwan reported that women exposed to second-hand smoke had a 3.65-fold greater risk of being diagnosed with COPD, and that the duration of exposure to second-hand smoke correlated positively with the severity of COPD. The population-attributable risk for COPD from exposure to second-hand smoke was 47.3%.[24] Because the prevalence of cigarette smoking among Taiwanese men is high (55%–60%) and is low in women (3%–4%), a large

number of Taiwanese nonsmoking women exposed to second-hand smoke seem to be at a greater risk of developing COPD. A recent prospective study conducted in 910 Chinese men and women for a period of 17 years reported that exposure to second-hand tobacco smoke was associated with a dose-dependent and 2.3-fold greater risk of COPD.[25]

However, not all studies have shown a positive association between second-hand tobacco smoke exposure and the risk of developing COPD.[26] More work needs to be done to study the true impact of second-hand smoke on COPD.

EXPOSURE TO INDOOR BIOMASS FUEL SMOKE

An estimated 50% of the world's population and 90% of the rural population of Africa and Asia use biomass fuels for cooking and heating purposes, accounting for more than 3 billion persons exposed to biomass smoke.[27] Biomass fuels include wood, animal dung, crop residues, dried twigs, dried grass, and fossil coal (**Fig. 4**). These fuels are cheap and easily available in rural settings, and are therefore widely used by poor people. Even modern homes in many developed countries are shifting their fuels from electricity and gas to biomass because of the increasing cost of cleaner fuels.[28]

Biomass fuels are inefficient because they not only produce less heat but also burn incompletely to release many noncombustible air pollutants. Crop residues are the least efficient, followed by animal dung and wood. Burning of biomass fuels produces more than 200 known chemical compounds, more than 90% of which can penetrate deep into the lungs.[29] These pollutants are classified into gaseous pollutants (carbon monoxide, sulfur dioxide, nitrogen dioxide) and particulate pollutants (PM10 and PM2.5, which are particles

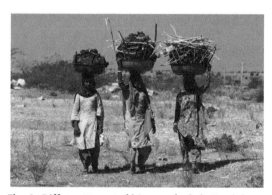

Fig. 4. Different types of biomass fuels (animal dung, wood, crop residues). (*From* Shutterstock, with permission. Available at: www.shutterstock.com.)

with a mass median aerodynamic diameter of 10 μm and 2.5 μm, respectively). These tiny particles are made up of black carbon, polyaromatic hydrocarbons, chlorinated dioxins, arsenic, lead, and transition metals such as nickel and vanadium. The indoor levels of PM10 in homes that use biomass fuel for cooking are often 5 to 50 times above the safety limits prescribed by the World Health Organization.[30] As many as 14 carcinogenic compounds, 6 cilia-toxic compounds and mucus-coagulating agents, and 4 cocarcinogenic or cancer-promoting agents have been identified in biomass fuel smoke.[31]

Women are typically exposed to high levels of biomass smoke pollutants for between 3 and 7 hours each day during cooking, often in poorly ventilated homes. On average, women spend 60,000 hours during their lifetime cooking near the biomass stove, during which period they inhale more than 25 million liters of highly polluted air.[32]

Two large meta-analyses investigated the association between exposure to biomass smoke and the risk of developing COPD. Hu and colleagues[33] analyzed 15 published studies and concluded that people exposed to biomass smoke had a 2.44-fold increased risk of COPD compared with those not exposed. Po and colleagues[34] analyzed 25 studies, and also reported a 2.4-fold increased odds of COPD among women exposed to biomass smoke. Of note, these odds are similar to those observed in chronic smokers who develop COPD. Compared with 1.1 billion smokers worldwide, 3 billion people are exposed to biomass smoke. It has therefore been argued that exposure to biomass smoke is probably a bigger risk factor for COPD than tobacco smoking from a global perspective.[32] The association between exposure to biomass smoke and COPD is seen in both developing and developed countries. Sood and colleagues[28] reported that exposure to wood smoke was associated with a 70% greater prevalence of COPD in New Mexico County in the United States. The reader is referred to the article by Sood and colleagues[28] for more information on the impact of biomass smoke on COPD.

Preliminary work from the author's laboratory indicates that subjects exposed to biomass smoke who develop COPD have a cellular and mediator inflammatory profile in the airways similar to that of tobacco smoke–induced COPD as evaluated by induced sputum.[35] Apart from greater small-airway obstruction in biomass smoke–induced COPD, the extent of physiologic impairment is similar to that of tobacco smoke–induced COPD.[36] More recently, the author compared the quality of life of patients with COPD caused by biomass smoke exposure and those with tobacco

smoke–induced COPD using the St George questionnaire, and observed that subjects with COPD from biomass smoke had the same degree of impairment in quality of life (unpublished observations by the author, September 2013). Dutta and colleagues[37] have recently demonstrated that biomass users showed greater amounts of inflammatory cells, cytokines (eg, interleukin-6, interleukin-8, tumor necrosis factor α), and oxidative stress in the induced sputum in comparison with women who use cleaner fuels.

Exposure to biomass smoke is now recognized as an important risk factor for COPD. Several interventional studies examining the impact of improved cooking stoves (reducing biomass smoke) have reported improvements in lung function, symptoms, and the prevalence of COPD.[38–40] However, more work is needed to better understand the impact of different interventions that reduce indoor biomass smoke on the burden of COPD.

OTHER INDOOR AIR POLLUTANTS

The other indoor air pollutant that could pose a significant risk for COPD in tropical countries is smoke from mosquito coils (**Fig. 5**). It has been shown that burning one mosquito coil over a period of 8 hours emits as much particulate matter and formaldehyde as that equivalent to 100 cigarettes and 51 cigarettes, respectively.[41] Smoke from the burning of mosquito coils may therefore pose a significant risk for the development of COPD, as these are widely used in many African and Asian countries to drive mosquitos away during sleeping hours. Moreover, mosquito-coil smoke has been shown to contain other harmful air pollutants, such as carbon monoxide, isoprene and benzene, and heavy

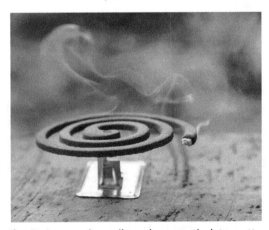

Fig. 5. A mosquito coil produces particulate matter equivalent to around 100 cigarettes. (*From* Shutterstock, with permission. Available at: www.shutterstock.com.)

metals such as lead, nickel, chromium, and tin. Smoke from mosquito coils has been shown to be a risk factor for lung cancer in Taiwan.[42] Animals exposed to mosquito-coil smoke have been shown to have significant histopathologic changes in the lung, such as loss of cilia, emphysema, metaplasia of epithelial cells, and morphologic alterations in alveolar macrophages.[43] Despite the concern over the risk of developing COPD from mosquito-coil smoke, very little research has been done on this aspect, even in countries where the use of these coils is common.

Other indoor air pollutants that are of potential risk in the development of COPD include cooking-oil smoke, kerosene smoke, incense smoke, pesticides, and volatile organic compounds from furnishings. However, there is very little information on these pollutants as potential risk factors for COPD.

OCCUPATIONAL COPD

Studies from developed countries indicate that the population-attributable fraction for COPD associated with occupational exposure varies between 9% and 31%.[44] A study from the United States estimated the population-attributable risk for COPD due to occupation to be 43%.[45] A prospective cohort study among Swiss workers reported that the population-attributable risk of COPD was 31% among smokers and 50% among nonsmokers in workers exposed to biological dusts.[46] The prevalence of occupational COPD is likely to be greater in developing countries because of the lack of stringent regulations at workplaces and the lack of adequate protective gear.

Several occupations are associated with an increased risk for COPD, and these are listed in **Box 1**.

Box 1
Occupations associated with COPD

- Dust exposures: coal mining, hard rock mining, concrete manufacturing, construction, tunneling, brick manufacturing, iron and steel founding, gold mining
- Animal farming: organic dust, ammonia, hydrogen sulfide, bacteria
- Crop farming: organic and inorganic dust
- Chemical exposure: plastic, textiles, rubber industry, leather manufacturing
- Diesel exhaust: trucking, transportation, automotive repair
- Road dust: sweeping

Farming

Farming is one of the most common and neglected occupations associated with an increased risk of COPD. Studies in crop farmers from Canada[47,48] and the United States[49] have reported higher prevalence of chronic bronchitis and lower lung function compared with controls. Lamprecht and colleagues[50] reported that 30.2% of the farmers in rural Austria showed evidence of poorly reversible mild airway obstruction and that 7.7% had moderate to severe COPD based on spirometry. Similar observations have been reported from Spain,[51] and more recently from the Philippines[52] and China.[53] In the Philippines, farming for more than 40 years was found to be associated with a 2.5-fold greater risk of COPD and was similar to the risk associated with smoking tobacco for more than 20 pack-years.[52] In China, the prevalence of COPD was found to be 24.3%, 20.8%, 17.9%, and 12.6% among fungus greenhouse farmers, poultry greenhouse farmers, flower greenhouse farmers, and vegetable greenhouse farmers, respectively,[53] although it is not known whether smoking was a major confounder in this study.

Several cross-sectional studies have shown that animal farming is also associated with a greater risk of COPD. Poultry farming,[54] pig farming,[55] and dairy farming[56] have been shown to be strongly associated with COPD. Poultry-farm workers **(Fig. 6)** are often exposed to total inhalable dust levels exceeding 10 mg/m^3 during most activities.[57] The composition of dust in animal farms ranges from wood dust to a complex mixture of organic material derived from feed, litter, fecal material, dander, feather, and microorganisms. A Norwegian study reported that livestock farmers had a 40% greater risk of COPD than crop farmers, and this was strongly associated with ambient levels of ammonia, hydrogen sulfide, and organic dusts.[58] Farmers rearing more than one type of livestock, for example, sheep, goats, and poultry, had a significantly higher risk of COPD than those rearing only 1 type. Multiple etiologic factors are linked to the risk of developing COPD at farm locations, including organic dusts, endotoxins, peptidoglycans, and gases. Feeding operations in situations of large animal confinement also contain a wide diversity of microbes such as gram-positive bacteria and archaebacteria.[59] It has been suggested that chronic exposure to these inhalants has a significant impact on local and systemic inflammatory responses that may underlie the development of chronic disease of the airways.[60]

Apart from organic dust, farmers are also exposed to significant amounts of inorganic soil

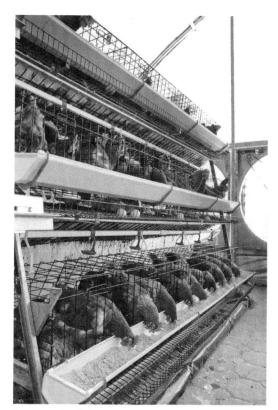

Fig. 6. Animal farming is an important occupation associated with COPD. (*From* Shutterstock, with permission. Available at: www.shutterstock.com.)

dust (**Fig. 7**). The highest dust exposures occur during soil = preparation activities (eg, plowing, disking, and planting). Tractors pulling soil-preparation equipment generate large dust clouds, with particle concentrations reaching levels of up to 20 mg/m^3, and sometimes even 100 mg/m^3.[61] Total respirable dust concentrations in tractor cans reach levels between 1 and 5 mg/m^3. It has

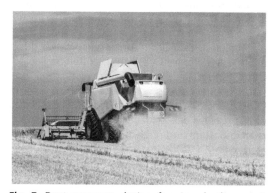

Fig. 7. Dust exposure during farming, both organic and inorganic, is a risk factor associated with COPD. (*From* Shutterstock, with permission. Available at: www.shutterstock.com.)

been shown that respirable quartz exposures in agriculture commonly exceed industrial standards. Silicates are the predominant inorganic fraction found in most soils, but in arid locations soil content is dominated by calcium carbonate and other soluble salts, whereas in warm humid climates soil dust is made up of oxides and hydroxides of iron and aluminum.[62]

Farming-induced COPD is poorly recognized across the world. Clinicians and policy makers need to be made aware of this association, so that early diagnosis and appropriate preventive strategies can be instituted. Farming-induced COPD can be prevented by controlling harmful exposures to organic dust, toxic gases, and chemicals on farms through improvements in animal-rearing techniques, ventilation of animal accommodation, careful drying and storage of animal feedstuffs, crops, and other products, and use of personal protective equipment.[63]

Other Occupations Associated with COPD

Mining and quarrying were the first occupations associated with significant reductions in lung function and the development of irreversible airflow obstruction. Coal mining has been shown to be associated with the risk of developing emphysema, 6 times more so than in nonminers.[64,65] Other mining activities that are generally characterized by silica exposure, such as gold, iron, and copper mining, and quarrying industries such as talc, potash, slate, and kaolin quarrying, have been reported to carry an increased risk of COPD.[66]

Petrochemical, mining, and steel industries are associated with chronic exposures to metals that are associated with an increased risk of COPD. A Danish study reported that cement and concrete workers have a higher risk of being hospitalized with COPD in comparison with gainfully employed men.[67] Occupations associated with exposure to diesel exhaust, such as transportation, trucking, construction, and vehicle mechanics, have been shown to be associated with an increased risk of COPD, but the evidence is weak.[68]

More recently, road sweepers from Pakistan have been shown to have a higher prevalence of COPD, which was proportional to the duration of exposure to road dust.[69]

In comparison with occupational asthma there is very little literature on the management and prevention of occupational COPD, and there are no published guidelines. The diagnosis of occupational COPD is infrequently made in clinical practice, and the clinician must therefore be attentive to all potential occupational causes in patients who have poorly reversible airway obstruction, especially among never-smokers.[70] Effective management should necessarily focus on medical treatment of already prevalent COPD and efforts to prevent and/or limit ongoing further damage via reduction of exposure.[70] The reader is referred to a review on this topic recently published in *Clinics in Chest Medicine*.[70]

OUTDOOR AIR POLLUTION

Outdoor air pollution, mainly from motor vehicular and industrial emissions, has been shown to be associated with various respiratory adverse effects, especially lung development in children aged 10 to 18 years.[71] The effects on adults are not clear, but women seem to be more affected than men.[72] In one of the largest published studies on the impact of traffic exposure on lung function in the United States, heavier traffic density was associated with greater decrements in lung function as evaluated by spirometry; when the distance from the main road was used as a parameter, the closer was the residence from the main road, the lower was the lung function.[72] Several biological mechanisms have been proposed to explain the harmful effects of ambient air pollutants, namely, increase in bronchial hyperresponsiveness, oxidative stress, airway inflammation, amplification of viral infections, and damage to ciliary activity of the airways.[73]

Few studies have investigated the effects of ambient air pollution on the risk of COPD prevalence. A German study of 4757 women living in the Rhine-Ruhr Basin reported that ambient PM10 levels were significantly associated with the risk of COPD. A 7-μg/m^3 increase in 5-year means of PM10 was associated with a 33% increased odds of contracting COPD. Moreover, women living within 100 m from the main road had 79% greater odds of presenting with COPD than those who lived more than 100 m away.[74] When the same cohort was followed up after 10 years, the prevalence of COPD had reduced as the levels of PM10 reduced.[75] A large cross-sectional study from Denmark showed a strong association between 35-year mean NO$_2$ levels and the risk of being hospitalized for COPD.[76]

A recent longitudinal cohort study from Vancouver, Canada, which examined the long-term exposure to elevated traffic-related air pollution with the risk of COPD hospitalization and mortality, reported that even a small increase in ambient black carbon air pollutants was associated with an increase in COPD hospitalizations and an increase in COPD mortality after adjustment for covariates.[77] A study from Rome, Italy reported that

patients with COPD had 5 times greater mortality associated with ambient PM10 and NO$_2$ levels in comparison with normal subjects. Moreover, pre-existing heart-conduction disorders and cerebrovascular diseases were found to have stronger effects in older men with COPD.[78]

Despite all the evidence, it remains unclear whether ambient air pollution may lead to a decline in lung function and subsequent development of COPD. Because few studies have confirmed COPD by spirometry and the published data are conflicting, a causal relationship between outdoor air pollution and COPD cannot be drawn at this stage.[73] A study from Nottingham, United Kingdom did not report any association between ambient levels of air pollutants and COPD.[79] A recent meta-analysis of 8 morbidity and 6 mortality studies reported that the evidence of chronic effects of air pollution on the prevalence and incidence of COPD among adults was suggestive but not conclusive, despite plausible biological mechanisms and good evidence that air pollution affects lung development in childhood and triggers exacerbations in COPD patients. The investigators recommend that larger studies with longer follow-up periods, specific definitions of COPD phenotypes, and more refined and source-specific exposure assessments are needed before any conclusive statement can be made.[80]

SUMMARY

Tobacco smoking is an important and preventable risk factor for the development and progression of COPD. Apart from the cigarette, several other devices are used to inhale tobacco smoke, many of which are in fact more harmful than cigarettes. However, tobacco smoking is not the only risk factor associated with COPD. Second-hand exposure to tobacco smoke has also been shown to be associated with the risk of COPD, although more robust evidence needs to be generated. Exposure to biomass smoke occurs in 50% of the world's population, especially in Africa and Asia, and is a major risk factor for COPD that is often neglected. Other indoor air pollutants are also important. Occupational causes contribute to up to 30% of COPD, and several occupations are associated with a greater risk of developing COPD. Farming is an important and neglected occupation associated with COPD. Cross-sectional studies have shown as association between outdoor air pollution and COPD, but more robust evidence is required.

A better understanding of the risk factors and their relative contribution to the development of COPD will help guide policy makers and health care providers to take appropriate interventional measures for primary as well as secondary prevention. Only then will the global burden of COPD be reduced.

REFERENCES

1. Oswald NC, Medvei VC. Chronic bronchitis: the effect of cigarette smoking. Lancet 1955;269:843–4.
2. Fletcher C, Peto R. The natural history of chronic airflow obstruction. BMJ 1977;1:645–8.
3. Kohansal R, Martinez-Camblor P, Agusti A, et al. The natural history of chronic airflow obstruction revisited: an analysis of the Framingham offspring cohort. Am J Respir Crit Care Med 2009;180:3–10.
4. Fairbairn AS, Reid DD. Air pollution and other local factors in respiratory disease. Br J Prev Soc Med 1958;12:94–103.
5. Phillips AM. The influence of environmental factors in chronic bronchitis. J Occup Med 1963;5:468–75.
6. Lundbäck B, Lindberg A, Lindström M, et al. Not 15 but 50% of smokers develop COPD? Report from the Obstructive Lung Disease in Northern Sweden Studies. Respir Med 2003;97(2):115–22.
7. Mannino DM, Buist AS, Petty TL, et al. Lung function and mortality in the United States: data from the First National Health and Nutrition Examination Survey follow up study. Thorax 2003;58(5):388–93.
8. Ezatti M, Lopez AD. Estimates of global mortality attributable to smoking in 2000. Lancet 2003; 362(9387):847–52.
9. Salvi SS, Barnes PJ. Chronic obstructive pulmonary disease in non-smokers. Lancet 2009;374: 733–43.
10. Lamprecht B, McBurnie MA, Vollmer WM, et al. COPD in never smokers: results from the population-based burden of obstructive lung disease study. Chest 2011;139(4):752–63.
11. Nicotine Addiction in Britain. A report of the Tobacco Advisory Group of the Royal College of Physicians. London: Royal College of Physicians; 2000.
12. Singh S, Soumya M, Saini A, et al. Breath carbon monoxide levels in different forms of smoking. Indian J Chest Dis Allied Sci 2011;53(1):25–8.
13. Raad D, Gaddam S, Schunemann HJ, et al. Effects of water-pipe smoking on lung function: a systemic review and meta-analysis. Chest 2011; 139(4):764–74.
14. Bartal M. COPD and tobacco smoke. Monaldi Arch Chest Dis 2005;63(4):213–5.
15. California Environment Protection Agency. Health effects of exposure to environmental tobacco smoke. Tob Control 1997;6:346–53.
16. Woodruff PG, Ellwanger A, Solon M, et al. Alveolar macrophage recruitment and activation by chronic secondhand smoke exposure in mice. COPD 2009; 6(2):86–94.
17. Goldklang MP, Marks SM, D'Armiento JM. Second hand smoke and COPD. Lessons from animal studies. Front Physiol 2013;4(30):1–8.
18. Slowik N, Ma S, He J, et al. The effect of second hand smoke exposure on markers of elastic degradation. Chest 2011;140(4):946–53.
19. Kalandidi A, Trichopoulos D, Hatzakis A, et al. Passive smoking and chronic obstructive lung disease. Lancet 1987;2(8571):1325–6.
20. Sandler DP, Comstock GW, Helsing KJ, et al. Deaths from all causes in non-smokers who lived with smokers. Am J Public Health 1989;79(2):163–7.
21. Simoni M, Baldacci S, Puntoni R, et al. Respiratory symptoms/diseases and environmental tobacco smoke (ETS) in never smoker Italian women. Respir Med 2007;101(3):531–8.
22. Yin P, Jiang CQ, Cheng KK, et al. Passive smoking exposure and risk of COPD among adults in China: The Guangzhou Biobank Cohort Study. Lancet 2007;370:751–7.
23. Eisner MD, Balmes J, Katz PP, et al. Lifetime environmental tobacco smoke exposure and the risk of COPD. Environ Health 2005;4:7.
24. Wu CF, Feng NH, Chong IW, et al. Second hand smoke and chronic bronchitis in Taiwanese women: a health care based study. BMC Public Health 2010;10:44.
25. He Y, Jiang B, Li LS, et al. Second hand smoke exposure predicted COPD and other tobacco-related mortality in a 17-year cohort study in China. Chest 2012;142(4):909–18.
26. Jaakkola MS, Jaakkola JJ. Effects of environmental tobacco smoke on respiratory health of adults. Scand J Work Environ Health 2002;28(Suppl 2): 52–70.
27. World resources institute, UNEP, UNDP, World Bank. 1998-99 world resources: a guide to global environment. Oxford (United Kingdom): Oxford University Press; 1998.
28. Sood A, Petersen H, Blanchette CM, et al. Wood smoke exposure and gene promoter methylation are associated with increased risk for COPD in smokers. Am J Respir Crit Care Med 2010;182(9): 1098–104.
29. Torres-Duque C, Maldonado D, Perez-Padilla R, et al. Biomass fuels and respiratory diseases: a review of the evidence. Proc Am Thorac Soc 2008; 5(5):577–90.
30. Kodgule R, Salvi S. Exposure to biomass smoke as a cause for airway disease in women and children. Curr Opin Allergy Clin Immunol 2012;12(1):82–90.
31. Balkrishnan K, Mehta S, Kumar P, et al. Indoor air pollution associated with household fuel use in India. India: ESMAP, World Bank; 2004.
32. Salvi S, Barnes PJ. Is exposure to biomass smoke the biggest risk factor for COPD globally? Chest 2010;138:3–6.

33. Hu G, Zhou Y, Tian J, et al. Risk of COPD from exposure to biomass smoke: a meta-analysis. Chest 2010;138(1):20–31.

34. Po JT, Fitzgerald JM, Carlsten C. Respiratory disease associated with solid biomass fuel exposure in rural women and children: systematic review and meta-analysis. Thorax 2011;66:232–9.

35. Brashier B, Vanjare N, Londhe J, et al. Comparison of airway cellular and mediator profiles between tobacco smoke-induced COPD and biomass fuel exposure-induced COPD in an Indian Population. Eur Respir J 2011;734.

36. Brashier B, Vanjare N, Vincent V, et al. Lung function differences in subjects with tobacco smoke-induced COPD (TS-COPD) and biomass smoke-induced COPD (BS-COPD) in an Indian population. Eur Respir J 2011;918.

37. Dutta A, Roychoudhury S, Chowdhury S, et al. Changes in sputum cytology, airway inflammation and oxidative stress due to chronic inhalation of biomass smoke during cooking in premenopausal rural Indian women. Int J Hyg Environ Health 2013;216(3):301–8.

38. Smith-Siversten T, Diaz E, Pope D, et al. Effect of reducing indoor air pollution on women's respiratory symptoms and lung function: the RESPIRE randomized trial, Guatemala. Am J Epidemiol 2009;170(2):211–20.

39. Romieu I, Riojas-Rodriguez H, Marron-Mares AT, et al. Improved biomass stove intervention in rural Mexico. Impact on the respiratory health of women. Am J Respir Crit Care Med 2009;180(7):649–56.

40. Chapman RS, He X, Blair AE, et al. Improvement in household cookstoves and risk of COPD in Xuanwei, China: Retrospective cohort study. BMJ 2005;331:1050.

41. Liu W, Zhang J, Hashim JH, et al. Mosquito coil emissions and health implications. Environ Health Perspect 2003;111(12):1454–60.

42. Chen SC, Wong RH, Shiu LJ, et al. Exposure to mosquito coil smoke may be a risk factor for lung cancer in Taiwan. J Epidemiol 2008;18(1):19–25.

43. Liu WK, Wong MH. Toxic effects of mosquito coil smoke on rats. II. Morphological changes of the respiratory system. Toxicol Lett 1987;39(2):231–9.

44. Trupin L, earnest G, San Pedro M, et al. The occupational burden of chronic obstructive pulmonary disease. Eur Respir J 2003;22:561–9.

45. Weinmann S, Vollmer WM, Breen V, et al. COPD and occupational exposures: a case control study. J Occup Environ Med 2008;50(5):561–9.

46. Mehta AJ, Miedinger D, Keidel D, et al. Occupational exposures to dusts, gases, and fumes and incidence of COPD in the Swiss cohort study on air pollution and lung and heart diseases in adults. Am J Respir Crit Care Med 2012;185:1292–300.

47. Dosman JA, Graham BL, Hall D, et al. Respiratory symptoms and pulmonary function in farmers. J Occup Med 1987;29(1):38–43.

48. Kennedy SM, Dimich-Ward H, Desjardins A, et al. Respiratory health among retired grain elevator workers. Am J Respir Crit Care Med 1994;150(1):59–65.

49. Gamsky TE, Schenker MB, McCurdy SA, et al. Smoking, respiratory symptoms and pulmonary function among a population of Hispanic farmworkers. Chest 1992;101(5):1361–8.

50. Lamprecht B, Schirnhofer L, Kaiser B, et al. Farming and the prevalence of non-reversible airways obstruction: results from a population based study. Am J Ind Med 2007;50(6):421–6.

51. Monso E. Bronchial colonization in chronic obstructive pulmonary disease: what's hiding under the rug. Arch Bronconeumol 2004;40(12):543–6.

52. Idolor LF, de Guia TS, Francisco NA, et al. Burden of obstructive lung disease in a rural setting in the Philippines. Respirology 2011;16(7):1111–8.

53. Liu S, Wen DL, Li LY, et al. Chronic pulmonary disease group of greenhouse farmers in Liaoning Province. Zhonghua Jie He He Hu Xi Za Zhi 2011;34(10):753–6.

54. Viegas S, Faisca VM, Dias H, et al. Occupational exposure to poultry dust and effects on the respiratory system in workers. J Toxicol Environ Health 2013;76(4–5):230–9.

55. Costa M, Teixeira PJ, Freitas PF. Respiratory manifestations and respiratory diseases: prevalence and risk factors among pig farmers in Braco de Norte, Brazil. J Bras Pneumol 2007;33(4):380–8.

56. Jouneau S, Boche A, Brinchault G, et al. On-site screening of farming-induced chronic obstructive pulmonary disease with the use of an electronic mini-spirometer: results of a pilot study in Britanny, France. Int Arch Occup Environ Health 2012;85(6):623–30.

57. Crook B, Easterbrook A, Stagg S. Exposure to dust and bioaerosols in poultry farming. Summary of observations and data. Health and Safety Laboratory. 2008. vii. Available at: http://www.hse.gov.uk/research/rrpdf/rr655.pdf. Accessed August 1, 2013.

58. Eduard W, Pearce N, Douwes J. Chronic bronchitis, COPD, and lung function in farmers: the role of biological agents. Chest 2009;136(3):716–25.

59. May S. Respiratory health effects of large animal farming environments. J Toxicol Environ Health 2012;15(8):524–41.

60. Sahlander K, Larsson K, Palmberg L. Altered innate immune response in farmers and smokers. Innate Immun 2010;16(1):27–38.

61. Nieuwenhuijsen MJ, Kruize H, Schenker MB. Exposure to dust, noise and pesticides, their determinants and the use of protective equipment among

California farm operators. Appl Occup Environ Hyg 1996;11:1217–25.

62. Schenker M. Exposures and health effects from inorganic agricultural dusts. Environ Health Perspect 2000;108(4):661–4.

63. Linaker C, Smedley J. Respiratory illness in agriculture workers. Occup Med 2002;52(8):451–9.

64. Kuempel ED, Wheeler MW, Smith RJ, et al. Contributions of dust exposure and cigarette smoking to emphysema severity in coal miners in the United States. Am J Respir Crit Care Med 2009;180(3):257–64.

65. Santo-Tomas LH. Emphysema and COPD in coal miners. Curr Opin Pulm Med 2011;17(2):123–5.

66. Becklake MR. Chronic airflow limitation: its relationship to work in dusty occupations. Chest 1985;88(4):608–17.

67. Molgaard EF, Hannerz H, Tuchsen F, et al. Chronic lower respiratory diseases among demolition and cement workers: a population-based register study. BMJ Open 2013;3(1). http://dx.doi.org/10.1136/bmjopen-2012-001938.

68. Hart JE, Eisen EA, Laden F. Occupational diesel exhaust exposure as a risk factor for COPD. Curr Opin Pulm Med 2012;18(2):151–4.

69. Anwar SK, Mehmood N, Nasim N, et al. Sweeper's lung disease: a cross sectional study of an overlooked illness among sweepers of Pakistan. Int J Chron Obstruct Pulmon Dis 2013;8:193–7.

70. Diaz-Guzman E, Aryal S, Mannino DM. Occupational COPD. An update. Clin Chest Med 2012;33:625–36.

71. Gauderman WJ, Avol E, Gilliland F, et al. The effect of air pollution on lung development from 10-18 years of age. N Engl J Med 2004;351:1057–67.

72. Kan H, Heiss G, Rose KM, et al. Traffic exposure and lung function in adults: the atherosclerosis risk in communities study. Thorax 2007;62:873–9.

73. Ko FW, Hui DS. Air pollution and COPD. Respirology 2012;17:395–401.

74. Schikowski T, Sugiri D, Ranft U, et al. Long-term air pollution exposure and living close to busy roads are associated with COPD in women. Respir Res 2005;6:152.

75. Schikowski T, Ranft U, Sugiri D, et al. Decline in air pollution and change in prevalence in respiratory symptoms and COPD in elderly women. Respir Res 2010;11:113.

76. Andersen ZH, Hvidberg M, Jensen SS, et al. COPD and long term exposure to traffic related air pollution: a cohort study. Am J Respir Crit Care Med 2011;183(4):455–61.

77. Gan WQ, Fitzgerald JM, Carlsten C, et al. Associations of ambient air pollution with COPD hospitalisation and mortality. Am J Respir Crit Care Med 2013;187(7):721–7.

78. Faustini A, Stafoggia M, Cappai G, et al. Short-term effects of air pollution in a cohort of patients with COPD. Epidemiology 2012;23(6):861–79.

79. Pujades-Rodriguez M, McKeever T, Lewis S, et al. Effect of traffic pollution on respiratory and allergic disease in adults: cross sectional and longitudinal analyses. BMC Pulm Med 2009;9:42.

80. Schikowski T, Mills IC, Andersen HR, et al. Ambient air pollution—a cause for COPD? Eur Respir J 2013. [Epub ahead of print].

Genetic Susceptibility

Stefan J. Marciniak, PhD, FRCP[a,b,*],
David A. Lomas, PhD, ScD, FRCP, FMedSci[c]

KEYWORDS

- Genetics • COPD • Emphysema • GWAS • SNP

KEY POINTS

- Approximately 20% of the population-attributable risk for chronic obstructive pulmonary disease (COPD) arises from family history.
- Early hypothesis-driven candidate gene approaches identified several genes contributing to risk for COPD, including components of the protease/antiprotease system and of the antioxidant pathway.
- More recent unbiased genome-wide association studies have gone on to reveal unanticipated genetic factors, for example, polymorphisms within the nicotinic acetyla choline receptor.
- The individual risk contributed by most genetic variants that predispose to COPD is small (odds ratios of less than 1.5), but current technological advances have rendered their analysis a tractable and therapeutically important question.

INTRODUCTION

Although most smokers will die of a smoking-related disorder, only 20% suffer from significant chronic obstructive pulmonary disease (COPD). Familial clustering suggests that heritable factors play an important role in the development of this disease.[1,2] In one large series, 18.6% of population-attributable risk for COPD could be accounted for by family history: patients with an affected parent having more severe disease, more frequent exacerbations, and a worse quality of life.[3] Similarly, in twin pairs the risk of developing COPD is higher for monozygotic than for dizygotic twins, with 60% of the individual susceptibility explained by genetic factors.[4] Both the airway and the emphysema components cluster independently, suggesting that different genetic factors play a role in the development of these 2 components of the disease.[5] Unsurprisingly, for a

disorder with a substantial heritable component, race and ethnicity seem to impact on the development of COPD. For example, in the COPDGene Study, 42% of affected African Americans were found to suffer severe early-onset COPD (age <55 years, forced expiratory volume in 1 second [FEV1] <50% predicted) compared with 14% of non-Hispanic whites.[6] In contrast, self-reported Hispanic ethnicity and Native American genetic ancestry have both been reported to be associated with significantly lower risks of developing COPD.[7]

Efforts to identify the genetic determinants of COPD have evolved as the available technologies have changed. The analysis of candidate genes yielded some successes that will be discussed later (in "Candidate Gene Approaches" section), but that approach also led to numerous blind alleys, with initial excitement followed by disappointment as associations proved impossible to reproduce. The analysis of large cohorts of patients in

This work was supported by the Medical Research Council (UK), British Lung Foundation, and Diabetes UK. S.J. Marciniak is an MRC Senior Clinical Fellow (G1002610).
[a] Division of Respiratory Medicine, Department of Medicine, Addenbrooke's Hospital, Cambridge CB2 0QQ, UK;
[b] Cambridge Institute for Medical Research (CIMR), University of Cambridge, Wellcome Trust/MRC Building, Hills Road, Cambridge CB2 0XY, UK; [c] University College London, 1st Floor, Maple House, 149 Tottenham Court Road, London W1T 7NF, UK
* Corresponding author. Cambridge Institute for Medical Research (CIMR), University of Cambridge, Wellcome Trust/MRC Building, Hills Road, Cambridge CB2 0XY, UK.
E-mail address: sjm20@cam.ac.uk

genome-wide association studies (GWAS) using microarray technology to assay up to a million single nucleotide polymorphisms (SNPs) in each case led to the unbiased identification of novel disease-associated loci. This approach is hypothesis-free and so has the potential to open novel avenues of research.

UNBIASED APPROACHES

Until recently, only mutations of the *SERPINA1* gene that are responsible for α_1-antitrypsin deficiency were unambiguously linked with the development of COPD. However, this disorder accounts for only 1% to 2% of cases of COPD and so other disease-associated alleles must exist. Recent large multinational GWAS have shed much light on this. In addition to validating the involvement of some candidate genes previously suspected of playing a role in the pathogenesis of COPD, these landmark studies have identified novel pathways that might plausibly lead to novel therapies for COPD.

SNPs in chromosome 15 at the α-nicotinic acetylcholine receptor *CHRNA3/5* locus (15q25.1, rs8034191, and rs1051730) were found to reach genome-wide significance and have subsequently been replicated in several independent studies.[8–13] This locus is significantly associated with pack-years of smoking, emphysema (by computed tomography [CT]), and airflow obstruction.[9,14] Notably, the C allele of the rs8034191 SNP was estimated to have a population attributable risk for COPD of 12.2% and has previously been identified in genome-wide association studies of lung cancer, being thought to be important in nicotine addiction.[8] Individuals who carry this SNP may require more cigarettes to satisfy nicotine addiction, may inhale more deeply, and may find it more difficult to withdraw from cigarette smoking. Indeed, it has been reported that the association of the *CHRNA3/5* locus is substantially mediated by smoking phenotype,[12] although this finding has been disputed.[14] However, *IREB2* is a gene in tight linkage disequilibrium with *CHRNA3/5* and has also been identified as a potential determinant of COPD.[9,15,16] This gene encodes an iron regulatory protein localized in epithelia that may plausibly affect oxidative stress responses in smoked-exposed lungs. These candidate genes are not mutually exclusive and it remains possible that both genes within the haplotype contribute to the disease phenotype.[12]

GWAS have also identified a locus at 4q22.1 containing the gene *FAM13A* to be significantly associated with COPD and lung function in multiple cohorts.[9,17] Although the function of *FAM13A* is unclear, another gene at 4q31 newly identified and replicated by GWAS as being associated with both COPD and lung function encodes hedgehog interacting protein, which appears to play a role in signaling that modulates lung development or remodeling.[8,18–20] Hedgehog interacting protein is expressed in pulmonary tissues but at lower levels in COPD-affected lungs, and disease-associated SNPs have been identified within the gene's promoter (rs6537296A and rs1542725C) that appear to reduce its transcription.[21] Other loci that have been identified using similar techniques include 2q35, 4q24, 5q33, 6p21, 15q23, and 19q13, although these require validation.[19,22] Other COPD-related phenotypes have also been linked with specific loci, for example, low body mass index in COPD is significantly association with SNP rs8050136 within the first intron of the fat mass and obesity-associated (*FTO*) gene,[23] whereas an SNP in *BICD1* (rs10844154 in 12p11.2) is associated with the presence and severity of emphysema on CT scan.[24]

CANDIDATE GENE APPROACHES
The Extracellular Matrix

Alveolar tissue consists of epithelial cells, capillaries, and extracellular matrix (ECM), the latter comprising a complex network of scaffolding proteins, principally elastin and collagen. The elastin filaments form from tropoelastin monomers that self-assemble into aggregates and then fuse with microfilaments. Multiple covalent cross-links between the lysines in neighboring filaments provide stability. Cutis laxa is a family of autosomal-dominant (OMIM #123700), X-linked (OMIM #304150), and recessive (OMIM #219100, 219200) human diseases characterized by excessively slack connective tissues. Several families with the milder autosomal-dominant form show early-onset pulmonary pathologic abnormality including emphysema,[25] particularly if inherited with the Z allele of α_1-antitrypsin.[26] Two groups independently identified separate mutations within the ELN (elastin) gene that cause mild cutis laxa and early-onset COPD.[27,28] The ELN gene maps to 7q11.23 in man, but as chromosome 7 has not been identified in linkage analysis as a site associated with COPD, it is likely that ELN mutations are a rare cause of this disease.

Elastin fibers bind other proteins including fibulins, which in turn bind multiple ECM components and the basement membrane. The fibulins are a family of 6 proteins, at least 2 of which are mutated in severe autosomal-recessive forms of cutis laxa and whose phenotype often includes early-onset emphysema.[29,30] A novel mutation in the fibulin-4 gene (FBLN4; 11q13) was recently identified in autosomal-recessive cutis laxa with developmental emphysema.[29] The mutation caused an amino acid substitution in an epidermal growth factor–like domain of FBLN-4, leading to very low levels of extracellular protein. In a consanguineous Turkish family, a homozygous mutation in the related fibulin-5 gene (FBLN5; 14q32.1) was also found to cause cutis laxa and emphysema complicated by recurrent pulmonary infections.[30] Once again, the mutation was located within an epidermal growth factor–like domain, suggesting these are critical for fibulins to maintain the integrity of the ECM within the lung. Interestingly, analogous mutations in fibrillin, which bare homology to the fibulins, cause Marfan syndrome. Moreover, mutations of fibrillin (FBN1; 15q21.1) have been described in neonatal Marfan with very early-onset emphysema.[31–33]

Menkes disease (OMIM #309400), characterized by abnormal hair and dysmorphic features, is caused by mutations in an intracellular copper transporter (ATP7A; Xq13.3). The clinical features are due to defective connective tissue synthesis thought to be the result of dysfunction of lysyl oxidase. This copper-dependent enzyme is required for proper cross-linking of both collagen and elastin fibers. A recent case report described a child with Menkes disease and severe bilateral pan-lobular emphysema who died at the age of 14 months.[34] Gene sequencing revealed a splice-site mutation in ATP7A, suggesting that proper ECM cross-linking is vital for stability of the lung parenchyma.

In contrast to animal models of COPD, mutations in collagen have not been identified in humans, but does not appear to be due to an incompatibility of mutated collagen with survival, as numerous collagen mutations have been described that cause other human diseases. Instead, it may reflect a more important role for elastin integrity in emphysema in humans than in mice. However, aberrant collagen synthesis has been implicated in COPD. The signaling molecule TGFβ1 enhances collagen synthesis in vivo, and polymorphisms in its gene (TGFB1; 19q13.1) have been associated with COPD,[35–39] although a recent, large study found no association between TGFB1 polymorphisms and the rate of lung function decline in smokers.[40] Intriguingly, the TGFβ1 gene maps to a locus on chromosome 19, which has high linkage (LOD 3.3) with FEV_1 in smokers.[36,41] However, as is frequently the case with polymorphism studies, the literature is unclear. For example, 2 TGFB1 SNPs, rs1800469 and rs1982073, were found to be independently associated with COPD in 2 studies,[35,38] but in another, they were only significant when analyzed as part of a haplotype (combination of alleles), whereas yet another SNP, rs6957, was significant in its own right.[39] Detailed analysis of the Boston Early-Onset COPD Study data revealed further complexity.[36] Although some alleles of TGFB1 were associated with FEV_1 (rs2241712, rs2241718, rs6957), there was a separate but partially overlapping set of alleles associated with airflow obstruction (rs2241712, rs1800469, rs1982073). TGFβ1 protein is inactive when first secreted owing to the presence of an inhibitory N-terminal propeptide. It is secreted associated with latent TGFβ1 binding proteins (LTBP), which share structural features with fibrillins and are assembled into the ECM. Mice with mutations in LTBP4 develop severe emphysema.[42] Intriguingly, the sole study that has addressed LTBP4 (19q13.1-q13.2) polymorphisms found an association with COPD in man.[38] More recently, genome-wide linkage analysis of pedigrees stratified by emphysema status (on CT scan) identified a region on chromosome 1p (LOD score = 2.99).[43] An intronic SNP in TGFB-receptor-3 at this locus was found to be associated with COPD status, FEV_1, and CT emphysema.

Taken together, these studies provide strong evidence in support of a crucial role for the loss of ECM integrity, in particular, the elastic components, in the development of COPD. It is therefore important to consider the enzymes implicated in degradation of the ECM.

Protease-Antiprotease Balance

The protease antiprotease theory has its roots in the observation that individuals with α_1-antitrypsin are particularly susceptible to COPD and in experimental models of emphysema from the 1960s. This theory suggests that the pathogenesis of COPD and emphysema is the result of an imbalance between enzymes that degrade the ECM within the lung and proteins that oppose this proteolytic activity. Many proteases play important roles in remodeling or inflammation within the lung. It is essential that they be controlled by antiproteases to protect against uncontrolled degradation of the ECM.

The best-understood example of genetically induced emphysema results from mutations in the α_1-antitrypsin gene (SERPINA1; 14q32.1). These mutations increase the protein's propensity to form ordered polymers, which are incapable of inhibiting its target enzyme, neutrophil elastase. This abnormal behavior leads to retention of the protein within hepatocytes as periodic acid Schiff–positive inclusions and results in plasma deficiency of an important protease inhibitor (OMIM #107400). It is now increasingly recognized that mutant α_1-antitrypsin can also form polymers within the interstitium and alveolar spaces of the lung. These polymers are chemotactic for neutrophils and so combine with the deficiency of α_1-antitrypsin to focus and amplify the inflammatory response within the lung.[44] In most Northern European populations the frequency of the most severe Z allele is about 1/2000. Classically, Z α_1-antitrypsin homozygotes carry the Glu342Lys mutation and suffer from early-onset emphysema when compared with normal MM α_1-antitrypsin individuals. The onset and progression of emphysema are markedly accelerated by cigarette smoking. Moreover, it appears that even a single allele of Z α_1-antitrypsin may increase the risk of COPD. In the longitudinal Copenhagen City Heart Study, the MZ α_1-antitrypsin genotype increased the rate of decline of FEV_1 by 19% compared with those who were MM homozygotes, causing a 30% increased risk of obstructive lung function and a 50% increased risk of physician-diagnosed COPD.[45] The authors found that the frequency of the MZ genotype in their Danish population was as high as 5% and so calculated that it would account for 2.4% of cases of COPD. This finding is in contrast to the ZZ genotype, which was causal in only 0.8% of cases. In meta-analysis, heterozygosity for the Z allele carried an odds ratio for COPD of 2.31.[46] In one study, the MZ (but not MS; the S allele has the Glu264Val mutation) α_1-antitrypsin genotype was associated with a rapid decline in FEV_1, which was even more marked if there was also a family history of COPD, suggesting an interaction with additional genetic factors.[47] A further meta-analysis combining 17 studies found a 3-fold increase in COPD in SZ α_1-antitrypsin heterozygotes and a small increase in MS α_1-antitrypsin heterozygotes. Other polymorphisms of the SERPINA1 gene do not appear to be associated with increased risk of developing COPD.[48]

Other pulmonary serine protease inhibitors may also be involved in the pathogenesis of COPD. Following earlier linkage studies demonstrating an association between chromosome 2q and COPD, expression profiling of genes within that locus identified SERPINE2 (2q33-q35) as being up-regulated during murine lung development and in the lungs of individuals with COPD.[49] The authors went on to demonstrate an association between SNPs in SERPINE2 and COPD. SERPINE2 SNPs were found to segregate with COPD in a large multicenter family-based study and to be associated with COPD in a case-control analysis.[50] However, another large study failed to replicate the association with COPD despite having adequate power.[51] The latter study included individuals with COPD with and without emphysema, whereas the studies by Demeo and colleagues[49] included a preponderance of patients with emphysema assessed for lung volume reduction surgery. Nevertheless, although these differences may reflect different COPD phenotypes, they illustrate the need to replicate the findings of genetic association studies in multiple populations before drawing firm conclusions. A recent study of Finish construction workers found that 3 SNPs within SERPINE2 (rs729631, rs975278, and rs6748795) were in tight linkage disequilibrium and so focused solely on one (rs729631),[52] which showed a significant association with panlobular emphysema, as seen with mutants of SERPINA1.

Because mutations of α_1-antitrypsin so clearly lead to emphysema, one might infer that its target, neutrophil elastase, is central to the pathogenesis of disease. However, mutations in this protease have not been shown to be important, despite being studied extensively in other conditions. Instead, most evidence implicates matrix metalloproteases (MMPs) in the pathogenesis of COPD. These MMPs are zinc-dependent endopeptidases involved in the degradation of many ECM components. An SNP of MMP9 (20q11) was associated with COPD in Japanese[53] and Chinese[54] populations; however, a further Japanese study found an association with emphysema distribution rather than COPD per se.[55] Another large study failed to show MMP9 association with COPD, but instead MMP1 (11q22) and MMP12 (11q22) polymorphisms were identified.[56] Further support for a role for MMP9, but not MMP1 polymorphisms, has also been published.[57] Tissue inhibitors of metalloproteinases inhibit the MMPs, but thus far, only one polymorphism in tissue inhibitors of metalloproteinases 2 (17q25) has been associated with COPD.[58] When more than 8000 individuals were analyzed, the minor allele of the promoter of MMP12 (rs2276109 [$-82A \rightarrow G$]) showed clear association with FEV_1 in a combined analysis of adult ever-smokers and children with asthma and with a reduced risk of COPD.[59] In a separate study, a haplotype containing this SNP in MMP-12 (rs652438 and rs2276109) was found to be associated with severe COPD (Global Initiative for Chronic Obstructive Lung Disease stages III and IV; 20078883). When expressed in cells in vitro, the COPD-associated A allele of rs652438 was 3-fold more proteolytically active than the G allele, suggesting that it might mediate enhanced ECM degradation.[60]

Reactive Oxygen Species

Cigarette smoke contains vast numbers of free radicals that impose an oxidative stress on the lung. Such stress is thought to induce damage through multiple mechanisms, including direct oxidation of cellular lipids and DNA, and through inactivation of key proteins such as α_1-antitrypsin. For this reason, much work has gone into assessing the role of endogenous antioxidant enzymes in protecting against smoke-induced lung damage.

Many toxins in cigarette smoke are subject to first-pass metabolism in the liver. Among the many enzymes involved, microsomal epoxide hydrolase (EPHX1; 1q42.1) has been intensely studied in the context of COPD. Several EPHX1 SNPs have been described that affect its activity. One of these leads to a 40% loss of in vitro activity (rs1051740 Tyr113His, the "slow" allele), whereas another increases activity by 25% (rs2234922 His139Arg, the "fast" allele). In 1997, the "slow" variant of EPHX1 was found to increase the risk of emphysema by a staggering odds ratio of 5.0 and of COPD by an odds ratio of 4.1.[61] Since then, numerous studies have attempted to reproduce this effect with varying success.[38,62–73] Recently, analysis of randomly selected white Danish individuals participating in the Copenhagen City Heart Study (n = 10,038) and the Copenhagen General Population Study (n = 37,022) for the rs1051740 and rs2234922 variants in the EPHX1 gene combined with a meta-analysis of 19 previous studies indicates that genetically reduced EPHX1 activity is not a major risk factor for COPD or asthma in the Danish population.[74]

Glutathione S-transferase (GST) comprises a large family of enzymes capable of catalyzing the conjugation of reduced glutathione to endogenous and xenobiotic electrophilic compounds. The GSTs are important in the detoxification of many compounds and are highly polymorphic. These polymorphisms have been linked to susceptibility to toxins and carcinogens. SNPs in GSTP1 have been associated with COPD,[75] the distribution of emphysema,[76] and more rapid decline in lung function.[77] However, the data should be interpreted with caution because one-third of the cohorts[77] have been used in multiple analyses[68] and there was a lack of Hardy-Weinberg equilibrium for GSTP1 in their population, suggesting either a systematic defect in genotyping or an unidentified bias in the selection of subjects. Moreover, no convincing association was found in other studies.[70,78] The null mutation of GSTM1 (1p13.1) has also been associated with COPD,[63] but others have failed to reproduce this finding.[71]

Heme-oxygenase catalyses the first step in heme degradation. Heme-oxygenase 1 (HMOX1; 22q13.1) is the inducible isoform that can be up-regulated by a wide range of stresses. Bile pigments generated by heme cleavage are thought to have antioxidant properties; thus, HMOX1 induction is protective during cellular oxidant injury and overexpression of HMOX1 in lung tissue protects against hyperoxia. The HMOX1 gene 5′-flanking region contains stretches of group-specific component (GC) repeats that are highly polymorphic in length. An early report found a higher proportion of long repeats in patients with COPD and also demonstrated that long repeats were associated with impaired promoter activity.[79] Attempts to reproduce this effect have had varied success.[64,77,80,81] Although HMOX1 GC-repeat length has not convincingly been shown to be associated with developing COPD, there are some data to support an association between the long allele and increased severity of disease,[81,82] although a recent study of smokers in the NHLBI Lung Health Study found no association between 5 HMOX1 SNPs and the decline of lung function.[83] Moreover, that study failed to detect evidence that the promoter polymorphisms affected regulation of the HMOX1 gene.

Superoxide dismutase (SOD) is an important antioxidant enzyme that catalyses the conversion of superoxide to oxygen and hydrogen peroxide. The extracellular isoform (SOD3; 4p15) is abundant in lung parenchyma. In the cross-sectional Copenhagen Heart Study, the R213G allele that results in higher plasma levels was associated with significantly less COPD in smokers.[84] A second study found similar results for the SOD3 isoenzyme, but not for other forms of SOD.[85]

While biologically very plausible, current genetic evidence fails to provide clear support for the involvement of detoxifying enzymes in the pathogenesis of COPD. Because the potential list of candidates to detoxify cigarette smoke remains long, it would be preferable if future studies were to take an unbiased approach to target identification rather than studying small numbers of candidate genes.

Inflammation

Tumor necrosis factor-α (TNF; 6p21) is a multifunctional cytokine whose levels are elevated in bronchoalveolar lavage, induced sputa, and biopsies from patients with COPD. It is a plausible candidate gene for susceptibility to inflammatory disease, especially as well-studied promoter polymorphisms clearly alter expression levels. Consequently, considerable effort has been invested into determining whether the promoter polymorphism in TNFα also predisposes smokers to COPD. Much interest was generated when an early study revealed an association (with a staggering odds ratio of greater than 10) between allele 2 and "bronchitis" in Taiwanese men.[86] This study is difficult to interpret as one-third of the men were "never smokers". Despite some supportive evidence,[87] many subsequent studies appeared to find little evidence that TNF polymorphisms are associated with, or modify, the progression of COPD.[68,73,88–97]

GC (4q12), also known as vitamin D binding globulin, is a multifunctional protein that enhances the neutrophil and monocyte chemotactic activity of complement component 5a. It is a highly polymorphic protein with more than 124 forms, although 3, Gc*1F, Gc*1S, and Gc2, make up the majority. Kueppers and colleagues[98] found Gc2 homozygotes to be protected from COPD. Others have seen this protective effect,[99,100] whereas Gc*1F homozygosity has been found to be associated with COPD.[101,102] However, a much larger recent study has failed to reproduce these associations.[103]

SUMMARY

Although environmental exposure to smoke remains the preeminent risk factor for developing COPD, the evidence that heredity plays a major role in an individual's risk is clear. The combination of GWAS and carefully conducted candidate gene approaches is helping to tease out those genetic variants responsible for the familial clustering of this disease, offering both the personalization of individual risk stratification and, more excitingly, the hope for rational therapeutic interventions based on a better understanding of the underlying molecular pathologic abnormality. The confusion surrounding many of the early (and some current) studies lies almost entirely with study power. Apart from the notable exception of SERPINA1, the contribution of individual genetic variants to risk of disease will prove to be small; for this reason, large stratified cohorts of well-phenotyped individuals are likely to prove invaluable. A recent large systematic review of all case control candidate genetic studies in COPD before 2008 concluded that although most such studies were underpowered to detect small genetic effects (OR 1.2–1.5), 4 genetic variants (or the 27 for which adequate data were available) remained significantly associated with COPD: the GSTM1 null variant (OR 1.45), rs1800470 in TGFB1 (0.73), rs1800629 in TNFα (OR 1.19), and rs1799896 in SOD3 (OR 1.97).[104] Such findings, combined with the hypothesis generating observations from GWAS, will direct COPD research for the next decade.

REFERENCES

1. Silverman EK, Chapman HA, Drazen JM, et al. Genetic epidemiology of severe, early-onset chronic obstructive pulmonary disease. Risk to relatives for airflow obstruction and chronic bronchitis. Am J Respir Crit Care Med 1998;157(6 Pt 1):1770–8.

2. McCloskey SC, Patel BD, Hinchliffe SJ, et al. Siblings of patients with severe chronic obstructive pulmonary disease have a significant risk of airflow obstruction. Am J Respir Crit Care Med 2001;164(8 Pt 1):1419–24.

3. Hersh CP, Hokanson JE, Lynch DA, et al. Family history is a risk factor for COPD. Chest 2011; 140(2):343–50.

4. Ingebrigtsen T, Thomsen SF, Vestbo J, et al. Genetic influences on chronic obstructive pulmonary disease - a twin study. Respir Med 2010; 104(12):1890–5.

5. Patel BD, Coxson HO, Pillai SG, et al. Airway wall thickening and emphysema show independent familial aggregation in chronic obstructive pulmonary disease. Am J Respir Crit Care Med 2008; 178(5):500–5.

6. Foreman MG, Zhang L, Murphy J, et al. Early-onset chronic obstructive pulmonary disease is associated with female sex, maternal factors, and African American race in the COPDGene Study. Am J Respir Crit Care Med 2011;184(4):414–20.

7. Bruse S, Sood A, Petersen H, et al. New Mexican Hispanic smokers have lower odds of chronic obstructive pulmonary disease and less decline in lung function than non-Hispanic whites. Am J Respir Crit Care Med 2011;184(11):1254–60.

8. Pillai SG, Ge D, Zhu G, et al. A genome-wide association study in chronic obstructive pulmonary disease (COPD): identification of two major susceptibility loci. PLoS Genet 2009;5(3):e1000421.

9. Pillai SG, Kong X, Edwards LD, et al. Loci identified by genome-wide association studies influence different disease-related phenotypes in chronic obstructive pulmonary disease. Am J Respir Crit Care Med 2010;182(12):1498–505.

10. Kaur-Knudsen D, Nordestgaard BG, Bojesen SE. CHRNA3 genotype, nicotine dependence, lung function and disease in the general population. Eur Respir J 2012;40(6):1538–44.

11. Hardin M, Zielinski J, Wan ES, et al. CHRNA3/5, IREB2, and ADCY2 are associated with severe chronic obstructive pulmonary disease in Poland. Am J Respir Crit Care Med 2012;47(2):203–8.

12. Siedlinski M, Tingley D, Lipman PJ, et al. Dissecting direct and indirect genetic effects on chronic obstructive pulmonary disease (COPD) susceptibility. Hum Genet 2013;132:431–41.

13. Wilk JB, Shrine NR, Loehr LR, et al. Genome-wide association studies identify CHRNA5/3 and HTR4 in the development of airflow obstruction. Am J Respir Crit Care Med 2012;186(7):622–32.

14. Lambrechts D, Buysschaert I, Zanen P, et al. The 15q24/25 susceptibility variant for lung cancer

and chronic obstructive pulmonary disease is associated with emphysema. Am J Respir Crit Care Med 2010;181(5):486–93.

15. DeMeo DL, Mariani T, Bhattacharya S, et al. Integration of genomic and genetic approaches implicates IREB2 as a COPD susceptibility gene. Am J Hum Genet 2009;85(4):493–502.

16. Chappell SL, Daly L, Lotya J, et al. The role of IREB2 and transforming growth factor beta-1 genetic variants in COPD: a replication case-control study. BMC Med Genet 2011;12:24.

17. Cho MH, Boutaoui N, Klanderman BJ, et al. Variants in FAM13A are associated with chronic obstructive pulmonary disease. Nat Genet 2010;42(3):200–2.

18. Wilk JB, Chen TH, Gottlieb DJ, et al. A genome-wide association study of pulmonary function measures in the Framingham Heart Study. PLoS Genet 2009;5(3):e1000429.

19. Repapi E, Sayers I, Wain LV, et al. Genome-wide association study identifies five loci associated with lung function. Nat Genet 2010;42(1):36–44.

20. Van Durme YM, Eijgelsheim M, Joos GF, et al. Hedgehog-interacting protein is a COPD susceptibility gene: the Rotterdam Study. Eur Respir J 2010;36(1):89–95.

21. Zhou X, Baron RM, Hardin M, et al. Identification of a chronic obstructive pulmonary disease genetic determinant that regulates HHIP. Hum Mol Genet 2012;21(6):1325–35.

22. Cho MH, Castaldi PJ, Wan ES, et al. A genome-wide association study of COPD identifies a susceptibility locus on chromosome 19q13. Hum Mol Genet 2012;21(4):947–57.

23. Wan ES, Cho MH, Boutaoui N, et al. Genome-wide association analysis of body mass in chronic obstructive pulmonary disease. Am J Respir Cell Mol Biol 2011;45(2):304–10.

24. Kong X, Cho MH, Anderson W, et al. Genome-wide association study identifies BICD1 as a susceptibility gene for emphysema. Am J Respir Crit Care Med 2011;183(1):43–9.

25. Callewaert B, Renard M, Hucthagowder V, et al. New insights into the pathogenesis of autosomal-dominant cutis laxa with report of five ELN mutations. Hum Mutat 2011;32(4):445–55.

26. Corbett E, Glaisyer H, Chan C, et al. Congenital cutis laxa with a dominant inheritance and early onset emphysema. Thorax 1994;49(8):836–7.

27. Urban Z, Gao J, Pope FM, et al. Autosomal dominant cutis laxa with severe lung disease: synthesis and matrix deposition of mutant tropoelastin. J Invest Dermatol 2005;124(6):1193–9.

28. Kelleher CM, Silverman EK, Broekelmann T, et al. A functional mutation in the terminal exon of elastin in severe, early-onset chronic obstructive pulmonary disease. Am J Respir Cell Mol Biol 2005; 33(4):355–62.

29. Hucthagowder V, Sausgruber N, Kim KH, et al. Fibulin-4: a novel gene for an autosomal recessive cutis laxa syndrome. Am J Hum Genet 2006;78(6): 1075–80.

30. Loeys B, Van Maldergem L, Mortier G, et al. Homozygosity for a missense mutation in fibulin-5 (FBLN5) results in a severe form of cutis laxa. Hum Mol Genet 2002;11(18):2113–8.

31. Revencu N, Quenum G, Detaille T, et al. Congenital diaphragmatic eventration and bilateral uretero-hydronephrosis in a patient with neonatal Marfan syndrome caused by a mutation in exon 25 of the FBN1 gene and review of the literature. Eur J Pediatr 2004;163(1):33–7.

32. Shinawi M, Boileau C, Brik R, et al. Splicing mutation in the fibrillin-1 gene associated with neonatal Marfan syndrome and severe pulmonary emphysema with tracheobronchomalacia. Pediatr Pulmonol 2005;39(4):374–8.

33. Tekin M, Cengiz FB, Ayberkin E, et al. Familial neonatal Marfan syndrome due to parental mosaicism of a missense mutation in the FBN1 gene. Am J Med GenetA 2007;143(8):875–80.

34. Grange DK, Kaler SG, Albers GM, et al. Severe bilateral panlobular emphysema and pulmonary arterial hypoplasia: unusual manifestations of Menkes disease. Am J Med GenetA 2005;139(2):151–5.

35. Wu L, Chau J, Young RP, et al. Transforming growth factor-beta1 genotype and susceptibility to chronic obstructive pulmonary disease. Thorax 2004;59(2): 126–9.

36. Celedon JC, Lange C, Raby BA, et al. The transforming growth factor-beta1 (TGFB1) gene is associated with chronic obstructive pulmonary disease (COPD). Hum Mol Genet 2004;13(15):1649–56.

37. Su ZG, Wen FQ, Feng YL, et al. Transforming growth factor-beta1 gene polymorphisms associated with chronic obstructive pulmonary disease in Chinese population. Acta Pharmacol Sin 2005; 26(6):714–20.

38. Hersh CP, Demeo DL, Lazarus R, et al. Genetic association analysis of functional impairment in chronic obstructive pulmonary disease. Am J Respir Crit Care Med 2006;173(9):977–84.

39. van Diemen CC, Postma DS, Vonk JM, et al. Decorin and TGF-beta1 polymorphisms and development of COPD in a general population. Respir Res 2006;7:89.

40. Ogawa E, Ruan J, Connett JE, et al. Transforming growth factor-beta1 polymorphisms, airway responsiveness and lung function decline in smokers. Respir Med 2007;101(5):938–43.

41. Silverman EK, Palmer LJ, Mosley JD, et al. Genomewide linkage analysis of quantitative spirometric phenotypes in severe early-onset chronic obstructive pulmonary disease. Am J Hum Genet 2002;70(5):1229–39.

42. Sterner-Kock A, Thorey IS, Koli K, et al. Disruption of the gene encoding the latent transforming growth factor-beta binding protein 4 (LTBP-4) causes abnormal lung development, cardiomyopathy, and colorectal cancer. Genes Dev 2002; 16(17):2264–73.

43. Hersh CP, Hansel NN, Barnes KC, et al. Transforming growth factor-beta receptor-3 is associated with pulmonary emphysema. Am J Respir Cell Mol Biol 2009;41(3):324–31.

44. Gooptu B, Lomas DA. Polymers and inflammation: disease mechanisms of the serpinopathies. J Exp Med 2008;205(7):1529–34.

45. Dahl M, Tybjaerg-Hansen A, Lange P, et al. Change in lung function and morbidity from chronic obstructive pulmonary disease in alpha1-antitrypsin MZ heterozygotes: a longitudinal study of the general population. Ann Intern Med 2002;136(4):270–9.

46. Hersh CP, Dahl M, Ly NP, et al. Chronic obstructive pulmonary disease in alpha1-antitrypsin PI MZ heterozygotes: a meta-analysis. Thorax 2004;59(10): 843–9.

47. Sandford AJ, Weir TD, Spinelli JJ, et al. Z and S mutations of the alpha1-antitrypsin gene and the risk of chronic obstructive pulmonary disease. Am J Respir Cell Mol Biol 1999;20(2):287–91.

48. Quint JK, Donaldson GC, Kumari M, et al. SERPINA1 11478G→A variant, serum alpha1-antitrypsin, exacerbation frequency and FEV1 decline in COPD. Thorax 2011;66(5):418–24.

49. Demeo DL, Mariani TJ, Lange C, et al. The SERPINE2 gene is associated with chronic obstructive pulmonary disease. Am J Hum Genet 2006;78(2):253–64.

50. Zhu G, Warren L, Aponte J, et al. The SERPINE2 gene is associated with chronic obstructive pulmonary disease in two large populations. Am J Respir Crit Care Med 2007;176(2):167–73.

51. Chappell S, Daly L, Morgan K, et al. The SERPINE2 gene and chronic obstructive pulmonary disease. Am J Hum Genet 2006;79(1):184–6.

52. Kukkonen MK, Tiili E, Hamalainen S, et al. SERPINE2 haplotype as a risk factor for panlobular type of emphysema. BMC Med Genet 2011;12:157.

53. Minematsu N, Nakamura H, Tateno H, et al. Genetic polymorphism in matrix metalloproteinase-9 and pulmonary emphysema. Biochem Biophys Res Commun 2001;289(1):116–9.

54. Zhou M, Huang SG, Wan HY, et al. Genetic polymorphism in matrix metalloproteinase-9 and the susceptibility to chronic obstructive pulmonary disease in Han population of south China. Chin Med J (Engl) 2004;117(10):1481–4.

55. Ito I, Nagai S, Handa T, et al. Matrix metalloproteinase-9 promoter polymorphism associated with upper lung dominant emphysema. Am J Respir Crit Care Med 2005;172(11):1378–82.

56. Joos L, He JQ, Shepherdson MB, et al. The role of matrix metalloproteinase polymorphisms in the rate of decline in lung function. Hum Mol Genet 2002; 11(5):569–76.

57. Tesfaigzi Y, Myers OB, Stidley CA, et al. Genotypes in matrix metalloproteinase 9 are a risk factor for COPD. Int J Chron Obstruct Pulmon Dis 2006; 1(3):267–78.

58. Hirano K, Sakamoto T, Uchida Y, et al. Tissue inhibitor of metalloproteinases-2 gene polymorphisms in chronic obstructive pulmonary disease. Eur Respir J 2001;18(5):748–52.

59. Hunninghake GM, Cho MH, Tesfaigzi Y, et al. MMP12, lung function, and COPD in high-risk populations. N Engl J Med 2009;361(27):2599–608.

60. Haq I, Lowrey GE, Kalsheker N, et al. Matrix metalloproteinase-12 (MMP-12) SNP affects MMP activity, lung macrophage infiltration and protects against emphysema in COPD. Thorax 2011; 66(11):970–6.

61. Smith CA, Harrison DJ. Association between polymorphism in gene for microsomal epoxide hydrolase and susceptibility to emphysema. Lancet 1997;350(9078):630–3.

62. Korytina GF, Ianbaeva DG, Viktorova TV. Role of polymorphic variants of cytochrome P450 genes (CYP1A1, CYP2E1) and microsomal epoxide hydrolase (mEPHX) in pathogenesis of cystic fibrosis and chronic respiratory tract diseases. Mol Biol (Mosk) 2003;37(5):784–92 [in Russian].

63. Cheng SL, Yu CJ, Chen CJ, et al. Genetic polymorphism of epoxide hydrolase and glutathione S-transferase in COPD. Eur Respir J 2004;23(6): 818–24.

64. Fu WP, Sun C, Dai LM, et al. Relationship between COPD and polymorphisms of HOX-1 and mEPH in a Chinese population. Oncol Rep 2007;17(2):483–8.

65. Hersh CP, Demeo DL, Lange C, et al. Attempted replication of reported chronic obstructive pulmonary disease candidate gene associations. Am J Respir Cell Mol Biol 2005;33(1):71–8.

66. Matheson MC, Raven J, Walters EH, et al. Microsomal epoxide hydrolase is not associated with COPD in a community-based sample. Hum Biol 2006;78(6):705–17.

67. Park JY, Chen L, Wadhwa N, et al. Polymorphisms for microsomal epoxide hydrolase and genetic susceptibility to COPD. Int J Mol Med 2005;15(3): 443–8.

68. Sandford AJ, Chagani T, Weir TD, et al. Susceptibility genes for rapid decline of lung function in the lung health study. Am J Respir Crit Care Med 2001;163(2):469–73.

69. Takeyabu K, Yamaguchi E, Suzuki I, et al. Gene polymorphism for microsomal epoxide hydrolase and susceptibility to emphysema in a Japanese population. Eur Respir J 2000;15(5):891–4.

70. Xiao D, Wang C, Du MJ, et al. Relationship between polymorphisms of genes encoding microsomal epoxide hydrolase and glutathione S-transferase P1 and chronic obstructive pulmonary disease. Chin Med J (Engl) 2004;117(5):661–7.

71. Yim JJ, Park GY, Lee CT, et al. Genetic susceptibility to chronic obstructive pulmonary disease in Koreans: combined analysis of polymorphic genotypes for microsomal epoxide hydrolase and glutathione S-transferase M1 and T1. Thorax 2000; 55(2):121–5.

72. Yoshikawa M, Hiyama K, Ishioka S, et al. Microsomal epoxide hydrolase genotypes and chronic obstructive pulmonary disease in Japanese. Int J Mol Med 2000;5(1):49–53.

73. Brogger J, Steen VM, Eiken HG, et al. Genetic association between COPD and polymorphisms in TNF, ADRB2 and EPHX1. Eur Respir J 2006; 27(4):682–8.

74. Lee J, Nordestgaard BG, Dahl M. EPHX1 polymorphisms, COPD and asthma in 47,000 individuals and in meta-analysis. Eur Respir J 2011;37(1): 18–25.

75. Ishii T, Matsuse T, Teramoto S, et al. Glutathione S-transferase P1 (GSTP1) polymorphism in patients with chronic obstructive pulmonary disease. Thorax 1999;54(8):693–6.

76. DeMeo DL, Hersh CP, Hoffman EA, et al. Genetic determinants of emphysema distribution in the national emphysema treatment trial. Am J Respir Crit Care Med 2007;176(1):42–8.

77. He JQ, Ruan J, Connett JE, et al. Antioxidant gene polymorphisms and susceptibility to a rapid decline in lung function in smokers. Am J Respir Crit Care Med 2002;166(3):323–8.

78. Rodriguez F, de la Roza C, Jardi R, et al. Glutathione S-transferase P1 and lung function in patients with alpha1-antitrypsin deficiency and COPD. Chest 2005;127(5):1537–43.

79. Yamada N, Yamaya M, Okinaga S, et al. Microsatellite polymorphism in the heme oxygenase-1 gene promoter is associated with susceptibility to emphysema. Am J Hum Genet 2000;66(1):187–95.

80. Nakayama K, Kikuchi A, Yasuda H, et al. Heme oxygenase-1 gene promoter polymorphism and decline in lung function in Japanese men. Thorax 2006;61(10):921.

81. Budhi A, Hiyama K, Isobe T, et al. Genetic susceptibility for emphysematous changes of the lung in Japanese. Int J Mol Med 2003;11(3):321–9.

82. Fu WP, Zhao ZH, Fang LZ, et al. Heme oxygenase-1 polymorphism associated with severity of chronic obstructive pulmonary disease. Chin Med J (Engl) 2007;120(1):12–6.

83. Tanaka G, Aminuddin F, Akhabir L, et al. Effect of heme oxygenase-1 polymorphisms on lung function and gene expression. BMC Med Genet 2011;12:117.

84. Juul K, Tybjaerg-Hansen A, Marklund S, et al. Genetically increased antioxidative protection and decreased chronic obstructive pulmonary disease. Am J Respir Crit Care Med 2006;173(8):858–64.

85. Young RP, Hopkins R, Black PN, et al. Functional variants of antioxidant genes in smokers with COPD and in those with normal lung function. Thorax 2006;61(5):394–9.

86. Huang SL, Su CH, Chang SC. Tumor necrosis factor-alpha gene polymorphism in chronic bronchitis. Am J Respir Crit Care Med 1997;156(5): 1436–9.

87. Cordoba-Lanus E, Baz-Davila R, de-Torres JP, et al. TNFA-863 polymorphism is associated with a reduced risk of chronic obstructive pulmonary disease: a replication study. BMC Med Genet 2011; 12:132.

88. Higham MA, Pride NB, Alikhan A, et al. Tumour necrosis factor-alpha gene promoter polymorphism in chronic obstructive pulmonary disease. Eur Respir J 2000;15(2):281–4.

89. Ishii T, Matsuse T, Teramoto S, et al. Neither IL-1beta, IL-1 receptor antagonist, nor TNF-alpha polymorphisms are associated with susceptibility to COPD. Respir Med 2000;94(9):847–51.

90. Ferrarotti I, Zorzetto M, Beccaria M, et al. Tumour necrosis factor family genes in a phenotype of COPD associated with emphysema. Eur Respir J 2003;21(3):444–9.

91. Patuzzo C, Gile LS, Zorzetto M, et al. Tumor necrosis factor gene complex in COPD and disseminated bronchiectasis. Chest 2000;117(5):1353–8.

92. Seifart C, Plagens A, Dempfle A, et al. TNF-alpha, TNF-beta, IL-6, and IL-10 polymorphisms in patients with lung cancer. Dis Markers 2005;21(3):157–65.

93. Chierakul N, Wongwisutikul P, Vejbaesya S, et al. Tumor necrosis factor-alpha gene promoter polymorphism is not associated with smoking-related COPD in Thailand. Respirology 2005;10(1):36–9.

94. Hegab AE, Sakamoto T, Saitoh W, et al. Polymorphisms of TNFalpha, IL1beta, and IL1RN genes in chronic obstructive pulmonary disease. Biochem Biophys Res Commun 2005;329(4):1246–52.

95. Tanaka G, Sandford AJ, Burkett K, et al. Tumour necrosis factor and lymphotoxin A polymorphisms and lung function in smokers. Eur Respir J 2007; 29(1):34–41.

96. Ruse CE, Hill MC, Tobin M, et al. Tumour necrosis factor gene complex polymorphisms in chronic obstructive pulmonary disease. Respir Med 2007; 101(2):340–4.

97. Papatheodorou A, Latsi P, Vrettou C, et al. Development of a novel microarray methodology for the study of SNPs in the promoter region of the TNF-alpha gene: their association with obstructive pulmonary disease in Greek patients. Clin Biochem 2007;40(12):843–50.

98. Kueppers F, Miller RD, Gordon H, et al. Familial prevalence of chronic obstructive pulmonary disease in a matched pair study. Am J Med 1977; 63(3):336–42.

99. Horne SL, Cockcroft DW, Dosman JA. Possible protective effect against chronic obstructive airways disease by the GC2 allele. Hum Hered 1990;40(3):173–6.

100. Schellenberg D, Pare PD, Weir TD, et al. Vitamin D binding protein variants and the risk of COPD. Am J Respir Crit Care Med 1998;157(3 Pt 1):957–61.

101. Ishii T, Keicho N, Teramoto S, et al. Association of Gc-globulin variation with susceptibility to COPD and diffuse panbronchiolitis. Eur Respir J 2001; 18(5):753–7.

102. Ito I, Nagai S, Hoshino Y, et al. Risk and severity of COPD is associated with the group-specific component of serum globulin 1F allele. Chest 2004;125(1): 63–70.

103. Kasuga I, Pare PD, Ruan J, et al. Lack of association of group specific component haplotypes with lung function in smokers. Thorax 2003;58(9):790–3.

104. Castaldi PJ, Cho MH, Cohn M, et al. The COPD genetic association compendium: a comprehensive online database of COPD genetic associations. Hum Mol Genet 2010;19(3):526–34.

Alpha1-antitrypsin Review

Robert A. Stockley, MD, DSc, FRCP

KEYWORDS

- Alpha1-antitrypsin deficiency • Neutrophils • Genetics • Emphysema • Therapy

KEY POINTS

- Alpha1-antitrypsin deficiency remains the commonest genetic cause of emphysema.
- The clinical penetrance is variable but is amplified by cigarette smoking.
- The pathophysiology reflects excessive tissue damage by neutrophil serine proteinases.
- Augmentation therapy with plasma-derived alpha1-antitrypsin is widely (but not uniformly) accepted, but efficacy has been difficult to prove by conventionally accepted outcomes.
- Understanding the genetic defects responsible and the mechanisms of deficiency provides prospects for future treatment strategies, including gene therapy.

The first description of alpha1-antitrypsin (AAT) deficiency (AATD) identified by paper electrophoresis was published in 1963 by Laurel and Eriksson.[1] As part of their publication they reported the first 5 individuals who had been identified, 3 of whom had recurrent chest problems and significant evidence of emphysema, the eldest being 42 years of age and 1 of whom also had a family history of emphysema. Because of this high prevalence of emphysema, particularly at a young age, subsequent studies of the family of these index cases identified nonindex cases with the deficiency and also pulmonary emphysema, confirming the inherited nature of the condition.

Because AAT was known to be an inhibitor of proteolytic enzymes, subsequent research was based on the hypothesis that an enzyme normally inhibited by AAT played a central role in the development of emphysema. Senior and colleagues[2] subsequently showed in an animal model that neutrophil elastase was able to reproduce these features of emphysema, as can proteinase 3,[3] another serine proteinase from the neutrophil. These observations led to the proteinase/antiproteinase theory of the mechanism of emphysema, in which proteolytic destruction of the lung interstitium (and particularly lung elastin) resulted in structural changes in the alveolar region, leading to the pathologic changes of emphysema. This concept has continued to dominate research into the pathophysiology of emphysema, exploring several potential mechanisms, namely deficiency of protective inhibitors, poor function of defective inhibitors, modulation of the function of inhibitors by oxidation or proteolytic cleavage, and overwhelming of the inhibitors by excessive inflammatory cell recruitment and/or activation releasing sufficient enzyme to exceed any protective inhibitors.

PREVALENCE

AAT of the Pi Z phenotype is thought to have originated some 2000 years ago in the Baltic region, thereafter becoming spread by Viking migration. The prevalence follows this migration in a dilutional manner and the incidence can vary from 1 in 1600 in some of the Baltic countries to approximately 1 in 5000 in the United States.

AAT is a 52-kDa single-chain glycoprotein with a sequence of 394 amino acids that is synthesized predominantly in the liver and functions as a serine proteinase inhibitor or serpin. The protein is encoded on the serpin a-1 gene and consists of 7 exons on the long arm of chromosome 14. Since the original discovery there have been more than

ADAPT Project, Lung Function & Sleep Department, Queen Elizabeth Hospital Birmingham, Ground Floor, Out-patients Area 3, Mindelsohn Way, Edgbaston, Birmingham B15 2WB, UK
E-mail address: rob.stockley@bham.ac.uk

Clin Chest Med 35 (2014) 39–50
http://dx.doi.org/10.1016/j.ccm.2013.10.001
0272-5231/14/$ – see front matter © 2014 Elsevier Inc. All rights reserved.

500 single-nucleotide polymorphisms reported at this gene locus, although many are associated with normal gene transcription, translation, and protein function. However, several mechanisms are recognized as being related to deficiency, including total absence of the gene, frame shift mutations that lead to premature stop codons, as well as point mutations that may lead to no production or production of abnormal AAT phenotypes.[4] The function of the protein depends on a methionine amino acid at position 358 that gives the protein its specificity for interlocking with the catalytic triad of serine proteinases and in particular neutrophil elastase.[5] This interlocking results in inactivation of both proteins and the formation of a stable complex. In the commonest severe Z type of AATD, the gene is normally transcribed and translated although a single point mutation leads to an amino acid change at position 342 (glu-lys). This change affects the mobility of the reactive center loop and produces a gap in beta sheet A. The reactive loop of one molecule can then insert itself into this gap, causing the so-called loop sheet polymerization[6] leading to accumulation of AAT in the hepatocytes, a reduction in secretion of AAT, and a retained tendency to form spontaneous polymers both in the serum and tissues (especially the lung). The most common phenotype of AAT is the normal M form. Affected individuals have 2 genes and these are usually expressed in a codominant form, thus heterozygotes are common (1%–3% of affected populations) such that MZ heterozygotes have partially reduced levels (approximately 60% of normal MM homozygotes) and SZ heterozygotes have levels approximately 40% of the normal MM homozygotes. The level of AAT may be key to the susceptibility to develop pulmonary emphysema (discussed later).

CLINICAL IMPACT

The classic presentation for individuals with AATD is early-onset basal panacinar emphysema (compared with the usual later onset apical centrilobular emphysema of chronic obstructive pulmonary disease [COPD]). For these reasons, initially testing for AAT was confined to such patients, leading to an acquisition bias that continued to support the clinical phenotype. Once these index individuals had been identified, family screening identified further deficient subjects as nonindex patients and, in general, these individuals have much less severe disease.[7] Subsequent testing also confirmed that never smokers also had less clinical evidence of lung disease[8] and more often presented later in life.[9]

However, in recent years testing has become more widespread and the variability of the age of presentation has become more apparent as well as variations in the clinical phenotype. Patients may present with bronchiectasis and no emphysema,[10] upper zone and centrilobular emphysema,[11] as well as the classic lower zone panacinar emphysema. There may be evidence of airways predominance with little emphysema,[12] which can be reflected in physiologic discordance with some patients having reduced gas transfer alone, and others reduced spirometry alone,[13] which at least partly reflects the emphysema distribution. However, in most cases, both physiologic measures are impaired. This discordance can also be seen within siblings, in whom there seems to be no concordance with spirometry but clearer concordance with both gas transfer and upper zone rather than lower zone emphysema as determined by lung densitometry.[14] This finding raises the possibility that the emphysema and gas transfer abnormalities are more closely linked to the AATD and that airways disease may reflect other modifying or epigenetic phenomena (discussed later).

Smoking plays a key role in the clinical impact of AATD. Patients who present earlier are nearly always smokers and smoking cessation can largely stabilize the disease. In addition, recurrent exacerbations also influence spirometric decline as well as gas transfer decline,[15] and reversibility of airways obstruction is associated with more rapid spirometric decline.[16] Recent studies have not shown a significant reduction in life expectancy in never smokers[17] and such patients often present at a later age.[8]

However, even in smoking individuals, the progression of lung disease can be widely variable. Recent studies have suggested that spirometry in individuals identified at birth remains normal until their 30s despite an increased prevalence of breathlessness.[18] Studies of never smokers have indicated that deterioration in gas transfer and lung densitometry can be identified even in this good-prognosis group in the early to late 20s, whereas spirometric change starts to occur in the 50s and 60s.[19] In addition, in cross-sectional data, the greatest rate of decline of forced expiratory volume in 1 second (FEV_1) occurs in the range of 35% to 60% predicted, whereas the greatest change in gas transfer occurs when the FEV_1 is lower.[16] Lung densitometry (which is a more direct measure of the emphysema process) seems to show steady progression throughout all stages of the disease,[20] suggesting that the disjunction with spirometry or gas transfer change reflects the parts of the lungs that are undergoing emphysematous change. Nevertheless, these features suggest that all individuals with AATD should be monitored on a regular basis to determine the nature and degree of progression in order that prognosis and the potential effects of therapy can be predicted and evaluated (discussed later).

Most patients with AATD are treated as for usual COPD with long-acting bronchodilators and inhaled corticosteroids. Many patients with AATD have a degree of reversibility (**Fig. 1**) and recurrent exacerbations,[21] although no formal trials of usual inhaled therapies have been performed in deficient patients. However, at least one small study has indicated that inhaled corticosteroids have some benefit.[22]

The continuous progression and young age in some individuals leads to lung transplantation being a viable option toward the end of the disease process. Survival data (especially over the period of 2–9 years after transplantation) suggests that this is improved[23] and is associated with an improvement in lung function and health status, although longer term survival is not necessarily better when patients are closely matched for physiologic impairment at baseline.[24]

Lung volume reduction surgery is rarely indicated because most patients have basal emphysema,[25] although studies are ongoing of nonsurgical lung volume reduction.

PATHOPHYSIOLOGY

The neutrophil, which is the main source of serine proteinases thought to cause the pathologic changes, is present in large numbers both in the airways[26] and the interstitium of patients with AATD.[27] Early studies suggested that failure to control elastase within the airways led to the stimulation of the neutrophil chemoattractant leukotriene B4 (LTB4) by alveolar macrophages.[28]

Studies of airway secretions from patients with AATD confirmed that LTB4 was the major recognized chemoattractant that influenced neutrophil migration.[29]

In an elegant series of experiments Campbell and colleagues[30] described the process of quantum proteolysis, whereby neutrophils migrating in the presence of connecting tissue release concentrations of serine proteinases in excess of the concentration of AAT even in individuals without deficiency. It was thought that this process was necessary to allow neutrophils to migrate through the interstitium of the lung by destroying the connective tissue in close proximity to the cell. This process showed little relationship to the AAT concentration until it decreased to less than 11 μM (Pi Z antitrypsin deficiency has an approximate concentration of 5 μM). At this point there was an exponential increase in the degree of damage seen in the presence of a migrating neutrophil. This concept has major implications concerning the risk of heterozygotes such as the MZ and SZ phenotypes, because in general these phenotypes have AAT plasma levels that are more than the critical 11 μM threshold (discussed later). More recently it has been recognized that polymers of AAT can be chemoattractants in their own right,[31] although they are also proinflammatory.[32] It has been suggested that these properties of the polymers may be more important in driving the neutrophilic infiltration into the lung than the effect of uninhibited elastase on LTB4. Whether this is true remains unresolved. However, AAT enters the lung mainly by diffusion from plasma and the interstitial concentration should be about 80% of that in plasma.[33] Larger proteins (including polymers) would be restricted in this diffusion, leading to a reversed plasma/lung gradient that would thus not act as a conventional chemoattractant. In addition, polymer formation is concentration

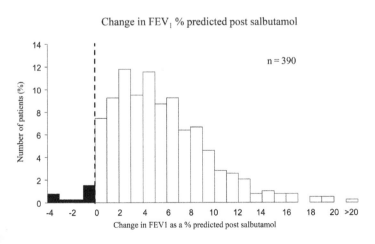

Change in FEV$_1$ % predicted post salbutamol

n = 390

Number of patients (%)

Change in FEV1 as a % predicted post salbutamol

Fig. 1. The change in FEV$_1$ as a percentage of predicted following inhalation of 400 mg of salbutamol expressed as the proportion of the population showing each change.

dependent and hence should not increase in the interstitium to more than that in plasma. However, there are potential caveats to this concept. First, lung cells have the potential to produce some AAT locally[34] and hence increase polymer formation in situ, establishing a gradient. As an alternative, the proinflammatory nature of polymers may increase local chemoattractant production, providing an alternative gradient. Nevertheless, polymers of AAT are in the interstitium of the lung and this chemoattractant property may be the reason that some neutrophils colocalize with the polymers[28] and, if so, are likely to cause even more local connective tissue destruction by retaining them (and their proteolytic activity) in situ. These concepts are summarized in **Fig. 2**.

There are other factors that may complicate the development of emphysema, including the role of uninhibited proteinases on cell apoptosis (which has also been implicated in the emphysema process)[35] and activation of other proteinases in the inflammation cascade and inactivation of cognate inhibitors.[36] In addition, MMP-9 (matrix metallo proteinase)[37] and IREB2 (iron responsive element binding protein)[38] have been implicated as further genetic modifiers in AATD, and, more recently, polymorphism of the tumor necrosis factor alpha gene has also been shown to amplify the inflammation and progression of lung function decline as well as influencing the clinical phenotype.[39]

Susceptibility of Other Phenotypes

Most information concerning AATD relates to studies of the Pi Z phenotype (usually Pi ZZ genotype) because this is the most common severe variant presenting with disease. There is limited literature on the null variants of AAT, although in a small series the patients seem (if anything) to have worse lung function than Pi Z subjects.[40]

The null variants have undetectable levels of AAT and hence no circulating polymers, suggesting that the level is more critical than polymers in the pathophysiology of AATD lung disease. This finding is consistent with the quantum proteolysis process described by Campbell and colleagues.[30]

With this last concept in mind, the in vitro studies of Campbell and colleagues[41] indicated that a prevailing plasma AAT concentration also showed this critical threshold for more extensive tissue damage in the presence of a degranulating neutrophil. For this reason the common MZ heterozygote carriers should not be at greater risk of developing emphysema than the normal MM individuals because their AAT levels are invariably more than this threshold. However, there is some controversy in the literature because MZ subjects have been reported as having evidence of increased elastase activity in 1 study,[42] are more likely to have slightly lower lung function as a group[43] and more severe COPD than MM subjects,[44] as well as greater hospitalization and mortality.[45] Although these data do not indicate the MZ as a susceptibility factor, they do suggest that, if a patient is going to develop COPD and also has the MZ phenotype, the disease may become more of a problem. However, these data mainly relate to known patients with COPD or subjects tested or detected as part of family screening, and as such represent a selection bias. The most robust data from epidemiologic studies suggested that, at worst, MZ subjects have a minimal decrease in FEV_1 compared with MM subjects.[46] Thus, in general, the MZ phenotype alone is not considered a risk factor.

The SZ phenotype is approximately 3 times as common as the Z phenotype, especially around the Mediterranean. The average AAT level in these individuals is about 14, although a proportion has levels less than the 11 μM threshold, suggesting

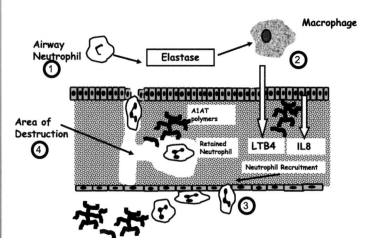

Fig. 2. Airway neutrophils release elastase (1) which remains active because of AAT deficiency. This stimulates macrophages and epithelial cells to release chemoattractants (2), which leads to neutrophil recruitment (3) and retention in the interstitium adjacent to polymers (4) enhancing tissue destruction. IL8, interleukin 8.

a theoretic susceptibility in some individuals. Meta analysis of published data provides credence to this possibility,[47] although again selection bias is likely to have influenced the results. However, patients with the SZ phenotype are more likely to have emphysema with the usual apical distribution of usual nondeficient COPD,[48] which is therefore not typical of the AATD phenotype.

Furthermore, despite the greater prevalence, few patients with COPD and the SZ phenotype have been identified (approximately one-fifth as many as patients with the Z phenotype [49]). Nevertheless, in some countries the SZ phenotype is considered appropriate for augmentation therapy.

Even less information is available for other partial deficiencies including the IZ, PZ, and FZ phenotypes. Although the FZ phenotype has comparable plasma AAT with the MZ phenotype, it is less functional.[50] The F variant has a reduced association rate constant for neutrophil elastase and binds it more slowly once the enzyme is released. This property could provide a mechanism to increase local elastase-induced tissue damage. However, few such subjects have been identified and studied to provide more certainty about the role of the F variant.

AUGMENTATION

Because of the proteinase/antiproteinase hypothesis it became accepted that augmentation of the AAT level would prove beneficial in protecting the lung from progressive damage. Studies in the 1980s showed that purified AAT given by the intravenous route increased and maintained AAT levels in the blood (beyond that of SZ heterozygotes and thus thought to remove the increased risk) and in the airways of deficient individuals, where it remained functional[51] and was subsequently shown to reduce inflammation, in particular the major neutrophil chemoattractant LTB4.[52] Although biochemical efficacy was therefore shown, clinical efficacy has been difficult to show. In the early days the FEV_1 was the gold standard outcome measure for studies in COPD. Power calculations indicated that it would be impossible to recruit and deliver a clinical trial of augmentation therapy with FEV_1 as the primary outcome.[53] For this reason no such trial was deemed feasible or has been undertaken. Evidence for efficacy therefore has come predominantly from indirect observational studies.

The US National Institutes of Health developed an AATD register and eventually analyzed outcomes in individuals who had received augmentation therapy (at least for 6 months) and those who had never received augmentation. Mortality over 5 years was greater in individuals who had never received such therapy. In addition, the decline in FEV_1 between the values of 35% and 60% predicted was also greater in individuals who had never received augmentation therapy.[54] This last observation has led to a general belief that augmentation therapy is only effective within this physiologic range, and in some countries augmentation is stopped once the FEV_1 decreases to less than 30% predicted. However, there are some problems with the interpretation of these data. First, in the health care systems in the United States, the least privileged individuals are unlikely to receive therapy and individuals of low social class have poorer outcomes for all health care issues. This trend is consistent with the observation that patients who had always or only partially received augmentation therapy seemed to have a similar outcome. Second, in all clinical trials it is easier to detect a benefit on the outcome measure if the outcome measure is highly prevalent and changing most rapidly. As indicated earlier, the FEV_1 decline in AATD is most rapid in the 35% to 60% predicted range, which may explain the positive data only in this range. Other observational studies have also shown some benefit on FEV_1 decline, namely comparing countries where augmentation therapy is available with those where it is not.[55] Sequential studies of decline in FEV_1 before and after therapy,[56] although it should be noted that FEV_1 decline is not linear and slows down later in the disease process,[16] which could explain the sequential change. In addition, meta-analysis from reported data on decline in FEV_1 in treated and untreated cohorts also suggests an overall benefit in terms of spirometric decline if augmentation was given.[57]

In recent years it has become accepted that FEV_1 is generally a poor surrogate of the emphysema process. Because emphysema is thought to be central to the pathophysiology of COPD in AATD, lung densitometry has become the outcome measure of choice. Data show that lung densitometry progresses in a linear fashion throughout the disease process.[20] It is the sensitive parameter to change[58] and thus power calculations for interventional studies with densitometry as an outcome are more favorable for this rare disease group. An initial study between Denmark and Holland confirmed that augmentation therapy had no benefit on spirometry but did show a trend ($P = .07$) for preservation of lung density and, by implication, stabilization of the emphysema process.[59] The subsequent Exacerbations and Computed Tomography as Lung Endpoints (EXACTLE) study was performed using more sophisticated scanning techniques with densitometry as a primary outcome. Again, the decline in lung densitometry in patients receiving augmentation was less than on placebo using the same analysis as the Danish/Dutch study, although again it failed to achieve statistical significance ($P = .07$), but there was a significant reduction in severe exacerbations requiring hospitalization.[60] Further analysis of the data from the EXACTLE trial did show a significant reduction in densitometry progression at the bases of the lung where the characteristic emphysema occurs,[61] and combining the data of these two trials in which densitometry was measured, even when biasing the data in favor of the earlier and hence less sophisticated trial, led to a highly significant difference between treatment and placebo, indicating preservation of lung density.[62]

Augmentation therapy is currently licensed in many countries as a weekly infusion, although other therapeutic regimens have been used; however, it is expensive[63] and this raises the possibility of providing augmentation through the inhaled route. However, deposition studies have shown that the inhaled route does not target the most affected emphysematous areas[64] and deposition is unlikely to occur in the alveolar region (as with most nebulized drug delivery). Even if such a deposition could be achieved, the integrity of the epithelial surface would restrict any movement of AAT into the interstitium[65] where the destruction is occurring. One possible caveat to this physiologic problem is that, if the chemoattractant (LTB4) is generated on the airway side of the lung, augmentation of the elastase inhibitory capacity at this site would lead to a reduction in free elastase activity and hence LTB4 production by local macrophages, and this in turn would lead to reduction in neutrophil migration and hence neutrophil-dependent connective tissue damage.

Nevertheless, the inhaled route may be of more benefit for individuals having recurrent exacerbations. About half the patients with AATD do not have a history of exacerbations but, in those who do, most have 1 or 2 per year (**Fig. 3**). These episodes usually include all 3 of the major symptoms of such episodes and occur throughout the year with some preponderance in the autumn and winter months (**Fig. 4**) Exacerbations in AATD are more inflammatory than those in usual COPD, with higher elastase activity,[66] and tend to last longer.[67] These episodes are related to the progressive reduction in FEV_1.[15] AAT by the inhaled route is predicted to result in a more rapid reduction in the local proteinase burden of these larger airways events and may therefore reduce the proteinase-generated inflammation and frequency, severity, and perhaps length of exacerbations. Such a trial is currently underway[68] and the results will be informative in terms of the frequency, severity, and pathophysiologic processes involved. At worst, the treatment may change episodes requiring treatment to less severe/symptomatic ones not requiring intervention (**Fig. 5**).

It would also be possible to give intravenous boluses of AAT at the start of an exacerbation, which may have the same (although less efficient) effect of increasing airways AAT by diffusion from plasma. However, this would require an ability to predict early whether the episode would be mild or severe; perhaps limiting to episodes at admission to hospital may prove most beneficial if length of stay or mortality were to be influenced. Nevertheless, at present, even if the overall efficacy of augmentation therapy is accepted, it is largely unknown whether all patients should receive such therapy or whether it is possible to identify a subset for whom it would be important and hence in whom there is likely to be a greater cost/benefit.

At best, effective augmentation therapy slows down the progression of emphysema and its physiologic markers. Thus, ideally all patients with

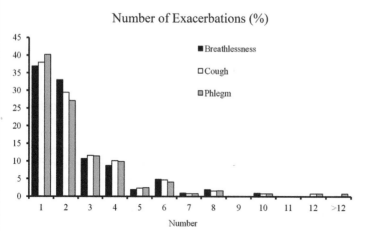

Number of Exacerbations (%)

■ Breathlessness
□ Cough
▣ Phlegm

Number

Fig. 3. The features and frequency of exacerbations is shown as a percentage of patients experiencing at least 1 episode per year.

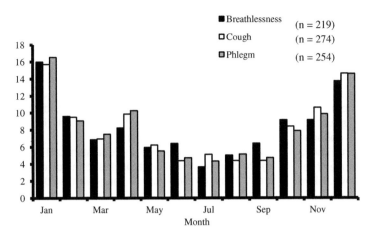

Month of Exacerbations (%)

■ Breathlessness (n = 219)
□ Cough (n = 274)
▨ Phlegm (n = 254)

Month

Fig. 4. Distribution of exacerbations throughout the year for patients with AATD.

AATD who are identified should be monitored so that the natural history in the absence of augmentation can be determined. For smokers this should be done after smoking cessation and in many such patients lung function stabilizes. In others there is a continual progression that may be within or greater than the normal aging decline. It seems logical therefore that, for individuals in whom the decline in either spirometry or gas transfer exceeds that expected as part of the normal aging process, augmentation therapy would be indicated and that the younger the individual the more important this would be to either stabilize disease or prolong the phase until transplantation becomes the only remaining option. In never smokers, the physiologic measurements at presentation related to the age would already provide good evidence of the rate of progression even though life expectancy in such individuals remains normal. In times of austerity, rationalization along

the lines of this approach may become critical for the prescription and funding of augmentation therapy.[69]

For Pi Z individuals without respiratory disease, less information is available of the benefits of augmentation therapy. Acute necrotizing panniculitis can respond dramatically[70] but it is unknown whether the vasculitis would also benefit from augmentation therapy, although this is also a proteinase-dependent process in some subjects.[71] The cirrhosis caused by liver damage from AAT retention is not expected to respond to or require augmentation therapy because the endogenous polymerization will still continue. Methods to silence gene transcription may prove protective to the liver but potentially amplify the lung damage. Mechanisms to enhance liver AAT secretion by preventing polymerization treat the liver and protect the lung if AAT function can be retained (discussed later).

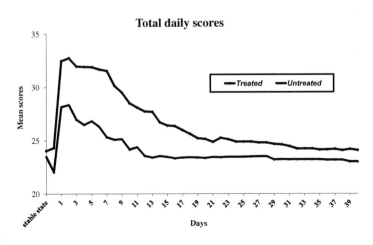

Total daily scores

—Treated —Untreated

Mean scores

Days

Fig. 5. Daily diary card score reflecting severity and duration of symptoms for exacerbations in AATD that did or did not require intervention (data are derived from Ref.[68]).

NEW TREATMENTS

There are many strategies that can potentially overcome the problems of AATD.

Recombinant A1AT

Because of the cost and limited supply of plasma-derived AAT, recombinant forms of protein have been generated. Initial studies produced nongly-cosylated proteins that result in more rapid clearance,[72] and potential problems with structural stability and exposure of immunogenic epitopes normally hidden. A glycosylated transgenic sheep protein induced immune responses because of impurities[73] that were impractical to remove. More recently a sialyzed version has been produced in a human neuronal cell line[74] and it remains to be seen whether this becomes a viable source.

Secretion Strategies

Because at least the Z form of AAT is translated normally, strategies to prevent retention in the hepatocytes would have 2 potential benefits. Release of AAT would reduce the endoplasmic stress in the hepatocytes and thus (potentially) prevent the development of cirrhosis and liver failure. At the same time, the increased secretion would raise the plasma concentration and potentially protect the lung from proteolytic damage. Chemical chaperones intended to stabilize the intermediate forms of Z AAT on the folding pathway were shown to work in animal studies[75] but have proved to be toxic and ineffective in humans.[76]

Small peptides can prevent intrahepatic polymerization in vitro,[77] although there is currently no identified method of delivering these compounds to the endoplasmic reticulum (ER) of hepatocytes. In addition, they inactivate the AAT,[78] which produces a null phenotype. This process would be expected to worsen the lung disease in such naturally occurring individuals.[40]

Gene Therapies

A variety of gene therapies have been explored. In general, these result in minimal and only transient expression and hence production of A1AT.[79] This approach would fail to influence the liver disease. The hepatocyte ER stress could be abrogated by the use of a silencing strategy using Si RNA.[80] This strategy would lead to a null phenotype but potentially can be combined with a transgenic approach leading to normal AAT production to protect the lung as well.[81] An alternative is to correct the gene defect using small DNA fragment technology.[82] However all these methods still depend on the development of effective transfer of gene-modifying agents into the hepatocytes before trials can be undertaken.

A further strategy is to deliver the gene to the lung in a way that minimizes any immune response to the vector and provides significant and sustained AAT production. This strategy would make repeated treatments less frequent and immune activation to the vector less likely. Such a strategy introducing the vector into the pleural space seems to fulfill these criteria in animal models.[83] Further studies including long-term safety in humans need to be undertaken.

In addition, transfection and/or a stem cell strategy to deliver normal hepatocytes to the diseased liver[84] may provide further long-term solutions, although again safety may be a major issue.

Drugs

Specific inhibitors of Neutrophil Elastase (NE) have been developed, although they have not been tested in AATD. Most have failed at the phase 2 development stage because of failure to improve lung function in usual COPD (an outcome that is improbable in phase 2 studies for such agents). Because AAT inhibits other serine proteinases released at the same time as NE (Pr3 and Cat G) having many similar effects on the lung and being increased in AATD,[85] it is possible that a highly selective NE inhibitor may not provide significant or total protection against serine proteolytic attack to the lung. However, in the absence of such a study, the direct role of elastase and, in particular, the contribution of other serine proteinases remains speculative.

In addition, alveolar repair could potentially progress ahead of alveolar damage. Retinoic acid receptor (RAR) gamma agonists are effective in animal models of emphysema.[86] However, this strategy proved ineffective in a 1-year study of patients with AATD[87] and further development is on hold.

Inhibitors of chemotaxis (CXCR 1 and 2 antagonists or particularly on LTB4 receptor antagonists) may have a potential role. These inhibitors would reduce neutrophil reflux and hence proteinase release in the lung. However, these agents have not been studied in AATD.

BIOMARKERS

Biomarkers of disease activity and hence determinants of future progression remain illusive in AATD as in usual COPD. However, the mechanism that leads to the development of emphysema has been accepted as destruction of lung connective tissue and specifically elastin by serine proteinases and most likely elastase. For this reason elastin degradation products have been proposed and extensively studied as appropriate markers. However, elastin is a widespread connective tissue and little is know about systemic turnover, although in the healthy lung it is minimal.[88] Thus systemic or secreted elastin peptides or cross-linking amino acids may reflect changes in other tissues or even diet. Nevertheless, recent studies have suggested that reassessment of these elastin products may still be useful as an indicator of emphysema progression and the effectiveness of specific, protective interventions.[89]

An alternative is to measure elastase directly, although, because of the presence of inhibitors both in the plasma and the airways, enzyme activity is often largely inhibited by the time samples are collected and analyzed. Such data do not inform about the activity at the point of release (ie, where the damage occurs). For this reason a footprint of the local activity would serve all potential needs. Recent studies of a specific cleavage product of fibrinogen may serve this purpose. The peptide is increased in AATD and correlates with physiologic impairment. In addition, it increases during exacerbations, which are known to influence physiologic decline, and responds positively to augmentation therapy.[90] Further validation is required but such an approach may prove invaluable in predicting physiologic decline and in short-term monitoring of drug efficacy.

SUMMARY

Since the identification in 1963, understanding of the molecular mechanism, natural history, clinical phenotype, and progression in AATD has improved from simple interpretation in the 1960s to mid-1990s. In general, outcomes are better than originally thought, clinical illness is not a given, and there is a clearer understanding of the expected role of augmentation therapy. However, because of the general rarity of the condition, it is essential that all such patients get referred to centers of excellence, monitored, and treated/not treated. These centers should be located alongside relevant transplant facilities. Nevertheless, further research is required to identify specific epigenetic factors that influence clinical phenotype, markers of progression, and treatment benefit.

REFERENCES

1. Laurell C, Eriksson S. The electrophoretic alpha 1-globulin pattern of serum in alpha 1-antitrypsin deficiency. Scand J Clin Lab Invest 1963;15: 132–40.
2. Senior RM, Tegner H, Kuhn C, et al. The induction of pulmonary emphysema with human leukocyte elastase. Am Rev Respir Dis 1977;116(3):469–75.
3. Kao RC, Wehner NG, Skubitz KM, et al. Proteinase 3. A distinct human polymorphonuclear leukocyte proteinase that produces emphysema in hamsters. J Clin Invest 1988;82(6):1963–73.
4. Dickens JA, Lomas DA. Why has it been so difficult to prove the efficacy of alpha-1-antitrypsin replacement therapy? Insights from the study of disease pathogenesis. Drug Des Devel Ther 2011;5:391–405.
5. Matheson NR, Gibson HL, Hallewell RA, et al. Recombinant DNA-derived forms of human alpha 1-proteinase inhibitor. Studies on the alanine 358 and cysteine 358 substituted mutants. J Biol Chem 1986;261(22):10404–9.
6. Lomas DA, Evans DL, Finch JT, et al. The mechanism of Z alpha 1-antitrypsin accumulation in the liver. Nature 1992;357(6379):605–7.
7. Seersholm N, Kok-Jensen A, Dirksen A. Survival of patients with severe alpha 1-antitrypsin deficiency with special reference to non-index cases. Thorax 1994;49(7):695–8.
8. Seersholm N, Kok-Jensen A. Clinical features and prognosis of life time non-smokers with severe alpha 1-antitrypsin deficiency. Thorax 1998;53(4): 265–8.
9. Campos MA, Alazemi S, Zhang G, et al. Clinical characteristics of subjects with symptoms of alpha1-antitrypsin deficiency older than 60 years. Chest 2009;135(3):600–8.
10. Rodriguez-Cintron W, Guntupalli WK, Fraire AE. Bronchiectasis and homozygous (P1ZZ) alpha 1-antitrypsin deficiency in a young man. Thorax 1995;50(4):424–5.
11. Parr DG, Stoel BC, Stolk J, et al. Pattern of emphysema distribution in α-1-antitrypsin deficiency influences lung function impairment. Am J Respir Crit Care Med 2004;170(11):1172–8.
12. Piras B, Ferrarotti I, Lara B, et al. Clinical phenotypes of Italian and Spanish patients with alpha-1-antitrypsin deficiency. Eur Respir J 2013;42(1): 54–64.
13. Holme J, Stockley RA. Radiologic and clinical features of COPD patients with discordant pulmonary physiology: lessons from a-1-antitrypsin deficiency. Chest 2007;132:909–15.
14. Wood AM, Needham M, Simmonds MJ, et al. Phenotypic differences in alpha 1 antitrypsin deficient sibling pairs may relate to genetic variation. COPD 2008;5:353–9.
15. Dowson LJ, Guest PJ, Stockley RA. Longitudinal changes in physiological, radiological, and health status measurements in alpha(1)-antitrypsin deficiency and factors associated with decline. Am J Respir Crit Care Med 2001;164:1805–9.

16. Dawkins PA, Dawkins CL, Wood AM, et al. Rate of progression of lung function impairment in alpha-1-antitrypsin deficiency. Eur Respir J 2009;33:1338–44.
17. Tanash HA, Nilsson PM, Nilsson JA, et al. Survival in severe alpha-1-antitrypsin deficiency (Pi ZZ). Respir Res 2010;11:44.
18. Bernspang E, Wollmer P, Sveger T, et al. Lung function in 30-year-old alpha-1-antitrypsin-deficient individuals. Respir Med 2009;103(6):861–5.
19. Holme J, Stockley JA, Stockley RA. Age related development of respiratory abnormalities in non-index a-1 antitrypsin deficient studies. Respir Med 2013;107(3):387–93.
20. Parr DG, Stoel BC, Stolk J, et al. Validation of computed tomographic lung densitometry for monitoring emphysema in α-1-antitrypsin deficiency. Thorax 2006;61:485–90.
21. Needham M, Stockley RA. Exacerbations in α-1-antitrypsin deficiency. Eur Respir J 2005;25:992–1000.
22. Corda L, Bertella E, La Piana GE, et al. Inhaled corticosteroids as additional treatment in alpha-1-antitrypsin-deficiency-related COPD. Respiration 2008;76(1):61–8.
23. Tanash HA, Riise GC, Hansson L, et al. Survival benefit of lung transplantation in individuals with severe alpha1-anti-trypsin deficiency (PiZZ) and emphysema. J Heart Lung Transplant 2011; 30(12):1342–7.
24. Stone H, Edgar RG, Stockley RA. Lung Transplantation in Alpha-1-Antitrypsin Deficiency. British Q19 Thoracic Society Winter Meeting. Thorax 2012; 67(suppl 2):A99.
25. Fishman A, Martinez F, Naunheim K, et al. A randomized trial comparing lung-volume-reduction surgery with medical therapy for severe emphysema. N Engl J Med 2003;348(21):2059–73.
26. Morrison HM, Kramps JA, Burnett D, et al. Lung lavage fluid from patients with alpha1-proteinase inhibitor deficiency or chronic obstructive bronchitis: anti-elastase function and cell profile. Clin Sci 1987;72:373–81.
27. Mahadeva R, Atkinson C, Li Z, et al. Polymers of Z alpha1-antitrypsin co-localize with neutrophils in emphysematous alveoli and are chemotactic in vivo. Am J Pathol 2005;166(2):377–86.
28. Hubbard RC, Fells G, Gadek J, et al. Neutrophil accumulation in the lung in alpha 1-antitrypsin deficiency. Spontaneous release of leukotriene B4 by alveolar macrophages. J Clin Invest 1991;88(3): 891–7.
29. Woolhouse IS, Bayley DL, Stockley RA. Sputum chemotactic activity in chronic obstructive pulmonary disease: effect of α1-antitrypsin deficiency and the role of leukotriene B4 and interleukin 8. Thorax 2002;57:709–14.
30. Liou TG, Campbell EJ. Quantum proteolysis resulting from release of single granules by human neutrophils: a novel, nonoxidative mechanism of extracellular proteolytic activity. J Immunol 1996; 157(6):2624–31.
31. Parmar JS, Mahadeva R, Reed BJ, et al. Polymers of alpha(1)-antitrypsin are chemotactic for human neutrophils: a new paradigm for the pathogenesis of emphysema. Am J Respir Cell Mol Biol 2002; 26(6):723–30.
32. Gooptu B, Ekeowa UI, Lomas DA. Mechanisms of emphysema in alpha1-antitrypsin deficiency: molecular and cellular insights. Eur Respir J 2009; 34(2):475–88.
33. Stockley RA. Long-term intervention studies: α1-antitrypsin substitution. In: Pauwels RA, Postma DS, Weiss ST, editors. Long-term intervention in chronic obstructive pulmonary disease. New York: Marcel Dekker; 2005. p. 445–62.
34. Dhami R, Zay K, Gilks B, et al. Pulmonary epithelial expression of human alpha1-antitrypsin in transgenic mice results in delivery of alpha1-antitrypsin protein to the interstitium. J Mol Med (Berl) 1999;77(4):377–85.
35. Morissette MC, Parent J, Milot J. Alveolar epithelial and endothelial cell apoptosis in emphysema: what we know and what we need to know. Int J Chron Obstruct Pulmon Dis 2009;4:19–31.
36. Sullivan AL, Stockley RA. Proteinases and COPD. In: Hansel TT, Barnes PJ, editors. Recent Advances in the Pathophysiology of COPD. Birkhäuser Verlag Basel/Switzerland; 2004. p. 75–99.
37. McAloon CJ, Wood AM, Gough SC, et al. Matrix metalloprotease polymorphisms are associated with gas transfer in alpha 1 antitrypsin deficiency. Ther Adv Respir Dis 2009;3:23–30.
38. Kim WJ, Wood AM, Barker AF, et al. Association of IREB2 and CHRNA3 polymorphisms with airflow obstruction in severe alpha-1 antitrypsin deficiency. Respir Res 2012;13(1):16.
39. Sapey E, Wood AM, Ahmad A, et al. TNF alpha rs361525 polymorphism is associated with increased local production and downstream inflammation in COPD. Am J Respir Crit Care Med 2010; 182(2):192–9.
40. Fregonese L, Stolk J, Frants RR, et al. Alpha-1 antitrypsin Null mutations and severity of emphysema. Respir Med 2008;102(6):876–84.
41. Campbell EJ, Campbell MA, Boukedes SS, et al. Quantum proteolysis by neutrophils: implications for pulmonary emphysema in alpha 1-antitrypsin deficiency. J Clin Invest 1999;104(3):337–44.
42. Weitz JI, Silverman EK, Thong B, et al. Plasma levels of elastase-specific fibrinopeptides correlate with proteinase inhibitor phenotype. Evidence for increased elastase activity in subjects with homozygous and

heterozygous deficiency of alpha 1-proteinase inhibitor. J Clin Invest 1992;89(3):766–73.

43. Sorheim IC, Bakke P, Gulsvik A, et al. Alpha(1)-antitrypsin protease inhibitor MZ heterozygosity is associated with airflow obstruction in two large cohorts. Chest 2010;138(5):1125–32.

44. Stockley RA. Alpha1-antitrypsin phenotypes in cor pulmonale due to chronic obstructive airways disease. Q J Med 1979;191:419–28.

45. Seersholm N, Wilcke JT, Kok-Jensen A, et al. Risk of hospital admission for obstructive pulmonary disease in alpha(1)-antitrypsin heterozygotes of phenotype PiMZ. Am J Respir Crit Care Med 2000; 161(1):81–4.

46. Dahl M, Tybjaerg-Hansen A, Lange P, et al. Change in lung function and morbidity from chronic obstructive pulmonary disease in alpha1-antitrypsin MZ heterozygotes: a longitudinal study of the general population. Ann Intern Med 2002; 136(4):270–9.

47. Dahl M, Hersh CP, Ly NP, et al. The protease inhibitor PI*S allele and COPD: a meta-analysis. Eur Respir J 2005;26(1):67–76.

48. Holme J, Stockley RA. CT Scan appearance, densitometry, and health status in protease inhibitor SZ α1-antitrypsin deficiency. Chest 2009; 136(5):1284–90.

49. Stockley RA, Stolk J, Dirksen A. Alpha-1-antitrypsin deficiency: the European experience. COPD 2013; 10(Suppl 1):50–3.

50. Cook L, Burdon JG, Brenton S, et al. Kinetic characterisation of alpha-1-antitrypsin F as an inhibitor of human neutrophil elastase. Pathology 1996; 28(3):242–7.

51. Gadek JE, Klein HG, Holland PV, et al. Replacement therapy of alpha 1-antitrypsin deficiency. Reversal of protease-antiprotease imbalance within the alveolar structures of PiZ subjects. J Clin Invest 1981;68(5):1158–65.

52. Stockley RA, Bayley DL, Unsal I, et al. The effect of augmentation therapy on bronchial inflammation in α1-antitrypsin deficiency. Am J Respir Crit Care Med 2002;165:1494–8.

53. Schluchter MD, Stoller JK, Barker AF, et al. Feasibility of a clinical trial of augmentation therapy for alpha(1)-antitrypsin deficiency. The Alpha 1-Antitrypsin Deficiency Registry Study Group. Am J Respir Crit Care Med 2000;161(3 Pt 1):796–801.

54. Survival and FEV1 decline in individuals with severe deficiency of alpha1-antitrypsin. The Alpha-1-Antitrypsin Deficiency Registry Study Group. Am J Respir Crit Care Med 1998;158(1):49–59.

55. Seersholm N, Wencker M, Banik N, et al. Does alpha1-antitrypsin augmentation therapy slow the annual decline in FEV1 in patients with severe hereditary alpha1-antitrypsin deficiency? Wissenschaftliche Arbeitsgemeinschaft zur Therapie von Lungenerkrankungen (WATL) alpha1-AT study group. Eur Respir J 1997;10(10):2260–3.

56. Wencker M, Fuhrmann B, Banik N, et al. Longitudinal follow-up of patients with alpha(1)-protease inhibitor deficiency before and during therapy with IV alpha(1)-protease inhibitor. Chest 2001;119(3): 737–44.

57. Chapman KR, Stockley RA, Dawkins C, et al. Augmentation therapy for alpha-1 antitrypsin deficiency: a meta-analysis. COPD 2009;6(3): 177–84.

58. Stolk J, Cooper BG, Stoel B, et al. Retinoid treatment of emphysema in patients on the Alpha-1 International Registry. The REPAIR study: study design, methodology and quality control of study assessments. Ther Adv Respir Dis 2010;4(6):319–32.

59. Dirksen A, Dijkman JH, Madsen F, et al. A randomized clinical trial of alpha(1)-antitrypsin augmentation therapy. Am J Respir Crit Care Med 1999;160(5 Pt 1):1468–72.

60. Dirksen A, Piitulainen E, Parr DG, et al. Exploring the role of CT densitometry: a randomised study of augmentation therapy in alpha-1-antitrypsin deficiency. Eur Respir J 2009;33:1345–53.

61. Parr DG, Dirksen A, Piitulainen E, et al. Exploring the optimum approach to the use of CT densitometry in a randomised placebo-controlled study augmentation therapy in alpha-1-antitrypsin deficiency. Respir Res 2009;10(1):75.

62. Stockley RA, Parr DG, Piitulainen E, et al. Therapeutic efficacy of alpha-1 antitrypsin augmentation therapy on the loss of lung tissue: an integrated analysis of 2 randomised clinical trials using computed tomography densitometry. Respir Res 2010;11:136.

63. Hay JW, Robin ED. Cost-effectiveness of alpha-1 antitrypsin replacement therapy in treatment of congenital chronic obstructive pulmonary disease. Am J Public Health 1991;81(4):427–33.

64. Stolk J, Camps J, Feitsma H, et al. Pulmonary deposition and disappearance of aerosolised secretory leucocyte protease inhibitor. Thorax 1995;50(6):645–50.

65. Gorin AB, Stewart PA. Differential permeability of endothelial and epithelial barriers to albumin flux. J Appl Physiol Respir Environ Exerc Physiol 1979; 47(6):1315–24.

66. Hill AT, Campbell EJ, Bayley DL, et al. Evidence for excessive bronchial inflammation during an acute exacerbation of COPD in patients with alpha-1-antitrypsin deficiency. Am J Respir Crit Care Med 1999;160:1968–75.

67. Vijayasaratha K, Stockley RA. Reported and unreported exacerbations of COPD: analysis by diary cards. Chest 2008;133:34–41.

68. International Study Evaluating the Safety and Efficacy of Inhaled, Human, Alpha-1 Antitrypsin (AAT) in Alpha-1 Antitrypsin Deficient Patients With Emphysema. 2010. ClinicalTrials.gov. NCT01217671.

69. Stockley RA, Vogelmeier C, Miravitlles M. Augmentation therapy for alpha1-antitrypsin deficiency: towards a personalised approach. Orphanet Journal of Rare Diseases 2013;8:149.

70. Pittelkow MR, Smith KC, Su WP. Alpha-1-antitrypsin deficiency and panniculitis. Perspectives on disease relationship and replacement therapy. Am J Med 1988;84(6A):80–6.

71. Morris H, Morgan MD, Wood AM, et al. ANCA-associated vasculitis is linked to carriage of the allele of alpha-1 antitrypsin and its polymers. Ann Rheum Dis 2011;70(10):1851–6.

72. Yu SD, Gan JC. Effects of progressive desialylation on the survival of human plasma alpha1-antitrypsin in rat circulation. Int J Biochem 1978;9(2): 107–15.

73. Spencer LT, Humphries JE, Brantly ML. Antibody response to aerosolized transgenic human alpha1-antitrypsin. N Engl J Med 2005;352(19): 2030–1.

74. Blanchard V, Liu X, Eigel S, et al. N-glycosylation and biological activity of recombinant human alpha1-antitrypsin expressed in a novel human neuronal cell line. Biotechnol Bioeng 2011;108(9): 2118–28.

75. Burrows JA, Willis LK, Perlmutter DH. Chemical chaperones mediate increased secretion of mutant alpha 1-antitrypsin (alpha 1-AT) Z: a potential pharmacological strategy for prevention of liver injury and emphysema in alpha 1-AT deficiency. Proc Natl Acad Sci U S A 2000;97(4):1796–801.

76. Teckman JH. Lack of effect of oral 4-phenylbutyrate on serum alpha-1-antitrypsin in patients with alpha-1-antitrypsin deficiency: a preliminary study. J Pediatr Gastroenterol Nutr 2004;39(1): 34–7.

77. Mallya M, Phillips RL, Saldanha SA, et al. Small molecules block the polymerization of Z alpha1-antitrypsin and increase the clearance of intracellular aggregates. J Med Chem 2007;50(22): 5357–63.

78. Lee C, Maeng JS, Kocher JP, et al. Cavities of alpha(1)-antitrypsin that play structural and functional roles. Protein Sci 2001;10(7):1446–53.

79. Flotte TR, Trapnell BC, Humphries M, et al. Phase 2 clinical trial of a recombinant adeno-associated viral vector expressing alpha1-antitrypsin: interim results. Hum Gene Ther 2011;22(10):1239–47.

80. Cruz PE, Mueller C, Cossette TL, et al. In vivo post-transcriptional gene silencing of alpha-1 antitrypsin by adeno-associated virus vectors expressing siRNA. Lab Invest 2007;87(9):893–902.

81. Mueller CG, Hess E. Emerging functions of RANKL in lymphoid tissues. Front Immunol 2012;3:261.

82. McNab GL, Ahmad A, Mistry D, et al. Modification of gene expression and increase in $\alpha 1$-antitrypsin ($\alpha 1$-AT) secretion after homologous recombination in $\alpha 1$-AT-deficient monocytes. Hum Gene Ther 2007;18:1171–7.

83. De BP, Heguy A, Hackett NR, et al. High levels of persistent expression of alpha1-antitrypsin mediated by the nonhuman primate serotype rh.10 adeno-associated virus despite preexisting immunity to common human adeno-associated viruses. Mol Ther 2006;13(1):67–76.

84. Yusa K, Rashid ST, Strick-Marchand H, et al. Targeted gene correction of alpha1-antitrypsin deficiency in induced pluripotent stem cells. Nature 2011;478(7369):391–4.

85. Sinden NJ, Stockley RA. Proteinase 3 activity in sputum from subjects with alpha-1-antitrypsin deficiency and COPD. Eur Respir J 2013;41(5): 1042–50.

86. Maden M. Retinoids have differing efficacies on alveolar regeneration in a dexamethasone-treated mouse. Am J Respir Cell Mol Biol 2006;35(2): 260–7.

87. Stolk J, Stockley RA, Stoel BC, et al. Randomized controlled trial for emphysema with a selective agonist of the gamma type retinoic acid receptor. Eur Respir J 2012;40:306–12.

88. Shapiro SD, Endicott SK, Province MA, et al. Marked longevity of human lung parenchymal elastic fibers deduced from prevalence of D-aspartate and nuclear weapons-related radiocarbon. J Clin Invest 1991;87(5):1828–34.

89. Turino GM, Lin YY, He J, et al. Elastin degradation: an effective biomarker in COPD. COPD 2012;9(4): 435–8.

90. Carter RI, Mumford RA, Treonze KM, et al. The fibrinogen cleavage product AαVal360, a specific marker of neutrophil elastase activity in vivo. Thorax 2011;66:686–91.

Chronic Obstructive Pulmonary Disease: Clinical Integrative Physiology

Denis E. O'Donnell, MD, FRCP(I), FRCP(C)[a],[*],
Pierantonio Laveneziana, MD, PhD[b], Katherine Webb, MSc[a],
J. Alberto Neder, MD, DSc[a]

KEYWORDS

- Chronic obstructive pulmonary disease • Small airways • Lung mechanics • Dyspnea • Exercise
- Cardiac output

KEY POINTS

- COPD is characterized by heterogeneous physiologic abnormalities that are not adequately represented by simple spirometry.
- Extensive peripheral airway dysfunction is often present in smokers with mild spirometric abnormalities and may have negative clinical consequences.
- Activity-related dyspnea and exercise intolerance in patients with mild airway obstruction are linked to increased ventilatory inefficiency and dynamic gas trapping during exercise.
- Progressive increases in dyspnea and activity restriction are explained, in many instances, by the consequences of progressive erosion of resting inspiratory capacity.
- Although restrictive mechanics and increasing neuromechanical uncoupling of the respiratory system contribute to exercise intolerance across the spectrum of COPD severity, coexistent cardiocirculatory impairment is also potentially important.

INTRODUCTION

Chronic obstructive pulmonary disease (COPD) is characterized by inflammatory injury to the intra-thoracic airways, lung parenchyma, and pulmonary vasculature in highly variable combinations. It follows that the measured physiologic abnormalities are equally heterogeneous and these, in turn, likely underscore the common clinical manifestations of this complex disease. Expiratory flow limitation (EFL) is a defining physiologic characteristic of COPD and represents the final expression of diverse derangements of respiratory mechanics. Spirometric measurement of reduced maximal expiratory flow rate is required for diagnosis of

COPD and can be used to follow the course of the disease. However, such measurements as forced expiratory volume in 1 second (FEV_1) are not useful in predicting the cardinal symptoms of the disease, dyspnea and exercise intolerance. This article reviews the respiratory mechanical and cardiocirculatory abnormalities across the spectrum of mild to severe COPD, at rest and during the stress of exercise.

MILD COPD
Clinical Relevance

It is well established that those with mild-to-moderate disease severity represent most patients

[a] Division of Respiratory and Critical Care Medicine, Department of Medicine, Queen's University, 102 Stuart Street, Kingston, Ontario K7L 2V6, Canada; [b] Service d'Explorations Fonctionnelles de la Respiration, de l'Exercice et de la Dyspnée Hôpital Universitaire Pitié-Salpêtrière (AP-HP), Laboratoire de Physio-Pathologie Respiratoire, Faculty of Medicine, Pierre et Marie Curie University (Paris VI), 47-83 Boulevard de l'Hôpital, 75013 Paris, France
[*] Corresponding author. Division of Respiratory and Critical Care Medicine, Department of Medicine, Kingston General Hospital, Queen's University, Richardson House, 102 Stuart Street, Kingston, Ontario K7L 2V6, Canada.
E-mail address: odonnell@queensu.ca

Clin Chest Med 35 (2014) 51–69
http://dx.doi.org/10.1016/j.ccm.2013.09.008
0272-5231/14/$ – see front matter © 2014 Elsevier Inc. All rights reserved.

with COPD, yet this subpopulation is understudied.[1,2] For the purpose of this review, mild COPD refers to spirometrically defined mild airway obstruction (ie, FEV_1 80%–100 % predicted), which need not be synonymous with early COPD. There is evidence from several population studies that, compared with nonsmoking healthy populations, smokers with mild COPD show increased mortality (including cardiovascular mortality),[3,4] increased hospitalizations, decreased health-related quality of life,[5–10] increased activity-related dyspnea, and reduced daily physical activity levels.[11–15] The underlying pathophysiologic linkages between mild COPD, dyspnea, and activity restriction have only recently become the subject of systematic study.[16–18]

Resting Physiologic Abnormalities in Mild COPD

A recent cross-sectional study of patients with COPD attests to the vast physiologic heterogeneity that exists even in those with mild airflow obstruction (**Fig. 1**).[19] Thus, in patients with a largely preserved FEV_1 there is wide variability in airways resistance (and conductance); pulmonary gas trapping; resting lung hyperinflation; and the

integrity of the alveolar-capillary gas exchanging interface. Quantitative computed tomography (CT) scans also confirm a broad range of structural abnormalities in mild COPD, which include emphysema, pulmonary gas trapping, airway wall thickening, and even vascular abnormalities.[20–22]

Small airways dysfunction

The small airways are believed to be the initial locus of inflammation in COPD, and refer to the membranous (<2 mm diameter) and respiratory bronchioles.[23] Previous studies have shown evidence of active inflammation and obliteration of peripheral airways in mild COPD.[23–25] McDonough and colleagues[25] have proposed that such loss of small airways precedes the development of centrilobular emphysema. Mucus hypersecretion as a result of chronic bronchitis can also result in extensive peripheral airway dysfunction.[24,25]

Hogg and colleagues[24] were the first to report that peripheral airway resistance, measured by retrograde catheters, was increased by up to four-fold in the excised lungs of smokers with mild emphysema compared with those of healthy control subjects. This increase occurred despite normal values of total airways resistance. With the progression of emphysema, the increasing

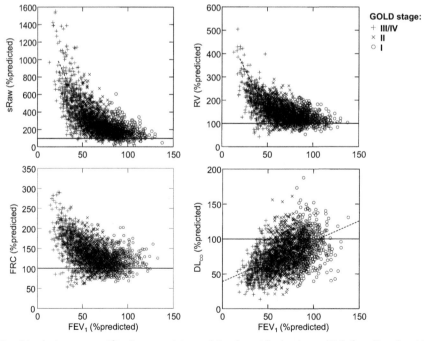

Fig. 1. Relationships between specific airway resistance (sRaw), residual volume (RV), functional residual capacity (FRC), and diffusing capacity of the lung (DL_{CO}) are shown against FEV_1 (all measurements expressed as % of predicted normal values). sRaw, RV, and FRC increased exponentially as FEV_1 decreased, and DL_{CO} decreased linearly as FEV_1 decreased. GOLD, Global Initiative on Obstructive Lung Disease. (*Modified from* Deesomchok A, Webb KA, Forkert L, et al. Lung hyperinflation and its reversibility in patients with airway obstruction of varying severity. COPD 2010;7(6):431; with permission.)

total airway resistance predominantly reflected the rise of peripheral airway resistance.[22] EFL, the hallmark of COPD, is present when the expired flows generated during spontaneous tidal breathing represent the maximal possible flow rates that can be achieved at that lung volume. EFL arises because of the combined effects of airway narrowing (caused by mucosal edema, mucus plugging, airway remodeling, and peribronchial fibrosis); reduced lung elastic recoil (reduced driving pressure for expiratory flow); and disrupted alveolar attachments, which predispose to dynamic airway collapse.[26–28] Corbin and colleagues[29] provided evidence that in smokers with mild airway obstruction, lung compliance increased in most subjects over a 4-year follow-up period: the increase in total lung capacity (TLC) correlated well with reduced static lung recoil pressure. Altered elastic properties of the lung potentially contribute to small airway dysfunction by reducing alveolar pressure gradients (particularly in panacinar emphysema) and by diminishing normal airway tethering.[28] The relative contribution of these factors to EFL in mild COPD varies from patient to patient and is difficult to quantify with any precision.[28]

The knowledge that extensive peripheral airways disease may exist in smokers with preserved spirometry and few respiratory symptoms has prompted the quest for sensitive tests of small airway function. These tests measure respiratory system resistance during tidal breathing or exploit the presence of nonuniform behavior of dynamic lung mechanics. The main physiologic manifestations of mild COPD as determined by such tests are summarized in **Box 1**. For instance, tidal esophageal pressure-derived measurements show increased frequency-dependence of dynamic lung compliance and resistance.[30] This behavior primarily reflects nonuniformity of mechanical time constants in the lung caused by regional changes in the compliance or resistance (or both) of alveolar units. Exaggerated frequency-dependence may also indicate the presence of delayed gas emptying in alveolar units

---

Box 1
Pathophysiology of mild COPD

- Increased peripheral airway resistance
- Maldistribution of ventilation
- Disruption of pulmonary gas exchange
- Premature airway closure
- Increased pulmonary gas trapping
- Increased airway hyperresponsiveness

---

that are slowly ventilated by collateral channels. Single-breath or multibreath nitrogen washout tests confirm maldistribution of ventilation and early airway closure.[31] Volume at isoflow during helium-oxygen and room air breathing indicates lack of a normal increase in flow during helium-oxygen in COPD and suggests that the major site of resistance is in the peripheral rather than central airways.[32,33] Forced and impulse oscillometry techniques measure respiratory system impedance. Typical abnormalities in mild COPD are increased respiratory system resistance; decreased reactance (increased elastance) at low oscillation frequencies; and increased resonant frequency.[34,35] Mid to low volume (effort-independent) maximal expiratory flow rates are often reduced below normal in smokers with a preserved FEV_1 and suggest small airway dysfunction.[36–38] Increased residual volume (RV) or RV/TLC ratio signifies increased pulmonary gas trapping caused by early airway closure, and provides indirect evidence of peripheral airways obstruction.[19,29]

Nonspecific increased airway hyperresponsiveness is a well-documented finding in most patients with mild COPD and is believed to reflect inflammation and the combined morphometric changes in the peripheral airways. Increased airway hyperresponsiveness is more frequently found in women (reflecting their naturally smaller airway diameter) and in both genders predicts accelerated decline of FEV_1 with time and increased all-cause and specific mortality.[39–43] In an important study by Riess and colleagues,[43] in 77 patients with mild-to-moderate COPD, airway hyperresponsiveness was inversely related to airway wall thickness in resected lungs, after accounting for lung elastic recoil and $FEV_1\%$ predicted.

Ventilation-perfusion abnormalities

The diffusing capacity of the lung for carbon monoxide (DL_{CO}) is reduced in some patients with mild COPD, suggesting alteration of the surface area for gas exchange (see **Fig. 1**).[19,37] Patients with mild COPD and smokers with normal lung function have evidence of small-vessel disease affecting mainly the muscular pulmonary arteries.[22,44–49] Increased intimal thickness and narrow vessel lumen are the main manifestations of vascular injury in these patients.[44–46] Abnormal features include muscle cell proliferation and deposition of extracellular matrix proteins in the intima of pulmonary muscular arteries.[44–49] A recent noninvasive CT assessment of the cross-sectional area (CSA) of segmental and subsegmental small vessels revealed that the percentage of CSA of arteries less than 5 mm² was significantly lower in subjects with the emphysema phenotype than in subjects with the bronchitis phenotype in all COPD Global Initiative on Obstructive Lung Disease (GOLD) stages.[22] In mild-to-moderate COPD, Barbera and colleagues[46,47] and Rodriguez-Roisin and colleagues[44] have demonstrated that significant alveolar ventilation (V_A)-to-perfusion (Q) mismatching and loss of protective hypoxic vasoconstriction can occur while breathing at rest. Thus, the resting alveolar-to-arterial oxygen tension gradient was abnormally widened (>15 mm Hg) in most of a small sample of patients with milder COPD who also had predominantly low regional V_A/Q ratios measured by multiple inert gas elimination techniques.[46,47]

Responses to Exercise in Mild COPD

High ventilatory requirements
In patients with mild COPD who report persistent activity-related dyspnea, peak oxygen uptake ($V'O_2$) measured during incremental exercise to tolerance has been shown to be diminished compared with healthy control subjects (**Fig. 2**).[15–18,50] One consistent abnormality has been the finding of higher than normal ventilation/carbon dioxide production slopes ($V'_E/V'CO_2$) during cycle and treadmill exercise.[15–18,50] Possible underlying causes of this increased ventilatory inefficiency include (1) increased physiologic dead space (DS) that fails to decline as normal during exercise, (2) altered set-point for $Paco_2$, and (3) a combination of the above. Future studies with measurement of $Paco_2$ are needed to determine if increased V_A/Q ratios are the main explanation. Significant arterial O_2 desaturation (>5%) has not been reported during incremental cycle exercise in symptomatic mild COPD.[15–18] Preservation of Pao_2 during exercise suggests that compensatory increases in ventilation (V'_E) in the setting of a normal increase in cardiac output ensure improved overall V_A/Q relations during exercise in mild-to-moderate COPD.[46–48] The lack of arterial O_2 desaturation during exercise also means that significant diffusion limitation of pulmonary O_2 transfer or intrapulmonary shunt are unlikely to be present to any significant degree. It remains plausible that in unfit patients, earlier lactate accumulation during physical exertion may provide an added stimulus to V'_E (by bicarbonate buffering and increased $V'CO_2$).[18] Finally, reduced oxidative capacity and reduced systemic O_2 delivery secondary to subclinical cardiocirculatory impairment, with an attendant early metabolic acidosis, may exist in some patients with mild COPD (see below).

Impairment of dynamic respiratory mechanics
We have proposed that the combination of increased ventilatory requirements, increased dynamic gas-trapping, and resultant restrictive mechanical constraints on tidal volume (V_T) expansion may contribute to reduced peak V'_E and peak $V'O_2$ in mild COPD.[15–18] The increased gas trapping during exercise reflects the combination of tachypnea and EFL: in alveolar units with slow mechanical time constants, expiratory time is insufficient to allow end-expiratory lung volume (EELV) to decline to its natural relaxation volume. To determine if mechanical factors represent the proximate limitation to exercise in mild COPD, Chin and colleagues[18] selectively stressed the respiratory system by adding DS to the breathing apparatus during exercise. Previous studies in younger healthy participants have shown that added DS (0.6 L) during exercise results in significant increases in peak V_T and V'_E and preservation of exercise capacity.[51–53] In mild COPD, the inability to further increase end-inspiratory lung volume (EILV), V_T, and V'_E at the peak of exercise in response to DS loading indicated that the respiratory system had reached its physiologic limits at end-exercise. This occurred in the presence of adequate cardiac reserve. Increased central chemostimulation during DS loading, in the face of such mechanical constraints on V_T expansion, caused an earlier onset of intolerable dyspnea in COPD but not in healthy control subjects.[18] Mechanical studies have also confirmed that dynamic lung compliance is decreased and pulmonary resistance, rest-to-peak changes in EELV, intrinsic positive end-expiratory pressures (PEEPi), and oxygen cost and work of breathing are all elevated in symptomatic mild COPD compared with healthy control subjects.[16,17]

Cardiocirculatory impairment
It is widely believed that the cardiovascular complications of COPD occur only in the advanced stage of the disease as a consequence of chronic hypoxemia (eg, pulmonary hypertension and cor pulmonale). More recently, however, several clinical and epidemiologic studies have shown cardiocirculatory abnormalities in patients in the early stages of COPD.[54–61] In fact, many patients with COPD have coexistent cardiovascular disease because smoking history is a common risk factor for both.[55,58,62,63] Notably, Lange and colleagues[4] recently showed that the presence of dyspnea in the setting of only mild airway obstruction was an independent predictor of cardiovascular mortality in a large Danish population. The Multiethnic Study of Atherosclerosis found that even in mild preclinical COPD, increases in airflow obstruction (as estimated by FEV_1/forced vital capacity ratio) and extent of emphysema (measured by CT) were linearly associated with reductions in

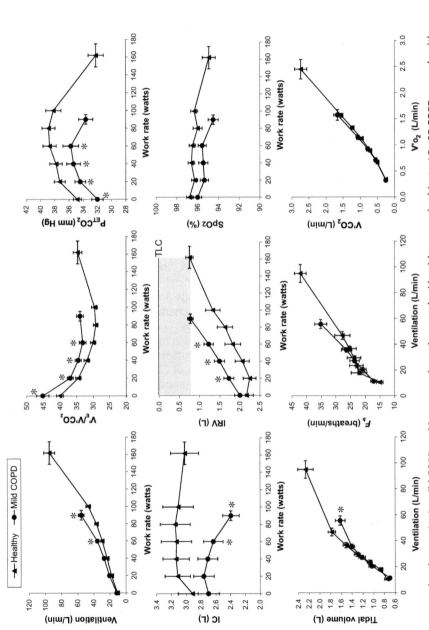

Fig. 2. Responses to incremental cycle exercise in mild COPD and in age- and gender-matched healthy normal subjects. *$P<.05$ COPD versus healthy group at standardized work rates or at peak exercise. Values are means ± SEM. F_b, breathing frequency; IC, inspiratory capacity; IRV, inspiratory reserve volume; $P_{ET}CO_2$, partial pressure of end-tidal carbon dioxide; SpO_2, oxygen saturation; $V'CO_2$, carbon dioxide production; $V'_E/V'CO_2$, ventilatory equivalent for carbon dioxide; $V'O_2$, oxygen consumption. (Reprinted with permission of the American Thoracic Society. Copyright © 2013 American Thoracic Society. Chin RC, Guenette JA, Cheng S, et al. Does the respiratory system limit exercise in mild COPD? Am J Respir Crit Care Med 2013;187(12):1319–20. Official Journal of the American Thoracic Society.)

left ventricular (LV) end-diastolic volume, stroke volume, and cardiac output measured by magnetic resonance imaging.[56,59] In the same study, pulmonary hyperinflation, as measured by RV or RV/TLC ratio, was associated with greater LV mass.[60] Malerba and colleagues[58] also found that minor emphysema determined by CT was related to impaired LV diastolic function and cardiac output.

The mechanisms underlying the cardiocirculatory abnormalities in mild COPD are unknown but they might include smoking-related pulmonary vascular damage,[22,49,61,64] impairments in nitric-oxide–induced vasodilatation,[65] simultaneous aging of the lungs and heart as indicated by "senile" emphysema and LV stiffness,[66] and negative central hemodynamic effects of exercise-related dynamic lung hyperinflation.[56,59,60] In fact, minor emphysema determined by CT imaging is associated with impaired LV diastolic function and cardiac output.[56] The pulmonary microvasculature, in particular, may become damaged early in the course of the disease because its endothelium is exquisitely sensitive to the deleterious effects of inflammation and hyperoxidative stress.[67,68] It is noteworthy that in the late 1950s, Liebow[69] suggested that alveolar destruction in emphysema is secondary to inflammation of the pulmonary microvasculature. Indirect support for this contention has been provided by Alford and colleagues[70] who found that smokers showing early signs of emphysema susceptibility had a greater heterogeneity in regional perfusion parameters by multidetector CT perfusion imaging than emphysema-free smokers and never-smokers. Thomashow and colleagues[61] found that markers of increased alveolar endothelial cell apoptosis were positively related to percent emphysema and inversely associated with pulmonary microvascular blood flow and diffusing capacity in patients with mild COPD. It is also remarkable that patients with early chronic heart failure[71] and mild COPD[72] have evidence of impaired cardiovascular autonomic regulation, decreased baroreceptor sensitivity, and heart rate variability suggesting common pathogenic pathways.

Skeletal muscle dysfunction

There is growing recognition that the peripheral skeletal muscles may show abnormalities in structure and function in mild COPD,[73–75] which might negatively impact on patients' exercise tolerance.[76] In fact, these patients report higher perceived leg effort ratings for a given metabolic demand compared with healthy control subjects.[15–18] Muscle biopsy studies also indicate that the general morphologic pattern of abnormalities form a continuum from mild-to-very severe COPD.[74,75] Unfitness

and detraining are certainly important contributors, because regular daily physical activity decreases early in the course of the disease[77] and resistance exercise training can restore muscle function back to normal.[78] The relevance of sustained inactivity to muscle atrophy in mild COPD was emphasized by the findings of Shrikrishna and colleagues[79] who reported a close association between cross-sectional area of rectus femoris (measured by ultrasound) with physical activity levels in patients with GOLD stage I. Active smoking seems to play a significant role because it has several negative effects on muscle bioenergetics and protein synthesis.[75] The relevance of systemic inflammation in muscle dysfunction remains conjectural in mild COPD.[68]

MODERATE-TO-SEVERE COPD

Concepts of the natural history of COPD are strongly influenced by the seminal longitudinal population study of Fletcher and Peto[80] who have charted the decline in FEV$_1$ with time in susceptible smokers. Much less information is available on the temporal evolution of complex mechanical abnormalities and of pulmonary gas exchange abnormalities. Clearly, disease progression is characterized by worsening of the heterogeneous physiologic derangements already outlined in mild COPD. Recent short-term longitudinal studies have confirmed marked variability in change of FEV$_1$, which ranges from stability over time to accelerated decline.[81,82] Researchers are only beginning to understand the potentially important influences on the individual rate of physiologic decline of factors, such as obesity,[83] exacerbation history,[84,85] presence of comorbidities (eg, cardiocirculatory disease),[86] and the overlap with asthma. Clinical subtypes of COPD with dominant mucus hypersecretion (chronic bronchitis), structural emphysema, and a mixture of both have been identified for many years but the relative importance of these differing pathologic and physiologic features of COPD in contributing to dyspnea and activity restriction is still unclear.[87]

Resting Physiologic Abnormalities in Moderate-to-Severe COPD

Progression of resting lung hyperinflation

One of the major consequences of worsening EFL is lung hyperinflation (**Fig. 3**). The (reduced) resting inspiratory capacity (IC) and IC/TLC ratio have been shown to be independent risk factors for all-cause and respiratory mortality, and are linked to risk of exacerbation, activity-related dyspnea, and exercise limitation.[88–91] The presence of lung hyperinflation means that elastic properties of the

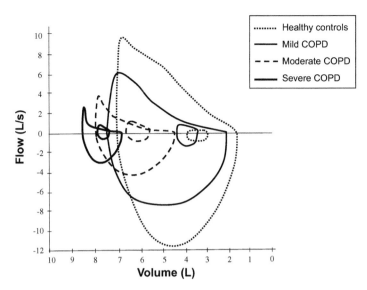

<table>
<tr><td>········ Healthy controls</td></tr>
<tr><td>—— Mild COPD</td></tr>
<tr><td>– – – Moderate COPD</td></tr>
<tr><td>—— Severe COPD</td></tr>
</table>

Fig. 3. Tidal flow-volume loops at rest are shown within their respective maximal loops. With worsening severity of disease, expiratory flow-limitation and static lung volumes increase. Resting inspiratory capacity progressively decreases with advancing disease so that tidal volume is closer to total lung capacity where elastic loading is increased.

lungs have changed (increased lung compliance) to such an extent that EELV fails to decline to the natural relaxation volume of the respiratory system. In flow-limited patients, resting EELV is also dynamically determined and varies with the prevailing breathing pattern and autonomic control of airway smooth muscle tone. This latter dynamic component of resting hyperinflation can be successfully manipulated by bronchodilator therapy.[92–98] Lung hyperinflation places the inspiratory muscles, especially the diaphragm, at a significant mechanical disadvantage by shortening its fibers, thereby compromising its force-generating capacity.[99] In patients with chronic lung hyperinflation, adaptive alterations in muscle fiber composition[100,101] and oxidative capacity[102] are believed to help preserve the functional strength and force-generating capacity of the diaphragm.[103]

Lung hyperinflation forces tidal breathing to take place nearer to the upper nonlinear extreme of the respiratory system's sigmoidal static pressure-volume relaxation curve where there is increased inspiratory threshold (auto-PEEP effect) and elastic loading of the inspiratory muscles.[104–107] High lung volumes in COPD attenuate increased airway resistance during resting breathing but this beneficial effect is negated if further "acute-on-chronic" dynamic hyperinflation (DH) occurs, for example, during physical activity[15,16,97,104,108–110] or during exacerbations.[84,111,112] In this latter circumstance, acute overloading and functional weakness of the inspiratory muscles may be linked to fatigue or even overt mechanical failure.[113]

Pulmonary gas exchange abnormalities

Among patients with COPD, those with predominant emphysema have high V_A/Q areas within the lungs, whereas those with predominant chronic bronchitis have low V_A/Q regions as a result of small airways distortion and mucus plugging.[44,45] The attendant abnormalities in arterial blood gases, if sustained, stimulate integrated compensatory adaptations over time. Thus, activation of neurohumoral, renal, and hemodynamic homeostatic mechanisms, together with modulation of the central respiratory controller, combine to preserve critical arterial oxygenation and acid-base status. Ultimately, in advanced COPD, the compensations may fail and reduced alveolar ventilation at a given $V'CO_2$ leads to CO_2 retention.[113] This occurs in the presence of abnormalities of the ventilatory control or as a result of critical respiratory muscle weakness (eg, nutritional and electrolytic deficiencies) and the negative mechanical effects of resting lung hyperinflation.

Responses to Exercise in Moderate-to-Severe COPD

Exercise limitation is multifactorial in COPD: peripheral muscle weakness and cardiocirculatory impairment undoubtedly contribute but increased central respiratory drive, dynamic mechanical impairment, and the associated dyspnea are major contributors, particularly in more advanced disease.[109,114–118]

Increased central respiratory drive

Ventilatory requirements progressively increase as COPD advances, primarily reflecting the consequences of worsening pulmonary gas exchange. Although the central drive to breathe during exercise steadily increases with worsening disease, VE/work rate slopes may not reflect this because of the increasing mechanical constraints imposed on the respiratory system. At the limits of exercise tolerance in severe COPD, central neural drive has been shown to increase to near maximal values in response to the increased chemostimulation.[117–119] Recently, the potential for added ventilatory stimulation from metoboreceptors in the active locomotor muscles has been emphasized.[120] Critical arterial hypoxemia can also stimulate ventilation by peripheral chemoreceptor activation. This mainly reflects the effect of a fall in mixed venous O_2 on alveolar units with low V_A/Q ratios. Decreased mixed venous O_2 occurs because increase in cardiac output (or peripheral blood flow) is not commensurate with the increase in $V'O_2$ of the active locomotor muscles.

Dynamic respiratory mechanics across the continuum of COPD

The progression of COPD is associated with increasing erosion of the resting IC caused by increasing lung hyperinflation (**Fig. 4**). The resting IC dictates the limits of V_T expansion during exercise in flow-limited patients with COPD.[97,108–110,121–125] Thus, the lower the resting IC, the lower the peak V_T, and thus V'_E, achieved during exercise (see **Fig. 4**; **Fig. 5**).[97,108–110,121–125] Exercise DH further reduces the already diminished resting IC.[121,124] When V_T reaches approximately

70% of the prevailing IC (or EILV reaches ~90% of the TLC at a minimal inspiratory reserve volume), there is an inflection or plateau in the V_T/V'_E relation (see **Fig. 5**).[97,108,110,121] This critical volume restriction represents a mechanical limit where further sustainable increases in V'_E are impossible.[97,108,110,121] The inability to further expand V_T is associated with tachypnea, the only strategy available in response to the increasing central respiratory drive. Increased breathing frequency has added detrimental effects on inspiratory muscle function including further elastic loading caused by DH, increased velocity of shortening of the inspiratory muscles with associated functional weakness, and decreased dynamic lung compliance.[117–119] With worsening mechanical abnormalities, tidal esophageal pressure swings increase and, with it, the work and O_2 cost of breathing required to achieve a given increase (**Fig. 6**) in V'_E steadily increases. Theoretically, these collective derangements of respiratory mechanics can predispose to inspiratory muscle fatigue.[126,127] However, the evidence that measurable fatigue develops in COPD is inconclusive[100,102] even at the limits of exercise tolerance.[128] This may reflect temporal adaptations of the respiratory muscles or that exercise in many patients with COPD is terminated by intolerable respiratory discomfort before physiologic maxima are attained.

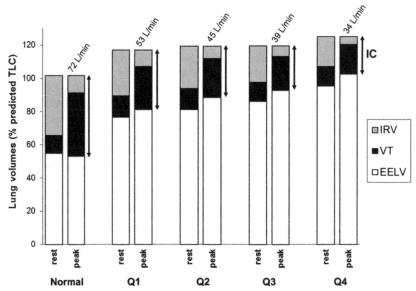

Fig. 4. Progressive hyperinflation, shown by increasing end-expiratory lung volume (EELV), is illustrated at rest and peak exercise as FEV_1 quartile worsens. Peak values of dynamic inspiratory capacity (IC), tidal volume (V_T), and ventilation (values shown above peak exercise bars) decreased with worsening severity, although similar peak ratings of dyspnea intensity were reached. Normative data are shown for comparison. IRV, inspiratory reserve volume; TLC, total lung capacity. (*From* O'Donnell DE, Guenette JA, Maltais F, et al. Decline of resting inspiratory capacity in COPD: the impact on breathing pattern, dyspnea, and ventilatory capacity during exercise. Chest 2012;141(3):758; with permission.)

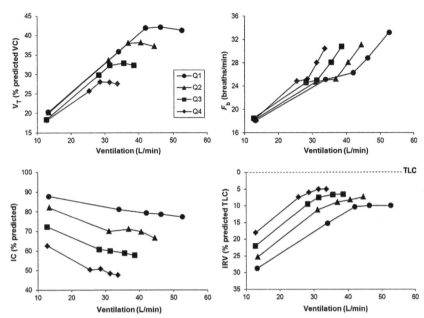

Fig. 5. Tidal volume (V_T), breathing frequency (F_b), dynamic inspiratory capacity (IC), and inspiratory reserve volume (IRV) are shown plotted against minute ventilation (V'_E) during constant work-rate exercise. Note the clear inflection (plateau) in the V_T/V'_E relationship, which coincides with a simultaneous inflection in the IRV. After this point, further increases in V'_E are accomplished by accelerating F. Data plotted are mean values at steady-state rest; isotime (ie, 2 minutes, 4 minutes); the V_T/V'_E inflection point; and peak exercise. TLC, total lung capacity; VC, vital capacity. (*From* O'Donnell DE, Guenette JA, Maltais F, et al. Decline of resting inspiratory capacity in COPD: the impact on breathing pattern, dyspnea, and ventilatory capacity during exercise. Chest 2012;141(3):759; with permission.)

Cardiocirculatory impairment

Acute-on-chronic hyperinflation may have deleterious effects on cardiac performance during exercise.[118,129–139] The resulting decreases in dynamic lung compliance with increasing levels of PEEPi require higher mean tidal intrathoracic pressure swings.[92,97] Increased intrathoracic pressure, in turn, decreases the gradient for venous return and leads to higher RV impedance. Of note, high right atrial pressures may contribute to decrease venous return but, conversely, can be beneficial in maintaining RV filling during expiration.[136] Juxta-alveolar capillary compression by high alveolar pressures also contributes to increased RV afterload.[136–139] Pulmonary vasoconstriction caused by hypoxemia and,

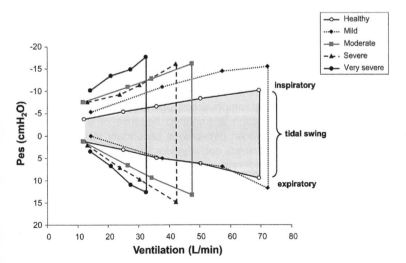

Fig. 6. Tidal esophageal pressure (Pes) swings are shown with varying severity of COPD and in age-matched healthy control subjects. As disease severity worsens, the amplitude of inspiratory and expiratory Pes increases for a given ventilation during exercise. The *shaded area* represents the tidal Pes swing in the healthy control subjects. (*Data from* Refs.[97,104,110] and unpublished data from the authors' laboratory, 2013.)

secondarily, hypercapnia and acid-base (acidosis) disturbances may further increase RV afterload. A recent prospective study with a large number of patients with COPD who underwent right heart catheterization during exercise found abnormal elevations in pulmonary artery pressures as a function of cardiac output, even in those without resting pulmonary hypertension.[140] In line with the concept that disturbed RV hemodynamics is relevant to cardiocirculatory impairment in COPD, exercise-related pulmonary hypertension has been closely related to impaired peripheral O_2 delivery in patients GOLD stages II to IV.[137] Combined effects of reduced RV preload and high afterload would then decrease stroke volume and cardiac output (**Fig. 7**).[54,56,140–144]

Impairment in LV diastolic filling is another consistent hemodynamic finding in advanced COPD,[56,142,143] even in patients without pulmonary hypertension.[145] Patients enrolled in the

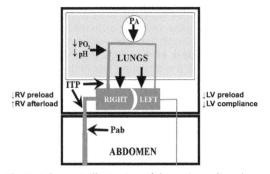

Fig. 7. Schematic illustration of dynamic cardiopulmonary interactions in patients with moderate-to-severe COPD presenting with expiratory flow limitation, intrinsic positive end-expiratory pressure, and lung hyperinflation. Hypercapnia-induced venous blood pooling, intra-abdominal compression of splanchnic vessels (particularly vena cava), and increased intrathoracic pressure (ITP) may have deleterious consequences on right ventricular (RV) preload. Increased ITP, pulmonary arteriolar vasoconstriction caused by alveolar hypoxia and respiratory acidosis, and juxtaalveolar capillary compression by supraphysiologic alveolar pressures (PA) might increase RV afterload. Hyperinflated lungs may also mechanically compress the heart, particularly the right chambers. Left ventricular (LV) stroke volume can be compromised by lower filling pressures, hypoxia-related myocardial stiffness, and decreased compliance caused by a leftward shift of the septum by the overdistended right ventricle. Large negative intrathoracic pressure with no change in lung volume at early inspiration can transitorily increase venous return and contribute to leftward shift of the septum. This chain of maladaptation is strongly modulated by fluid status, exercise, and comorbidities, especially chronic heart failure. Pab, abdominal pressure.

National Emphysema Treatment Trial, for instance, had elevated cardiac diastolic pressures and pulmonary capillary wedge pressures without systolic dysfunction,[146] which were improved with lung-volume reduction surgery.[146–148] Of note, LV filling rather than distensibility has been more closely associated with hyperinflation[56,59,143] suggesting that reduced preload might underlie LV diastolic dysfunction in COPD.[141,148,149] Tachycardia, a common finding in COPD, is likely to further reduce time for diastolic filling. The combination of increased RV dimensions and pressures with low end-diastolic LV volumes may heighten the transseptal pressure gradient. This would flatten or even displace the intraventricular septum toward the LV cavity thereby decreasing its compliance and filling.[150,151] Calcium-mediated abnormalities of myocardial relaxation induced by chronic hypoxemia may also contribute to impaired LV compliance.[152] The heart in the cardiac fossa can also be directly compressed by the overdistended lungs. Recent data confirm there is an inverse relationship between lung hyperinflation and cardiac size[60,143,148] more likely reflecting a combination of impaired LV filling and direct heart compression.

The functional impact of improving the negative cardiopulmonary interactions in COPD has been recently explored. In addition to lung-volume reduction surgery,[146–148,153] noninvasive positive pressure ventilation,[154,155] heliox,[130,156–158] and bronchodilators[129,159] have all been found to ameliorate the hemodynamic responses to exertion. Interestingly, some of these interventions had positive effects on peripheral muscle blood flow and $\dot{V}O_2$ kinetics.[130,156,157] These studies suggest that cardiocirculatory dysfunction might contribute to exercise impairment in advanced COPD. However, improvements secondary to those interventions occurred in parallel with decreases in work of breathing, DH, and dyspnea. It is difficult, therefore, to ascertain the relative contributions of increasing muscle blood flow to enhance patients' functional capacity.

Collectively, the bulk of evidence obtained in patients with advanced disease with a predominant emphysema phenotype indicates that LV function is impaired because of small LV end-diastolic dimensions secondary to increased RV afterload and dysfunctional ventricular interdependence. Although these abnormalities are particularly pronounced on exertion or during acute exacerbations, they might be present at rest in severely hyperinflated patients with end-stage disease. Concomitant intrinsic myocardial disease, a common feature in elderly patients with moderate-to-severe disease,[160] is expected to further magnify exercise intolerance but clinical or experimental evidence to support this assertion is still lacking.

Skeletal muscle dysfunction

There is a long-standing interest in investigating the mechanisms and consequences of skeletal muscle dysfunction in COPD.[161] This is clinically relevant because loss of fat-free mass is a marker of disease severity and negative prognosis, particularly in patients with a predominantly emphysematous phenotype.[161] The same muscle morphologic and functional abnormalities observed in mild COPD are found in patients with advanced COPD albeit at a greater extent.[162–164] The putative relationships between proinflammatory/hyperoxidative stresses, nutritional abnormalities, neurohumoral disturbances, hypoxemia, and muscle loss were more convincingly demonstrated in patients with end-stage COPD.[165] Patients who develop peripheral muscle fatigue after exercise are more likely to benefit from exercise training,[166] although this is not a sine qua non.[161] The relative contribution of muscle dysfunction to exercise limitation in COPD is difficult to ascertain because multiple physiologic abnormalities are simultaneously present at different degrees in individual patients.

PHYSIOLOGIC MECHANISMS OF DYSPNEA IN COPD

Most patients with COPD experience dyspnea during daily activities.[117,124,167] As COPD progresses, dyspnea intensity ratings become progressively higher at any given V'_E, power output, or metabolic load (**Fig. 8**).[108] At the breakpoint of exercise healthy individuals report that their breathing requires more work or effort.[104] However, patients with COPD additionally report the sense of unsatisfied inspiration ("can't get enough air in").[97,104,110] These distinct qualitative dimensions of dyspnea likely have different neurophysiologic mechanisms. Increased sense of effort in COPD is related to the increased motor drive to respiratory muscles.[117,118,167–171] Contractile muscle effort is increased for any given V'_E in COPD because of the increased intrinsic mechanical (elastic/threshold) loading and functional muscle weakness, in part caused by resting and DH during exercise.[117,118,167–171] In this circumstance, greater neural drive or electrical activation of the muscle is required to generate a given force.[117,118,167–171] There is evidence that the amplitude of central motor command output to the respiratory muscles is sensed by neural interconnections (ie, central corollary discharge) between cortical motor and

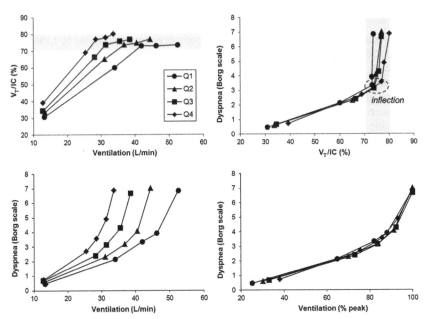

Fig. 8. Interrelationships are shown between exertional dyspnea intensity, the tidal volume/inspiratory capacity (V_T/IC) ratio, and ventilation. After the V_T/IC ratio plateaus (ie, the V_T inflection point), dyspnea rises steeply to intolerable levels. The progressive separation of dyspnea/minute ventilation (V'_E) plots with worsening quartile is abolished when ventilation is expressed as a percentage of the peak value. Data plotted are mean values at steady-state rest; isotime (ie, 2 minutes, 4 minutes); the V_T/V'_E inflection point; and peak exercise. (*From* O'Donnell DE, Guenette JA, Maltais F, et al. Decline of resting inspiratory capacity in COPD: the impact on breathing pattern, dyspnea, and ventilatory capacity during exercise. Chest 2012;141(3):760; with permission.)

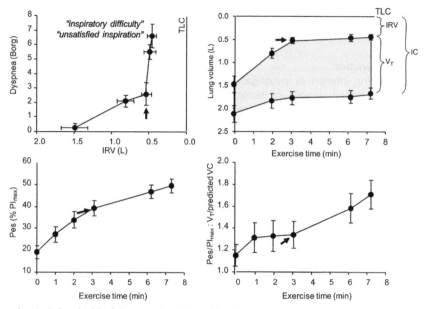

Fig. 9. The mechanical threshold of dyspnea is indicated by the abrupt rise in dyspnea after a critical "minimal" inspiratory reserve volume (IRV) is reached, which prevents further expansion of tidal volume (V_T) during exercise in COPD. Beyond this dyspnea/IRV inflection point during exercise, respiratory effort (tidal esophageal pressure swings as a fraction of the maximum inspiratory pressure [Pes/PI_{max}]) and the effort-displacement ratio continue to rise. *Arrows* indicate the dyspnea/IRV inflection point. Values are means $\pm$ SEM. IC, inspiratory capacity; TLC, total lung capacity; VC, vital capacity. (*Modified from* O'Donnell DE, Hamilton AL, Webb KA. Sensory-mechanical relationships during high-intensity, constant-work-rate exercise in COPD. J Appl Physiol 2006;101(4):1028; with permission.)

medullary centers in the brain and the somatosensory cortex.[117,118,167–171]

The neurophysiologic underpinnings of unsatisfied inspiration may be different.[117,118,167–171] The V_T/V'_E inflection point during exercise marks the point where dyspnea intensity sharply increases toward end-exercise and the dominant descriptor selected by patients changes from increased effort to unsatisfied inspiration.[110] The V_T inflection represents the onset of a widening disparity between increasing central neural drive and the mechanical/muscular response of the respiratory system (**Fig. 9**).[97,110] Dyspnea intensity seems to be more closely correlated with the change in EILV or inspiratory reserve volume during exercise than the change in EELV (ie, DH) per se (see **Fig. 9**).[97,108,110,121] Dyspnea intensity ratings also correlate well with indices of neuromechanical uncoupling, such as the ratio of V_T expansion to respired effort (relative to maximal possible effort). When vigorous inspiratory efforts become unrewarded, affective distress (anxiety, fear, panic) is evoked and is a major component of exertional dyspnea.[53,117,118,167–171]

SUMMARY

COPD is characterized by diverse physiologic derangements that are not adequately represented by simple spirometry. The human respiratory system has enormous reserve and develops effective compensatory strategies to fulfill its primary function of maintaining blood gas homeostasis even in the face of extensive injury to the small airways, lung parenchyma, and its microvasculature. These physiologic adaptations together with behavioral modification (eg, activity avoidance) can result in a prolonged preclinical phase (and late diagnosis) in susceptible smokers. In patients with spirometrically defined mild airway obstruction who report more persistent activity-related dyspnea, there is usually evidence of increased peripheral airways resistance and nonuniform behavior of dynamic respiratory mechanics. Increased dyspnea and exercise intolerance in this group is explained, at least in part, by increased ventilatory inefficiency and dynamic gas trapping during exercise. Additionally, there is new evidence that peripheral muscle dysfunction and cardiocirculatory impairment may variably contribute to exercise intolerance in patients with mild airway obstruction. As the disease progresses increasing dyspnea and activity restriction is explained by the combined effects of worsening respiratory mechanics and pulmonary gas exchange. Thus, the intensity and quality of dyspnea during physical activity is explained by the growing disparity between the increased central neural drive to breathe (augmented by pulmonary gas exchange and metabolic abnormalities) and the reduced ability of the respiratory muscles to respond because of increased intrinsic mechanical loading and the effects of lung hyperinflation. The progressive erosion of the resting IC with time means progressively earlier mechanical limitation and ever-increasing neuromechanical uncoupling of the respiratory system, which together with the effects of impaired cardiocirculatory function lead to earlier onset of intolerable dyspnea during physical activity.

REFERENCES

1. Murray CJ, Lopez AD. Global mortality, disability, and the contribution of risk factors: Global Burden of Disease Study. Lancet 1997;349(9063):1436–42.
2. Buist AS, McBurnie MA, Vollmer WM, et al. International variation in the prevalence of COPD (the BOLD Study): a population-based prevalence study. Lancet 2007;370(9589):741–50.
3. Mannino DM, Buist AS, Petty TL, et al. Lung function and mortality in the United States: data from the First National Health and Nutrition Examination Survey follow up study. Thorax 2003;58(5):388–93.
4. Lange P, Marott JL, Vestbo J, et al. Prediction of the clinical course of chronic obstructive pulmonary disease, using the new GOLD classification: a study of the general population. Am J Respir Crit Care Med 2012;186(10):975–81.
5. Maleki-Yazdi MR, Lewczuk CK, Haddon JM, et al. Early detection and impaired quality of life in COPD GOLD stage 0: a pilot study. COPD 2007;4(4):313–20.
6. Antonelli-Incalzi R, Imperiale C, Bellia V, et al. Do GOLD stages of COPD severity really correspond to differences in health status? Eur Respir J 2003;22(3):444–9.
7. Ferrer M, Alonso J, Morera J, et al. Chronic obstructive pulmonary disease stage and health-related quality of life. The Quality of Life of Chronic Obstructive Pulmonary Disease Study Group. Ann Intern Med 1997;127(12):1072–9.
8. Jones PW. Health status measurement in chronic obstructive pulmonary disease. Thorax 2001;56(11):880–7.
9. Jones PW, Harding G, Berry P, et al. Development and first validation of the COPD assessment test. Eur Respir J 2009;34(3):648–54.
10. Decramer M, Rennard S, Troosters T, et al. COPD as a lung disease with systemic consequences: clinical impact, mechanisms, and potential for early intervention. COPD 2008;5(4):235–56.
11. Watz H, Waschki B, Boehme C, et al. Extrapulmonary effects of chronic obstructive pulmonary disease on physical activity: a cross-sectional study. Am J Respir Crit Care Med 2008;177(7):743–51.
12. Pitta F, Troosters T, Spruit MA, et al. Characteristics of physical activities in daily life in chronic obstructive pulmonary disease. Am J Respir Crit Care Med 2005;171(9):972–7.
13. Walker PP, Burnett A, Flavahan PW, et al. Lower limb activity and its determinants in COPD. Thorax 2008;63(8):683–9.
14. Steuten LM, Creutzberg EC, Vrijhoef HJ, et al. COPD as a multicomponent disease: inventory of dyspnoea, underweight, obesity and fat free mass depletion in primary care. Prim Care Respir J 2006;15(2):84–91.
15. Guenette JA, Jensen D, Webb KA, et al. Sex differences in exertional dyspnea in patients with mild COPD: physiological mechanisms. Respir Physiol Neurobiol 2011;177(3):218–27.
16. Ofir D, Laveneziana P, Webb KA, et al. Mechanisms of dyspnea during cycle exercise in symptomatic patients with GOLD stage I chronic obstructive pulmonary disease. Am J Respir Crit Care Med 2008;177(6):622–9.
17. O'Donnell DE, Laveneziana P, Ora J, et al. Evaluation of acute bronchodilator reversibility in patients with symptoms of GOLD stage I COPD. Thorax 2009;64(3):216–23.
18. Chin RC, Guenette JA, Cheng S, et al. Does the respiratory system limit exercise in mild COPD? Am J Respir Crit Care Med 2013;187(12):1315–23.
19. Deesomchok A, Webb KA, Forkert L, et al. Lung hyperinflation and its reversibility in patients with airway obstruction of varying severity. COPD 2010;7(6):428–37.
20. Yuan R, Hogg JC, Pare PD, et al. Prediction of the rate of decline in FEV(1) in smokers using quantitative computed tomography. Thorax 2009;64(11):944–9.
21. Rambod M, Porszasz J, Make BJ, et al. Six-minute walk distance predictors, including CT scan measures, in the COPDGene cohort. Chest 2012;141(4):867–75.
22. Matsuoka S, Washko GR, Dransfield MT, et al. Quantitative CT measurement of cross-sectional area of small pulmonary vessel in COPD: correlations with emphysema and airflow limitation. Acad Radiol 2010;17(1):93–9.
23. Hogg JC, Macklem PT, Thurlbeck WM. Site and nature of airway obstruction in chronic obstructive lung disease. N Engl J Med 1968;278(25):1355–60.
24. Hogg JC, Chu F, Utokaparch S, et al. The nature of small-airway obstruction in chronic obstructive pulmonary disease. N Engl J Med 2004;350(26):2645–53.
25. McDonough JE, Yuan R, Suzuki M, et al. Small-airway obstruction and emphysema in chronic

obstructive pulmonary disease. N Engl J Med 2011;365(17):1567–75.

26. Mitzner W. Emphysema: a disease of small airways or lung parenchyma? N Engl J Med 2011;365(17):1637–9.

27. Black LF, Hyatt RE, Stubbs SE. Mechanism of expiratory airflow limitation in chronic obstructive pulmonary disease associated with 1-antitrypsin deficiency. Am Rev Respir Dis 1972;105(6):891–9.

28. Leaver DG, Tatterfield AE, Pride NB. Contributions of loss of lung recoil and of enhanced airways collapsibility to the airflow obstruction of chronic bronchitis and emphysema. J Clin Invest 1973;52(9):2117–28.

29. Corbin RP, Loveland M, Martin RR, et al. A four-year follow-up study of lung mechanics in smokers. Am Rev Respir Dis 1979;120(2):293–304.

30. Woolcock AJ, Vincent NJ, Macklem PT. Frequency dependence of compliance as a test for obstruction in the small airways. J Clin Invest 1969;48(6):1097–106.

31. Buist AS, Vollmer WM, Johnson LR, et al. Does the single-breath N2 test identify the smoker who will develop chronic airflow limitation? Am Rev Respir Dis 1988;137(2):293–301.

32. Hutcheon M, Griffin P, Levison H, et al. Volume of isoflow. A new test in detection of mild abnormalities of lung mechanics. Am Rev Respir Dis 1974;110(4):458–65.

33. Dosman J, Bode F, Urbanetti J, et al. The use of a helium-oxygen mixture during maximum expiratory flow to demonstrate obstruction in small airways in smokers. J Clin Invest 1975;55(5):1090–9.

34. Coe CI, Watson A, Joyce H, et al. Effects of smoking on changes in respiratory resistance with increasing age. Clin Sci (Lond) 1989;76(5):487–94.

35. Crim C, Celli B, Edwards LD, et al. Respiratory system impedance with impulse oscillometry in healthy and COPD subjects: ECLIPSE baseline results. Respir Med 2011;105(7):1069–78.

36. Fry DL, Hyatt RE. Pulmonary mechanics. A unified analysis of the relationship between pressure, volume and gasflow in the lungs of normal and diseased human subjects. Am J Med 1960;29:672–89.

37. Gelb AF, Gold WM, Wright RR, et al. Physiologic diagnosis of subclinical emphysema. Am Rev Respir Dis 1973;107(1):50–63.

38. Knudson RJ, Burrows B, Lebowitz MD. The maximal expiratory flow-volume curve: its use in the detection of ventilatory abnormalities in a population study. Am Rev Respir Dis 1976;114(5):871–9.

39. Rijcken B, Schouten JP, Weiss ST, et al. The distribution of bronchial responsiveness to histamine in symptomatic and in asymptomatic subjects. A population-based analysis of various indices of responsiveness. Am Rev Respir Dis 1989;140(3):615–23.

40. Rijcken B, Schouten JP, Weiss ST, et al. The relationship between airway responsiveness to histamine and pulmonary function level in a random population sample. Am Rev Respir Dis 1988;137(4):826–32.

41. Buist AS, Connett JE, Miller RD, et al. Chronic obstructive pulmonary disease early intervention trial (lung health study). Baseline characteristics of randomized participants. Chest 1993;103(6):1863–72.

42. Anthonisen NR, Connett JE, Kiley JP, et al. Effects of smoking intervention and the use of an inhaled anticholinergic bronchodilator on the rate of decline of FEV1. The Lung Health Study. JAMA 1994;272(19):1497–505.

43. Riess A, Wiggs B, Verburgt L, et al. Morphologic determinants of airway responsiveness in chronic smokers. Am J Respir Crit Care Med 1996;154(5):1444–9.

44. Rodriguez-Roisin R, Drakulovic M, Rodriguez DA, et al. Ventilation-perfusion imbalance and chronic obstructive pulmonary disease staging severity. J Appl Physiol 2009;106(6):1902–8.

45. Wagner PD, Dantzker DR, Dueck R, et al. Ventilation-perfusion inequality in chronic obstructive pulmonary disease. J Clin Invest 1977;59(2):203–16.

46. Barbera JA, Riverola A, Roca J, et al. Pulmonary vascular abnormalities and ventilation-perfusion relationships in mild chronic obstructive pulmonary disease. Am J Respir Crit Care Med 1994;149(2 Pt 1):423–9.

47. Barbera JA, Ramirez J, Roca J, et al. Lung structure and gas exchange in mild chronic obstructive pulmonary disease. Am Rev Respir Dis 1990;141(4 Pt 1):895–901.

48. Peinado VI, Barbera JA, Ramirez J, et al. Endothelial dysfunction in pulmonary arteries of patients with mild COPD. Am J Physiol 1998;274(6 Pt 1):L908–13.

49. Santos S, Peinado VI, Ramirez J, et al. Characterization of pulmonary vascular remodelling in smokers and patients with mild COPD. Eur Respir J 2002;19(4):632–8.

50. O'Donnell DE, Maltais F, Porszasz J, et al. Lung function and exercise impairment in patients with GOLD stage I and II COPD. Am J Respir Crit Care Med 2012;185:A5875.

51. McParland C, Mink J, Gallagher CG. Respiratory adaptations to dead space loading during maximal incremental exercise. J Appl Physiol 1991;70(1):55–62.

52. Syabbalo NC, Zintel T, Watts R, et al. Carotid chemoreceptors and respiratory adaptations to dead space loading during incremental exercise. J Appl Physiol 1993;75(3):1378–84.

53. O'Donnell DE, Hong HH, Webb KA. Respiratory sensation during chest wall restriction and dead space loading in exercising men. J Appl Physiol 2000;88(5):1859–69.

54. Vonk-Noordegraaf A, Marcus JT, Holverda S, et al. Early changes of cardiac structure and function in COPD patients with mild hypoxemia. Chest 2005; 127(6):1898–903.

55. Mannino DM, Doherty DE, Sonia Buist A. Global Initiative on Obstructive Lung Disease (GOLD) classification of lung disease and mortality: findings from the Atherosclerosis Risk in Communities (ARIC) study. Respir Med 2006;100(1):115–22.

56. Barr RG, Bluemke DA, Ahmed FS, et al. Percent emphysema, airflow obstruction, and impaired left ventricular filling. N Engl J Med 2010;362(3): 217–27.

57. Sabit R, Bolton CE, Fraser AG, et al. Sub-clinical left and right ventricular dysfunction in patients with COPD. Respir Med 2010;104(8):1171–8.

58. Malerba M, Ragnoli B, Salameh M, et al. Sub-clinical left ventricular diastolic dysfunction in early stage of chronic obstructive pulmonary disease. J Biol Regul Homeost Agents 2011;25(3):443–51.

59. Grau M, Barr RG, Lima JA, et al. Percent emphysema and right ventricular structure and function: the MESA Lung and MESA-RV Studies. Chest 2013;144:136–44.

60. Smith BM, Kawut SM, Bluemke DA, et al. Pulmonary hyperinflation and left ventricular mass: the Multi-Ethnic Study of Atherosclerosis COPD Study. Circulation 2013;127(14):1503–11, 1511e1–6.

61. Thomashow MA, Shimbo D, Parikh MA, et al. Endothelial microparticles in mild COPD and emphysema: the MESA COPD Study. Am J Respir Crit Care Med 2013;188:60–8.

62. Sin DD, Wu L, Man SF. The relationship between reduced lung function and cardiovascular mortality: a population-based study and a systematic review of the literature. Chest 2005;127(6):1952–9.

63. Iwamoto H, Yokoyama A, Kitahara Y, et al. Airflow limitation in smokers is associated with subclinical atherosclerosis. Am J Respir Crit Care Med 2009; 179(1):35–40.

64. Barr RG. The epidemiology of vascular dysfunction relating to chronic obstructive pulmonary disease and emphysema. Proc Am Thorac Soc 2011;8(6): 522–7.

65. Barbera JA, Peinado VI, Santos S, et al. Reduced expression of endothelial nitric oxide synthase in pulmonary arteries of smokers. Am J Respir Crit Care Med 2001;164(4):709–13.

66. Cheng S, Fernandes VR, Bluemke DA, et al. Age-related left ventricular remodeling and associated risk for cardiovascular outcomes: the Multi-Ethnic Study of Atherosclerosis. Circ Cardiovasc Imaging 2009;2(3):191–8.

67. Voelkel NF, Cool CD. Pulmonary vascular involvement in chronic obstructive pulmonary disease. Eur Respir J Suppl 2003;46:28s–32s.

68. Sinden NJ, Stockley RA. Systemic inflammation and comorbidity in COPD: a result of "overspill" of inflammatory mediators from the lungs? Review of the evidence. Thorax 2010;65(10):930–6.

69. Liebow AA. Pulmonary emphysema with special reference to vascular changes. Am Rev Respir Dis 1959;80(1, Part 2):67–93.

70. Alford SK, van Beek EJ, McLennan G, et al. Heterogeneity of pulmonary perfusion as a mechanistic image-based phenotype in emphysema susceptible smokers. Proc Natl Acad Sci U S A 2010; 107(16):7485–90.

71. Tjeerdsma G, Szabo BM, van Wijk LM, et al. Autonomic dysfunction in patients with mild heart failure and coronary artery disease and the effects of add-on beta-blockade. Eur J Heart Fail 2001;3(1):33–9.

72. Haider T, Casucci G, Linser T, et al. Interval hypoxic training improves autonomic cardiovascular and respiratory control in patients with mild chronic obstructive pulmonary disease. J Hypertens 2009;27(8):1648–54.

73. Guder G, Brenner S, Angermann CE, et al. GOLD or lower limit of normal definition? A comparison with expert-based diagnosis of chronic obstructive pulmonary disease in a prospective cohort-study. Respir Res 2012;13(1):13.

74. Orozco-Levi M, Coronell C, Ramirez-Sarmiento A, et al. Injury of peripheral muscles in smokers with chronic obstructive pulmonary disease. Ultrastruct Pathol 2012;36(4):228–38.

75. van den Borst B, Slot IG, Hellwig VA, et al. Loss of quadriceps muscle oxidative phenotype and decreased endurance in patients with mild-to-moderate COPD. J Appl Physiol 2013;114: 1319–28.

76. Diaz AA, Morales A, Diaz JC, et al. CT and physiologic determinants of dyspnea and exercise capacity during the six-minute walk test in mild COPD. Respir Med 2013;107(4):570–9.

77. Van Remoortel H, Hornikx M, Demeyer H, et al. Daily physical activity in subjects with newly diagnosed COPD. Thorax 2013;68:962–3.

78. Vogiatzis I, Zakynthinos SG. The physiological basis of rehabilitation in chronic heart and lung disease. J Appl Physiol 2013;115:16–21.

79. Shrikrishna D, Patel M, Tanner RJ, et al. Quadriceps wasting and physical inactivity in patients with COPD. Eur Respir J 2012;40(5):1115–22.

80. Fletcher C, Peto R. The natural history of chronic airflow obstruction. Br Med J 1977;1(6077):1645–8.

81. Celli BR, Thomas NE, Anderson JA, et al. Effect of pharmacotherapy on rate of decline of lung function in chronic obstructive pulmonary

disease: results from the TORCH study. Am J Respir Crit Care Med 2008;178(4):332–8.

82. Tashkin DP, Celli B, Senn S, et al. A 4-year trial of tiotropium in chronic obstructive pulmonary disease. N Engl J Med 2008;359(15):1543–54.

83. O'Donnell DE, Deesomchok A, Lam YM, et al. Effects of BMI on static lung volumes in patients with airway obstruction. Chest 2011;140(2):461–8.

84. Parker CM, Voduc N, Aaron SD, et al. Physiological changes during symptom recovery from moderate exacerbations of COPD. Eur Respir J 2005;26(3):420–8.

85. Pitta F, Troosters T, Probst VS, et al. Physical activity and hospitalization for exacerbation of COPD. Chest 2006;129(3):536–44.

86. Barnes PJ, Celli BR. Systemic manifestations and comorbidities of COPD. Eur Respir J 2009;33(5):1165–85.

87. Burrows B, Niden AH, Fletcher CM, et al. Clinical types of chronic obstructive lung disease in London and in Chicago. A study of one hundred patients. Am Rev Respir Dis 1964;90:14–27.

88. Tantucci C, Donati P, Nicosia F, et al. Inspiratory capacity predicts mortality in patients with chronic obstructive pulmonary disease. Respir Med 2008;102(4):613–9.

89. Zaman M, Mahmood S, Altayeh A. Low inspiratory capacity to total lung capacity ratio is a risk factor for chronic obstructive pulmonary disease exacerbation. Am J Med Sci 2010;339(5):411–4.

90. Albuquerque AL, Nery LE, Villaca DS, et al. Inspiratory fraction and exercise impairment in COPD patients GOLD stages II-III. Eur Respir J 2006;28(5):939–44.

91. Casanova C, Cote C, de Torres JP, et al. Inspiratory-to-total lung capacity ratio predicts mortality in patients with chronic obstructive pulmonary disease. Am J Respir Crit Care Med 2005;171(6):591–7.

92. Belman MJ, Botnick WC, Shin JW. Inhaled bronchodilators reduce dynamic hyperinflation during exercise in patients with chronic obstructive pulmonary disease. Am J Respir Crit Care Med 1996;153(3):967–75.

93. Celli B, ZuWallack R, Wang S, et al. Improvement in resting inspiratory capacity and hyperinflation with tiotropium in COPD patients with increased static lung volumes. Chest 2003;124(5):1743–8.

94. Guenette JA, Raghavan N, Harris-McAllister V, et al. Effect of adjunct fluticasone propionate on airway physiology during rest and exercise in COPD. Respir Med 2011;105(12):1836–45.

95. O'Donnell DE, Fluge T, Gerken F, et al. Effects of tiotropium on lung hyperinflation, dyspnoea and exercise tolerance in COPD. Eur Respir J 2004;23(6):832–40.

96. O'Donnell DE, Forkert L, Webb KA. Evaluation of bronchodilator responses in patients with "irreversible" emphysema. Eur Respir J 2001;18(6):914–20.

97. O'Donnell DE, Hamilton AL, Webb KA. Sensory-mechanical relationships during high-intensity, constant-work-rate exercise in COPD. J Appl Physiol 2006;101(4):1025–35.

98. O'Donnell DE, Lam M, Webb KA. Spirometric correlates of improvement in exercise performance after anticholinergic therapy in chronic obstructive pulmonary disease. Am J Respir Crit Care Med 1999;160(2):542–9.

99. Laghi F, Tobin MJ. Disorders of the respiratory muscles. Am J Respir Crit Care Med 2003;168(1):10–48.

100. Levine S, Kaiser L, Leferovich J, et al. Cellular adaptations in the diaphragm in chronic obstructive pulmonary disease. N Engl J Med 1997;337(25):1799–806.

101. Mercadier JJ, Schwartz K, Schiaffino S, et al. Myosin heavy chain gene expression changes in the diaphragm of patients with chronic lung hyperinflation. Am J Physiol 1998;274(4 Pt 1):L527–34.

102. Orozco-Levi M, Gea J, Lloreta JL, et al. Subcellular adaptation of the human diaphragm in chronic obstructive pulmonary disease. Eur Respir J 1999;13(2):371–8.

103. Similowski T, Yan S, Gauthier AP, et al. Contractile properties of the human diaphragm during chronic hyperinflation. N Engl J Med 1991;325(13):917–23.

104. O'Donnell DE, Bertley JC, Chau LK, et al. Qualitative aspects of exertional breathlessness in chronic airflow limitation: pathophysiologic mechanisms. Am J Respir Crit Care Med 1997;155(1):109–15.

105. Mead J. Respiration: pulmonary mechanics. Annu Rev Physiol 1973;35:169–92.

106. Roussos C, Macklem PT. The respiratory muscles. N Engl J Med 1982;307(13):786–97.

107. Smith TC, Marini JJ. Impact of PEEP on lung mechanics and work of breathing in severe airflow obstruction. J Appl Physiol 1988;65(4):1488–99.

108. O'Donnell DE, Guenette JA, Maltais F, et al. Decline of resting inspiratory capacity in COPD: the impact on breathing pattern, dyspnea, and ventilatory capacity during exercise. Chest 2012;141(3):753–62.

109. O'Donnell DE, Revill SM, Webb KA. Dynamic hyperinflation and exercise intolerance in chronic obstructive pulmonary disease. Am J Respir Crit Care Med 2001;164(5):770–7.

110. Laveneziana P, Webb KA, Ora J, et al. Evolution of dyspnea during exercise in chronic obstructive pulmonary disease: impact of critical volume constraints. Am J Respir Crit Care Med 2011;184(12):1367–73.

111. O'Donnell DE, Parker CM. COPD exacerbations. 3: Pathophysiology. Thorax 2006;61(4):354–61.

112. Stevenson NJ, Walker PP, Costello RW, et al. Lung mechanics and dyspnea during exacerbations of chronic obstructive pulmonary disease. Am J Respir Crit Care Med 2005;172(12):1510–6.

113. O'Donnell DE, D'Arsigny C, Fitzpatrick M, et al. Exercise hypercapnia in advanced chronic obstructive pulmonary disease: the role of lung hyperinflation. Am J Respir Crit Care Med 2002; 166(5):663–8.

114. Diaz O, Villafranca C, Ghezzo H, et al. Role of inspiratory capacity on exercise tolerance in COPD patients with and without tidal expiratory flow limitation at rest. Eur Respir J 2000;16(2):269–75.

115. Marin JM, Carrizo SJ, Gascon M, et al. Inspiratory capacity, dynamic hyperinflation, breathlessness, and exercise performance during the 6-minute-walk test in chronic obstructive pulmonary disease. Am J Respir Crit Care Med 2001;163(6): 1395–9.

116. Puente-Maestu L, Garcia de Pedro J, Martinez-Abad Y, et al. Dyspnea, ventilatory pattern, and changes in dynamic hyperinflation related to the intensity of constant work rate exercise in COPD. Chest 2005;128(2):651–6.

117. Laveneziana P, Parker CM, O'Donnell DE. Ventilatory constraints and dyspnea during exercise in chronic obstructive pulmonary disease. Appl Physiol Nutr Metab 2007;32(6):1225–38.

118. Laveneziana P, Wadell K, Webb K, et al. Exercise limitation in chronic obstructive pulmonary disease. Am J Respir Crit Care Med 2008;4(4):258–69.

119. O'Donnell DE, Laveneziana P. Physiology and consequences of lung hyperinflation in COPD. Eur Respir Rev 2006;15(100):61–7.

120. Gagnon P, Bussieres JS, Ribeiro F, et al. Influences of spinal anesthesia on exercise tolerance in patients with chronic obstructive pulmonary disease. Am J Respir Crit Care Med 2012;186(7):606–15.

121. Guenette JA, Webb KA, O'Donnell DE. Does dynamic hyperinflation contribute to dyspnoea during exercise in patients with COPD? Eur Respir J 2012; 40:322–9.

122. O'Donnell DE, Bredenbroker D, Brose M, et al. Physiological effects of roflumilast at rest and during exercise in COPD. Eur Respir J 2012;39(5): 1104–12.

123. O'Donnell DE, Casaburi R, Vincken W, et al. Effect of indacaterol on exercise endurance and lung hyperinflation in COPD. Respir Med 2011;105(7): 1030–6.

124. O'Donnell DE, Travers J, Webb KA, et al. Reliability of ventilatory parameters during cycle ergometry in multicentre trials in COPD. Eur Respir J 2009;34(4): 866–74.

125. Paoletti P, De Filippis F, Fraioli F, et al. Cardiopulmonary exercise testing (CPET) in pulmonary emphysema. Respir Physiol Neurobiol 2011;179:167–73.

126. Bye PT, Esau SA, Levy RD, et al. Ventilatory muscle function during exercise in air and oxygen in patients with chronic air-flow limitation. Am Rev Respir Dis 1985;132(2):236–40.

127. Sinderby C, Spahija J, Beck J, et al. Diaphragm activation during exercise in chronic obstructive pulmonary disease. Am J Respir Crit Care Med 2001;163(7):1637–41.

128. Mador MJ, Kufel TJ, Pineda LA, et al. Diaphragmatic fatigue and high-intensity exercise in patients with chronic obstructive pulmonary disease. Am J Respir Crit Care Med 2000;161(1):118–23.

129. Laveneziana P, Palange P, Ora J, et al. Bronchodilator effect on ventilatory, pulmonary gas exchange, and heart rate kinetics during high-intensity exercise in COPD. Eur J Appl Physiol 2009;107(6): 633–43.

130. Laveneziana P, Valli G, Onorati P, et al. Effect of heliox on heart rate kinetics and dynamic hyperinflation during high-intensity exercise in COPD. Eur J Appl Physiol 2011;111(2):225–34.

131. Travers J, Laveneziana P, Webb KA, et al. Effect of tiotropium bromide on the cardiovascular response to exercise in COPD. Respir Med 2007;101(9): 2017–24.

132. Chiappa GR, Borghi-Silva A, Ferreira LF, et al. Kinetics of muscle deoxygenation are accelerated at the onset of heavy-intensity exercise in patients with COPD: relationship to central cardiovascular dynamics. J Appl Physiol 2008;104(5):1341–50.

133. Montes de Oca M, Rassulo J, Celli BR. Respiratory muscle and cardiopulmonary function during exercise in very severe COPD. Am J Respir Crit Care Med 1996;154(5):1284–9.

134. Saito S, Miyamoto K, Nishimura M, et al. Effects of inhaled bronchodilators on pulmonary hemodynamics at rest and during exercise in patients with COPD. Chest 1999;115(2):376–82.

135. Vassaux C, Torre-Bouscoulet L, Zeineldine S, et al. Effects of hyperinflation on the oxygen pulse as a marker of cardiac performance in COPD. Eur Respir J 2008;32(5):1275–82.

136. Boerrigter B, Trip P, Bogaard HJ, et al. Right atrial pressure affects the interaction between lung mechanics and right ventricular function in spontaneously breathing COPD patients. PloS One 2012; 7(1):e30208.

137. Boerrigter BG, Bogaard HJ, Trip P, et al. Ventilatory and cardiocirculatory exercise profiles in COPD: the role of pulmonary hypertension. Chest 2012; 142(5):1166–74.

138. Ranieri VM, Dambrosio M, Brienza N. Intrinsic PEEP and cardiopulmonary interaction in patients with COPD and acute ventilatory failure. Eur Respir J 1996;9(6):1283–92.

139. Tyberg JV, Grant DA, Kingma I, et al. Effects of positive intrathoracic pressure on pulmonary and

systemic hemodynamics. Respir Physiol 2000; 119(2–3):171–9.

140. Hilde JM, Skjørten I, Hansteen V, et al. Haemodynamic responses to exercise in patients with COPD. Eur Respir J 2013;41(5):1031–41.

141. Jorgensen K, Muller MF, Nel J, et al. Reduced intrathoracic blood volume and left and right ventricular dimensions in patients with severe emphysema: an MRI study. Chest 2007;131(4):1050–7.

142. Watz H, Waschki B, Magnussen H. Emphysema, airflow obstruction, and left ventricular filling. N Engl J Med 2010;362(17):1638–9 [author reply: 1640–1].

143. Watz H, Waschki B, Meyer T, et al. Decreasing cardiac chamber sizes and associated heart dysfunction in COPD: role of hyperinflation. Chest 2010; 138(1):32–8.

144. Orr R, Smith LJ, Cuttica MJ. Pulmonary hypertension in advanced chronic obstructive pulmonary disease. Curr Opin Pulm Med 2012;18(2):138–43.

145. Funk GC, Lang I, Schenk P, et al. Left ventricular diastolic dysfunction in patients with COPD in the presence and absence of elevated pulmonary arterial pressure. Chest 2008;133(6):1354–9.

146. Criner GJ, Scharf SM, Falk JA, et al. Effect of lung volume reduction surgery on resting pulmonary hemodynamics in severe emphysema. Am J Respir Crit Care Med 2007;176(3):253–60.

147. Criner GJ, Cordova F, Sternberg AL, et al. The National Emphysema Treatment Trial (NETT). Part II: lessons learned about lung volume reduction surgery. Am J Respir Crit Care Med 2011;184(8): 881–93.

148. Jorgensen K, Houltz E, Westfelt U, et al. Effects of lung volume reduction surgery on left ventricular diastolic filling and dimensions in patients with severe emphysema. Chest 2003;124(5):1863–70.

149. Jorgensen K, Houltz E, Westfelt U, et al. Left ventricular performance and dimensions in patients with severe emphysema. Anesth Analg 2007; 104(4):887–92.

150. Vonk Noordegraaf A, Marcus JT, Roseboom B, et al. The effect of right ventricular hypertrophy on left ventricular ejection fraction in pulmonary emphysema. Chest 1997;112(3):640–5.

151. Mitchell JR, Whitelaw WA, Sas R, et al. RV filling modulates LV function by direct ventricular interaction during mechanical ventilation. Am J Physiol Heart Circ Physiol 2005;289(2):H549–57.

152. Larsen KO, Lygren B, Sjaastad I, et al. Diastolic dysfunction in alveolar hypoxia: a role for interleukin-18-mediated increase in protein phosphatase 2A. Cardiovasc Res 2008;80(1):47–54.

153. Lammi MR, Ciccolella D, Marchetti N, et al. Increased oxygen pulse after lung volume reduction surgery is associated with reduced dynamic hyperinflation. Eur Respir J 2012;40(4):837–43.

154. Carrascossa CR, Oliveira CC, Borghi-Silva A, et al. Haemodynamic effects of proportional assist ventilation during high-intensity exercise in patients with chronic obstructive pulmonary disease. Respirology 2010;15(8):1185–91.

155. Oliveira CC, Carrascosa CR, Borghi-Silva A, et al. Influence of respiratory pressure support on hemodynamics and exercise tolerance in patients with COPD. Eur J Appl Physiol 2010;109(4):681–9.

156. Chiappa GR, Queiroga F Jr, Meda E, et al. Heliox improves oxygen delivery and utilization during dynamic exercise in patients with chronic obstructive pulmonary disease. Am J Respir Crit Care Med 2009;179(11):1004–10.

157. Vogiatzis I, Habazettl H, Aliverti A, et al. Effect of helium breathing on intercostal and quadriceps muscle blood flow during exercise in COPD patients. Am J Physiol Regul Integr Comp Physiol 2011;300(6):R1549–59.

158. Queiroga F Jr, Nunes M, Meda E, et al. Exercise tolerance with helium-hyperoxia versus hyperoxia in hypoxaemic patients with COPD. Eur Respir J 2013;42:362–70.

159. Berton DC, Barbosa PB, Takara LS, et al. Bronchodilators accelerate the dynamics of muscle O_2 delivery and utilisation during exercise in COPD. Thorax 2010;65(7):588–93.

160. Le Jemtel TH, Padeletti M, Jelic S. Diagnostic and therapeutic challenges in patients with coexistent chronic obstructive pulmonary disease and chronic heart failure. J Am Coll Cardiol 2007; 49(2):171–80.

161. Laveneziana P, Palange P. Physical activity, nutritional status and systemic inflammation in COPD. Eur Respir J 2012;40(3):522–9.

162. Donaldson AV, Maddocks M, Martolini D, et al. Muscle function in COPD: a complex interplay. Int J Chron Obstruct Pulmon Dis 2012;7:523–35.

163. Levine S, Bashir MH, Clanton TL, et al. COPD elicits remodeling of the diaphragm and vastus lateralis muscles in humans. J Appl Physiol 2013;114: 1235–45.

164. Meyer A, Zoll J, Charles AL, et al. Skeletal muscle mitochondrial dysfunction during chronic obstructive pulmonary disease: central actor and therapeutic target. Exp Physiol 2013;98(6):1063–78.

165. Debigare R, Maltais F. The major limitation to exercise performance in COPD is lower limb muscle dysfunction. J Appl Physiol 2008;105(2):751–3 [discussion: 755–7].

166. Burtin C, Saey D, Saglam M, et al. Effectiveness of exercise training in patients with COPD: the role of muscle fatigue. Eur Respir J 2012;40(2): 338–44.

167. O'Donnell DE, Laveneziana P. Dyspnea and activity limitation in COPD: mechanical factors. COPD 2007;4(3):225–36.

168. O'Donnell DE, Banzett RB, Carrieri-Kohlman V, et al. Pathophysiology of dyspnea in chronic obstructive pulmonary disease: a roundtable. Proc Am Thorac Soc 2007;4(2):145–68.

169. O'Donnell DE, Laveneziana P. The clinical importance of dynamic lung hyperinflation in COPD. COPD 2006;3(4):219–32.

170. O'Donnell DE, Ora J, Webb KA, et al. Mechanisms of activity-related dyspnea in pulmonary diseases. Respir Physiol Neurobiol 2009;167(1):116–32.

171. Parshall MB, Schwartzstein RM, Adams L, et al. An Official American Thoracic Society statement: update on the mechanisms, assessment, and management of dyspnea. Am J Respir Crit Care Med 2012;185(4):435–52.

Cellular and Molecular Mechanisms of Chronic Obstructive Pulmonary Disease

Peter J. Barnes, FRS, FMedSci

KEYWORDS

- Inflammation • Macrophage • Neutrophil • Oxidative stress • Cytokine • Chemokine
- Autoantibody • Nuclear factor-κB

KEY POINTS

- Chronic inflammation in peripheral airways and lung parenchyma in patients with chronic obstructive pulmonary disease (COPD) may underlie progressive airways obstruction, may flare up during infective exacerbations, and extend into the systemic circulation to contribute to comorbidities.
- Several cells are involved in COPD inflammation, including macrophages, epithelial cells, dendritic cells, neutrophils, eosinophils, and T and B lymphocytes.
- These inflammatory and structural cells release many inflammatory mediators that contribute to the pathophysiology of COPD, including lipid mediators, cytokines, chemokines, and growth factors.
- Oxidative stress, including defective antioxidant defenses, plays a key role in the mechanisms of COPD, with activation of inflammatory genes, cellular senescence, autoimmunity, and corticosteroid resistance.
- There are several abnormal disease processes in COPD that may reveal novel therapeutic targets, including accelerated aging, defective phagocytosis, and failure to resolve inflammation and repair.

INTRODUCTION

Chronic obstructive pulmonary disease (COPD) involves chronic inflammation of the lung, particularly in peripheral airways and parenchyma, which increases during acute exacerbations. It is also associated with systemic inflammation, which may contribute to or worsen several comorbidities and may be derived from overspill from the peripheral lung.[1] It is important to understand the nature of this inflammatory response in order to develop effective antiinflammatory treatments for COPD in the future.[2]

COPD is an obstructive disease of the lungs that slowly progresses over many decades, leading to death from respiratory failure unless patients die of comorbidities, such as cardiovascular disease and lung cancer, before this stage. Although the commonest cause of COPD is chronic cigarette smoking, some patients, particularly in developing countries, develop the disease from inhalation of smoke from burning biomass fuels or other inhaled irritants.[3] However, only about 25% of smokers develop COPD, suggesting that there may be genetic, epigenetic, or host factors that predispose to its development, although these have not yet been identified.

PATHOLOGY

The progressive airflow limitation in COPD is caused by 2 major pathologic processes: remodeling and narrowing of small airways and destruction of the lung parenchyma with consequent destruction of the alveolar attachments of these airways as a result of emphysema. These

National Heart and Lung Institute, Imperial College, Dovehouse Street, London SW3 6LY, UK
E-mail address: p.j.barnes@imperial.ac.uk

Clin Chest Med 35 (2014) 71–86
http://dx.doi.org/10.1016/j.ccm.2013.10.004

pathologic changes are caused by chronic inflammation in the lung periphery, which increases as the disease progresses.[4] Even in mild disease there is obstruction and loss of small airways.[5] Analysis of serial computed tomography scans suggests that small airway obstruction usually precedes the development of emphysema.[6] The small airway obstruction and loss of alveolar attachments result in airway closure and air trapping and hyperinflation. These changes worsen on exercise, resulting in exertional dyspnea, the major symptom of COPD.

COPD AS AN INFLAMMATORY DISEASE

There is a characteristic pattern of inflammation with increased numbers of macrophages, T lymphocytes, and B lymphocytes, together with increased numbers of neutrophils in the lumen.[7–9] The inflammatory response in COPD involves both innate and adaptive immune responses, which are linked through the activation of dendritic cells.[10] Multiple inflammatory mediators derived from inflammatory cells and structural cells of the airways and lungs are increased in COPD.[11] A similar pattern of inflammation and mediator expression is seen in smokers without airflow limitation, but in COPD this inflammation seems to be amplified and further increased during acute exacerbations precipitated by bacterial or viral infection. The molecular basis for the amplification of inflammation is not yet fully understood but may be, at least in part, determined by genetic and epigenetic factors. Cigarette smoke and other irritants inhaled into the respiratory tract may activate surface macrophages and airway epithelial cells to release multiple chemotactic mediators, particularly chemokines, which attract circulating neutrophils, monocytes, and lymphocytes into the lungs.[12] This inflammation persists even when smoking is stopped, suggesting that there are self-perpetuating mechanism, although these have not yet been elucidated.[13] It is possible that memory T cells, bacterial colonization, or autoimmunity may drive the persistent inflammation in patients with COPD.

INFLAMMATORY CELLS

The inflammation of COPD lungs involves both innate immunity (neutrophils, macrophages, eosinophils, mast cells, natural killer cells, gamma delta T cells, and dendritic cells) and adaptive immunity (T and B lymphocytes) but also involves the activation of structural cells, including airway and alveolar epithelial cells, endothelial cells, and fibroblasts.

EPITHELIAL CELLS

Epithelial cells are activated by cigarette smoke and other inhaled irritants, such as biomass fuel smoke, to produce inflammatory mediators, including tumor necrosis factor (TNF) alpha, interleukin (IL)-1 beta, IL-6, granulocyte-macrophage colony–stimulating factor (GM-CSF), and CXCL8 (IL-8). Epithelial cells in small airways may also be an important source of transforming growth factor (TGF) beta which then induces local fibrosis. Vascular endothelial growth factor (VEGF) seems to be necessary to maintain alveolar cell integrity, and blockade of VEGF receptors (VEGFR2) in rats induces apoptosis of alveolar cells and an emphysemalike disorder.[14] Airway epithelial cells are also important in defense of the airways, with mucus production from goblet cells, and secretion of antioxidants, antiproteases, and defensins. It is possible that cigarette smoke and other noxious agents may impair these responses of the airway epithelium, increasing susceptibility to infection. The airway epithelium in chronic bronchitis and COPD often shows squamous metaplasia, which may result from increased proliferation of basal airway epithelial cells but the nature of the growth factors involved in epithelial cell proliferation, cell cycle, and differentiation in COPD are not yet certain. Epithelial growth factor receptors (EGFR) show increased expression in airway epithelial cells of patients with COPD and may contribute to basal cell proliferation, resulting in squamous metaplasia and an increased risk of bronchial carcinoma.[15]

MACROPHAGES

Macrophages play a key role in the pathophysiology of COPD and may orchestrate the chronic inflammatory response (**Fig. 1**).[16] There is a marked increase (5-fold to 10-fold) in the numbers of macrophages in airways, lung parenchyma, bronchoalveolar lavage (BAL) fluid, and sputum in patients with COPD. Macrophages are localized to sites of alveolar wall destruction in patients with emphysema and there is a correlation between macrophage numbers in the parenchyma and severity of emphysema.[17] Macrophages may be activated by cigarette smoke extract to release inflammatory mediators, including TNF-α, CXCL1, CXCL8, CCL2 (MCP-1), LTB$_4$, and reactive oxygen species (ROS), providing a cellular mechanism that links smoking with inflammation in COPD. Alveolar macrophages also secrete elastolytic enzymes, including MMP-2; MMP-9; MMP-12; cathepsins K, L, and S; and neutrophil elastase taken up from neutrophils.[18] Alveolar macrophages from

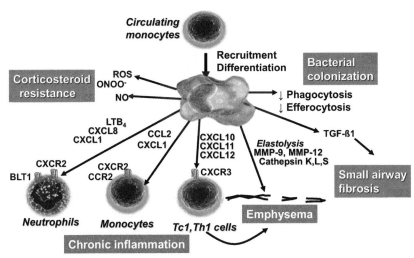

Fig. 1. Central role of alveolar macrophages in COPD. Alveolar macrophages are derived from circulating mono-cytes that differentiate within the lung. They secrete many inflammatory proteins that may orchestrate the inflammatory process in COPD. Neutrophils may be attracted by CXCL8, CXCL1, and leukotriene B₄ (LTB₄); mono-cytes by CCL2, and Tc1; and Th1 lymphocytes by CXCL10, CXC11, and CXCL12. Release of elastolytic enzymes including matrix metalloproteinases (MMP) and cathepsins causes elastolysis, which contributes to emphysema together with cytotoxic T cells. Release of TGF-β1 may induce fibrosis of small airways. Macrophages generate reactive oxygen species (ROS) and nitric oxide (NO), which together form peroxynitrite (ONOO⁻) and may contribute to corticosteroid resistance. Defective bacterial phagocytosis may lead to bacterial colonization.

patients with COPD secrete more inflammatory proteins and have a greater elastolytic activity at baseline than those from normal smokers and this is further increased by exposure to cigarette smoke.[18] Macrophages show this difference even when maintained in culture for 3 days and therefore seem to be intrinsically different from the macro-phages of normal smokers and nonsmoking normal control subjects.[18]

There may be different phenotypes of macro-phage that may be differently activated and with different responses. The murine M1 of classically activated macrophages are proinflammatory, whereas M2 or alternatively activated macro-phages are more antiinflammatory, release IL-10, and show marked phagocytic activity.[19] However, these distinctions are less clear in human macro-phages and the surface markers of these phe-notypes less distinct. In general, it is likely that M1-like macrophages predominate in COPD, but further studies are needed.

The predominant elastolytic enzyme secreted by alveolar macrophages in patients with COPD is MMP-9. Most of the inflammatory proteins that are upregulated in COPD macrophages are regu-lated by the transcription factor nuclear factor kappa B (NF-κB), which is activated in alveolar macrophages of patients with COPD, particularly during exacerbations.[20] The increased numbers of macrophages in the lungs of smokers and pa-tients with COPD are caused by increased

recruitment of monocytes from the circulation in response to the monocyte-selective chemokines CCL2 and CXCL1, which are increased in sputum and BAL of patients with COPD.[21] Monocytes from patients with COPD show a greater chemotactic response to CXCL1 than cells from normal smokers and nonsmokers, but this is not explained by an increase in its receptor CXCR2.[22] Although all monocytes express CCR2, the receptor for CCL2, only ~30% of monocytes express CXCR2. Mac-rophages also release CXCL9, CXCL10, and CXCL11, which are chemotactic for CD8⁺ Tc1 and CD4⁺ Th1 cells, via interaction with the chemokine receptor CXCR3 expressed on these cells.[23] Macrophages from patients with COPD release more inflammatory proteins than macro-phages from normal smokers and nonsmokers, indicating increased activation.[24]

Corticosteroids are ineffective in suppressing inflammation, including cytokines, chemokines, and proteases, in patients with COPD.[25] In vitro, the release of CXCL8, TNF-α, and MMP-9 macro-phages from normal subjects and normal smokers are inhibited by corticosteroids, whereas cortico-steroids are ineffective in macrophages from patients with COPD.[24] The reasons for resistance to corticosteroids in COPD may be the marked reduction in activity of histone deacetylase (HDAC) 2,[26,27] which is recruited to activated in-flammatory genes by glucocorticoid receptors to switch off inflammatory genes. The reduction in

HDAC activity in macrophages is correlated with increased secretion of cytokines like TNF-α and CXCL8, and reduced response to corticosteroids. The reduction of HDAC2 activity in patients with COPD may be mediated through oxidative stress and peroxynitrite formation.[28]

Both alveolar macrophages and monocyte-derived macrophages from patients with COPD also show reduced phagocytic uptake of bacteria and this may be a factor in determining chronic colonization of the lower airways by bacteria such as *Haemophilus influenzae* or *Streptococcus pneumoniae*.[29] COPD macrophages are also defective in taking up apoptotic cells and this may contribute to the failure to resolve inflammation in COPD.[30] The nature of this defect in phagocytosis is not fully understood, but it seems to be caused by a defect in microtubular function that is required for phagocytosis rather than any abnormality of recognition of the phagocytosed particles.[31] The bacterial colonization of lower airways may predispose to increased acute exacerbations and also to the increased risk of developing community-acquired pneumonia in patients with COPD.[32]

NEUTROPHILS

Increased numbers of activated neutrophils are found in sputum and BAL fluid of patients with COPD,[33] although few neutrophils are seen airway wall and lung parenchyma, likely reflecting their rapid transit through these tissues. Neutrophil numbers in induced sputum correlate with COPD disease severity.[33] Smoking has a direct stimulatory effect on granulocyte production and release from the bone marrow and survival in the respiratory tract, possibly mediated by GM-CSF and granulocyte colony-stimulating factor (G-CSF) released from lung macrophages. Neutrophil recruitment to the airways and parenchyma involves initial adhesion to endothelial cells via E-selectin, which is upregulated on endothelial cells in the airways of patients with COPD. Adherent neutrophils migrate into the respiratory tract under the direction of various neutrophil chemotactic factors, including LTB$_4$, CXCL1, CXCL5 (ENA-78), and CXCL8, which are increased in COPD airways.[21] These chemotactic mediators may be derived from alveolar macrophages, T cells, and epithelial cells, but the neutrophil may be a major source of CXCL8. Neutrophils recruited to the airways of patients with COPD are activated because there are increased concentrations of granule proteins, such as myeloperoxidase (MPO), and human neutrophil lipocalin, in the sputum supernatant.[34] Neutrophils secrete serine proteases, including neutrophil elastase,

cathepsin G, and proteinase-3, as well as matrix metalloproteinase (MMP) 8 and MMP-9, which may contribute to alveolar destruction. Airway neutrophilia is linked to mucus hypersecretion because neutrophil elastase, cathepsin G, and proteinase-3 are potent stimulants of mucus secretion from submucosal glands and goblet cells. There is a marked increase in neutrophil numbers in the airways in acute exacerbations of COPD accounting for the increased purulence of sputum, which may reflect increased production of neutrophil chemotactic factors, including LTB$_4$ and CXCL8.[35,36] Neutrophils from patients with COPD show marked abnormalities in chemotactic response, with increased migration but reduced accuracy,[37] reminiscent of the abnormal monocyte chemotactic responses.[38]

EOSINOPHILS

Although eosinophils are the predominant leukocyte in asthma, their role in COPD is less certain. Increased numbers of eosinophils have been described in the airways and BAL of patients with stable COPD, whereas other investigators have not found increased numbers in airway biopsies, BAL, or induced sputum.[39] The presence of eosinophils in patients with COPD predicts a response to corticosteroids and may indicate co-existing asthma.[40,41] Increased numbers of eosinophils have been reported in bronchial biopsies and BAL fluid during acute exacerbations of chronic bronchitis.[42–44] The levels of eosinophil basic proteins in induced sputum are as increased in COPD as in asthma, despite the absence of eosinophils, suggesting that they may have degranulated and are no longer recognizable by microscopy.[34] Perhaps this is caused by the high levels of neutrophil elastase that have been shown to cause degranulation of eosinophils.[45]

DENDRITIC CELLS

Dendritic cell plays a central role in the linking of the innate to the adaptive immune response. The airways and lungs contain a rich network of dendritic cells that are localized near the surface, so that they are ideally located to signal the entry of foreign substances that are inhaled. Dendritic cells can activate a variety of other inflammatory and immune cells, including macrophages, neutrophils, and T and B lymphocytes, so dendritic cells may play an important role in the pulmonary response to cigarette smoke and other inhaled noxious agents. Dendritic cells seem to be activated in the lungs of patients with COPD[46] and are linked to disease severity.[47]

T LYMPHOCYTES

There is an increase in the total numbers of T lymphocytes in lung parenchyma, peripheral airways, and central airways of patients with COPD, with the greater increase in $CD8^+$ than $CD4^+$ cells.[4,23] There is a correlation between the numbers of T cells and the amount of alveolar destruction and the severity of airflow obstruction. Furthermore, the only significant difference in the inflammatory cell infiltrate in asymptomatic smokers and smokers with COPD is an increase in T cells, mainly $CD8^+$ (Tc1), in patients with COPD. There is also an increase in the absolute number of $CD4^+$ (Th1) T cells, albeit in smaller numbers, in the airways of smokers with COPD and these cells express activated STAT-4, a transcription factor that is essential for activation and commitment of the Th1 lineage.[48] $CD4^+$ Th17 cells, which secrete IL-17A and IL-22, are also increased in airways of patients with COPD and may play a role in orchestrating neutrophilic inflammation.[49,50] Th17 cells may be regulated by IL-6 and IL-23 released from alveolar macrophages. $CD4^+$ and $CD8^+$ T cells in the lungs of patients with COPD show increased expression of CXCR3, a receptor activated by the chemokines CXCL9, CXCL10, and CXCL11, all of which are increased in COPD.[51] There is increased expression of CXCL10 by bronchiolar epithelial cells and this could contribute to the accumulation of $CD4^+$ and $CD8^+$ T cells, which preferentially express CXCR3.[52] $CD8^+$ cells are typically increased in airway infections and it is possible that the chronic bacterial colonization of the lower respiratory tract of patients with COPD is responsible for this inflammatory response.

Autoimmune mechanisms may also be involved. Cigarette-induce lung injury may uncover previously sequestered autoantigens, or cigarette smoke may damage lung interstitial and structural cells and make them antigenic.[8] Oxidative stress may result in the formation of carbonylated proteins that are antigenic, and several anticarbonylated protein antibodies have been found in the circulation of patients with COPD, particularly in severe disease.[53] Antiendothelial antibodies have also been detected.[53,54] Autoantibodies may cause cell damage through the binding of complement, which is increased in the lungs of patients with COPD.

$CD8^+$ cells cause cytolysis and apoptosis of alveolar epithelial cells through release of perforins, granzyme B, and TNF-α, and there is an association between $CD8^+$ cells and apoptosis of alveolar cells in emphysema.[55] There is evidence for immunologic senescence in COPD with increased numbers of T cells with no expression of the costimulatory receptor CD28 ($CD4/CD28^{null}$, $CD8/CD28^{null}$ cells) and these cells release increased amounts of perforins and granzyme B.[56,57]

MEDIATORS OF INFLAMMATION

Many inflammatory mediators have now been implicated in COPD, including lipids, free radicals, cytokines, chemokines, and growth factors.[11] These mediators are derived from inflammatory and structural cells in the lung and interact with each other in a complex manner. Because so many mediators are involved, it is unlikely that blocking a single mediator will have much clinical impact. Similar mediators in the lungs of patients with COPD may also be increased in the circulation and this systemic inflammation may underlie and potentiate comorbidities, as discussed later.

Lipid Mediators

The profile of lipid mediators in exhaled breath condensates of patients with COPD shows an increase in prostaglandins and leukotrienes.[58] There is a significant increase in prostaglandin E_2 and prostaglandin $F_{2\alpha}$ and an increase in LTB_4 but not cysteinyl-leukotrienes. This pattern is different from that seen in asthma, in which increases in thromboxane and cysteinyl-leukotrienes have been shown. The increased production of prostanoids in COPD is likely to be secondary to the induction of cyclo-oxygenase-2 (COX2) by inflammatory cytokines, and increased expression of COX2 is described in alveolar macrophages of patients with COPD. LTB_4 concentrations are also increased in induced sputum and further increased in sputum and exhaled breath condensate during acute exacerbations.[35] LTB_4 is a potent chemoattractant of neutrophils, acting through high-affinity BLT_1 receptors. A BLT_1-receptor antagonist reduces the neutrophil chemotactic activity of sputum by approximately 25%.[59] BLT_1-receptors were recently identified on T lymphocytes and there is evidence that LTB_4 is also involved in recruitment of T cells.

Cytokines

Cytokines are the mediators of chronic inflammation and several have been implicated in COPD.[60,61] There is an increase in concentration of TNF-α in induced sputum in stable COPD with a further increase during exacerbations.[33,36] TNF-α production from peripheral blood monocytes is also increased in patients with COPD and has been implicated in the cachexia and skeletal muscle apoptosis in some patients with severe disease. TNF-α is a potent activator of NF-κB and this may amplify the inflammatory response. However, anti-TNF therapies have not proved to be effective in patients with COPD and may have serious adverse effects. IL-1β and IL-6 are other proinflammatory cytokines that may amplify the inflammation in COPD and may be important for systemic circulation. IL-1β and the related cytokine IL-18 may be produced via the activation of the NLRP3 inflammasome by cellular stress, including bacterial infections.[62] IL-17, and other Th17 cytokines, are also increased in COPD sputum and airways and may play a role in orchestrating neutrophilic inflammation in the lungs.[49,63]

Chemokines

Several chemokines have been implicated in COPD and have been of particular interest because chemokine receptors are G protein–coupled receptors, for which small molecule receptor antagonists have been developed.[12] CXCL8 concentrations are increased in induced sputum of patients with COPD and increase further during exacerbations.[33,36] CXCL8 is secreted from macrophages, T cells, epithelial cells, and neutrophils. CXCL8 activates neutrophils via low-affinity specific receptors CXCR1, and is chemotactic for neutrophils via high-affinity receptors CXCR2, which are also activated by related CXC chemokines, such as CXCL1. CXCL1 concentrations are markedly increased in sputum and BAL fluid of patients with COPD and this chemokine may be more important as a chemoattractant than CXCL8, acting via CXCR2, which are expressed on neutrophils and monocytes.[21] CXCL1 induces significantly more chemotaxis of monocytes of patients with COPD compared with those of normal smokers and this may reflect increased turnover and recovery of CXCR2 in monocytes of patients with COPD.[22] CXCL5 shows a marked increase in expression in airway epithelial cells during exacerbations of COPD and this is accompanied by a marked upregulation of epithelial CXCR2.

CCL2 is increased in concentration in COPD sputum and BAL fluid[21] and plays a role in monocyte chemotaxis via activation of CCR2. CCL2 seems to cooperate with CXCL1 in recruiting monocytes into the lungs. The chemokine CCL5 (RANTES) is also expressed in airways of patients with COPD during exacerbations and activates CCR5 on T cells and CCR3 on eosinophils, which may account for the increased eosinophils and T cells in the walls of large airways that have been reported during exacerbations of chronic bronchitis. As discussed earlier, CXCR3 are upregulated on Tc1 and Th1 cells of patients with COPD with increased expression of their ligands CXCL9, CXCL10, and CXCL11.[51]

Growth Factors

TGF-β1 is expressed in alveolar macrophages and airway epithelial cells of patients with COPD and is released from epithelial cells of small airways. TGF-β is released in a latent from and activated by various factors, including MMP-9 and oxidative stress. TGF-β may play an important role in the characteristic peribronchiolar fibrosis of small airways, either directly or through the release of connective tissue growth factor. Alveolar macrophages produce TGF-α in greater amounts than TGF-β and this may be a major endogenous activator of EGFR that play a key role in regulating mucus secretion in response to many stimuli, including cigarette smoke. Cigarette smoke activates TNF-α-converting enzyme on airway epithelial cells, which results in the shedding of TGF-α and the activation of EGFR, resulting in increased mucus secretion.[64]

VEGF is a major regulator of vascular growth and is likely to be involved in the pulmonary vascular remodeling that occurs as a result of hypoxic pulmonary vasoconstriction in severe COPD. There is increased expression of VEGF in pulmonary vascular smooth muscle of patients with mild and moderate COPD, but paradoxically a reduction in expression in severe COPD with emphysema. Inhibition of VEGF receptors using a selective inhibitor induces apoptosis of alveolar endothelial cells in rats, resulting in emphysema, and this seems to be driven by oxidative stress.[65]

PROTEASES

The increase in elastase activity in patients with COPD may contribute to the development of emphysema and to neutrophilic inflammation through the generation of chemotactic peptides such as Pro-Gly-Pro (matrikines). Human neutrophil elastase not only has elastolytic activity but is also a potent stimulant of mucus secretion in the airways. MMP9 seems to be the predominant elastolytic enzyme in COPD and is secreted from macrophages, neutrophils, and epithelial cells. MMP9 causes elastolysis but also stimulates neutrophilic inflammation through the generation of N-acetyl-PGP (Proline-Glycine-Proline).[66] MMP9 activation has been implicated in skin wrinkling and in arterial stiffness, which are indicators of COPD comorbidity.

OXIDATIVE STRESS

Oxidative stress occurs when ROS are produced in excess of the antioxidant defense mechanisms and result in harmful effects, including damage to lipids, proteins, and DNA. Oxidative stress is a critical feature in COPD.[67] Inflammatory and structural cells, including neutrophils, macrophages, and epithelial cells that are activated in the airways of patients with COPD, produce ROS. Superoxide anions (O_2^-) are generated by nicotinamide adenine dinucleotide phosphate hydrogen (NADPH) oxidase and converted to hydrogen peroxide (H_2O_2) by superoxide dismutases. H_2O_2 is then converted to water by catalase. O_2^- and H_2O_2 may interact in the presence of free iron to form the highly reactive hydroxyl radical (OH). O_2^- may also combine with NO to form peroxynitrite, which also generates OH. Oxidative stress leads to the oxidation of arachidonic acid and the formation of a new series of prostanoid mediators called isoprostanes, which may exert significant functional effects, including bronchoconstriction and plasma exudation.[68] Peroxynitrite is also increased in the breath of patients with COPD.[69] Nitric oxide may be increased in peripheral lung of patients with COPD and seems to be linked to increased expression of inducible and neural NO synthases (NOS2, NOS1).[69,70]

The normal production of oxidants is counteracted by several antioxidant mechanisms in the human respiratory tract, including catalase, superoxide dismutase (SOD), and glutathione, formed by the enzyme gamma-glutamyl cysteine ligase, and glutathione synthetase. In the lung, intracellular antioxidants are expressed at low levels and are not induced by oxidative stress, whereas the major antioxidants are extracellular. Extracellular antioxidants, particularly glutathione peroxidase, are markedly upregulated in response to cigarette smoke and oxidative stress. Extracellular antioxidants also include the dietary antioxidants vitamin C (ascorbic acid) and vitamin E (alpha-tocopherol), uric acid, lactoferrin, and extracellular SOD3, which is highly expressed in human lung. Most antioxidants are regulated by the transcription factor nuclear erythroid-2–related factor-2 (Nrf2), which is activated by oxidative stress. However, in COPD lungs and cells, Nrf2 is not appropriately activated despite high levels of oxidative stress in the lungs[71,72] and this may be related to increased acetylation caused by decreased HDAC2.[73]

ROS have wide-ranging effects on the airways and parenchyma and increase the inflammatory response (**Fig. 2**). ROS activate NF-κB, which switches on multiple inflammatory genes resulting in amplification of the inflammatory response. Oxidative stress results in activation of histone acetyltransferase activity, which opens up the chromatin structure and is associated with increased transcription of multiple inflammatory genes.[74] Oxidative stress may also impair the function of antiproteases such as alpha$_1$-antitrypsin and SLPI, and thereby accelerates the breakdown of elastin in lung parenchyma. Oxidative stress markedly reduces HDAC2 activity and expression, through activation of phosphoinositide-3-kinase-delta (PI3Kδ) and

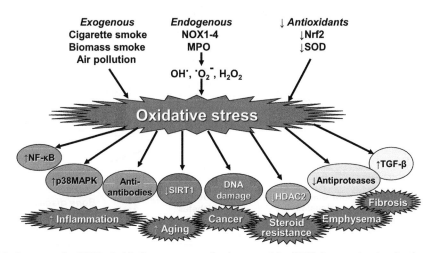

Fig. 2. Oxidative stress in COPD. Oxidative stress may be increased in COPD by a reduction in the transcription factor Nrf2, activation of NADPH oxidases (NOX), MPO, and reduced superoxide dismutase (SOD). Oxidative stress is a key driving mechanisms in COPD through activation of the proinflammatory transcription factor nuclear factor-κB (NF-κB), p38 mitogen-activated protein kinase (MAPK), generation of autoantibodies to carbonylated proteins, reduced sirtuin-1 (SIRT1), DNA damage, reduced histone deacetylase (HDAC)-2, reduced antiproteases, and increased TGF-β.

peroxynitrite-induced nitration of tyrosine resides. This process amplifies inflammation further and prevents corticosteroids from inactivating activated inflammatory genes. Through similar mechanisms, oxidative stress reduces the expression and activity of sirtuin-1, a key repair molecule that is implicated in aging. The reduction in sirtuin-1 in COPD lungs and cells may underlie the accelerated aging response seen in COPD.[75] Oxidative stress may also predispose to lung cancer, through the activation of growth factors and via DNA damage.[76] Oxidative stress leads to formation of carbonylated proteins, which may be antigenic and stimulate the development of autoantibodies in patients with COPD.[53]

There is also evidence for systemic oxidative stress in patients with COPD with an increase in lipid peroxidation products and decreased antioxidant capacity. Furthermore, circulating neutrophils release more ROS than neutrophils from normal smokers and nonsmokers.[77] Systemic oxidative stress increases further during acute exacerbations.[78]

SYSTEMIC INFLAMMATION IN COPD

Patients with COPD, particularly when the disease is severe and during exacerbations, have evidence of systemic inflammation, measured either as increased circulating cytokines, chemokines, and acute phase proteins, or as abnormalities in circulating cells (**Fig. 3**).[79,80] Smoking may cause systemic inflammation (for example, increased total leukocyte count) but in patients with COPD the degree of systemic inflammation is greater. It is still uncertain whether these systemic markers of inflammation are a spill-over from inflammation in the peripheral lung, are a parallel abnormality, or are related to some comorbid disease that then has effects on the lung. In any case, the components of this systemic inflammation may account for the systemic manifestations of COPD and may worsen comorbid diseases. In a large population study, systemic inflammation (increased C-reactive protein [CRP], fibrinogen, and leukocytes) was associated with a 2-fold to 4-fold increased risk of cardiovascular disease, diabetes, lung cancer, and pneumonia, but not with depression.[81] Using 6 inflammatory markers (CRP, IL-6, CXCL8, fibrinogen, TNF-α, and leukocytes), 70% of patients with COPD had some components of systemic inflammation and 16% had persistent inflammation.[82] Patients with persistent systemic inflammation had increased mortality and more frequent exacerbations. Systemic inflammation seems to relate to accelerated decline in lung function and is increased further during exacerbations.[83]

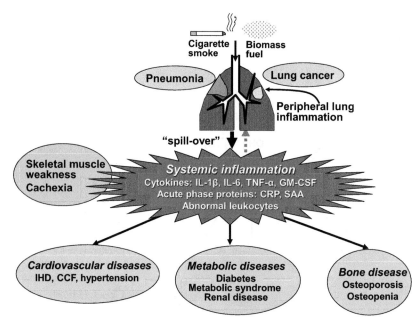

Fig. 3. Systemic inflammation and comorbidities in COPD. Patients with COPD have peripheral lung inflammation that may extend into the systemic circulation, leading to skeletal muscle weakness and cachexia and increasing propensity to cardiovascular, metabolic, and bone diseases. There is an increase in circulating cytokines, including IL-1β, IL-6, TNF-α, and GM-CSF, as well as acute phase proteins, such as C-reactive protein (CRP), serum amyloid A (SAA), and abnormal leukocytes. Peripheral lung inflammation may also increase the risk of developing lung cancer and community-acquired pneumonia. CCF, congestive cardiac failure; IHD, ischemic heart disease.

Acute Phase Proteins

CRP is an acute phase protein that is increased in plasma of patients with COPD, particularly during acute infective exacerbations. In stable COPD, plasma concentrations are related to all-cause mortality in mild to moderate patients,[84] but not in severe or very severe patients.[85] However, although CRP is related to forced expiratory volume in 1 second (FEV_1) in cross-sectional studies, there is no association with progressive decline of FEV_1 in longitudinal studies.[86] CRP is also increased in exacerbations of COPD, whether because of viral or bacterial causes,[83] and a high concentration of CRP 2 weeks after an exacerbation predicts the likelihood of recurrent exacerbation.[87] CRP in plasma is produced by the liver in response to circulating IL-6 and therefore may be a biomarker of systemic inflammation rather than directly contributing to comorbid diseases.

Plasma fibrinogen concentrations are increased in patients with COPD with frequent exacerbations.[78,88] An increased plasma fibrinogen in a population is related to worse FEV_1 and increased risks of hospitalization for COPD.[89] Serum amyloid A (SAA) is another acute phase protein released by circulating proinflammatory cytokines from liver, but, unlike CRP, also from inflamed tissue. It has been identified by proteomic analysis of plasma as showing an increase during acute exacerbations of COPD and its concentrations are correlated with the severity of exacerbations.[90] SAA binds to gram-negative bacteria and is part of the innate defense mechanism against bacterial infections, but it also has proinflammatory effects, including activation of epithelial cells, neutrophils, monocytes, and Th17 cells to release proinflammatory mediators and inhibit the effects of antiinflammatory lipoxins.[91] SAA activates Toll-like receptor (TLR) 2, resulting in activation of NF-κB.[92] SAA also binds to the receptor for advanced glycation end products (RAGE) and soluble RAGE concentrations are reduced in plasma of patients with COPD and are related to disease severity.[93]

Surfactant protein-D (SP-D) is a glycoprotein member of the collectin family and is secreted mainly by type II pneumocytes and Clara cells and plays a role in innate defense against microorganisms. Serum SP-D concentrations are increased in smokers and in patients with COPD but are weakly correlated with disease severity.[94] Serum SP-D is further increased transiently during exacerbations. Serum SP-D is also increased in other lung diseases, including asthma, pulmonary fibrosis, and pneumonia, and so has poor specificity. Although SP-D in serum is increased in COPD, its concentrations are reduced in BAL fluid, suggesting that it may translocate from lung to systemic circulation.[95] The reduced concentration of SP-D in BAL fluid may be caused by oxidative damage of the quaternary structure, so it is not detectable by immunoassay.

Cytokines

IL-6 is consistently increased in the systemic circulation of patients with COPD, particularly during exacerbations, and may account for the increase in circulating acute phase proteins such CRP and SAA.[96] The functional effects of circulating IL-6, apart from increasing acute phase proteins, are not certain but there is evidence that they may be associated with skeletal muscle weakness. In an aging population with or without airway obstruction, plasma IL-6 concentrations are related to decreased muscle strength measured by quadriceps strength and exercise capacity.[97] In rats, infusion of IL-6 induces both cardiac failure and skeletal muscle weakness.[98] Increased circulating IL-6 concentrations are associated with several comorbid diseases, including ischemic heart disease, diabetes, and osteoporosis.

Plasma TNF-α and its soluble receptor (sTNFR75) are increased in patients with COPD,[99] and TNF-α is also released from circulating cells in patients with COPD with cachexia.[100] Circulating TNF-α seems to be related, at least in part, to hypoxaemia.[101] Increased systemic TNF-α has been implicated as a mechanism of cachexia and skeletal muscle weakness in patients with COPD. Chronic administration of TNF-α in animals results in cachexia, anemia, leukocytosis, and infiltration of neutrophils into organs such as heart, liver, and spleen.[102]

IL-1β has also been linked to cachexia, but increased plasma concentrations or decreased concentrations of its endogenous antagonist IL-1 receptor antagonist have not been found in COPD, although there is an association between COPD and a polymorphism of the IL-1β gene.[99]

CXCL8 and other CXC chemokines play an important role in neutrophil and monocyte recruitment in patients with COPD. Circulating CXCL8 concentrations are also increased in patients with COPD and have been related to muscle weakness.[103]

DEFECTIVE RESOLUTION OF INFLAMMATION AND REPAIR

The reason why inflammation persists in patients with COPD even after long-term smoking cessation is currently unknown, but if the molecular and cellular mechanisms for impaired resolution could be identified this may provide a novel approach to COPD therapy. A major mechanism of airway obstruction in COPD is loss of elastic recoil caused by proteolytic destruction of lung parenchyma, so it is unlikely that this could be reversible by drug therapy. However, it might be possible to reduce the rate of progression by preventing the inflammatory and enzymatic disease process. In a similar way, the peribronchiolar fibrosis of small airways may not be reversible, but its progression may be halted by antifibrotic therapies.

Proresolving Lipid Mediators

Resolution of inflammation is an active process that may be facilitated by several endogenous proresolving mediators, including lipoxins, E-series resolvins, D-series protectins, and maresins, all of which are derived from polyunsaturated fatty acids and act on distinct receptors.[104] These mediators promote the resolution of neutrophilic inflammation by preventing neutrophil recruitment and enhancing neutrophil removal by efferocytosis. Endogenous mediators or stable structural analogues that activate the same receptors may have therapeutic potential in promoting resolution of inflammation in COPD. Maresin-1 is the most potent proresolving mediator that stimulates macrophage efferocytosis so a stable analogue of this mediator may be useful in COPD.[105]

Accelerated Aging

There is growing evidence that emphysema may be caused by accelerated aging of the lungs and it is hypothesized that accelerated aging may be caused by defective function of endogenous antiaging molecules, such as sirtuins and Forkhead box type O (FOXO) proteins, as a result of increased oxidative stress in the lung.[106] Sirtuin-1 (SIRT1) is markedly reduced in the peripheral lung of patients with COPD and in vitro this is mimicked by oxidative stress, which reduces activity and expression of SIRT1 resulting in increased expression of MMP9.[75] Resveratrol, a chemical found in red wine and derived from the skin of red fruits, is a weak sirtuin activator and prolongs the lifespan of several species, including mice. Resveratrol also suppresses the inflammatory response of macrophages from patients with COPD and epithelial cells, which is resistant to the effects of corticosteroids.[107,108] Resveratrol has poor bioavailability, which prompted a search for orally available and more potent sirtuin activators. An oral sirtuin activator, SRT2172, reverses the effects of cigarette smoking on MMP9 activity and inflammation in mice exposed to cigarette smoke.[75]

The pathway linking oxidative stress to reduced SIRT1 expression involved PI3K and activation of

mammalian target of rapamycin (mTOR), which is inhibited by rapamycin and indirectly by metformin, both of which have been shown to have antiaging effects and to extend lifespan.[109] Through further understanding of the molecular pathways of cellular senescence in COPD it may be possible to identify novel targets and therapies to prevent disease progression and associated comorbidities.

Telomere shortening is associated with aging and there is evidence for reduced telomere length in lung and circulating cells from patients with COPD compared with normal smokers. This finding is associated with increased senescence and reduced telomerase activity in pulmonary endothelial cells of patients with COPD, which is linked to increased release of inflammatory mediators, such as IL-6, CXCL8, and CCL2.[110]

Airway Fibrosis

Increasing small airway fibrosis is an important mechanism of disease progression in COPD and is presumed to result from chronic inflammation, suggesting that effective antiinflammatory treatments should prevent fibrosis. Fibrosis may be mediated via the activation of fibroblasts by fibrogenic mediators, such as TGF-β, connective tissue growth factor (CTGF), and endothelin, which are secreted from epithelial cells and macrophages.[111] There are currently no effective antifibrotic therapies and no evidence that fibrosis can be reversed in COPD. Peroxisome proliferator-activated receptor gamma activators, such as rosiglitazone and pioglitazone, also have antifibrotic effects and may inhibit TGF-β signaling pathways in pulmonary fibroblasts.[112] Endothelin-1 is also profibrotic and several endothelin receptor antagonists have been found to be effective in inhibiting pulmonary fibrosis in animal models.[113]

IMPLICATIONS FOR FUTURE THERAPY

Inflammation is a driving mechanism for the progression of COPD, exacerbations, and probably associated comorbidities, including cardiovascular disease and lung cancer, which are the major causes of death among patients with COPD. However, this inflammatory process is largely resistant to the antiinflammatory effects of corticosteroids, although they are still widely used in the management of COPD, resulting in significant morbidity from side effects.

Reversal of Corticosteroid Resistance

This poor clinical response to corticosteroids in COPD reflects resistance to the antiinflammatory effects of corticosteroids and may be explained by a reduction in HDAC2 as a result of oxidative and nitrative stress.[114] A reduction in HDAC2 activity and expression increases histone acetylation, with increased expression of inflammatory genes and reduction in the antiinflammatory effects of corticosteroids. The reduction in HDAC2 also results in increased acetylation of the glucocorticoid receptor, which prevents it from inhibiting NF-κB–driven inflammation.[27] A novel therapeutic strategy is reversal of this corticosteroid resistance through increasing the expression and activity of HDAC2 and this may be achieved with several existing and developing drugs.

Low concentrations of oral theophylline increase HDAC2 expression and activity in alveolar macrophages from patients with COPD and thus restore steroid responsiveness in these cells.[115] Mice exposed to cigarette smoke develop a steroid-resistant pulmonary inflammation that is suppressed by adding low-dose oral theophylline to the corticosteroid.[116] In patients with COPD, a low dose of oral theophylline combined with an inhaled corticosteroid was more effective in reducing inflammation in sputum than either drug alone.[117] This action of theophylline is independent of phosphodiesterase (PDE) inhibition and seems to be mediated by direct inhibition of oxidant stress–activated PI3Kδ.[116] Clinical trials with low-dose theophylline combined with corticosteroids are now underway. The tricyclic antidepressant nortriptyline also increases HDAC2 and reverses corticosteroid resistance by directly inhibiting PI3Kδ.[118] Oxidative stress is a major mechanism leading to corticosteroid resistance in COPD through reduced HDAC2. The antioxidant sulforaphane, increases HDAC2 and reverses corticosteroid resistance in mice exposed to cigarette smoke and in macrophages from patients with COPD.[72] Curcumin (diferuloylmethane), found in turmeric spice used in curry, also increases HDAC2 after it has been reduced by oxidative stress, and at concentrations lower than required for antioxidant effects.[119] Macrolides, including nonantibiotic macrolides, also reverse corticosteroid resistance through inhibiting PI3K signaling.[120]

New Antiinflammatory Therapies

There is an unmet need for safe and effective antiinflammatory treatments for COPD, but it has proved difficult to develop such drugs, despite the discovery of several logical targets.[2] Blocking individual cytokines with blocking antibodies or blocking chemokine receptors has so far proved to be disappointing in clinical studies. Broad-spectrum antiinflammatory treatments, such as PDE4 and proinflammatory kinase inhibitors, have often been poorly tolerated with side effects that limit the dose that can be used. For example, a PDE4 inhibitor, roflumilast, has significant antiinflammatory effects in COPD cells and animal models of COPD but the dose in patients with COPD is limited by side effects, so the therapeutic benefit is marginal.[121] It may be necessary to develop potent inhaled drugs in order to reduce systemic exposure and side effects, but it has proved difficult to discover inhibitors with high local potency that are retained within the lungs. If systemic inflammation is derived from peripheral lung inflammation, inhaled antiinflammatory treatments should reduce systemic inflammation and may therefore reduce or treat comorbidities.

New Pathways

There may be several coexisting mechanisms that interact in complex ways, so targeting a single pathway or mediator may not be effective in treating COPD, unless specific responder phenotypes are identified. It is important to identify the molecular mechanisms that underlie susceptibility so that only a minority of smokers develop COPD. So far, genome-wide association studies of COPD have been disappointing, but this may be because the studies include all types of COPD. It is also likely that epigenetic mechanisms such as DNA methylation play an important role in disease susceptibility and these have yet to be explored.

As discussed earlier, there may be new disease processes, such as autoimmunity, defective phagocytosis, ineffective repair mechanisms, and cellular senescence, that may be targeted in the future, and there are several novel drugs in development.

The Need for Biomarkers

Clinical studies to show the effects of new drugs on disease progression are challenging because large numbers of patients studied over long periods (3 years) are necessary. It is important to identify biomarkers of disease activity or surrogate measurements that predict the clinical efficacy of antiinflammatory treatments in patients with COPD. Analysis of sputum parameters (cells, mediators, enzymes) or exhaled biomarkers (lipid mediators, ROS) may be useful as biomarkers of inflammation.[122]

Disease Phenotypes

It has long been recognized that COPD includes several different clinical and pathophysiologic phenotypes, but so far it has been different to link any phenotype to a differential response to therapy. For example, roflumilast seems to work more effectively in a phenotype defined by disease severity, frequent exacerbations, and mucus hypersecretion, which may be a surrogate for neutrophilic inflammation.[123] Biomarkers that predict responsiveness to particular treatments are needed, particularly as treatments become more specific, such as targeting specific proteins. Patients with early disease seem to decline more rapidly may show better responses to therapy, whereas the focus of treatment currently is on patients with late disease who have the most symptoms. If effective and safe antiinflammatory therapies are developed for COPD it may be more useful to introduce these early in the course of the disease to prevent disease progression and possibly to reduce the burden of concomitant comorbidities. This approach is akin to the therapy for systemic hypertension and hypercholesterolemia in which treatment is given to prevent future risk.

Treating Acute Exacerbations

Because exacerbations represent a flare-up of the inflammation seen in stable disease, effective antiinflammatory treatments should also be able to reduce the intensity, duration, and consequences of an acute exacerbation.[124] This application of novel antiinflammatory therapies may be important, although it is challenging to test a novel antiinflammatory therapy in the management of an acute exacerbation. However, because such a treatment may be expected to be of only a few days' duration, this may make it possible to use therapies that would have side effects if used long-term.

REFERENCES

1. Barnes PJ. Chronic obstructive pulmonary disease: effects beyond the lungs. PLoS Med 2010;7: e1000220.
2. Barnes PJ. New anti-inflammatory treatments for chronic obstructive pulmonary disease. Nat Rev Drug Discov 2013;12(7):543–59.
3. Salvi SS, Barnes PJ. Chronic obstructive pulmonary disease in non-smokers. Lancet 2009;374: 733–43.
4. Hogg JC, Chu F, Utokaparch S, et al. The nature of small-airway obstruction in chronic obstructive pulmonary disease. N Engl J Med 2004;350:2645–53.
5. McDonough JE, Yuan R, Suzuki M, et al. Small-airway obstruction and emphysema in chronic obstructive pulmonary disease. N Engl J Med 2011;365:1567–75.
6. Galban CJ, Han MK, Boes JL, et al. Computed tomography-based biomarker provides unique signature for diagnosis of COPD phenotypes and disease progression. Nat Med 2012;18:1711–5.
7. Barnes PJ. Immunology of asthma and chronic obstructive pulmonary disease. Nat Rev Immunol 2008;8:183–92.
8. Cosio MG, Saetta M, Agusti A. Immunologic aspects of chronic obstructive pulmonary disease. N Engl J Med 2009;360:2445–54.
9. Brusselle GG, Joos GF, Bracke KR. New insights into the immunology of chronic obstructive pulmonary disease. Lancet 2011;378:1015–26.
10. Van Pottelberge GR, Bracke KR, Joos GF, et al. The role of dendritic cells in the pathogenesis of COPD: liaison officers in the front line. COPD 2009;6: 284–90.
11. Barnes PJ. Mediators of chronic obstructive pulmonary disease. Pharmacol Rev 2004;56:515–48.
12. Donnelly LE, Barnes PJ. Chemokine receptors as therapeutic targets in chronic obstructive pulmonary disease. Trends Pharmacol Sci 2006;27: 546–53.
13. Gamble E, Grootendorst DC, Hattotuwa K, et al. Airway mucosal inflammation in COPD is similar in smokers and ex-smokers: a pooled analysis. Eur Respir J 2007;30:467–71.
14. Petrache I, Natarajan V, Zhen L, et al. Ceramide upregulation causes pulmonary cell apoptosis and emphysema-like disease in mice. Nat Med 2005; 11:491–8.
15. de Boer WI, Hau CM, van Schadewijk A, et al. Expression of epidermal growth factors and their receptors in the bronchial epithelium of subjects with chronic obstructive pulmonary disease. Am J Clin Pathol 2006;125:184–92.
16. Barnes PJ. Macrophages as orchestrators of COPD. COPD 2004;1:59–70.
17. Meshi B, Vitalis TZ, Ionescu D, et al. Emphysematous lung destruction by cigarette smoke. The effects of latent adenoviral infection on the lung inflammatory response. Am J Respir Cell Mol Biol 2002;26:52–7.
18. Russell RE, Thorley A, Culpitt SV, et al. Alveolar macrophage-mediated elastolysis: roles of matrix metalloproteinases, cysteine, and serine proteases. Am J Physiol Lung Cell Mol Physiol 2002; 283:L867–73.
19. Gordon S, Pluddemann A. Tissue macrophage heterogeneity: issues and prospects. Semin Immunopathol 2013;35(5):533–40.
20. Caramori G, Romagnoli M, Casolari P, et al. Nuclear localisation of p65 in sputum macrophages but not in sputum neutrophils during COPD exacerbations. Thorax 2003;58:348–51.
21. Traves SL, Culpitt S, Russell RE, et al. Elevated levels of the chemokines GRO-alpha and MCP-1

in sputum samples from COPD patients. Thorax 2002;57:590–5.

22. Traves SL, Smith SJ, Barnes PJ, et al. Specific CXC but not CC chemokines cause elevated monocyte migration in COPD: a role for CXCR2. J Leukoc Biol 2004;76:441–50.

23. Grumelli S, Corry DB, Song LX, et al. An immune basis for lung parenchymal destruction in chronic obstructive pulmonary disease and emphysema. PLoS Med 2004;1:75–83.

24. Culpitt SV, Rogers DF, Shah P, et al. Impaired inhibition by dexamethasone of cytokine release by alveolar macrophages from patients with chronic obstructive pulmonary disease. Am J Respir Crit Care Med 2003;167:24–31.

25. Keatings VM, Jatakanon A, Worsdell YM, et al. Effects of inhaled and oral glucocorticoids on inflammatory indices in asthma and COPD. Am J Respir Crit Care Med 1997;155:542–8.

26. Ito K, Ito M, Elliott WM, et al. Decreased histone deacetylase activity in chronic obstructive pulmonary disease. N Engl J Med 2005;352: 1967–76.

27. Ito K, Yamamura S, Essilfie-Quaye S, et al. Histone deacetylase 2-mediated deacetylation of the glucocorticoid receptor enables NF-kappaB suppression. J Exp Med 2006;203:7–13.

28. Barnes PJ. Role of HDAC2 in the pathophysiology of COPD. Annu Rev Physiol 2009;71:451–64.

29. Taylor AE, Finney-Hayward TK, Quint JK, et al. Defective macrophage phagocytosis of bacteria in COPD. Eur Respir J 2010;35:1039–47.

30. Hodge S, Hodge G, Scicchitano R, et al. Alveolar macrophages from subjects with chronic obstructive pulmonary disease are deficient in their ability to phagocytose apoptotic airway epithelial cells. Immunol Cell Biol 2003;81:289–96.

31. Donnelly LE, Barnes PJ. Defective phagocytosis in airways disease. Chest 2012;141:1055–62.

32. Mullerova H, Chigbo C, Hagan GW, et al. The natural history of community-acquired pneumonia in COPD patients: a population database analysis. Respir Med 2012;106:1124–33.

33. Keatings VM, Collins PD, Scott DM, et al. Differences in interleukin-8 and tumor necrosis factor-alpha in induced sputum from patients with chronic obstructive pulmonary disease or asthma. Am J Respir Crit Care Med 1996;153:530–4.

34. Keatings VM, Barnes PJ. Granulocyte activation markers in induced sputum: comparison between chronic obstructive pulmonary disease, asthma and normal subjects. Am J Respir Crit Care Med 1997;155:449–53.

35. Biernacki WA, Kharitonov SA, Barnes PJ. Increased leukotriene B4 and 8-isoprostane in exhaled breath condensate of patients with exacerbations of COPD. Thorax 2003;58:294–8.

36. Aaron SD, Angel JB, Lunau M, et al. Granulocyte inflammatory markers and airway infection during acute exacerbation of chronic obstructive pulmonary disease. Am J Respir Crit Care Med 2001; 163:349–55.

37. Sapey E, Stockley JA, Greenwood H, et al. Behavioral and structural differences in migrating peripheral neutrophils from patients with chronic obstructive pulmonary disease. Am J Respir Crit Care Med 2011;183:1176–86.

38. Traves SL, Smith SJ, Barnes PJ, et al. Specific CXC but not CC chemokines cause elevated monocyte migration in COPD: a role for CXCR2. J Leukoc Biol 2004;76:441–50.

39. Turato G, Zuin R, Saetta M. Pathogenesis and pathology of COPD. Respiration 2001;68:117–28.

40. Brightling CE, Monteiro W, Ward R, et al. Sputum eosinophilia and short-term response to prednisolone in chronic obstructive pulmonary disease: a randomised controlled trial. Lancet 2000;356: 1480–5.

41. Papi A, Romagnoli M, Baraldo S, et al. Partial reversibility of airflow limitation and increased exhaled NO and sputum eosinophilia in chronic obstructive pulmonary disease. Am J Respir Crit Care Med 2000;162:1773–7.

42. Saetta M, Distefano A, Maestrelli P, et al. Airway eosinophilia in chronic bronchitis during exacerbations. Am J Respir Crit Care Med 1994;150: 1646–52.

43. Saetta M, Di Stefano A, Maestrelli P, et al. Airway eosinophilia and expression of interleukin-5 protein in asthma and in exacerbations of chronic bronchitis. Clin Exp Allergy 1996;26: 766–74.

44. Zhu J, Qiu YS, Majumdar S, et al. Exacerbations of bronchitis: bronchial eosinophilia and gene expression for interleukin-4, interleukin-5, and eosinophil chemoattractants. Am J Respir Crit Care Med 2001;164:109–16.

45. Liu H, Lazarus SC, Caughey GH, et al. Neutrophil elastase and elastase-rich cystic fibrosis sputum degranulate human eosinophils in vitro. Am J Physiol 1999;276:L28–34.

46. Van Pottelberge GR, Bracke KR, Demedts IK, et al. Selective accumulation of Langerhans-type dendritic cells in small airways of patients with COPD. Respir Res 2010;11:35.

47. Freeman CM, Martinez FJ, Han MK, et al. Lung dendritic cell expression of maturation molecules increases with worsening chronic obstructive pulmonary disease. Am J Respir Crit Care Med 2009;180:1179–88.

48. Di Stefano A, Caramori G, Capelli A, et al. STAT4 activation in smokers and patients with chronic obstructive pulmonary disease. Eur Respir J 2004;24:78–85.

49. Di Stefano A, Caramori G, Gnemmi I, et al. T helper type 17-related cytokine expression is increased in the bronchial mucosa of stable chronic obstructive pulmonary disease patients. Clin Exp Immunol 2009;157:316–24.

50. Pridgeon C, Bugeon L, Donnelly L, et al. Regulation of IL-17 in chronic inflammation in the human lung. Clin Sci (Lond) 2011;120:515–24.

51. Costa C, Rufino R, Traves SL, et al. CXCR3 and CCR5 chemokines in the induced sputum from patients with COPD. Chest 2008;133:26–33.

52. Saetta M, Mariani M, Panina-Bordignon P, et al. Increased expression of the chemokine receptor CXCR3 and its ligand CXCL10 in peripheral airways of smokers with chronic obstructive pulmonary disease. Am J Respir Crit Care Med 2002; 165:1404–9.

53. Kirkham PA, Caramori G, Casolari P, et al. Oxidative stress-induced antibodies to carbonyl-modified protein correlate with severity of chronic obstructive pulmonary disease. Am J Respir Crit Care Med 2011;184:796–802.

54. Karayama M, Inui N, Suda T, et al. Antiendothelial cell antibodies in patients with COPD. Chest 2010;138:1303–8.

55. Majo J, Ghezzo H, Cosio MG. Lymphocyte population and apoptosis in the lungs of smokers and their relation to emphysema. Eur Respir J 2001; 17:946–53.

56. Lambers C, Hacker S, Posch M, et al. T cell senescence and contraction of T cell repertoire diversity in patients with chronic obstructive pulmonary disease. Clin Exp Immunol 2009;155:466–75.

57. Hodge G, Mukaro V, Reynolds PN, et al. Role of increased CD8/CD28(null) T cells and alternative co-stimulatory molecules in chronic obstructive pulmonary disease. Clin Exp Immunol 2011;166: 94–102.

58. Montuschi P, Kharitonov SA, Ciabattoni G, et al. Exhaled leukotrienes and prostaglandins in COPD. Thorax 2003;58:585–8.

59. Beeh KM, Kornmann O, Buhl R, et al. Neutrophil chemotactic activity of sputum from patients with COPD: role of interleukin 8 and leukotriene B4. Chest 2003;123:1240–7.

60. Barnes PJ. Cytokine networks in asthma and chronic obstructive pulmonary disease. J Clin Invest 2008;118:3546–56.

61. Barnes PJ. The cytokine network in COPD. Am J Respir Cell Mol Biol 2009;41:631–8.

62. Birrell MA, Eltom S. The role of the NLRP3 inflammasome in the pathogenesis of airway disease. Pharmacol Ther 2011;130:364–70.

63. Doe C, Bafadhel M, Siddiqui S, et al. Expression of the T helper 17-associated cytokines IL-17A and IL-17F in asthma and COPD. Chest 2010;138: 1140–7.

64. Fahy JV, Dickey BF. Airway mucus function and dysfunction. N Engl J Med 2010;363:2233–47.

65. Tuder RM, Yoshida T, Arap W, et al. State of the art. Cellular and molecular mechanisms of alveolar destruction in emphysema: an evolutionary perspective. Proc Am Thorac Soc 2006;3:503–10.

66. O'Reilly P, Jackson PL, Noerager B, et al. N-alpha-PGP and PGP, potential biomarkers and therapeutic targets for COPD. Respir Res 2009;10:38.

67. Kirkham PA, Barnes PJ. Oxidative stress in COPD. Chest 2013;144(1):266–73.

68. Montuschi P, Barnes PJ, Roberts LJ. Isoprostanes: markers and mediators of oxidative stress. FASEB J 2004;18:1791–800.

69. Osoata GO, Hanazawa T, Brindicci C, et al. Peroxynitrite elevation in exhaled breath condensate of COPD and its inhibition by fudosteine. Chest 2009;135:1513–20.

70. Brindicci C, Kharitonov SA, Ito M, et al. Nitric oxide synthase isoenzyme expression and activity in peripheral lungs of COPD patients. Am J Respir Crit Care Med 2010;181:21–30.

71. Malhotra D, Thimmulappa R, Navas-Acien A, et al. Decline in NRF2 regulated antioxidants in COPD lungs due to loss of its positive regulator DJ-1. Am J Respir Crit Care Med 2008;178:592–604.

72. Malhotra D, Thimmulappa RK, Mercado N, et al. Denitrosylation of HDAC2 by targeting Nrf2 restores glucocorticosteroid sensitivity in macrophages from COPD patients. J Clin Invest 2011; 121(11):4289–302.

73. Mercado N, Thimmulappa R, Thomas CM, et al. Decreased histone deacetylase 2 impairs Nrf2 activation by oxidative stress. Biochem Biophys Res Commun 2011;406:292–8.

74. Tomita K, Barnes PJ, Adcock IM. The effect of oxidative stress on histone acetylation and IL-8 release. Biochem Biophys Res Commun 2003; 301:572–7.

75. Nakamaru Y, Vuppusetty C, Wada H, et al. A protein deacetylase SIRT1 is a negative regulator of metalloproteinase-9. FASEB J 2009;23:2810–9.

76. Adcock IM, Caramori G, Barnes PJ. Chronic obstructive pulmonary disease and lung cancer: new molecular insights. Respiration 2011;81: 265–84.

77. Rahman I, Morrison D, Donaldson K, et al. Systemic oxidative stress in asthma, COPD, and smokers. Am J Respir Crit Care Med 1996;154: 1055–60.

78. Groenewegen KH, Postma DS, Hop WC, et al. Increased systemic inflammation is a risk factor for COPD exacerbations. Chest 2008;133:350–7.

79. Gan WQ, Man SF, Senthilselvan A, et al. Association between chronic obstructive pulmonary disease and systemic inflammation: a systematic review and a meta-analysis. Thorax 2004;59:574–80.

80. van Eeden SF, Sin DD. Chronic obstructive pulmonary disease: a chronic systemic inflammatory disease. Respiration 2008;75:224–38.

81. Thomsen M, Dahl M, Lange P, et al. Inflammatory biomarkers and comorbidities in chronic obstructive pulmonary disease. Am J Respir Crit Care Med 2012;186(10):982–8.

82. Agusti A, Edwards LD, Rennard SI, et al. Persistent systemic inflammation is associated with poor clinical outcomes in COPD: a novel phenotype. PLoS One 2012;7:e37483.

83. Hurst JR, Donaldson GC, Perea WR, et al. Utility of plasma biomarkers at exacerbation of chronic obstructive pulmonary disease. Am J Respir Crit Care Med 2006;174:867–74.

84. Dahl M, Vestbo J, Lange P, et al. C-reactive protein as a predictor of prognosis in chronic obstructive pulmonary disease. Am J Respir Crit Care Med 2007;175:250–5.

85. de Torres JP, Pinto-Plata V, Casanova C, et al. C-reactive protein levels and survival in patients with moderate to very severe COPD. Chest 2008; 133:1336–43.

86. Fogarty AW, Jones S, Britton JR, et al. Systemic inflammation and decline in lung function in a general population: a prospective study. Thorax 2007; 62:515–20.

87. Perera WR, Hurst JR, Wilkinson TM, et al. Inflammatory changes, recovery and recurrence at COPD exacerbation. Eur Respir J 2007;29: 527–34.

88. Donaldson GC, Seemungal TA, Patel IS, et al. Airway and systemic inflammation and decline in lung function in patients with COPD. Chest 2005; 128:1995–2004.

89. Dahl M, Tybjaerg-Hansen A, Vestbo J, et al. Elevated plasma fibrinogen associated with reduced pulmonary function and increased risk of chronic obstructive pulmonary disease. Am J Respir Crit Care Med 2001;164:1008–11.

90. Bozinovski S, Hutchinson A, Thompson M, et al. Serum amyloid A is a biomarker of acute exacerbations of chronic obstructive pulmonary disease. Am J Respir Crit Care Med 2008;177:269–78.

91. Bozinovski S, Uddin M, Vlahos R, et al. Serum amyloid A opposes lipoxin A(4) to mediate glucocorticoid refractory lung inflammation in chronic obstructive pulmonary disease. Proc Natl Acad Sci U S A 2012;109:935–40.

92. Cheng N, He R, Tian J, et al. Cutting edge: TLR2 is a functional receptor for acute-phase serum amyloid A. J Immunol 2008;181:22–6.

93. Sukkar MB, Wood LG, Tooze M, et al. Soluble RAGE is deficient in neutrophilic asthma and COPD. Eur Respir J 2012;39:721–9.

94. Sin DD, Leung R, Gan WQ, et al. Circulating surfactant protein D as a potential lung-specific biomarker of health outcomes in COPD: a pilot study. BMC Pulm Med 2007;7:13.

95. Winkler C, Atochina-Vasserman EN, Holz O, et al. Comprehensive characterisation of pulmonary and serum surfactant protein D in COPD. Respir Res 2011;12:29.

96. Bhowmik A, Seemungal TA, Sapsford RJ, et al. Relation of sputum inflammatory markers to symptoms and lung function changes in COPD exacerbations. Thorax 2000;55(2):114–20.

97. Yende S, Waterer GW, Tolley EA, et al. Inflammatory markers are associated with ventilatory limitation and muscle dysfunction in obstructive lung disease in well functioning elderly subjects. Thorax 2006; 61:10–6.

98. Janssen SP, Gayan-Ramirez G, Van den BA, et al. Interleukin-6 causes myocardial failure and skeletal muscle atrophy in rats. Circulation 2005;111: 996–1005.

99. Broekhuizen R, Grimble RF, Howell WM, et al. Pulmonary cachexia, systemic inflammatory profile, and the interleukin 1beta -511 single nucleotide polymorphism. Am J Clin Nutr 2005;82:1059–64.

100. de Godoy I, Donahoe M, Calhoun WJ, et al. Elevated TNF-alpha production by peripheral blood monocytes of weight- losing COPD patients. Am J Respir Crit Care Med 1996;153:633–7.

101. Takabatake N, Nakamura H, Abe S, et al. The relationship between chronic hypoxemia and activation of the tumor necrosis factor-alpha system in patients with chronic obstructive pulmonary disease. Am J Respir Crit Care Med 2000;161: 1179–84.

102. Tracey KJ, Wei H, Manogue KR, et al. Cachectin/tumor necrosis factor induces cachexia, anemia, and inflammation. J Exp Med 1988;167:1211–27.

103. Spruit MA, Gosselink R, Troosters T, et al. Muscle force during an acute exacerbation in hospitalised patients with COPD and its relationship with CXCL8 and IGF-I. Thorax 2003;58:752–6.

104. Serhan CN. Novel lipid mediators and resolution mechanisms in acute inflammation: to resolve or not? Am J Pathol 2010;177:1576–91.

105. Serhan CN, Yang R, Martinod K, et al. Maresins: novel macrophage mediators with potent antiinflammatory and proresolving actions. J Exp Med 2009;206:15–23.

106. Ito K, Barnes PJ. COPD as a disease of accelerated lung aging. Chest 2009;135:173–80.

107. Culpitt SV, Rogers DF, Fenwick PS, et al. Inhibition by red wine extract, resveratrol, of cytokine release by alveolar macrophages in COPD. Thorax 2003; 58:942–6.

108. Donnelly LE, Newton R, Kennedy GE, et al. Anti-inflammatory effects of resveratrol in lung epithelial cells: molecular mechanisms. Am J Physiol Lung Cell Mol Physiol 2004;287(4):L774–83.

109. Sharp ZD. Aging and TOR: interwoven in the fabric of life. Cell Mol Life Sci 2011;68:587–97.

110. Amsellem V, Gary-Bobo G, Marcos E, et al. Telomere dysfunction causes sustained inflammation in chronic obstructive pulmonary disease. Am J Respir Crit Care Med 2011;184:1358–66.

111. de Boer WI, van Schadewijk A, Sont JK, et al. Transforming growth factor beta1 and recruitment of macrophages and mast cells in airways in chronic obstructive pulmonary disease. Am J Respir Crit Care Med 1998;158:1951–7.

112. Sime PJ. The antifibrogenic potential of PPAR-gamma ligands in pulmonary fibrosis. J Investig Med 2008;56:534–8.

113. Fonseca C, Abraham D, Renzoni EA. Endothelin in pulmonary fibrosis. Am J Respir Cell Mol Biol 2011; 44:1–10.

114. Barnes PJ, Adcock IM. Glucocorticoid resistance in inflammatory diseases. Lancet 2009; 342:1905–17.

115. Cosio BG, Tsaprouni L, Ito K, et al. Theophylline restores histone deacetylase activity and steroid responses in COPD macrophages. J Exp Med 2004;200:689–95.

116. To Y, Ito K, Kizawa Y, et al. Targeting phosphoinositide-3-kinase-delta with theophylline reverses corticosteroid insensitivity in COPD. Am J Respir Crit Care Med 2010;182:897–904.

117. Ford PA, Durham AL, Russell RE, et al. Treatment effects of low dose theophylline combined with an inhaled corticosteroid in COPD. Chest 2010;137: 1338–44.

118. Mercado N, To Y, Ito K, et al. Nortriptyline reverses corticosteroid insensitivity by inhibition of PI3K-δ. J Pharmacol Exp Ther 2011;337:465–70.

119. Meja KK, Rajendrasozhan S, Adenuga D, et al. Curcumin restores corticosteroid function in monocytes exposed to oxidants by maintaining HDAC2. Am J Respir Cell Mol Biol 2008;39:312–23.

120. Kobayashi Y, Wada H, Rossios C, et al. A novel macrolide/fluoroketolide, solithromycin (CEM-101), reverses corticosteroid insensitivity via phosphoinositide 3-kinase pathway inhibition. Br J Pharmacol 2013;169:1024–34.

121. Chong J, Poole P, Leung B, et al. Phosphodiesterase 4 inhibitors for chronic obstructive pulmonary disease. Cochrane Database Syst Rev 2011;(5):CD002309.

122. Barnes PJ, Chowdhury B, Kharitonov SA, et al. Pulmonary biomarkers in chronic obstructive pulmonary disease. Am J Respir Crit Care Med 2006; 174:6–14.

123. Rennard SI, Calverley PM, Goehring UM, et al. Reduction of exacerbations by the PDE4 inhibitor roflumilast–the importance of defining different subsets of patients with COPD. Respir Res 2011; 12:18.

124. Hansel TT, Barnes PJ. New drugs for exacerbations of chronic obstructive pulmonary disease. Lancet 2009;374:744–55.

Role of Infections

Kamen Rangelov, MD[a], Sanjay Sethi, MD[b],*

KEYWORDS

- Infection in COPD • Airway colonization • Chronic infection • New strain exacerbations
- Pneumonia and COPD • Innate immunity in COPD • Virulence factors • Vicious-circle hypothesis

KEY POINTS

- Infection and chronic obstructive pulmonary disease (COPD) can be regarded as comorbid conditions, because infections contribute the progression of COPD, and COPD alters the susceptibility and manifestations of lung infections.
- The underlying mechanism of acute exacerbations of COPD is acquisition of new strains of bacteria and viruses. A complex host-pathogen interaction then determines the clinical manifestations and outcomes of such acquisition.
- COPD predisposes to community-acquired pneumonia and alters its cause, treatment, and outcomes.
- Several lines of evidence now suggest that chronic airway infection by bacteria is prevalent in COPD, and by triggering a chronic inflammatory response contributes to progression of disease.
- Lung innate immune defenses are impaired in COPD, making these patients more susceptible to infection. Respiratory pathogens prevalent in COPD use various mechanisms to evade host responses and thereby cause acute and persistent infections.

INTRODUCTION

The role of infection in chronic obstructive pulmonary disease (COPD) was first postulated in 1953 by Stuart-Harris and colleagues[1] in what is now known as the British hypothesis. They speculated that the decline in the lung function in COPD was the result of mucus hypersecretion and recurrent bacterial infections. In the next 2 decades, several studies were performed to confirm the hypothesis. In some of these studies, sputum microbiology was used to compare the rate of bacterial infection in patients with chronic bronchitis at baseline and during exacerbations, as well as in comparison with individuals without COPD.[2–7] Some differences in bacterial infection related to disease state were found; for example, Smith and colleagues[2,3,8] found increased colonization with

Haemophilus influenzae in patients with severe COPD compared with mild COPD. However, for the most part, differences in the rate of bacterial isolation from sputum at stable state (ie, colonization) versus at acute exacerbation (ie, infection) were not seen in these studies. Advanced molecular biology techniques to differentiate bacterial strains within species had not been developed and were therefore not available to these investigators. Other investigators examined this hypothesis by using serologic studies to determine levels of antibacterial antibodies in patients with chronic bronchitis. These results were also confusing and contradictory and were confounded by the use of laboratory strains as an antigen (discussed in Ref.[9]). In 1977, Fletcher and colleagues[10] published a landmark study that showed

Funding Sources: S. Sethi, supported by VA Merit Review and NHLBI. K. Rangelov, Nil.
Conflict of Interest: The authors declare no conflict of interest.
[a] Pulmonary and Critical Care Medicine, University at Buffalo, SUNY, 3435 Main Street, Buffalo, NY 14214, USA;
[b] Pulmonary, Critical Care, and Sleep Medicine, VA Western New York Healthcare System, University at Buffalo, The State University of New York, 3495 Bailey Avenue, Buffalo, NY 14215, USA
* Corresponding author.
E-mail address: ssethi@buffalo.edu

that frequency of exacerbations and mucus hypersecretion did not result in faster decline of lung function in patients with COPD. By the early 1980s, because of these observations and the appreciation of the importance of tobacco smoke in COPD pathogenesis, the British hypothesis was rejected, and bacterial infection was relegated to an epiphenomenon in this disease.[7]

The role of viral infection in COPD exacerbations was also extensively investigated in the 1960s and 1970s with viral cultures and serology at exacerbation.[3,5,8] Because of the lack of confounding by chronic colonization and serologic cross reactivity, about 30% of exacerbations were confirmed to be of viral origin. Following 20 to –30 years of scant investigation, the role of infection has been revisited in the last 2 decades with new molecular biology, immunology, and microbiology techniques.[11] Understanding of infection in COPD, both in the acute and chronic settings, has consequently developed substantially, as discussed later (**Fig. 1**).

ACUTE INFECTION

Acute infections in COPD are clinically recognized either as exacerbations or as episodes of pneumonia. The differentiation between the two presentations is based on the presence (pneumonia) or absence (exacerbation) of lung parenchymal involvement, which presents as an infiltrate on chest radiology. Although pneumonia has been always considered to be a more significant acute infection, exacerbations occur with much greater frequency and also have serious consequences in COPD. As the British hypothesis was being largely discredited, the importance of exacerbations in COPD was also minimized. They came to

be regarded as self-resolving viral illness of little consequence (chest colds) for which no specific therapy was available and that were part of the natural course of the disease. The last 2 decades have seen considerable revision in this point of view, because data have emerged that exacerbations do contribute to the loss of quality of life and lung function in COPD and account for as much as half the cost of care of COPD. Furthermore, bacterial infection contributes to exacerbations, specific therapies are of benefit, and prevention of exacerbations is possible and is an important therapeutic goal in COPD.

Causes of Exacerbations

Exacerbations of COPD are airway inflammatory events that are induced by infection in most instances. The aggravating infection can be viral, bacterial, or a combination of viral and bacterial infections. Although there are episodes that are induced by poorly understood noninfectious factors, infections likely account for about 80% of exacerbations (**Table 1**).

Virus

The role of viruses in exacerbation was established in older studies (as discussed earlier) by viral culture and serology. Understanding of viral exacerbations has recently been expanded by the use of molecular diagnostic techniques and with the development of a human experimental model of rhinoviral exacerbations. The most common viruses detected in airway secretions at exacerbation are rhinovirus, influenza, respiratory syncytial virus (RSV), parainfluenza, and adenovirus. A recent systematic review found that viruses were detected in 34.1% of exacerbations.[12] More recent studies using molecular detection of virus

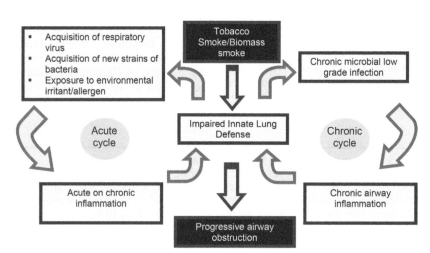

Fig. 1. Acute and chronic infection cycles in the pathogenesis of COPD.

Table 1
Microbial pathogens in COPD

Microbe	Role in Exacerbations	Role in Stable Disease
Bacteria		
H influenzae	20%–30% of exacerbations	Major pathogen
Streptococcus pneumoniae	10%–15% of exacerbations	Minor role
Moraxella catarrhalis	10%–15% of exacerbations	Minor role
Pseudomonas aeruginosa	5%–10% of exacerbations, prevalent in advanced disease	Likely important in advanced disease
Enterobacteriaceae	Isolated in advanced disease, pathogenic significance undefined	Undefined
Haemophilus haemolyticus	Isolated frequently, unlikely cause	Unlikely
Haemophilus parainfluenzae	Isolated frequently, unlikely cause	Unlikely
Staphylococcus aureus	Isolated infrequently, unlikely cause	Unlikely
Viruses		
Rhinovirus	20%–25% of exacerbations	Unlikely
Parainfluenza	5%–10% of exacerbations	Unlikely
Influenza	5%–10% of exacerbations	Unlikely
Respiratory syncytial virus	5%–10% of exacerbations	Controversial
Coronavirus	5%–10% of exacerbations	Unlikely
Adenovirus	3%–5% of exacerbations	Latent infection seen, pathogenic significance undefined
Human metapneumovirus	3%–5% of exacerbations	Unlikely
Atypical Bacteria		
Chlamydophila pneumoniae	3%–5% of exacerbations	Commonly detected, pathogenic significance undefined
Mycoplasma pneumoniae	1%–2%	Unlikely
Fungi		
Pneumocystis jiroveci	Undefined	Commonly detected, pathogenic significance undefined

From Sethi S, Murphy TF. Infection in the pathogenesis and course of chronic obstructive pulmonary disease. N Engl J Med 2008;359:2356; with permission.

by polymerase chain reaction (PCR) techniques have found viruses in up to half of all exacerbations.[13] The human experimental model of rhinoviral exacerbations was described in a study in which 13 subjects with COPD and 13 control subjects were nasally inoculated with a low dose of rhinovirus.[14] An increased neutrophilic inflammatory response in the lower airway, and more prominent lower respiratory symptoms and airway obstruction, were found in COPD compared with controls. An impaired interferon response to the infection was seen in patients with COPD. This work confirms the viral causation of exacerbations and has provided insights into susceptibility and pathogenic mechanisms involved in viral exacerbations.

Bacteria

In contrast with the role of viruses, the role of bacteria as a cause of exacerbations has been controversial and was not fully appreciated until recently. At present, pathogens clearly implicated in COPD exacerbations are nontypeable H influenzae, Streptococcus pneumoniae, Moraxella catarrhalis, and Pseudomonas aeruginosa. Whether Staphylococcus aureus and gram-negative enteric bacteria (Enterobacteriaceae), which are frequently isolated from sputum in COPD, are causative for exacerbations or are only capable of airway colonization is unclear at present.

Previous studies that defined bacterial pathogens isolated from sputum only at a species level were unable to fully appreciate the dynamic nature of bacterial infection in COPD. In a longitudinal prospective cohort study in patients with COPD, when bacterial strains in sputum were characterized by molecular techniques, combined with a careful analysis of host immune and immunologic responses, an important mechanism that likely underlies exacerbations caused by the 4 major pathogens listed earlier was found (**Fig. 2**).[15] The risk of having an exacerbation was increased by more than 2-fold with respiratory tract acquisition of strains of these bacterial pathogens that were new to the patient. In this initial study, 33% of the visits within a month of new strain acquisition were associated with an exacerbation compared with 15.4% without a new strain.[16] Subsequent analyses from this study have now shown that the incidence of exacerbations at a visit with a new strain isolated from sputum is 40% to 50%, and that this holds true for each of the 4 major pathogens (nontypeable *H influenzae*, *S pneumoniae*, *M catarrhalis*, and *P aeruginosa*).[17–19] Additional support for this mechanism for exacerbations comes from various observations. Exacerbation-associated strains of *H influenzae* are more inflammatory in in vitro and animal models than strains associated with colonization, showing that clinical implications of bacterial acquisition correlate with strain virulence.[20] Strain-specific host immune

response and a vigorous neutrophilic inflammatory response distinguish new strain exacerbations from those without new strains.[21]

Whether an increase in bacterial concentration (load) in the airway of a preexisting (colonizing) strain can be an additional independent mechanism of exacerbations is controversial. When bacterial sputum concentrations from our longitudinal cohort study were analyzed, either no differences or small differences were found between stable disease and exacerbation, and the small differences were no longer seen once new strain acquisition was taken into account.[21] In contrast, Rosell and colleagues[22] showed in pooled analysis of their data from bronchoscopic protected brush specimens that 54% of the patients with COPD exacerbation had pathogenic bacteria present in their airway secretions at significant concentrations compared with 29% of the patients with stable COPD. Intracellular *H influenzae* was found in bronchial mucosal biopsies in 87% of intubated patients with COPD exacerbation, compared with 33% of the patients with stable COPD.[23] Garcha and colleagues,[24] using quantitative PCR, found higher sputum bacterial loads at exacerbation than at stable state. However, these studies that have shown higher bacterial loads in sputum at exacerbation have not taken into account bacterial strain variation in their specimens.

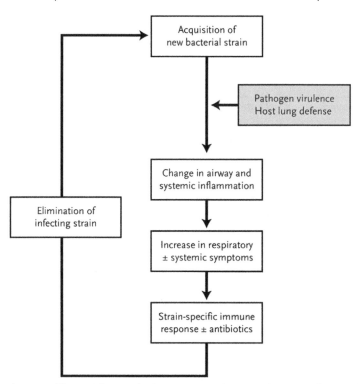

Fig. 2. Proposed mechanism of bacterial exacerbations in COPD. (*From* Sethi S, Murphy TF. Infection in the pathogenesis and course of chronic obstructive pulmonary disease. N Engl J Med 2008;359:2357; with permission.)

Coinfection with virus and bacteria

A few recent studies have examined the impact of simultaneous or sequential bacterial and viral infection at exacerbation. Papi and colleagues[25] examined 64 patients with COPD exacerbation requiring hospital admission; 25% had combined bacterial and viral infections, and these patients had more severe symptoms and longer hospitalization. Presence of cold symptoms and *H influenzae* in sputum has also been associated with more symptoms and a larger decrease in lung function than when either is present alone.[26] In the rhinoviral human experimental model discussed earlier, as many as 60% of patients with COPD developed a secondary bacterial infection with a greater inflammatory response and duration of symptoms.[27] However, the severity of the exacerbations was mild and none of the patients required steroids or antibiotics.

It is likely that viral infection predisposes the susceptible host to bacterial coinfection and vice versa.[28,29] In cultured airway epithelial cells, Sajjan and colleagues[29] found that infection with *H influenzae* increased expression of intercellular adhesion molecule (ICAM)-1 and Toll-like receptor (TLR)-3, receptors for rhinovirus and its double-stranded RNA. In contrast, in another experimental model, Avadhanula and colleagues[28] found increased bacterial adhesion to respiratory epithelial cells after viral infection. In the human rhinovirus experimental model, degradation of antimicrobial peptides such as elafin by neutrophil elastase could explain the occurrence of secondary bacterial infection.[27]

In summary, bacterial and viral infections play a critical role in COPD exacerbations. Application of molecular diagnostic techniques to exacerbations is likely to further enhance understanding of infectious episodes. The role of opportunistic bacterial pathogens in causing exacerbations still needs to be defined.

Community-acquired Pneumonia

Epidemiology

Community-acquired pneumonia (CAP) is a major cause of morbidity and mortality worldwide, with incidence of 2.6 to 11 per 1000 adults.[30,31] Mortality can reach 20%, with 14.9% of the mortality risk attributed to smoking, second only to age.[32] In a multivariate analysis, COPD was an independent risk factor for developing severe CAP, with an odds ratio (OR) of 1.91.[33] Evaluation of COPD subgroups revealed that severe COPD on home oxygen and severe COPD exacerbations requiring hospitalization were independent risk factors for developing CAP.[34] Merino-Sanchez and

colleagues[35] observed a 12.6% incidence of pneumonia in 596 patients with COPD over 3 years, with 55% of the cases with Pneumonia Severity Index (PSI) of 4 and 5. The mortality for a PSI of 5 was 35.7%. In 2 European studies, hospitalized patients with CAP with and without COPD were compared. Although mortality differences between the groups were not seen, patients with COPD experienced more severe pneumonia, higher rates of readmission, and recurrent pneumonia. Lower serum tumor necrosis factor alpha (TNF-α) and interleukin-6 levels were seen in the COPD group, suggesting an impaired inflammatory response in these patients.[36,37] Higher mortality with CAP in COPD has been observed in other studies, reiterating the importance of early recognition and appropriate management in this high-risk population.[38–40]

Causes of CAP in COPD

S pneumoniae remains the most common cause of CAP in COPD. However, because of alterations in the lung microbiome in COPD, pathogens such as *H influenzae*, *M catarrhalis*, and *P aeruginosa* may play a larger role in the development of CAP in these patients. Moreover, patients with COPD are exposed to frequent antibiotic courses and they are more likely to be infected with antibiotic-resistant pathogens, making empiric antibiotic choices challenging.[41] In a study of hospitalized patients with COPD with CAP, more infections attributable to *P aeruginosa* were observed.[42] However, the use of respiratory specimens to determine the microbiological cause of CAP in COPD is challenging, because chronic colonization with CAP-associated pathogens is common in COPD.

Role of inhaled corticosteroids

Inhaled corticosteroids (ICS), in combination with long acting beta agonists (LABA), are widely used in COPD, and reduce the frequency of exacerbations and daily symptoms in these patients.[43] However, the benefits come at a cost of increased risk of pneumonia. This increased risk was originally observed in the TORCH (Toward a Revolution in COPD Health) study, in which the ICS/LABA group had a higher probability (19.6%) of developing pneumonia over the course of 3 years.[43] A recent meta-analysis of 24 randomized controlled trials of ICS in COPD confirmed these results with a calculated relative risk of developing pneumonia at 1.56, and a number needed to harm of 60.[44–46] However, mortality was no different from the use of a LABA alone. The association between ICS use and pneumonia should be interpreted with caution. None of these trials were specifically designed to assess the risk of pneumonia, most episodes lack radiological confirmation, and COPD exacerbations may have been misdiagnosed as pneumonia. Mechanisms underlying this association have not been examined, but corticosteroid-induced impairment of local immune response to microbial pathogens is likely responsible.

Antimicrobial therapy in COPD and CAP

In outpatients with CAP, the presence of COPD as a comorbid condition places them in a high-risk group, and treatment with a respiratory fluoroquinolone or a β-lactam plus a macrolide is recommended.[47] Monotherapy with a macrolide or doxycycline is not appropriate in these patients. Because antibiotic use is common in these patients, a review of antibiotic use in the previous 3 months should guide empiric choice, and antibiotic classes used in the previous 3 months should be avoided. Among inpatients with CAP and COPD, the same choices are applicable. However, in patients requiring intensive care admission, combination therapy is always recommended, with a β-lactam and a respiratory fluoroquinolone or a macrolide. If *Pseudomonas* is suspected (previous *Pseudomonas* isolation, bronchiectasis, malnutrition, recent broad-spectrum antibiotic exposure), an antipseudomonal regimen is recommended.

CHRONIC INFECTION

In contrast with the (almost) sterile airways of a healthy lung, the lower airway of patients with COPD is frequently colonized with bacteria.[48,49] Although a wide variety of pathogens can be isolated, the two most common are *H influenzae* and *P aeruginosa* (see **Table 1**). Until recently, the presence of these bacteria was regarded as colonization, implying an innocuous process in the airway without sequelae. A growing body of evidence now suggests that this colonization in stable COPD, via complex interactions with the host immune-inflammatory system, could contribute to COPD pathogenesis and progression.

Vicious-circle Hypothesis

Similar to bronchiectasis and cystic fibrosis, the host-pathogen interaction in stable COPD is well described by the vicious-circle hypothesis (**Fig. 3**). Repeated insults to the lung, such as smoking and environmental exposures, lead to impairment of the host immune defenses, thus allowing bacterial colonization. The bacteria cause subclinical inflammatory response in the airway, resulting in further damage to the innate lung defense and persistence of chronic bacterial infection. This process accelerates during acute exacerbations.

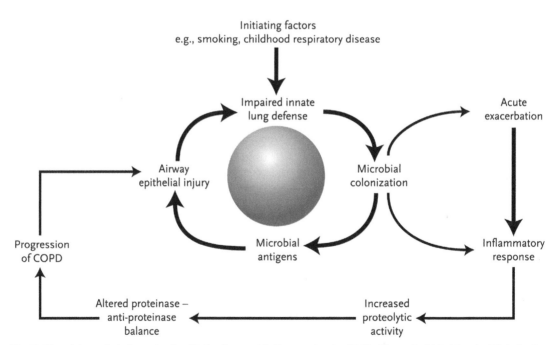

Fig. 3. The vicious-circle hypothesis of infection and inflammation in COPD. (*From* Sethi S, Murphy TF. Infection in the pathogenesis and course of chronic obstructive pulmonary disease. N Engl J Med 2008;359:2361; with permission.)

Evidence to Support Chronic Infection

Colonization is defined by the absence of damaging effects to the host related to the presence of a pathogen and the absence of a specific immune response. There are several parts of the body where such colonization is seen (eg, skin, colon) and is essential for health. The microbial pathogens that colonize these surfaces constitute a microbiome. Recent advances in research technologies, especially high-throughput genomic characterization, have made it possible to characterize the microbiome. The healthy lung is sterile by standard culture techniques. Even with molecular techniques, the microbiome of the healthy lung is sparse and transient, composed primarily of oral flora that are microaspirated and cleared.[50] In contrast, in a third of patients with COPD, potential respiratory pathogens can be retrieved by culture of lower airway samples.[49,51] An abundant microbiome can be found by molecular techniques in COPD lungs.[52] Unlike other body surfaces, like the skin and gut mucosa, the lung is not well equipped to handle a microbiome. Therefore, microbial presence in the lower airways in COPD is harmful.

Several studies have described excess inflammation in stable patients with COPD when colonized with bacterial pathogens.[51,53–56] The airway inflammation associated with bacterial colonization is predominantly neutrophilic. Studies comparing sputum samples from colonized and noncolonized patients have found higher levels of TNF-α, interleukin-8, interleukin-6, leukotriene B4, neutrophil myeloperoxidase, and elastase, and lower levels of the antiprotease secretory leukocyte protease inhibitor.[53,54,56,57] Bronchoscopic sampling of the lower airway with bronchoalveolar lavage showed increased levels of neutrophils, TNF-α, interleukin-8, matrix metalloproteinase 9, and endotoxin in association with bacterial colonization.[49,51,58] Although several mediators contribute to COPD pathogenesis, interleukin-8 in particular has been associated with increased exacerbation frequency, longer recovery periods, worsening airway obstruction, and development of bronchiectasis.[58,59] Bacterial (M catarrhalis) acquisition, even without an increase in symptoms of an exacerbation, has been associated with increases in proteolytic activity and a reduction in antiproteolytic defense, resulting in worsening of the protease/antiprotease imbalance that is thought to cause progressive lung damage in COPD.[56] The inflammatory profile seen with bacterial colonization is similar to that seen with bacterial exacerbations, implying that colonization is a low-grade infection.

Following exacerbations of COPD, specific immune responses, both systemic and mucosal, to the infecting strain are often observed. Similar observations have now been described following colonization.[18,19] This active immune response supports the presence of chronic infection in COPD. Furthermore, with M catarrhalis, a differential immune response is seen with colonization, which is accompanied by a stronger mucosal immune response, compared with a stronger systemic immune response accompanying exacerbations.[18] Whether the nature of the immune response dictates the clinical expression of infection or vice versa is not clear.

The potential contribution of viral and atypical pathogens to chronic infection in COPD has been controversial. Latent adenoviral infection of the lungs, in the form of integration of portions of adenoviral DNA into cellular DNA, was found to enhance the inflammatory response to tobacco smoke, and thereby was thought to contribute to COPD pathogenesis.[60] Initial studies showed that such adenoviral integration was more common in COPD than in controls; however, subsequent studies have not supported this observation. Latent RSV infection has been described in COPD by one group of investigators, but has not been found by others.[61,62] The presence and contribution of chronic chlamydial lung infection in COPD remains similarly controversial, with inconsistent observations from various investigators.

Besides the direct microbiological evidence of infection and its consequences, other indirect lines of evidence of chronic infection in COPD have emerged from radiological and pathologic studies. In a pathologic study of small airways of patients with COPD, the extent of formation of lymphoid aggregates predominantly composed of B cells had the best correlation with the degree of airflow obstruction.[63] It is likely that these aggregates represent a local host immune response to chronic microbial infection. Furthermore, this pathologic finding was replicated in a mouse model of chronic inflammation in the lungs induced by repeated instillation of nontypeable H influenzae lysate.[64]

Widespread use of high resolution computed tomography scans has revealed that bronchiectasis develops in a substantial proportion of patients with COPD. In a comprehensive study of 92 patients with stable moderate or severe disease, 57.5% had bronchiectasis, and its presence was related to worse lung function, hospital admission in the past year, and chronic bronchitic symptoms.[65] Repeated sputum cultures in these patients linked chronic colonization with potential bacterial pathogens (predominantly nontypeable

H influenzae and *P aeruginosa*) with the presence of bronchiectasis.[65]

In summary, these various lines of investigation support the paradigm of a vicious circle of infection and inflammation in COPD. However, COPD is a heterogeneous disease and it is likely that in 30% to 50% of these patients chronic infection plays a prominent role, these being the ones with chronic colonization, bronchiectasis, and/or chronic bronchitis. Future longitudinal natural history studies or studies with interventions that decrease bacterial colonization and measure disease progression are needed to prove the vicious-circle hypothesis.

Mechanism of Increased Susceptibility to Infection in COPD

Although infection is a comorbid condition in COPD and much has been learned about the incidence and consequences of infection in this disease, understanding of the mechanisms underlying increased susceptibility to infection seen in COPD is still in its early stages. Alterations in both the host and pathogen can contribute to establishment of acute and chronic infections, and both play a role in COPD. Disruptions in the host that increase susceptibility to infection can be categorized into changes in innate or adaptive lung defense. Pathogen alterations include host defense evasion mechanisms.

Host Defects: Innate Immunity

The healthy lung possesses a multilayered, redundant, and highly efficient innate defense system that allows it to maintain an almost pathogen-free environment in spite of being constantly exposed to a variety of microbes through inhalation and microaspiration. This innate immune system of the lung has 3 components: mechanical barrier, humoral, and cellular response systems. This nonspecific immunity is the first line of defense against viruses, bacteria, and other particulates. It recognizes antigenic ligands entering the airway via pattern-recognition receptors and triggers series of responses resulting in complement activation and phagocytosis. The end result is elimination of the antigen or its presentation on the surface of the macrophages and activation of the adaptive immunity. In patients with COPD, several innate responses are impaired, leading to increased susceptibility to infection.

Mucociliary clearance
The mucociliary clearance is the first barrier to noxious agents, by effectively trapping and clearing inhaled and microaspirated microbial pathogens. Both normal mucus and a normal ciliary apparatus are required for effective mucociliary clearance. Abnormal mucus (such as in cystic fibrosis) and a dysfunctional ciliary apparatus (such as in ciliary dyskinesia) are associated with acute and chronic bronchial infection. Augmented mucus production can be regarded as a defensive response to particulate or microbial exposure. However, when the exposure is chronic, and inflammation and ciliary dysfunction are also present, it could worsen mucociliary clearance.

Smoking disrupts mucociliary clearance, not only by augmenting mucus production but also by inducing structural abnormalities in the ciliary apparatus.[66] Studies in moderate to heavy smokers have shown longer lung clearance times, although the degree of impairment is variable.[67,68] Further deterioration in mucociliary clearance is seen with development of chronic bronchitis and airway obstruction in smokers.[69–71] Patients with COPD have hypertrophy and hyperplasia of their airway goblet cells and increased mucus stores.[72,73] In tissue and animal models, exposure to *S pneumoniae* and *H influenzae* results in further upregulation of mucin production.[74,75] Neutrophilic inflammation also worsens mucociliary function, mediated by increased mucus production, reduced ciliary beating, and altered viscoelastic properties of mucus.

Immunoglobulin A
Immunoglobulin (Ig) A, especially polymeric secretory IgA, plays an important role in innate defense by coating the bacterial pathogen, thereby interfering with its ability to interact with the mucosal surface (immune exclusion). IgA can also neutralize infectious agents and could act as an opsonin assisting in pathogen elimination. Localized areas of IgA deficiency in the large and small airways are seen in COPD that were associated with squamous metaplasia. Polymeric IgG receptor expression, a receptor required for transcytosis of the IgA molecule from the basolateral to the apical surface of the epithelial cell, was reduced in these areas.[76] These changes in IgA could be an important mechanism of infection susceptibility in COPD.

Antimicrobial peptides
Antimicrobial polypeptides abundant in the airway surface lining fluid have antimicrobial and immunoregulatory functions. One major group, the cationic polypeptides, includes lysozyme, lactoferrin, defensins, the cathelicidins (LL-37), and secretory leukocyte protease inhibitor (SLPI).[77–82] Another important group, the collectins, include surfactant protein-A (SP-A), surfactant protein-D

(SP-D), and mannose-binding lectin.[83] Complex and dynamic alterations in various antimicrobial polypeptides have been described in COPD, both in the stable state and during exacerbations.

Deficiencies of SLPI and lysozyme in the stable state have been associated with more frequent exacerbations.[84,85] Decreased serum mannose-binding lectin has been linked with exacerbation frequency in COPD, but this has not been a consistent observation.[86] Lower airway concentrations of SP-A and SP-D are seen in smokers, with further decreases in association with emphysema.[87,88] Lower levels of beta-defensin 2 and Clara Cell Protein 16 (CC16) and increased levels of elafin and SLPI in sputum supernatants in stable COPD have been observed.[89] Decreased levels of beta-defensin 2 in the central airways, but not in the distal airways, of smokers with COPD were found in a study of resected lung specimens.[90]

Dynamic changes in antimicrobial peptides have also been described with exacerbations of COPD. SLPI levels decrease significantly at the time of such exacerbations, which return to baseline after resolution.[78] Lysozyme and lactoferrin levels decrease and LL-37 levels increase with both

colonization and infective exacerbations with H influenzae and M catarrhalis.[78] In a human model of rhinoviral infection, impaired elafin and SLPI responses following rhinoviral infection were associated with secondary bacterial infection.[27]

Macrophage function

Key cellular components on innate lung defense are alveolar macrophages and airway epithelial cells. Phagocytic and cytokine responses of alveolar macrophages to bacterial pathogens are crucial for dealing with small pathogen inocula, without invoking potentially damaging inflammatory and adaptive immune responses. Alveolar macrophages from patients with COPD show impaired ability to phagocytose H influenzae and M catarrhalis, but not S pneumoniae or inert microspheres. This impairment is correlated with worsening lung function (**Fig. 4**).[91] Alveolar macrophages from patients with COPD also have a less robust cytokine response to bacterial proteins, specifically outer membrane protein P6 and lipo-oligosaccharide (endotoxin) of H influenzae.[92–94] Following exposure to rhinovirus, alveolar macrophages showed decreased cytokine responses to bacterial

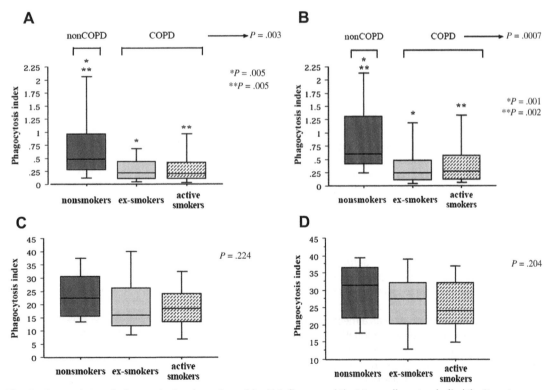

Fig. 4. Comparison of phagocytosis of nontypeable *H influenzae* (*A*), *Moraxella catarrhalis* (*B*), *Streptococcus pneumoniae* (*C*), and latex microspheres (*D*) by human alveolar macrophages from healthy controls, current smokers with COPD, and ex-smokers with COPD. (*Modified from* Berenson CS, Kruzel RL, Eberhardt E, et al. Phagocytic dysfunction of human alveolar macrophages and severity of chronic obstructive pulmonary disease. J Infect Dis 2013; with permission.)

lipopolysaccharide and lipoteichoic acid,[95] which could explain the increased susceptibility to bacterial infection after viral infection in COPD.

These decrements in macrophage function are likely secondary to several mechanisms, including reduction in pattern-recognition receptors such as Toll-like receptors TLR2 and TLR4, reduction in scavenger receptors such as macrophage receptor with collagenous structure (MARCO), or alteration in subpopulations of macrophages in the airway.[96–98] TLR2 has been found to be downregulated in smokers, patients with COPD, and farmers exposed to organic dust.[96,99,100] TLR4 downregulation is associated with the development of emphysema and worse airflow limitation in smokers.[101] Polymorphism T399I of the TLR4 gene has been associated with development of COPD phenotype in smokers.[102]

Pathogen Mechanisms

Tissue invasion

H influenzae was traditionally regarded as an extracellular pathogen. However, molecular detection techniques have shown this pathogen in the bronchial epithelium and inside subepithelial macrophages in COPD.[23,48] These tissue bacteria could be shielded from the actions of antibiotics and antibodies, and therefore could be more resistant to eradication. Molecular detection often detects *H influenzae* in airway secretions and lung samples when cultures are negative, which could be explained by such tissue invasion.

Biofilm formation

Biofilms are bacteria encased with an extracellular matrix, which is usually composed of polysaccharides produced and secreted by bacteria. Bacteria in the core of the film, which is predominantly anaerobic, are in a low metabolic state. Antibiotic penetration into biofilms is limited, requiring up to 1000 times higher concentrations to achieve eradication.[103] Parts of the biofilm can detach and cause distant infection. Pathogens common in COPD, including *H influenzae*, *M catarrhalis*, and *P aeruginosa*, are capable of biofilm formation. Furthermore, smoke exposure has been shown to increase biofilm formation.[104] *P aeruginosa* in cystic fibrosis is the prototypical example of biofilm formation as a mechanism of persistence in the lung. Whether bacterial biofilms are present in COPD airways is not yet known.[105] Mucoid *P aeruginosa* and some strains of *H influenzae* persist clinically for long periods in spite of repeated antibiotic exposure, which is reminiscent of cystic fibrosis.

Antigenic alteration

Pathogens can evade the host immune response by alteration of their surface proteins, which are targets of the host immune system. The P2 outer membrane protein of *H influenzae*, which is a major target of bactericidal antibodies in COPD, shows extensive antigenic variation among strains of this pathogen.[106] Serial persistent isolates of *H influenzae* in COPD show diminution of high-molecular-weight adhesin expression, which could represent another immune evasion mechanism.[107]

FUTURE DIRECTIONS

The role of infection in COPD is an evolving topic with extensive ongoing research trying to better understand host-pathogen interactions and find suitable targets for intervention. Although exacerbation pathogenesis is better understood now, much still needs to be learned about pathogen virulence and causal overlap. The vicious-circle hypothesis exposes the complex interactions between smoking, innate immunity, and respiratory pathogens. Augmentation and modulation of the innate and adaptive host immunity as well as formulation of novel antibacterial agents and vaccines are paramount in future research and development in COPD.

REFERENCES

1. Stuart-Harris CH, Pownall M, Scothorne CM, et al. The factor of infection in chronic bronchitis. Q J Med 1953;22:121–32.
2. Smith CB, Golden CA, Kanner RE, et al. *Haemophilus influenzae* and *Haemophilus parainfluenzae* in chronic obstructive pulmonary disease. Lancet 1976;1:1253–5.
3. Smith CB, Golden C, Klauber MR, et al. Interactions between viruses and bacteria in patients with chronic bronchitis. J Infect Dis 1976;134:552–61.
4. Gump DW, Phillips CA, Forsyth BR, et al. Role of infection in chronic bronchitis. Am Rev Respir Dis 1976;113:465–73.
5. McHardy VU, Inglis JM, Calder MA, et al. A study of infective and other factors in exacerbations of chronic bronchitis. Br J Dis Chest 1980;74:228–38.
6. Fagon JY, Chastre J. Severe exacerbations of COPD patients: the role of pulmonary infections. Semin Respir Infect 1996;11:109–18.
7. Tager I, Speizer FE. Role of infection in chronic bronchitis. N Engl J Med 1975;292:563–71.
8. Smith CB, Golden C, Kanner R, et al. Association of viral and *Mycoplasma pneumoniae* infections with acute respiratory illness in patients with chronic obstructive pulmonary diseases. Am Rev Respir Dis 1980;121:225–32.

9. Murphy TF, Sethi S. Bacterial infection in chronic obstructive pulmonary disease. Am Rev Respir Dis 1992;146:1067–83.

10. Fletcher F, Peto R. The natural history of chronic airflow obstruction. Br Med J 1977;1:1645–8.

11. Sethi S, Murphy TF. Infection in the pathogenesis and course of chronic obstructive pulmonary disease. N Engl J Med 2008;359:2355–65.

12. Mohan A, Chandra S, Agarwal D, et al. Prevalence of viral infection detected by PCR and RT-PCR in patients with acute exacerbation of COPD: a systematic review. Respirology 2010;15:536–42.

13. Kherad O, Kaiser L, Bridevaux PO, et al. Upper-respiratory viral infection, biomarkers, and COPD exacerbations. Chest 2010;138:896–904.

14. Mallia P, Message SD, Gielen V, et al. Experimental rhinovirus infection as a human model of chronic obstructive pulmonary disease exacerbation. Am J Respir Crit Care Med 2011;183:734–42.

15. Sethi S, Sethi R, Eschberger K, et al. Airway bacterial concentrations and exacerbations of chronic obstructive pulmonary disease. Am J Respir Crit Care Med 2007;176(4):356–61.

16. Sethi S, Evans N, Grant BJ, et al. New strains of bacteria and exacerbations of chronic obstructive pulmonary disease. N Engl J Med 2002;347:465–71.

17. Murphy TF, Brauer AL, Sethi S, et al. *Haemophilus haemolyticus*: a human respiratory tract commensal to be distinguished from *Haemophilus influenzae*. J Infect Dis 2007;195:81–9.

18. Murphy TF, Brauer AL, Grant BJ, et al. *Moraxella catarrhalis* in chronic obstructive pulmonary disease: burden of disease and immune response. Am J Respir Crit Care Med 2005;172:195–9.

19. Murphy TF, Brauer AL, Eschberger K, et al. *Pseudomonas aeruginosa* in chronic obstructive pulmonary disease. Am J Respir Crit Care Med 2008;177:853–60.

20. Chin CL, Manzel LJ, Lehman EE, et al. *Haemophilus influenzae* from patients with chronic obstructive pulmonary disease exacerbation induce more inflammation than colonizers. Am J Respir Crit Care Med 2005;172:85–91.

21. Sethi S, Wrona C, Eschberger K, et al. Inflammatory profile of new bacterial strain exacerbations of chronic obstructive pulmonary disease. Am J Respir Crit Care Med 2008;177:491–7.

22. Rosell A, Monso E, Soler N, et al. Microbiologic determinants of exacerbation in chronic obstructive pulmonary disease. Arch Intern Med 2005;165:891–7.

23. Bandi V, Apicella MA, Mason E, et al. Nontypeable *Haemophilus influenzae* in the lower respiratory tract of patients with chronic bronchitis. Am J Respir Crit Care Med 2001;164:2114–9.

24. Garcha DS, Thurston SJ, Patel AR, et al. Changes in prevalence and load of airway bacteria using quantitative PCR in stable and exacerbated COPD. Thorax 2012;67:1075–80.

25. Papi A, Bellettato CM, Braccioni F, et al. Infections and airway inflammation in chronic obstructive pulmonary disease severe exacerbations. Am J Respir Crit Care Med 2006;173:1114–21.

26. Wilkinson TM, Hurst JR, Perera WR, et al. Effect of interactions between lower airway bacterial and rhinoviral infection in exacerbations of COPD. Chest 2006;129:317–24.

27. Mallia P, Footitt J, Sotero R, et al. Rhinovirus infection induces degradation of antimicrobial peptides and secondary bacterial infection in chronic obstructive pulmonary disease. Am J Respir Crit Care Med 2012;186:1117–24.

28. Avadhanula V, Rodriguez CA, Devincenzo JP, et al. Respiratory viruses augment the adhesion of bacterial pathogens to respiratory epithelium in a viral species- and cell type-dependent manner. J Virol 2006;80:1629–36.

29. Sajjan US, Jia Y, Newcomb DC, et al. *H. influenzae* potentiates airway epithelial cell responses to rhinovirus by increasing ICAM-1 and TLR3 expression. FASEB J 2006;20:2121–3.

30. Marston BJ, Plouffe JF, File TM Jr, et al. Incidence of community-acquired pneumonia requiring hospitalization. Results of a population-based active surveillance Study in Ohio. The Community-Based Pneumonia Incidence Study Group. Arch Intern Med 1997;157:1709–18.

31. Vinogradova Y, Hippisley-Cox J, Coupland C. Identification of new risk factors for pneumonia: population-based case-control study. Br J Gen Pract 2009;59:e329–38.

32. Naucler P, Darenberg J, Morfeldt E, et al. Contribution of host, bacterial factors and antibiotic treatment to mortality in adult patients with bacteraemic pneumococcal pneumonia. Thorax 2013;68:571–9.

33. Ishiguro T, Takayanagi N, Yamaguchi S, et al. Etiology and factors contributing to the severity and mortality of community-acquired pneumonia. Intern Med 2013;52:317–24.

34. Mullerova H, Chigbo C, Hagan GW, et al. The natural history of community-acquired pneumonia in COPD patients: a population database analysis. Respir Med 2012;106:1124–33.

35. Merino-Sanchez M, Alfageme-Michavila I, Reyes-Nunez N, et al. Prognosis in patients with pneumonia and chronic obstructive pulmonary disease. Arch Bronconeumol 2005;41:607–11 [in Spanish].

36. Crisafulli E, Menendez R, Huerta A, et al. Systemic inflammatory pattern of patients with community-acquired pneumonia with and without COPD. Chest 2013;143:1009–17.

37. Liapikou A, Polverino E, Ewig S, et al. Severity and outcomes of hospitalised community-acquired

pneumonia in COPD patients. Eur Respir J 2012; 39:855–61.

38. Arancibia F, Bauer TT, Ewig S, et al. Community-acquired pneumonia due to gram-negative bacteria and *Pseudomonas aeruginosa*: incidence, risk, and prognosis. Arch Intern Med 2002;162: 1849–58.

39. Torres A, Dorca J, Zalacain R, et al. Community-acquired pneumonia in chronic obstructive pulmonary disease: a Spanish multicenter study. Am J Respir Crit Care Med 1996;154:1456–61.

40. Rello J, Rodriguez A, Torres A, et al. Implications of COPD in patients admitted to the intensive care unit by community-acquired pneumonia. Eur Respir J 2006;27:1210–6.

41. Desai H, Richter S, Doern G, et al. Antibiotic resistance in sputum isolates of *Streptococcus pneumoniae* in chronic obstructive pulmonary disease is related to antibiotic exposure. COPD 2010;7: 337–44.

42. Restrepo MI, Mortensen EM, Pugh JA, et al. COPD is associated with increased mortality in patients with community-acquired pneumonia. Eur Respir J 2006;28:346–51.

43. Calverley PM, Anderson JA, Celli B, et al. Salmeterol and fluticasone propionate and survival in chronic obstructive pulmonary disease. N Engl J Med 2007;356:775–89.

44. Singh S, Loke YK. An overview of the benefits and drawbacks of inhaled corticosteroids in chronic obstructive pulmonary disease. Int J Chron Obstruct Pulmon Dis 2010;5:189–95.

45. Singh S, Amin AV, Loke YK. Long-term use of inhaled corticosteroids and the risk of pneumonia in chronic obstructive pulmonary disease: a meta-analysis. Arch Intern Med 2009;169:219–29.

46. Spencer S, Karner C, Cates CJ, et al. Inhaled corticosteroids versus long-acting beta(2)-agonists for chronic obstructive pulmonary disease. Cochrane Database Syst Rev 2011;(12):CD007033.

47. Mandell LA, Wunderink RG, Anzueto A, et al. Infectious Diseases Society of America/American Thoracic Society consensus guidelines on the management of community-acquired pneumonia in adults. Clin Infect Dis 2007;44(Suppl 2):S27–72.

48. Murphy TF, Brauer AL, Schiffmacher AT, et al. Persistent colonization by *Haemophilus influenzae* in chronic obstructive pulmonary disease. Am J Respir Crit Care Med 2004;170:266–72.

49. Sethi S, Maloney J, Grove L, et al. Airway inflammation and bronchial bacterial colonization in chronic obstructive pulmonary disease. Am J Respir Crit Care Med 2006;173:991–8.

50. Charlson ES, Bittinger K, Haas AR, et al. Topographical continuity of bacterial populations in the healthy human respiratory tract. Am J Respir Crit Care Med 2011;184:957–63.

51. Soler N, Ewig S, Torres A, et al. Airway inflammation and bronchial microbial patterns in patients with stable chronic obstructive pulmonary disease. Eur Respir J 1999;14:1015–22.

52. Cabrera-Rubio R, Garcia-Nunez M, Seto L, et al. Microbiome diversity in the bronchial tracts of patients with chronic obstructive pulmonary disease. J Clin Microbiol 2012;50:3562–8.

53. Bresser P, Out TA, van Alphen L, et al. Airway inflammation in nonobstructive and obstructive chronic bronchitis with chronic *Haemophilus influenzae* airway infection. Comparison with noninfected patients with chronic obstructive pulmonary disease. Am J Respir Crit Care Med 2000;162:947–52.

54. Banerjee D, Khair OA, Honeybourne D. Impact of sputum bacteria on airway inflammation and health status in clinical stable COPD. Eur Respir J 2004; 23:685–91.

55. Hill AT, Campbell EJ, Hill SL, et al. Association between airway bacterial load and markers of airway inflammation in patients with stable chronic bronchitis. Am J Med 2000;109:288–95.

56. Parameswaran GI, Wrona CT, Murphy TF, et al. *Moraxella catarrhalis* acquisition, airway inflammation and protease-antiprotease balance in chronic obstructive pulmonary disease. BMC Infect Dis 2009;9:178.

57. Zhang M, Li Q, Zhang XY, et al. Relevance of lower airway bacterial colonization, airway inflammation, and pulmonary function in the stable stage of chronic obstructive pulmonary disease. Eur J Clin Microbiol Infect Dis 2010;29:1487–93.

58. Tumkaya M, Atis S, Ozge C, et al. Relationship between airway colonization, inflammation and exacerbation frequency in COPD. Respir Med 2007; 101:729–37.

59. Patel IS, Vlahos I, Wilkinson TM, et al. Bronchiectasis, exacerbation indices, and inflammation in chronic obstructive pulmonary disease. Am J Respir Crit Care Med 2004;170:400–7.

60. Retamales I, Elliott WM, Meshi B, et al. Amplification of inflammation in emphysema and its association with latent adenoviral infection. Am J Respir Crit Care Med 2001;164:469–73.

61. Falsey AR, Formica MA, Hennessey PA, et al. Detection of respiratory syncytial virus in adults with chronic obstructive pulmonary disease. Am J Respir Crit Care Med 2006;173:639–43.

62. Wilkinson TM, Donaldson GC, Johnston SL, et al. Respiratory syncytial virus, airway inflammation, and FEV1 decline in patients with chronic obstructive pulmonary disease. Am J Respir Crit Care Med 2006;173:871–6.

63. Hogg JC, Chu F, Utokaparch S, et al. The nature of small-airway obstruction in chronic obstructive pulmonary disease. N Engl J Med 2004;350:2645–53.

64. Moghaddam SJ, Clement CG, De la Garza MM, et al. *Haemophilus influenzae* lysate induces aspects of the chronic obstructive pulmonary disease phenotype. Am J Respir Cell Mol Biol 2008;38:629–38.

65. Martinez-Garcia MA, Soler-Cataluna JJ, Donat-Sanz Y, et al. Factors associated with bronchiectasis in chronic obstructive pulmonary disease patients. Chest 2011; 140(5):1130–7.

66. Verra F, Escudier E, Lebargy F, et al. Ciliary abnormalities in bronchial epithelium of smokers, ex-smokers, and nonsmokers. Am J Respir Crit Care Med 1995;151:630–4.

67. Foster WM, Langenback EG, Bergofsky EH. Disassociation in the mucociliary function of central and peripheral airways of asymptomatic smokers. Am Rev Respir Dis 1985;132:633–9.

68. Koblizek V, Tomsova M, Cermakova E, et al. Impairment of nasal mucociliary clearance in former smokers with stable chronic obstructive pulmonary disease relates to the presence of a chronic bronchitis phenotype. Rhinology 2011;49:397–406.

69. Smaldone GC, Foster WM, O'Riordan TG, et al. Regional impairment of mucociliary clearance in chronic obstructive pulmonary disease. Chest 1993;103:1390–6.

70. Vastag E, Matthys H, Zsamboki G, et al. Mucociliary clearance in smokers. Eur J Respir Dis 1986; 68:107–13.

71. Wanner A, Salathe M, O'Riordan TG. Mucociliary clearance in the airways. Am J Respir Crit Care Med 1996;154:1868–902.

72. Innes AL, Woodruff PG, Ferrando RE, et al. Epithelial mucin stores are increased in the large airways of smokers with airflow obstruction. Chest 2006; 130:1102–8.

73. Ma R, Wang Y, Cheng G, et al. MUC5AC expression up-regulation goblet cell hyperplasia in the airway of patients with chronic obstructive pulmonary disease. Chin Med Sci J 2005;20:181–4.

74. Ha U, Lim JH, Jono H, et al. A novel role for IkappaB kinase (IKK) alpha and IKKbeta in ERK-dependent up-regulation of MUC5AC mucin transcription by *Streptococcus pneumoniae*. J Immunol 2007;178:1736–47.

75. Chen R, Lim JH, Jono H, et al. Nontypeable *Haemophilus influenzae* lipoprotein P6 induces MUC5AC mucin transcription via TLR2-TAK1-dependent p38 MAPK-AP1 and IKKbeta-IkappaBalpha-NF-kappaB signaling pathways. Biochem Biophys Res Commun 2004;324: 1087–94.

76. Polosukhin VV, Cates JM, Lawson WE, et al. Bronchial secretory immunoglobulin a deficiency correlates with airway inflammation and progression of chronic obstructive pulmonary disease. Am J Respir Crit Care Med 2011;184:317–27.

77. Ganz T. Defensins: antimicrobial peptides of vertebrates. C R Biol 2004;327:539–49.

78. Parameswaran GI, Sethi S, Murphy TF. Effects of bacterial infection on airway antimicrobial peptides and proteins in chronic obstructive pulmonary disease. Chest 2011;140(3):611–7.

79. Tjabringa GS, Rabe KF, Hiemstra PS. The human cathelicidin LL-37: a multifunctional peptide involved in infection and inflammation in the lung. Pulm Pharmacol Ther 2005;18:321–7.

80. Dajani R, Zhang Y, Taft PJ, et al. Lysozyme secretion by submucosal glands protects the airway from bacterial infection. Am J Respir Cell Mol Biol 2005;32:548–52.

81. Ellison RT 3rd, Giehl TJ. Killing of gram-negative bacteria by lactoferrin and lysozyme. J Clin Invest 1991;88:1080–91.

82. Fitch PM, Roghanian A, Howie SE, et al. Human neutrophil elastase inhibitors in innate and adaptive immunity. Biochem Soc Trans 2006;34:279–82.

83. Crouch EC. Structure, biologic properties, and expression of surfactant protein D (SP-D). Biochim Biophys Acta 1998;1408:278–89.

84. Taylor D, Cripps A, Clancy R. A possible role for lysozyme in determining acute exacerbation in chronic bronchitis. Clin Exp Immunol 1995;102: 406–16.

85. Gompertz S, Bayley DL, Hill SL, et al. Relationship between airway inflammation and the frequency of exacerbations in patients with smoking related COPD. Thorax 2001;56:36–41.

86. Yang IA, Seeney SL, Wolter JM, et al. Mannose-binding lectin gene polymorphism predicts hospital admissions for COPD infections. Genes Immun 2003;4:269–74.

87. Betsuyaku T, Kuroki Y, Nagai K, et al. Effects of ageing and smoking on SP-A and SP-D levels in bronchoalveolar lavage fluid. Eur Respir J 2004; 24:964–70.

88. Honda Y, Takahashi H, Kuroki Y, et al. Decreased contents of surfactant proteins A and D in BAL fluids of healthy smokers. Chest 1996;109:1006–9.

89. Tsoumakidou M, Bouloukaki I, Thimaki K, et al. Innate immunity proteins in chronic obstructive pulmonary disease and idiopathic pulmonary fibrosis. Exp Lung Res 2010;36:373–80.

90. Pace E, Ferraro M, Minervini MI, et al. Beta defensin-2 is reduced in central but not in distal airways of smoker COPD patients. PLoS One 2012;7: e33601.

91. Berenson CS, Kruzel RL, Eberhardt E, et al. Phagocytic dysfunction of human alveolar macrophages and severity of chronic obstructive pulmonary disease. J Infect Dis 2013. [Epub ahead of print].

92. Hodge S, Hodge G, Ahern J, et al. Smoking alters alveolar macrophage recognition and phagocytic ability: implications in chronic obstructive

pulmonary disease. Am J Respir Cell Mol Biol 2007; 37:748–55.

93. Berenson CS, Garlipp MA, Grove LJ, et al. Impaired phagocytosis of nontypeable *Haemophilus influenzae* by human alveolar macrophages in chronic obstructive pulmonary disease. J Infect Dis 2006;194:1375–84.

94. Berenson CS, Wrona CT, Grove LJ, et al. Impaired alveolar macrophage response to *Haemophilus* antigens in chronic obstructive lung disease. Am J Respir Crit Care Med 2006;174:31–40.

95. Oliver BG, Lim S, Wark P, et al. Rhinovirus exposure impairs immune responses to bacterial products in human alveolar macrophages. Thorax 2008;63: 519–25.

96. Droemann D, Goldmann T, Tiedje T, et al. Toll-like receptor 2 expression is decreased on alveolar macrophages in cigarette smokers and COPD patients. Respir Res 2005;6:68.

97. Harvey CJ, Thimmulappa RK, Sethi S, et al. Targeting Nrf2 signaling improves bacterial clearance by alveolar macrophages in patients with COPD and in a mouse model. Sci Transl Med 2011;3:78ra32.

98. Kunz LI, Lapperre TS, Snoeck-Stroband JB, et al. Smoking status and anti-inflammatory macrophages in bronchoalveolar lavage and induced sputum in COPD. Respir Res 2011;12:34.

99. Macredmond RE, Greene CM, Dorscheid DR, et al. Epithelial expression of TLR4 is modulated in COPD and by steroids, salmeterol and cigarette smoke. Respir Res 2007;8:84.

100. Sahlander K, Larsson K, Palmberg L. Daily exposure to dust alters innate immunity. PLoS One 2012;7:e31646.

101. Lee SW, Kim DR, Kim TJ, et al. The association of down-regulated toll-like receptor 4 expression with airflow limitation and emphysema in smokers. Respir Res 2012;13:106.

102. Speletas M, Merentiti V, Kostikas K, et al. Association of TLR4-T399I polymorphism with chronic obstructive pulmonary disease in smokers. Clin Dev Immunol 2009;2009:260286.

103. Hoiby N, Ciofu O, Johansen HK, et al. The clinical impact of bacterial biofilms. Int J Oral Sci 2011;3: 55–65.

104. Goldstein-Daruech N, Cope EK, Zhao KQ, et al. Tobacco smoke mediated induction of sinonasal microbial biofilms. PLoS One 2011;6:e15700.

105. Starner TD, Zhang N, Kim G, et al. *Haemophilus influenzae* forms biofilms on airway epithelia: implications in cystic fibrosis. Am J Respir Crit Care Med 2006;174:213–20.

106. Hiltke TJ, Sethi S, Murphy TF. Sequence stability of the gene encoding outer membrane protein P2 of nontypeable *Haemophilus influenzae* in the human respiratory tract. J Infect Dis 2002;185:627–31.

107. Cholon DM, Cutter D, Richardson SK, et al. Serial isolates of persistent *Haemophilus influenzae* in patients with chronic obstructive pulmonary disease express diminishing quantities of the HMW1 and HMW2 adhesins. Infect Immun 2008;76(10): 4463–8.

Comorbidities and Systemic Effects of Chronic Obstructive Pulmonary Disease

Gourab Choudhury, MBBS, MRCP(UK)*,
Roberto Rabinovich, MBBS, MD, PhD,
William MacNee, MBChB, MD, FRCP(G), FRCP(E)

KEYWORDS

- Chronic obstructive pulmonary disease • Comorbidities • Systemic effects • Inflammation
- Management strategy

KEY POINTS

- Definitive types of systemic effects and co-morbidities have been seen in COPD patients.
- There are possible contributory mechanisms to these effects.
- There are clinical implications of these co-morbidities in the cohort.
- Novel therapies reduce the burden of observed effects.

INTRODUCTION

Chronic obstructive pulmonary disease (COPD) is a major cause of morbidity and mortality worldwide. It has been projected to move from the sixth to the third most common cause of death worldwide by 2020, while rising from fourth to third in terms of morbidity within the same time frame.[1]

The prevalence of COPD in the general population is estimated to be around 1% of the adult population, but rises sharply among those 40 years and older. The prevalence continues to climb appreciably higher with age.[2]

COPD is known primarily to affect the lung structure and function, resulting in emphysematous destruction of lung tissue and large and small airway disease that occur in varying proportion and severity within individuals.[3]

Besides the lung abnormalities, COPD is now recognized to be a condition that has an impact on other organs, the so-called systemic effects and comorbidities of COPD.[4–6] Conventionally, comorbidity has been defined as a disease coexisting with the primary disease of interest. In COPD, however, the definition becomes more perplexing, as certain coexisting illnesses may be a consequence of the patients' underlying COPD when it could termed as more of a systemic effect.

It is as yet unclear whether these associations are a consequence of shared risk factors such as cigarette smoking or poor physical activity, or whether COPD is a true causal factor. Nevertheless, these extrapulmonary features of COPD add to the challenge and burden of assessing and managing the disease.

This article reviews the types, possible mechanisms, and clinical implications of these systemic effects and comorbidities on COPD patients.

CLASSIFICATION

Table 1 lists the systemic effects and comorbidities associated with COPD. **Table 2** summarizes the results of a PubMed search investigating the prevalence of COPD and comorbidities in various studies performed in the past.

CARDIOVASCULAR DISEASE

COPD is now well known to be a risk factor for the development of atherosclerosis and consequent cardiovascular complications.[7,8]

ELEGI and COLT Laboratories, Queen's Medical Research Institute, 47 Little France Crescent, EH16 4TJ Edinburgh, UK
* Corresponding author.
E-mail address: gchoudhu@staffmail.ed.ac.uk

Clin Chest Med 35 (2014) 101–130
http://dx.doi.org/10.1016/j.ccm.2013.10.007

chestmed.theclinics.com

Table 1
Observed systemic effects and comorbidities in the COPD population

Systemic Effects of COPD[4-6]	Comorbidities in COPD[4-6]
Muscle dysfunction	Cardiovascular disease
Cachexia	Lung cancer
Anemia	Osteoporosis
Muscle dysfunction	Diabetes
Autonomic dysfunction	Psychological issues: anxiety/depression
Systemic inflammation	Obstructive sleep apnea

Prevalence

Cardiovascular disease is undoubtedly the most significant nonrespiratory contributor to both morbidity and mortality in COPD.

In a large cohort of patients with COPD admitted to a Veterans Administration Hospital or clinic, the prevalence of coronary artery disease was 33.6%, appreciably higher than the 27.1% prevalence seen in a matched cohort without COPD.[9] In the Lung Health Study,[10] which assessed deaths and hospitalizations over a 5-year period in a cohort of COPD patients, mortality in 5887 patients aged 35 to 46 years with COPD with mild to moderate airways obstruction was 2.5%, of whom 25% died of cardiovascular complications. Moreover, in these patients with relatively mild COPD, cardiovascular disease accounted for 42% of the first hospitalization and 44% of the second hospitalization over a follow-up period of 5 years. By comparison, only 14% of the hospitalizations in this cohort were from respiratory causes.

Divo and colleagues[11] looked at 1664 patients with COPD over 4 years to evaluate COPD comorbidities and mortality risk. Using a multivariate analysis, they generated a COPD comorbidity index (COPD-specific comorbidity test) based on the comorbidities that increase mortality risk. The prevalence of coronary artery disease in this study was unsurprisingly highest at 30.2%, with congestive heart failure (HF) and dysrhythmias making up another 15.7% and 13% of the cases, respectively, and correlated strongly with the association for increased risk of death ($P<.05$).

Holguin and colleagues[12] assessed the prevalence of COPD deaths in United States between 1979 and 2001, and found approximately 47 million hospital discharges (8.5% of all hospitalizations in adults) with a primary or secondary diagnosis of COPD (21% and 79%, respectively). The reported hospital mortality in this cohort was related to heart disease in 43%, taking the major

share for the cause of death, compared with 37% related to respiratory failure and another 25% related to pneumonia.

Forced expiratory volume in 1 second (FEV_1) is also known to be an independent predictor of cardiovascular complications in COPD patients. In the Lung Health Study, for every 10% decrease in FEV_1, cardiovascular mortality increased by approximately 28% and nonfatal coronary events increased by approximately 20% in mild to moderate COPD.[10] Even a moderate reduction of expiratory flow volumes multiplies the risk of cardiovascular morbidity and sudden cardiac deaths by 2 to 3 times, independent of other risk factors.[13-16]

COPD patients also have shown evidence of atherosclerotic plaque burden as assessed by increased carotid intimal medial thickening (CIMT),[17] and are associated with increased cardiovascular and all-cause mortality.[18]

Pathogenesis

The pathogenesis of atherosclerosis in COPD is multifactorial.[19] **Box 1** summarizes the potential mechanisms that have been linked directly or indirectly to the cardiovascular complications seen in this cohort. **Fig. 1** summarizes the presumed mechanisms for cardiovascular disease in COPD patients.

Inflammation

Inflammation is considered to be a potential pathogenic mechanism in atherosclerosis. Recent studies, however, indicate that sustained systemic inflammation occurs only in a proportion of patients with COPD, and its relationship to the development of cardiovascular disease has as yet not been fully established.[20] Patients with COPD and coexistent cardiovascular disease nevertheless tend to have higher systemic levels of biomarkers, such as interleukin (IL)-6 and fibrinogen, than those without this comorbidity.[21] In addition, systemic inflammation increases exacerbations of COPD when there is an increased risk of cardiovascular events.[22,23]

The specific cellular mechanisms by which systemic inflammation plays a role in the pathogenesis of cardiovascular disease are complex. However, studies have revealed the importance of inflammation in atherosclerotic plaque initiation, development, and rupture (see **Fig. 1**).[24,25]

[18]F-Fluorodeoxyglucose positron emission tomography imaging has also shown direct evidence of inflammation in the vascular wall of the aorta, presumably associated with atherosclerotic plaques, in patients with COPD when compared with smoking control subjects.[26]

Table 2
Data from various studies (PubMed search) looking at the prevalence of COPD and comorbidities

First Author	Journal	Type of Study	Patient Size (n)	Cardiac (%)	Hypertension (%)	Diabetes (%)	Psychiatric (%)	Cancer (%)	Osteoporosis (%)
van Manen et al	J Clin Epidemiol	Observational	1145	13	23	5	9	6	—
Almagro et al	Chest	Retrospective matched cohort	2699	22	—	—	10	4	—
Sidney et al	Chest	Retrospective matched cohort	45,966	18	18	2	—	—	—
Schnell et al	BMC Pulm Med	Cross-Sectional	995	12.7	—	—	20.6	16.5	16.9
Feary et al	Thorax	Cross-Sectional	29,870	28	—	12.2	—	—	—

— signifies no data available.

Systemic inflammation is discussed in more details later in this article.

Hypoxia

Patients with COPD are subjected to hypoxia: either sustained hypoxia in patients with severe disease, or intermittent hypoxia during exercise or exacerbations. There are several effects of hypoxia that can influence atherogenesis, including systemic inflammation and oxidative stress, upregulation of cell-adhesion molecules, and hemodynamic stress.[27–29] Animal studies have shown hypoxia to be a contributor to atherosclerosis in the presence of dyslipidemia, as increased lipid peroxidation, a marker of oxidative stress, and reduced levels of the antioxidant superoxide dismutase are found in the myocardial tissue of rats exposed to hypoxic environments.[30,31]

Hypoxia also induces hemodynamic stress, increasing the heart rate and cardiac index,[32] and affects the renal circulation, reducing renal blood flow and activating the renin-angiotensin system, resulting in increased peripheral vasoconstriction and oxidative stress.[33] Respiratory failure in patients with COPD is also associated with activation of the sympathetic nervous system,[34] which is associated with an increased risk for cardiovascular disease.[35]

Effect of cigarette smoking

Chronic cigarette smoking is an independent risk factor for the development of cardiovascular complications in COPD patients.[36] Possible mechanisms include increased systemic oxidative stress, altered nitric oxide (NO) bioavailability, endothelial dysfunction, and influence on the levels of other major risk factors, such as blood pressure.[37–39]

However, studies have also shown that independent of current smoking, plasma levels of fibrinogen and other markers of coagulation are significantly higher in patients with stable COPD than in healthy subjects.[40,41] This amplified procoagulant activity in COPD may principally be a consequence of inflammation, initiating the coagulation cascade by promoting tissue factor gene expression in endothelial cells, hence contributing to increased thrombotic events.[42]

Polycythemia

Secondary polycythemia is a known complication of COPD, and occurs mainly as a result of chronic hypoxemia. A prospective study by Cote and colleagues,[43] however, had shown that only 6% of their 683 COPD patients developed secondary polycythemia, perhaps because the development of polycythemia in COPD has been less common in recent times, and is thought to be due to more effective management of hypoxia in COPD such as the use of long-term oxygen therapy (LTOT) in patients who meet the criteria.

However, when present in COPD polycythemia can contribute to the development of pulmonary hypertension and pulmonary endothelial dysfunction with reduced cerebral and coronary blood flow, thus adding to the pathogenic cascade.[44]

Hypercapnic acidosis

Respiratory acidosis resulting from hypercapnia is a well-known occurrence in patients with COPD, particularly in the advanced phase. A recent study

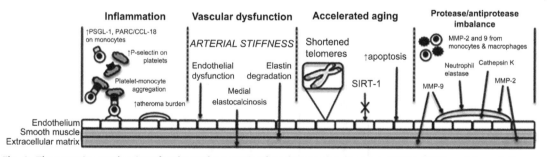

Fig. 1. The putative mechanisms for the pathogenesis of cardiovascular disease in COPD. MMP, matrix metalloproteinase; PARC/CCL-18, pulmonary and activation-regulated chemokine CC chemokine ligand 18; PSGL, P-selectin glycoprotein ligand 1; SIRT, sirtuin 1. (*From* Maclay JD, MacNee W. Cardiovascular disease in COPD: mechanisms. Chest 2013;143(3):798–807. http://dx.doi.org/10.1378/chest.12-0938; with permission.)

by Minet and colleagues[45] has shown that respiratory acidosis could be one of the potent mechanisms behind endothelial dysfunction, adding to the burden of cardiovascular complications.

Abnormalities in vascular endothelial function/vessel wall

Some,[46,47] but not all studies[48] have demonstrated abnormal endothelial function in COPD patients in comparison with smokers who have not developed COPD.

Arterial stiffness can be assessed using carotid-femoral pulse-wave velocity (PWV), a measure that is predictive of cardiovascular events in healthy individuals and in patients with ischemic heart disease.[49] Arterial stiffness is increased in COPD patients in comparison with healthy smokers[50,51] and is associated with the FEV_1 percent predicted emphysema and systemic inflammation,[52] and may result from increased elastolysis in the vessel wall.[53]

Common Cardiovascular Complications

HF is common in COPD patients, and COPD is common in HF patients. In a survey of COPD patients in primary care, 20% had previously unrecognized HF,[54] which is associated with a worse prognosis in COPD patients.[55]

A study of 186 consecutive patients with left ventricular systolic dysfunction in an HF clinic found that 39% had COPD diagnosed by spirometry, and those patients with HF and severe COPD had a worse prognosis than the HF patients with mild to moderate COPD or normal lung function.[56] Higher mortality was again reported among patients with COPD when compared with individuals without lung disease in a study of 4132 patients hospitalized with cardiac failure in Norway.[57]

In another prospective prognostic study performed as part of the EchoCardiography and Heart Outcome Study (ECHOS), 532 patients admitted with a clinical diagnosis of HF were studied.[58] The prevalence of COPD in these patients was found to be 35% and was associated with a worse prognosis.

COPD is indeed a predictor of mortality in HF.[30] Studies have shown 5-year survival in HF patients with COPD to be as low as 31%, compared with 71% in its absence.[57] HF in COPD patients has often been postulated to be secondary to increased intrathoracic pressure–induced impaired low-pressure ventricular filling, as is expected with hyperinflated lungs in this population.[59] However, Barr and colleagues[60] have shown that computed tomography (CT)-quantified emphysema scores negatively correlated with ventricular filling even in a group without COPD

and minor emphysema, in whom hyperinflation is unlikely to play a role. The investigators hypothesized that endothelial dysfunction associated with emphysema could contribute to impaired left ventricular filling and the consequent failure cascade.

Patients with COPD also have increased risk for cardiac arrhythmias.[61] Following surgery for non–small cell lung carcinoma, patients with spirometric evidence of COPD had an increased risk for supraventricular tachycardia, and were found to be refractory to first-line treatment.[62] Atrial fibrillation (AF) is also more common in COPD following coronary artery bypass grafting.[63] In a study conducted in Finland on 738 patients with COPD, AF was found to be an independent predictor of increased mortality and poor health-related quality of life (HRQoL) in comparison with the general population.[64]

Coronary artery disease is also common and is undertreated in patients with COPD.[65] In a group of healthy Japanese men, CIMT (a surrogate measure strongly associated with atherosclerotic plaque burden) was significantly increased in individuals who smoked and had airflow limitation compared with matched smokers and non-smokers.[17] This finding suggests that smokers with a spirometric-based diagnosis of COPD may have evidence of subclinical atherosclerosis independent of cigarette smoking.

The presence of COPD in patients with myocardial infarction (MI) is also associated with a poorer prognosis. In a study of 14,703 patients with acute MI, all-cause mortality was 30% in patients with COPD versus 19% in those without COPD.[66] Campo and colleagues[14] assessed 11,118 consecutive patients with ST-elevation MI (STEMI) stratified according to the presence or absence of COPD. At the 3-year follow-up, COPD was found to be an independent predictor of mortality (hazard ratio [HR] 1.4, 95% confidence interval [CI] 1.2–1.6). Hospital readmissions from recurrent MI (10% vs 6.9%, $P<.01$) and HF (10% vs 6.9%, $P<.01$) were significantly more frequent in patients with COPD when compared with those without. Also hospital readmission for COPD was found to be a strong independent risk factor for recurrence of MI (HR 2.1, 95% CI 1.4–3.3) and HF (HR 5.8, 95% CI 4.6–7.5).

In a study of exacerbations of COPD from the United Kingdom Health Improvement Database, the incidence rate of MI was 1.1 per 100 patient-years, with a 2.27-fold increased risk of MI 1 to 5 days after exacerbation.[67]

In another prospective study, 242 COPD patients admitted to hospital with an exacerbation were studied to observe the prevalence of MI following hospitalization.[22] Twenty-four patients (10%) were found to have elevated troponin, among whom 20 (8.3%; 95% CI 5.1%–12.5%) had chest pain and/or serial electrocardiographic changes, in keeping with MI. Overall, 1 in 12 patients met the criteria for MI.

Interventions to Reduce Cardiovascular Complications

Smoking cessation
A recent meta-analysis assessing the impact of smoking has shown a decline of acute coronary syndrome risk in 30 of 35 estimates with a 10% (95% CI 6–14, $P<.001$) pooled relative risk reduction, supporting the fact that smoking is an independent risk factor toward development of cardiovascular complications.[68] Smoking cessation therefore unsurprisingly remains one of the primary cornerstones of cardiovascular risk management.

Effective management of COPD
It is well known that for every 10% decrease in FEV_1, cardiovascular mortality increases by about 28%, and nonfatal coronary events increase by about 20% in mild to moderate COPD.[16] Therefore, early detection and effective management of the disease is of importance in reducing the associated complications of this condition.

The use of current medications to treat COPD, however, has not been shown to be definitive toward reduction of cardiovascular events. Whereas observational studies have suggested that inhaled corticosteroids (ICS) may potentially confer benefit on cardiovascular events or mortality,[69] randomized controlled trials (RCTs) have failed to show any significant effect of ICS therapy on MI or cardiovascular death. The use of long-acting inhaled β-agonists does not appear to produce an increased risk of cardiovascular deaths.[70] The long-acting antimuscarinic, tiotropium, appears to confer an increased risk of cardiovascular death when used in a higher dose in the Respimat inhaler but not in the Handihaler formulation,[71] which may even be associated with a decrease in cardiovascular mortality.[72]

Cardiovascular drugs
Medications currently associated with cardiovascular risk reduction, such as β-blockers (BB), angiotensin-converting enzyme (ACE) inhibitors, statins, and angiotensin II receptor blockers (ARBs), have been shown in retrospective pharmacoepidemiologic studies to have an impact on the clinical outcome of COPD patients by reducing the cardiovascular events and mortality.[73–75] These observational studies, however, suffer

from immortal time bias, and prospective studies are required to definitively assess the benefits of these drugs in this population.

BB are known to improve survival of patients within a large spectrum of cardiovascular diseases, including ischemic heart disease and HF.[76–80] In a large observational study involving 2230 COPD patients, the association of BB usage with all-cause mortality and risk of exacerbation was studied.[81] Use of BB was found to be associated with a reduction in mortality as well as the risk of exacerbations in a broad spectrum of patients with COPD with concurrent cardiovascular disease. Importantly in a subgroup analyses, including patients with COPD but without overt cardiovascular disease, but with hypertension as the main remaining indication for the prescription of BB, similar outcomes were noted. This result further indicates the potential protective benefit of BB in COPD even in those with no known history of heart disease.

However, BB have been underprescribed in patients with COPD cardiovascular disease,[82] largely because of the potential to worsen airflow limitation and consequent theoretical respiratory side effects (namely bronchospasm).

A recent meta-analysis of studies in COPD patients has shown that cardioselective BB, given as a single dose or for longer duration, produced no change in FEV_1 or respiratory symptoms when compared with placebo, and did not affect the FEV_1-guided treatment response to β2-agonists.[83]

Another recent study also explored the association between BB therapy and outcomes in patients hospitalized with acute exacerbations of COPD with underlying ischemic heart disease, HF, or hypertension. The study accounted for the problem of immortal time bias, and found no improvement or worse mortality in COPD patients using BB.[84] Judicious use of BB may therefore be warranted in patients with severe COPD and respiratory failure on LTOT in whom the use of BB was associated, in one study, with increased mortality.[85]

Similarly, statins, ACE inhibitors, and ARBs are also widely used for the treatment and prevention of cardiovascular disease, and their potential role in other disease states has become increasingly recognized. Mortensen and colleagues[86] studied the association of prior outpatient use of statins and ACE inhibitors on mortality for subjects of 65 years or older who were hospitalized with acute COPD exacerbations. A total of 11,212 subjects with a mean age of 74.0 years were studied in this group, of whom 32.0% were using ACE inhibitors or ARBs, the use of which was associated with significant reduction in 90-day mortality (odds ratio [OR] 0.55, 95% CI 0.46–0.66). A similar pharmacoepidemiologic study done by Mancini and colleagues[75] suggested that statins in combination with either ACE inhibitors or ARBs improved cardiovascular and pulmonary outcomes not only in the high-risk but also in the low-risk COPD populations.

SKELETAL MUSCLE EFFECTS

A striking systemic consequence of COPD is the reduction in peripheral muscle mass, resulting in muscle wasting and dysfunction. Muscle dysfunction, with or without evidence of atrophy, can be defined physiologically as the failure to achieve the basic muscle functions of strength and resistance, the latter being inversely related to an increase in the fatigability of the muscle.

Reduced quadriceps strength in COPD is associated with reduced exercise capacity,[87,88] compromised health status,[89] increased need for health care resources,[90] and mortality independent of airflow obstruction.[91] Skeletal muscle weakness, particularly quadriceps weakness, has also recently been shown to be a feature of early disease,[92] and its development is likely to be multifactorial with inflammation and oxidative stress[93] being the predominant factors, coupled with physical inactivity.[94,95] Several other factors such as protein synthesis/degradation imbalance and hypoxia have also been postulated to explain the initiation and the progression of muscle wasting in COPD patients.[88,96]

Prevalence

Eighteen percent to 36% of COPD patients present with net loss of muscle mass, which is responsible for weight loss in 17% to 35% of such patients.[97] However, muscle wasting is also present in 6% to 21% of patients of normal weight.[98] The reductions in mass and cross-sectional area of limb muscles of COPD patients have been linked to the impaired muscle strength seen in these patients. When limb-muscle strength is normalized per unit of mass or cross-sectional area, no differences can be observed between control subjects and COPD patients, suggesting that atrophy is indeed an important causative factor in the reduced limb-muscle strength and endurance in COPD.[97] Hence, it could be argued that muscle wasting is a better predictor of HRQoL and survival than is body weight.[99]

Unintentional loss of muscle mass, unsurprisingly, has a significant impact on the quality of life, and can be associated with premature death.[100]

Fig. 2 illustrates the various pathophysiologic changes that are observed in skeletal muscles of COPD patients and the possible mechanisms implicated.

Pathophysiologic Changes Associated with Muscle Dysfunction/Wasting

Fiber redistribution results in an increase in the number of type IIx muscle fibers,[101,102] which, in turn, is associated with significant muscle atrophy.[102]

Alterations in muscle bioenergetics in skeletal limb muscle of COPD patients correlate with exercise tolerance. For example, the early lactate release that occurs during exercise, the increased phosphate/phosphocreatine relationship during submaximal exercise, and the reduced activity of oxidative enzymes in these patients all indicate a change in muscle bioenergetics.[103]

Altered capillary structuration has also been found in the skeletal muscle of COPD patients. Electron and optic microscopy studies show reduced capillary density and the number of contacts between capillaries and fibers in skeletal muscles of COPD patients.[104]

Factors Contributing to Muscle Dysfunction

Several factors, such as protein synthesis/degradation imbalance, hypoxia, inactivity, inflammation, and oxidative stress, have been proposed to explain the initiation and the progression of muscle wasting in COPD.[96,97] Mitochondrial dysfunction, apoptosis, and oxidative stress have all also been implicated to the wasting and dysfunction observed in COPD.

Mitochondrial dysfunction is manifested as reduced citrate synthase activity that correlates with time to fatigue of the muscle,[105] while reduced mitochondrial oxidative phosphorylation and coupling have been associated with reduced muscle mass and endurance.[106]

Other factors that contribute to this muscle dysfunction include the following.

- Abnormal protein metabolism. A substantial proportion of COPD patients is characterized by low fat-free mass with altered muscle and plasma amino acid levels, suggesting abnormal protein metabolism.[107] The signaling pathways that govern muscle hypertrophy and/or atrophy have yet to be fully defined. However, several key factors have been identified. **Fig. 3** summarizes the salient pathways governing skeletal muscle metabolism. Marked activation of the ubiquitin-proteasome pathway is found in muscle of patients with COPD, and is thought to be one of the key factors in muscle atrophy and dysfunction as seen in COPD patients.[108,109]

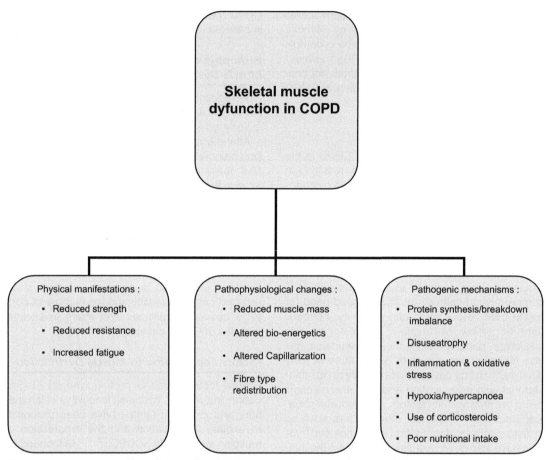

Fig. 2. The common manifestations and underlying pathophysiologic changes of skeletal muscle dysfunction in COPD patients.

- Poor nutritional intake and unmatched calorie expenditure are further factors contributing to muscle wasting in COPD patients. Chronic usage of oral corticosteroids is also a well-known contributor to myopathy in this group.[110] Previous studies have shown that the histology of steroid-induced myopathy in patients with COPD is of global myopathy affecting both type IIa and IIb fibers, and type I fibers to a lesser extent.[111] However, administration of corticosteroids for relatively short periods of time, for example during an exacerbation, has not been shown to cause any significant deleterious effect on the skeletal muscle of COPD patients.[112]
- Hypoxia is implicated in mitochondrial biogenesis, oxidative stress, inflammation, and autophagy. It results in enhanced cytokine production by macrophages, contributing to the activation of the tumor necrosis factor (TNF) system. Significant inverse correlations between partial pressure of arterial oxygen and circulating TNF-α and soluble TNF-receptor levels have been reported in patients with COPD,[113] limiting the production of energy and possibly affecting the protein synthesis also.[114]
- Hypercapnic acidosis can inhibit the oxidative enzymes, further contributing to protein degradation and the process of muscle wasting.[115]
- Inflammation, as in cardiovascular complications, is another mechanism contributing to skeletal muscle dysfunction in COPD patients. Relatively fewer data are currently available on the concentration of cytokines in muscle of COPD patients, the most studied being TNF-α. High levels of TNF-α protein in serum have been associated with quadriceps weakness,[116] and COPD patients with low fat-free mass (FFM) are reported to show high mRNA levels of TNF-α in the quadriceps, together with lower body mass index (BMI).[117] Of interest, high levels of C-reactive protein (CRP) have been found to be inversely related to the distance covered in a 6-minute walking test in COPD patients,

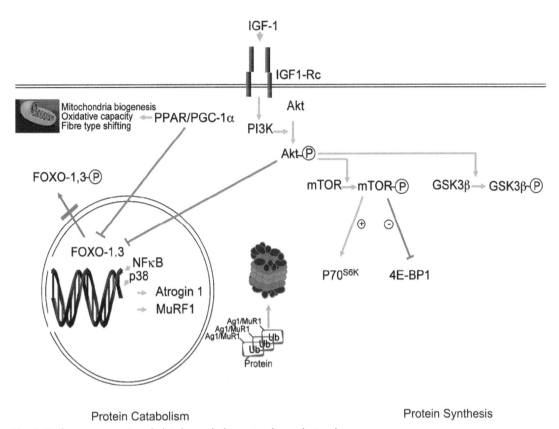

Fig. 3. Pathways governing skeletal muscle hypertrophy and atrophy.

suggesting a role for chronic inflammation in these patients.[118]

Interventions to Improve Skeletal Muscle Dysfunction

- Exercise training is the single most important therapeutic intervention to treat muscle dysfunction/wasting in patients with COPD.[119] Improving exercise tolerance by enhancing muscle strength, with consequent improved endurance and reduced fatigue, have all proved to be very effective.[119] Exercise training improves body weight by improving FFM, enhancing oxygen delivery to the muscle mitochondria and fiber-type redistribution.[119,120]
- Oxygen therapy and consequent correction of hypoxia in suitable candidates have also been shown to improve the mitochondrial oxidative capacity in COPD patients.[120,121]
- Smoking cessation is likely to be an important aspect in improving muscle dysfunction. Chronic smoking has been associated with diverse mitochondrial respiratory chain (MRC) dysfunction in lymphocytes. In a study

of MRC function in peripheral lymphocytes of 10 healthy chronic smokers before and after cessation of smoking,[122] smokers showed a significant decrease in complex IV MRC activity and respiration compared with control lymphocytes, which returned to normal values after cessation of tobacco smoking.
- Other novel therapies such as the antioxidant N-acetylcysteine[123] and peroxisome proliferator-activated receptors (such as polyunsaturated fatty acids)[120,124] are potential interventions that may improve muscle insufficiency in COPD patients, and are currently in the process of being tried and tested.

OSTEOPOROSIS

Osteoporosis is a systemic skeletal disorder characterized by low bone mineral density (BMD) and microarchitectural changes, leading to impaired bone strength and increased risk of fracture.[4]

Low BMI, advanced age, female sex, chronic use of oral corticosteroids, and endocrinologic disorders such as hyperthyroidism and primary hyperparathyroidism have all been implicated as risk factors in the development of osteoporosis in the general population.[125] Predictably, osteoporosis is a well-recognized comorbidity of COPD patients and is an important area of consideration for therapeutic interventions.[126]

The most commonly used tool to measure BMD is dual-energy x-ray absorptiometry (DEXA), which is used to define osteoporosis and provides a useful estimate of fracture risk.[127] The T score is one of the principal parameters used to measure BMD, and is calculated by subtracting the mean BMD of a young-adult reference population from the patient's BMD and dividing it by the standard deviation of the reference population. According to the World Health Organization (WHO), a T score greater than −1 is accepted as normal, T scores between −1 and −2.5 are classified as osteopenia, and T scores of less than −2.5 are defined as osteoporosis.[127]

Prevalence of Osteoporosis in COPD

The prevalence of osteoporosis in COPD varies between 4% and 59%, depending on the diagnostic methods used and the severity of the COPD population.[128]

A recent systematic review calculated an overall mean prevalence of osteoporosis of 35% from 14 articles by measuring BMD in a COPD population. The individuals in these studies had a mean age of 63 and a mean FEV_1 percent predicted of 47%.[128]

More than half of the patients with COPD recruited for the large TORCH (Toward a Revolution in COPD Health) trial (6000 patients) had osteoporosis or osteopenia as determined by DEXA scan.[129]

In another cross-sectional study, the prevalence of osteoporosis was 75% in patients with Global Initiative for Chronic Obstructive Lung Disease (GOLD) stage IV disease, and strongly correlated with reduced FFM.[130,131] Another important finding in this study was that the prevalence rate was high even for males, with an even higher incidence in postmenopausal women.

Another large cohort of 1634 COPD subjects was studied longitudinally with 259 smoker and 186 nonsmoker controls[132] in a study evaluating CT bone attenuation of the thoracic and lumber vertebrae, the extent of emphysema and coronary artery calcification on CT scans, and clinical parameters and outcomes. Bone attenuation was lower in the COPD patients than in control subjects, and correlated positively with FEV_1 ($P = .014$), FEV_1/forced vital capacity ratio ($P<.001$), FFM index ($P<.001$), and CRP ($P<.001$), and negatively with the extent of emphysema ($P<.001$). Lower CT bone attenuation was also found to be associated with higher exacerbation ($P = .022$) and hospitalization rates ($P = .002$).

In a Norwegian cross-sectional study of 1004 consecutively admitted COPD patients attending a 4-week rehabilitation program, the prevalence of vertebral deformities was found to be significantly higher in COPD patients than in the control group ($P<.0001$).[133] An increase in severity of airflow limitation from GOLD stage II to stage III was associated with an almost 2-fold increase in the average number of vertebral deformities. Of note, significant differences between COPD patients and controls were also found for pack-years ($P<.0001$), and use of calcium/vitamin D ($P<.0001$) and oral corticosteroids ($P<.0001$).

Potential Contributors to Osteoporosis in COPD

Corticosteroids
Oral glucocorticosteroids (OGCS) have both direct adverse effects on bone and indirect effects attributable to muscle weakening and atrophy.[134] OGCS are known to cause a decrease in vascular endothelial growth factor, skeletal angiogenesis, bone hydration, and strength.[135] These effects are both dose-dependent and duration-dependent. Fewer adverse effects are seen in episodic usage of OGCS in comparison with continuous use, but lower continuous doses have fewer detrimental effects on bone than frequent high-dose therapy,[136] because systemic usage of corticosteroids can cause rapid bone loss within the first few months of treatment, followed by a slower 2% to 5% loss per year with chronic use.[137] However, ICS have not been shown to aggravate the bone mineral loss in COPD patients.[138]

Inflammation
Studies suggest that COPD and associated systemic inflammation is a risk factor for osteoporosis independent of other potentiators such as age and oral corticosteroid therapy.[50,139] In a Chinese study, the presence of systemic inflammation was associated with a greater likelihood of low BMD, and multivariate logistic regression analysis showed that TNF-α and IL-6 were independent predictors of low BMD.[139] Both these factors are known to stimulate osteoclasts and increase bone resorption through receptor activator of nuclear factor (NF)-κB ligand (RANKL)-mediated bone resorption in vitro.[50,140] In addition, many other cytokines have been found to interact with the osteoprotegerin/RANKL system, supporting the concept that inflammatory mediators possibly contribute to the regulation of bone remodeling in COPD patients.[141]

Calcification paradox

Mounting data support a calcification paradox, whereby reduced BMD is associated with increased vascular calcification. Furthermore, BMD is more prevalent in older persons with lower BMI.[142] Therefore, although BMI and coronary artery calcification (CAC) exhibit a positive relationship in younger persons, it is predicted that in older persons and/or those at risk for osteoporosis, an inverse relationship between BMI and CAC may apply. Kovacic and colleagues[142] studied 9993 subjects who underwent percutaneous coronary intervention. Index lesion calcification (ILC) was analyzed with respect to BMI. In multivariable modeling, BMI was an independent inverse predictor of moderate to severe ILC (OR 0.967, 95% CI 0.953–0.980; $P<.0001$).

Therapeutic Interventions

Prevention and treatment of osteoporosis involves both pharmacologic and nonpharmacologic interventions.

Nonpharmacologic measures

Nonpharmacologic interventions include simple measures such as smoking cessation, and alcohol consumption in moderation along with good nutrition. As discussed earlier, exercise training, particularly weight-bearing and strengthening exercise performed at least 3 times per week, may be effective for maintaining skeletal health, given the association of reduced physical activity with bone loss and fracture in elderly COPD patients.[136,143,144]

Pharmacologic measures

COPD patients, with or without diagnosed osteoporosis, should be encouraged to take calcium (1000 mg/d) and vitamin D (800 IU/d) supplements routinely, as these have been shown to reduce the risk of fracture in this cohort.[126,136]

Definitive therapy is recommended in documented fragility hip or vertebral (clinical or morphometric) fracture; or T score lower than −2.5; or with less marked bone loss (T score between −1 and −2.5) and 1 major criterion (use of systemic corticosteroids [3 months/year], major fragility fracture [spine-hip] and so forth).[128,139] An oral bisphosphonate, such as alendronate and risedronate, is currently considered as the first line of treatment of osteoporosis together with vitamin D and calcium supplementation.[145,146] Bisphosphonates act by inhibiting bone resorption, and have also been shown to prevent osteoblast and osteocyte apoptosis.[145]

Anabolic drugs such as the human parathyroid hormone (PTH) analogue teriparatide (PTH_{1-34}) are also being increasingly used to treat osteoporosis in COPD patients, particularly in postmenopausal women and men with advanced osteoporosis. These agents act by stimulating bone formation through effects on osteoblasts and osteocytes, and therefore have great relevance predominantly in OGCS-induced osteoporosis.[134,147]

Efforts should be made to detect and treat low BMD in COPD patients to minimize fracture risk. Bone densitometry is widely available and should be used to screen patients at risk of low BMD, particularly those with low BMI, as current rates of detection and treatment of osteoporosis are low. Lehouck and colleagues[126] have suggested a more aggressive approach to the diagnosis and management of low BMD in COPD, and this should be widely implemented to minimize the risk of osteoporotic complications.[148] In this context the term FRAX has been described.[126] FRAX is a computer-based algorithm (http://www.shef.ac.uk/FRAX) that offers models for assessment of fracture likelihood in both men and women from the evidence provided from clinical risk factors such as age, sex, BMI, prior fragility fracture, smoking status, ethanol abuse, and prior use of corticosteroids. With FRAX, the 10-year fracture probability can be derived using these clinical risk factors, alone or in conjunction with femoral neck BMD, to enhance fracture-risk prediction and to differentiate the patients who will benefit most from definitive treatment.[149] It is hoped that FRAX will become an increasingly used tool in the future, but for the moment the identification of patients who need antiresorptive treatment remains based on clinical history, BMD, and prevalent fracture status.

NUTRITIONAL EFFECTS IN COPD

Nutritional abnormalities are also a common problem in COPD patients. There are 3 types of nutritional abnormality that occur in this population: semistarvation (low BMI with normal or above-normal FFM index), muscle atrophy (normal or above-normal BMI with low FFM index), and cachexia (low BMI with low FFM index).[150]

Prevalence and Implications

Weight loss has been reported in about 50% of patients with severe COPD and, although less common, it is still observed in about 10% to 15% of mild to moderate COPD.[5]

Several studies have shown an association between malnutrition and impaired pulmonary status in patients with COPD.[151] Poor nutritional status and consequent weight loss in these patients is known to be associated increased gas trapping, lower diffusing capacity, and lower exercise tolerance compared with their normal nourished counterparts.[152] Impairment of skeletal muscle function along with reduction in diaphragmatic mass, with a decrease in strength and endurance of the respiratory muscle that could occur in a malnourished state, have all been implicated in causing these adverse effects on pulmonary function.

Loss of skeletal muscle bulk is the main contributor to weight loss in COPD, with loss of fat mass contributing to a lesser extent.[153] It is important to recognize that if nutritional assessment includes only body weight and unintentional weight loss, some patients with normal BMI would go undetected despite being depleted of FFM.[154,155] In a cross-sectional study[154] involving 300 COPD patients requiring LTOT, 17% of patients had a low BMI, whereas the prevalence of FFM depletion was 2 times higher (around 38%).

This finding is of therapeutic importance, as improving the nutrition in COPD patients can lead to improvement in anthropometric measures and muscle strength, thus resulting in improved and better quality of life and survival rates in these patients. Post hoc analysis of COPD patients who gain weight has suggested a decrease in mortality.[156] At least one study has reported improved immune function as a result of nutritional support.[157]

Factors Contributing to Nutritional Depletion

The cause of nutritional abnormalities in COPD patients seems to be multifactorial, as with other systemic effects.[5,158] **Box 2** lists the important contributory mechanisms.

Therapeutic Interventions

Dietary intervention following a proper nutritional assessment remains one of the primary cornerstones in the management of this condition.

A meta-analysis of 13 RCTs on the effects of nutritional support in stable COPD patients[151]

Box 2
Factors governing the nutritional depletion in COPD

- Poor nutritional intake particularly during exacerbations
- Increased metabolic rate associated with breathing problems resulting from abnormal respiratory dynamics
- Drugs such as β2-agonists increasing metabolic rate
- Chronic systemic inflammation

---

showed significant improvements in favor of nutritional support for body weight ($P<.001$; in 11 studies) and grip strength ($P<.050$; in 4 studies) associated with greater increases in mean total protein and energy intakes following the intervention.

Similar results have been produced by Ferreira and colleagues,[152] who assessed 17 RCTs from the Cochrane Airways Review Group Trials Register. The meta-analysis showed that nutritional supplementation produced significant weight gain in patients with COPD, especially in those who were malnourished. In the 11 RCTs that studied 325 undernourished patients, there was a mean difference of 1.65 kg (95% CI 0.14–3.16) in favor of supplementation. Nourished patients, however, may not respond to supplemental feeding to the same degree as their undernourished counterparts (1 RCT with 71 participants: standardized mean difference [SMD] of 0.27, 95% CI −0.20–0.73).

Ferreira and colleagues[152] found a significant change from baseline in FFM index (overall SMD 0.57, 95% CI 0.04–1.09), which became even more significant in undernourished patients (3 RCTs, 125 participants: SMD 1.08, 95% CI 0.70–1.47). This study also emphasized the significant improvement in respiratory muscle strength and HRQoL that occurs in undernourished patients following a nutritional intervention.

This nutritional intervention can be in the form of oral supplementation, enteral nutrition, or, in some extreme cases, parenteral nutrition.[158] A diet rich in protein and fat content is desirable, as an increase in fat calories with a decrease in carbohydrate calories helps to limit the amount of carbon dioxide production while still maintaining an adequate intake of protein for lean muscle mass.[158,159]

In addition, the diet of these patients should include a good supply of vitamins, minerals, and antioxidants. In this context, ω-3 fatty acid has been shown to be of some value in combating the anti-inflammatory properties of TNF-α.[158,160] Therefore, this could potentially be of novel therapeutic benefit in achieving good nutritional status in these patients.

OBESITY AND OBSTRUCTIVE SLEEP APNEA IN COPD

The prevalence of obesity, defined as BMI greater than 30 kg/m^2, has multiplied during the last decades, and varies from 10% to 20% in most European countries to 32% in the United States.[161] It plays a major role in the development of the metabolic syndrome, and has been identified as an important risk factor for chronic diseases such as type 2 diabetes mellitus and cardiovascular disease. A link between obesity and COPD is also being increasingly recognized.[162] The risk of developing obesity is increased in patients with COPD as a result of physical inactivity in daily life in these patients in comparison with healthy age-matched controls.[163] In addition, patients with COPD who receive repeated courses of systemic OGCS are at increased risk of truncal obesity as a result of steroid-mediated redistribution of stored energy and the stimulatory effect on intake.[164]

As discussed previously, low BMI is associated with increased all-cause and COPD-related mortality, unrelated to disease severity.[154] By contrast, the relative risk for mortality seems somewhat decreased in overweight and obese patients with COPD, particularly in GOLD stage 3 to 4, imparting a sort of protective effect, the so-called obesity paradox, as mortality is increased in those with disease of GOLD stage 1 to 2 with obesity traits.[156,165]

Chronic low-grade inflammation is also a hallmark of obesity, insulin resistance, and type 2 diabetes.[166,167] Besides the presence of chronic airflow obstruction, low-grade systemic inflammation could therefore be one of the common mechanisms that may be responsible for the observed mortality and morbidity in obese COPD patients.

In this context, mention should also be made of obstructive sleep apnea (OSA). OSA syndrome (ie, OSA and excessive daytime sleepiness) affects at least 4% to 5% of middle-aged persons.[168] Well-recognized risk factors include excess body weight, nasal congestion, alcohol, smoking, and menopause in women.[169]

Epidemiologic studies have shown that 20% of patients with OSA also have COPD, whereas 10% of patients with COPD have OSA independent of disease severity.[170–172] Such bidirectional interplay between OSA and COPD has been given the term overlap syndrome.[172] Possible shared mechanistic links include increased parasympathetic tone, hypoxemia-related reflex bronchoconstriction/vasoconstriction, irritation of upper airway neural receptors, altered nocturnal neurohormonal secretion, proinflammatory mediators, within-breath and interbreath interactions between upper and lower airways, and lung volume–airway dependence.[172]

Management of OSA and COPD

It is currently unclear whether long-term positive airway pressure therapy for COPD patients without OSA affects outcomes. In one such study,

122 COPD patients hospitalized with respiratory failure were randomized to LTOT versus noninvasive nocturnal ventilation (positive airway pressure) plus oxygen therapy. There was an improvement in HRQoL and reduction in length of stay in the intensive care unit in the noninvasive ventilation group, but no difference in mortality or subsequent hospitalizations was found.[173]

Thus the overlap syndrome represents a condition with important phenotypic characterization, and clarifies the frequent association, symptomatic load, and mortality consequences noted. However, the use of positive airway pressure in overlap syndrome needs further assessment.

ANEMIA IN COPD

As discussed earlier, in severe COPD, polycythemia with a raised hematocrit is known to be a common phenomenon. However, just as for other chronic conditions, COPD could also be associated with anemia.

The WHO defines anemia as a disease associated with low hemoglobin (males <13.0 g/dL and females <12 g/dL).[174]

Prevalence

Key findings of studies of anemia in COPD are summarized in **Table 3**.

A study by Rutten and colleagues[177] in the Netherlands involved 321 patients with COPD admitted for pulmonary rehabilitation, and found anemia in 20% of the patients and polycythemia in another 8%. There was no difference in disease-related outcomes or other comorbidities in the patients with and without anemia. However, after adjustment for confounders, anemia was found to be an independent determinant for higher CRP levels and lower BMD.

Low blood count can also be defined by hematocrit (<39% in men and <36% in women). In a French study involving severe COPD patients who required LTOT, a reduced hematocrit level was associated with increased mortality, whereas a raised hematocrit level was protective, independent of other markers of mortality.[176]

Pathogenesis

The anemia of chronic illness is typically a normocytic anemia and is most commonly observed in patients with infectious disease, and inflammatory or neoplastic diseases.

COPD fulfills the criteria of a chronic, inflammatory, multisystem disease that would be expected to result in anemia. John and colleagues[175] studied 101 COPD patients and determined the

Table 3
PubMed search: anemia/anemia AND COPD OR chronic obstructive pulmonary disease in title/abstract

Authors,[Ref.] Year	Journal	Study Type	Prevalence (%)	Outcome	Comment
John et al,[175] 2005	Chest	Prospective (N = 101)	13/101 = 13	No outcome data EPO resistance?	Outpatients
John et al, 2006	Int J Cardiol	Retrospective hospital records (N = 312)	23	No outcome data	COPD hospitalized
Cote et al,[43] 2007	Eur Respir J	Prospective cohort (N = 677)	116/677 = 17	Independent predictor dyspnea	COPD outpatients
Chambellan et al,[176] 2005	Chest	Retrospective database (N = 2524)	M: 12.6, F: 8.2	Hb as outcome predictor	LTOT
Krishnan et al, 2006	BMC Pulm Med	Post hoc analysis from general population (N = 495)	7.5	Anemia associated with worse HRQoL	No outcome
Schonhofer et al, 1998	Crit Care Med	Prospective 20 anemic adults (10 COPD)	—	Correction of Hb improves breathing pattern and efficacy	No outcome
Kollert et al, 2011	IJCP	Retrospective hospital record database (N = 326)	14.7	Determinants of anemia: pH, Pao$_2$	No outcome
Boutou et al, 2011	Respiration	Prospective, 283 stable COPD	10	Association with dyspnea and exercise capacity	Good patient selection
Rasmussen et al, 2010	Clin Epidemiol	Retrospective hospital records (N = 222)	42/222 = 18	Increased mortality at 90 d	Mechanically ventilated
Markoulaki et al, 2011	Eur J Intern Med	Prospective observational 93 acute exacerbated COPD	NA	Hb decreased, EPO increased	No outcome
Similkowski et al, 2006	Eur Respir J	NA	10–15	Mechanisms of anemia Therapeutic implications	Review
Barnes & Celli,[6] 2009	Eur Respir J	NA	15–30	Impaired functional capacity Mortality predictor	Review

Abbreviations: EPO, erythropoietin; Hb, hemoglobin; HRQoL, health-related quality of life; LTOT, long-term oxygen therapy; NA, no data available; Pao$_2$, partial pressure of oxygen in arterial blood.

prevalence of anemia and its relationship to body mass and weight loss, inflammatory parameters, and erythropoietin levels. Anemia was diagnosed in 13 patients (12.8%). These patients showed elevated erythropoietin levels and had increased systemic inflammation markers (raised CRP) in comparison with the nonanemic patients. This finding raises the possibility that erythropoietin resistance, as is possible in the COPD cohort, is potentially mediated by chronic inflammation.

Management

As for any other anemia of chronic disease, treatment of the underlying disease is the therapeutic approach of choice for anemia in COPD.[178]

The level of hemoglobin is strongly and independently associated with increased functional dyspnea and poorer exercise tolerance, and is therefore an important contributor to poor quality of life.[43] Schönhofer and colleagues[179] demonstrated that correction of anemia with blood transfusions (among 20 patients with severe COPD) significantly reduced disease-related elevations in minute ventilation and work of breathing, suggesting that anemia correction may be beneficial in alleviating dyspnea and improving exercise capacity. Therefore, blood transfusion in selected cases may be necessary, as erythropoietin is unlikely to work in this cohort because of end-organ resistance. Iron supplements, likewise, are unlikely to be useful and possibly could have a deleterious effect by adding to the burden of systemic oxidative stress.[6]

Autonomic Dysfunction

The autonomic nervous system (ANS) controls physiologic processes such as regulation of the airway smooth muscle tone, fluid transport through the airway epithelium, capillary permeability, bronchial circulation, and release of mediators from inflammatory cells.[180] Autonomic dysfunction (AD) is a known phenomenon in COPD patients,[181] and may be an important factor in the pathogenesis of the disease because of the multiple parameters that are under control of the ANS such as the arterial and cardiac baroreceptors,[182] the bronchopulmonary C fibers, and pulmonary stretch receptors, which are capable of triggering ventilation, bronchomotor, and cardiovascular effects.[183,184]

Recurrent hypoxemia, hypercapnea, increased intrathoracic pressure swings resulting from airway obstruction, increased respiratory effort, and systemic inflammation along with the use of β-sympathomimetics have all been implicated as trigger factors for AD as observed in COPD.[181]

Prevalence and Clinical Implications

Tug and colleagues[185] assessed the prevalence of AD according to disease severity in 35 stable COPD patients. Sympathetic system (SS) was evaluated with sympathetic skin response (SSR), and QT- and QTc-interval (milliseconds) analyses. The parasympathetic system was evaluated with the variations in heart-rate interval. AD was detected in 20 patients (57%), parasympathetic dysfunction (PD) in 14 (40%), mixed-type dysfunction in 5 (14%), and sympathetic dysfunction (SD) in only 1 patient (3%). For the 12 patients with mild COPD, there were cases of isolated SD in 1 patient (8.5%), isolated PD in 5 (42%), and AD in 6 (50%). For the 23 moderate to severe COPD patients, mixed AD was detected in 5 patients (22%), isolated PD in 9 (39%), and AD in 14 (61%).

This imbalance in the autonomic nervous activity can contribute to airway narrowing via an effect on the airway smooth muscle, bronchial vessels, and mucous glands in the bronchial wall, and therefore could add to disease progression and severity.

Correction of hypoxia and control of the systemic inflammation seem reasonable target strategies that may help to improve health status in COPD patients.

LUNG CANCER AND COPD

With a shared common environmental risk factor in exposure to cigarette smoke, it is understandable why lung cancer is one of the most frequent comorbidities and one of the commonest causes of death in COPD patients.

Prevalence

Previous studies have shown that COPD is an independent risk factor for the development of lung cancer and that having moderate to severe COPD can increase the risk of developing lung cancer up to almost 5-fold.[186,187]

Thirty-eight percent of deaths in individuals with mild to moderate airflow limitation in the Lung Health Study died of lung cancer.[10] In addition to these 57 deaths, another 35 participants were diagnosed with the disease but survived to the end of follow-up.

An inverse correlation between the degree of airflow obstruction and the risk for lung cancer was demonstrated in an analysis of 22-year follow-up data of 5402 participants from the first National Health and Nutrition Examination Survey (NHANES I), including a total of 113 cases of lung cancer.[188] Tockman and colleagues[189] and

Skillrud and colleagues[190] have previously demonstrated that the incidence of lung cancer increased in individuals with COPD as their FEV_1 declined, a relationship that withstood correction for lifetime cigarette smoke dosage.

Fig. 4 summarizes the inverse relationship observed between lung cancer and lung function values as seen in COPD patients.[188] Unsurprisingly, lung cancer along with cardiovascular diseases comprises two-thirds of all deaths in COPD patients.[191]

Recent studies also indicate that emphysema and airflow limitation are risk factors for lung cancer, independent of exposure to cigarette smoke.[192] Cross-sectional studies have shown that after allowing for cigarette-smoke exposure, reduced FEV_1 (as seen in COPD) is the single most important risk factor for lung cancer, and that these 2 diseases are linked by more than smoking exposure alone.[188,193]

An Italian study has also shown that airflow limitation is primarily a risk factor for squamous cell lung cancer (95% CI 1.63–18.5; P = .006), whereas symptoms of chronic bronchitis without COPD is a risk factor (risk greater than 4-fold) for adenocarcinoma of the lung. In a subset analysis, the association of concurrent bronchitic symptoms and COPD imparted a 3-fold increased risk for squamous cell carcinoma of the lung, further consolidating the link between these 2 conditions.[194]

Pathogenesis and Clinical Implications of Lung Cancer in COPD

The pathogenic mechanism linking these conditions remains unclear, although like other comorbidities in COPD it seems to be multifactorial.

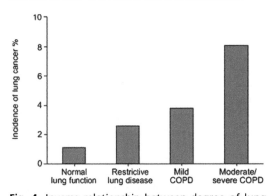

Fig. 4. Inverse relationship between degree of lung function obstruction and incidence of lung cancer. (*Reproduced* with permission of the European Respiratory Society. Sin DD, Anthonisen NR, Soriano JB, et al. Mortality in COPD: role of comorbidities. Eur Respir J 2006;28(6);1250; http://dx.doi.org/10.1183/09031936.00133805.)

Inflammation and oxidative stress seem to play important roles. The process of epithelial-to-mesenchymal transition (EMT), in which cells undergo a switch from an epithelial phenotype to a mesenchymal phenotype, is an important phenomenon that occurs in both patients with lung cancer and COPD patients.[195,196]

Studies have also shown that inflammation directly promotes EMT by inducing the expression of E-cadherin transcriptional repressors, which could explain the connecting link between these 2 conditions.[187,196] An exaggerated inflammatory response, leading to aberrant airway epithelial and matrix remodeling characterized by excessive growth factor release and elevated matrix metalloproteinases (MMP), has also been postulated as a possible mechanism connecting the 2 conditions.[197,198]

NF-κB activation has also been suggested as a link between inflammation and lung cancer.[199] Synergistic effects of latent infection and cigarette smoking cause chronic airway inflammation through enhanced expression of cytokines and adhesion molecules, possibly through NF-κB–mediated activation.[200,201] Some of the cytokines can also inhibit apoptosis, interfering with cellular repair and promoting angiogenesis.[202]

Retrospective studies have also suggested that reducing pulmonary inflammation with ICS or systemic inflammation with statin therapy may reduce the risk of lung cancer in COPD patients, adding further support for a role for inflammation as a common link in both of these conditions.[203,204]

Studies have also suggested specific candidate gene loci as potential genetic links connecting lung cancer and COPD.[205,206] The genes identified in these studies suggest that this common genetic susceptibility may be mediated through receptors expressed on the bronchial epithelium that implicate common molecular pathways underlying both COPD and lung cancer.

The transcription factor, nuclear factor erythroid 2-related factor 2 (Nrf2), which regulates multiple antioxidant and detoxifying genes, has been shown to be downregulated in COPD lungs[207] and may contribute to the increased susceptibility of COPD patients to lung cancer, because Nrf2 plays an important role in defense against carcinogens in tobacco smoke by regulating the expression of several detoxifying enzymes.[208] Epidermal growth factor receptor (EGFR), which promotes epithelial proliferation, also has increased expression in the lungs of COPD patients, which could promote carcinogenesis.[209]

As the increased risk of lung cancer in COPD may be a reflection of increased inflammation and oxidative stress in the lungs, anti-inflammatory therapies or antioxidants should hypothetically diminish the risk of lung cancer.

PSYCHOLOGICAL EFFECTS IN COPD

Anxiety and depression are common in patients with COPD, and have an impact on the psychosocial aspects of the management of this disease. Prognostic studies involving patients with COPD have mostly focused on physiologic variables, with less attention given to the psychological aspects of the disease.

Prevalence

The prevalence of generalized anxiety disorder in COPD patients ranges between 10% and 33%, and that of panic attacks or panic disorder between 8% and 67%.[210] Disease severity in COPD has not clearly been associated with the magnitude of anxiety/depression.[211,212]

Estimates of the prevalence of depression and depressive symptoms vary in COPD patients, ranging from 6% to 60%.[213–215] Hanania and colleagues[216] studied the prevalence and determinants of depression in COPD patient in the ECLIPSE study. The study cohort consisted of 2118 subjects with COPD, 335 smokers without COPD (smokers), and 243 nonsmokers without COPD (nonsmokers). A total of 26%, 12%, and 7% of COPD, smokers, and nonsmokers, respectively, suffered from depression. Using a multivariate logistic regression model, increased fatigue, higher score for St George's Respiratory Questionnaire for COPD patients, younger age, female sex, history of cardiovascular disease, and current smoking status were all significantly associated with depression in this cohort.

Clinical Implications

Depression in COPD might result from a vicious cycle of sedentary lifestyle, smoking habits, and poor nutritional and health status. There is increasing evidence that inflammation itself could be a mediator of depression in COPD patients.[217] Depressive symptoms were found to be strong predictors of mortality (OR 1.9, 3.6, and 2.7, respectively), independent of other markers of disease severity and risk factors, in COPD patients in 3 studies,[218–220] whereas one other study found no association between mortality and depression after adjustment for disease severity.[221]

Therefore, the effect of depression on function in COPD patients and the early recognition and treatment of symptoms remain inherent important aspects in the management of this cohort.

DIABETES AND METABOLIC SYNDROME IN COPD

Prevalence and Pathogenesis

Studies have shown prevalence rates for diabetes of between 1% and 16% in patients with COPD.[222,223] Large population studies have also shown that there is an increased prevalence of diabetes among COPD patients (risk ratio [RR] 1.5–1.8), even in patients with mild disease.[6,224]

Poulain and colleagues[225] looked at a cohort of 28 male patients with COPD, and divided patients according to their body habitus. The study showed that presence of obesity, particularly abdominal obesity, was associated with metabolic and inflammatory abnormalities that are typically associated with the development of cardiovascular diseases and diabetes, such as increased levels of insulin, TNF-α, and IL-6, and may mediate insulin resistance by blocking signaling through the insulin receptor. This finding further cements the common inflammatory pathway theory in the pathogenesis of the systemic effects of COPD.

Rana and colleagues[224] also performed a prospective cohort study in which they looked at the relationship of COPD and asthma with the development of type 2 diabetes. During 8 years of follow-up, a total of 2959 new cases of type 2 diabetes were documented. The risk was significantly higher for patients with COPD than for those without (multivariate RR 1.8, 95% CI 1.1–2.8), but this was not the case among the asthmatics. This finding would further corroborate the fact that COPD is potentially a risk factor for the development of diabetes.

Management and Clinical Implications

Hyperglycemia, especially during acute exacerbations of COPD, is associated with poorer outcomes of acute noninvasive ventilation,[226] longer inpatient stay, and higher rates of in-hospital mortality.[148,227] Therefore, it is important to identify underlying hyperglycemic status in COPD patients to reduce the burden of morbidity and mortality as well as unnecessary utilization of health care resources.

The metabolic syndrome is a complex disorder and an emerging clinical challenge, recognized clinically by the findings of abdominal obesity, elevated triglycerides, atherogenic dyslipidemia, elevated blood pressure, and high blood glucose and/or insulin resistance.[228] It is also associated with a prothrombotic state and a proinflammatory state. Patients with COPD often have 1 or more components of the metabolic syndrome,[228] which are, at least in part, independent of treatment with steroids and/or physical inactivity.[229]

Clini and colleagues[230] also postulated that the metabolic syndrome was more likely to be present in COPD patients, as augmented levels of circulatory proinflammatory proteins from both the lung and adipose tissue (adipokines) overlap in these patients. This coexistence perhaps rests on several factors including the presence of physical inactivity, systemic inflammation partly related to smoking habit, sedentary lifestyle, airway inflammation, adipose tissue, and inflammatory marker activation, among others.

Apart from the risks per se from high glucose level already described, COPD patients with hyperglycemia are likely to have more than one species of bacteria grown from sputum, suggesting impaired immunity.[148] Although some nondiabetic COPD patients have hyperglycemia induced by systemic corticosteroids during exacerbations, this is more likely in the context of diabetes,

therefore oral hypoglycemic medications or insulin may be a necessity.

Preventive measures include lifestyle advice including dietary guidance, and regular screening of those at higher risk, given the higher prevalence and adverse clinical impact of diabetes on COPD patients. This approach would potentially enable earlier diagnosis and prevention of complications.

There should also be more focus on global interventions intended at altering factors such as physical deconditioning and obesity, as such an approach may help slow the metabolic complications seen in COPD patients, particularly those with features of the metabolic syndrome.

SYSTEMIC INFLAMMATION IN COPD

As described earlier, systemic inflammation is a well-established occurrence in COPD patients.

Table 4
Mediators of systemic inflammation in COPD

	Mediators	Actions
Cytokines	Interleukin (IL)-6	Cardiovascular and skeletal muscle dysfunction[6,21]
	Tumor necrosis factor (TNF)-α	Metabolic and skeletal muscle dysfunction (SMD)[113,114,139]
	IL-1β	Cachexia in COPD[6]
	CXCL8 (IL-8) and other CXC chemokines	Neutrophil and monocyte recruitment and also contributes to SMD[6]
	Adipokines such as leptins	Possible role in cachexia in COPD[6]
Acute-phase proteins	C-reactive protein	Raised in infective exacerbations potentiates cardiovascular effects and SMD[4,118]
	Fibrinogen	Cardiovascular complications[40,41]
	Surfactant protein D	Derived from lung tissue; is a good marker of lung inflammation[248]
	Serum amyloid A (SA-A)	Released by circulating proinflammatory cytokines, SA-A levels are raised during acute exacerbations of COPD and its concentrations are correlated with the severity of exacerbation[6,249]
Circulating cells	Neutrophils	Inverse correlation between neutrophil numbers in the circulation and FEV_1,[250] increased turnover in smokers,[6] enhanced production of reactive oxygen species[251]
	Monocytes	Increase macrophage accumulation in the lungs with defective phagocytic property,[6] increase matrix metalloproteinase-9 production compared with nonsmokers[252]
	Lymphocytes	Increased apoptosis of peripheral T lymphocytes from COPD patients, with increased expression of Fas, TNF-α, and transforming growth factor β,[6,253] increase in apoptosis of $CD8^+$ T cells in COPD[254]
	Natural killer (NK) cells	Reduction of cytotoxic and phagocytic function of circulating NK cells has been reported in COPD[6,255]

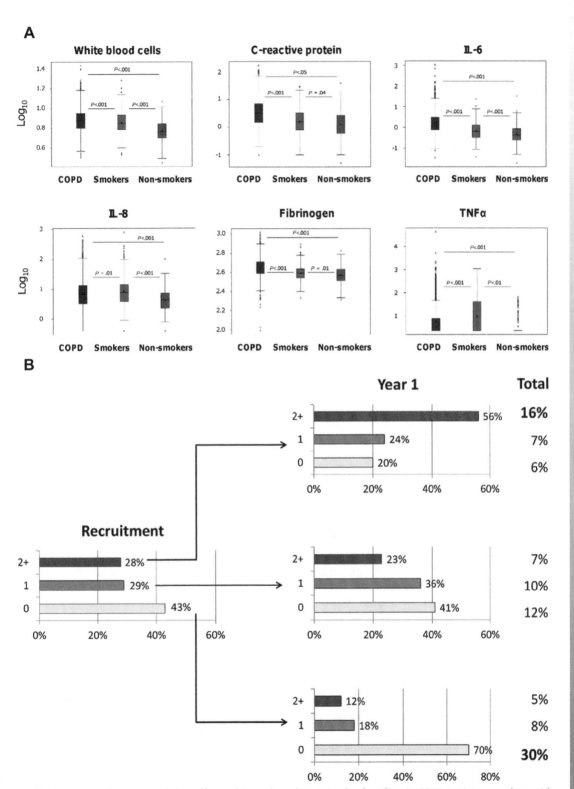

Fig. 5. (*A*) Box plot (log scale) of the different biomarkers determined at baseline in COPD patients, smokers with normal lung function (S), and nonsmokers (NS). IL, interleukin; TNF, tumor necrosis factor. (*B*) Proportion of patients with no, 1, or 2 (or more) biomarkers (white blood cell count, C-reactive protein, interleukin-6, and fibrinogen) in the upper quartile of the COPD distribution, at baseline (*left bars*) and after 1 year of follow-up (*right bars*). (*From* Agusti A, Edwards LD, Rennard SI, et al. Persistent systemic inflammation is associated with poor clinical outcomes in COPD: a novel phenotype. PLoS One 2012;7(5):e37483.)

Numerous studies have provided evidence of systemic inflammation in COPD patients, as shown by the presence of inflammatory mediators such as acute-phase proteins, as well as markers of oxidative stress and immune responses that are increased in the peripheral blood in COPD patients in comparison with smokers who have not developed the disease.[231–233]

However, the presence of systemic inflammation is poorly defined in COPD patients; most studies have been cross-sectional and indicate that not all COPD patients have a systemic inflammatory response. Systemic inflammation, as already discussed, is a known risk factor for developing many of the conditions described conventionally as comorbidities of COPD.[222,231,234,235] Smoking, a major cause of airway inflammation in COPD, is known to be associated with systemic inflammation, and is a potential link between the pulmonary and systemic inflammation in COPD and its comorbidities.[232,236–240] Smoking and reduced FEV_1 also have been found to have an additive effect on systemic inflammatory markers.[241]

While increasing evidence suggests that the systemic inflammatory pathway provides the common link between COPD and its comorbidities,[234,236,239,242] the mechanisms by which the systemic inflammation arises are unclear. There is much debate around whether the systemic inflammation in COPD arises from a spill-over of inflammatory mediators from lung inflammation,[6,231,243] or whether the systemic inflammation in COPD represents a systemic component of the disease that develops in parallel with, or before, pulmonary inflammation.[231,243] The absence of a relationship between inflammatory biomarkers in the sputum and blood of COPD patients has provided some evidence against the spill-over theory.[231,237,244] Smoking, lung hyperinflation, tissue hypoxia, skeletal muscle, bone marrow stimulation, immunologic disorders, and infections are all cited as possible sources of systemic inflammation as seen in COPD.[231,242,245]

Several studies and meta-analyses have shown that in patients with stable COPD there are often elevated levels of systemic inflammatory markers, such as increased circulating leukocytes, CRP, IL-6, IL-8, fibrinogen, and TNF-α.[233,234,245–247] **Table 4** summarizes the various inflammatory mediators as described in COPD.

However, the prevalence of systemic inflammation in COPD has not been well studied, and many of the earlier published data are derived from short-term, cross-sectional studies with small sample sizes.[256] These studies show a wide intersubject validation in systemic biomarkers.

Moreover, there is no agreed consensus on the type, number, and value of inflammatory biomarkers needed to define systemic inflammation. These cross-sectional studies are unable to fully establish the relationship between biomarkers and key health outcomes, owing to the chronic nature of COPD and its comorbidities. Data from the Evaluation of COPD Longitudinally to Identify Predictive Surrogate Endpoints (ECLIPSE) study[257] in more than 2000 COPD patients, control smokers, and nonsmokers assessed longitudinally over 3 years was used to evaluate systemic inflammatory biomarkers. Many systemic inflammatory biomarkers were found to be reproducible over time, with fibrinogen being the most repeatable.[258] As shown in other studies, differences in several biomarkers can be shown between COPD subjects and control smokers and nonsmokers, including peripheral white blood cell count, IL-6, CRP, and fibrinogen, despite large variability within each group (**Fig. 5**A), whereas others such as IL-8 and TNF-α appear to be higher in smokers than in COPD patients.[20] When the proportion of COPD patients with 0, 1, or 2 (or more) of these biomarkers (white blood cell count, high-sensitivity CRP, IL-6, and fibrinogen) were in the upper quartile of the COPD distribution, 28% of patients had 2 or more of these biomarkers elevated at the time of recruitment and 56% of these subjects still had 2 or more systemic inflammatory biomarkers elevated at 1 year (see **Fig. 5**B), whereas 43% of patients had no raised systemic inflammatory biomarkers at baseline and 70% of these patients still had none of the systemic biomarkers elevated at 1 year. Thus, from this study and according to this definition, approximately 16% of COPD patients have sustained systemic inflammation. Those patients with sustained systemic

Systemic Manifestations Associated with COPD

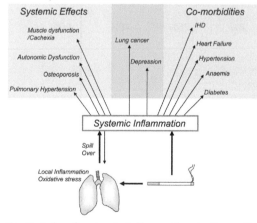

Fig. 6. Role of systemic inflammation in the pathogenesis of COPD.

inflammation were more breathless, with poorer exercise capacity, higher exacerbation rate, and higher mortality. Those patients with sustained systemic inflammation had a higher prevalence of cardiovascular disease. This study therefore suggests that there may be a systemic inflamed COPD phenotype of COPD, which can be described as a phenotype of COPD because it only occurs in a percentage of patients, is stable over time, and is associated with clinical and functional characteristics and poor clinical outcomes. It is possible that targeting these individuals with appropriate treatment may improve outcomes.

Vanfleteren and colleagues[259] looked at 213 COPD patients with the aim of clustering 13 clinically identified comorbidities, and to characterize the comorbidity clusters in terms of clinical outcomes and systemic inflammation. A total of 97.7% of all patients had 1 or more comorbidities and 53.5% had 4 or more comorbidities. Five comorbidity clusters were identified: (1) less comorbidity, (2) cardiovascular, (3) cachectic, (4) metabolic, and (5) psychological. An increased inflammatory state was observed only for TNF receptors in the metabolic cluster and for IL-6 in the cardiovascular cluster, suggesting a role for low-grade systemic inflammation in the pathogenesis of COPD comorbidities.

Fig. 6 summarizes the interrelation between inflammation and the comorbidities and systemic effects as observed in COPD, although some of the effects described as systemic could also be interchangeably described as comorbidity, as described earlier.

SUMMARY

The extrapulmonary effects of COPD are truly multifarious, and have an adverse effect on function and outcomes in COPD.

Fig. 7 summarizes the impact of comorbidities on all-cause mortality in COPD patients.

The clinical management of this condition should therefore be directed toward identifying and treating these extrapulmonary effects, which may lead to improved outcomes for this condition. Novel therapies particularly targeted toward the inflammation associated with COPD should be developed.

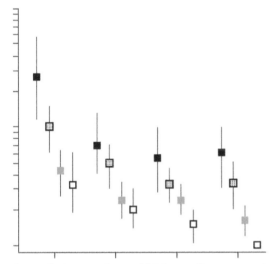

Fig. 7. The impact of comorbidities on all-cause mortality in COPD patients. Prediction of all-cause mortality within 5 years of COPD patients by modified GOLD category and the presence of no (▨), 1 (□), 2 (▨), or 3 (■) comorbid diseases (diabetes, hypertension, or cardiovascular disease). The reference group (normal) was subjects with normal lung function for each comorbid disease. Models were adjusted for age, sex, race, smoking status, education level, and body mass index. Subjects were from the Atherosclerosis Risk in Communities Study during 1986 to 1989 and the Cardiovascular Health Study during 1989 to 1990. GOLD 3/4: forced expiratory volume in 1 second (FEV_1)/forced vital capacity (FVC) <0.70 and FEV_1 <50% predicted; GOLD 2: FEV_1/FVC <0.70 and FEV_1 ≥50 to <80% predicted; GOLD 1: FEV_1/FVC <0.70 and FEV_1 ≥80% predicted; restricted (R): FEV_1/FVC ≥0.70 and FVC <80% predicted; GOLD 0: presence of respiratory symptoms in the absence of any lung function abnormality and no lung disease. (*Reproduced* with permission of the European Respiratory Society. Mannino DM, Thorn D, Swensen A, et al. Prevalence and outcomes of diabetes, hypertension and cardiovascular disease in COPD. Eur Respir J 2008;32(4):967; http://dx.doi.org/10.1183/09031936. 00012408.)

REFERENCES

1. Murray CJ, Lopez AD. Alternative projections of mortality and disability by cause 1990-2020: Global Burden of Disease Study. Lancet 1997; 349:1498–504.
2. Chapman KR, Mannino DM, Soriano JB, et al. Epidemiology and costs of chronic obstructive pulmonary disease. Eur Respir J 2006;27:188–207. http://dx.doi.org/10.1183/09031936.06.00024505.
3. Celli BR, MacNee W, Agusti A, et al. Standards for the diagnosis and treatment of patients with COPD: a summary of the ATS/ERS position paper. Eur Respir J 2004;23(6):932–46.
4. MacNee W. Systemic inflammatory biomarkers and co-morbidities of chronic obstructive pulmonary disease. Ann Med 2012;45:291–300.
5. Agusti AG. Systemic effects of chronic obstructive pulmonary disease. Proc Am Thorac Soc 2005; 2(4):367–70 [discussion: 371–2].
6. Barnes PJ, Celli BR. Systemic manifestations and comorbidities of COPD. Eur Respir J 2009;33:

1165–85. http://dx.doi.org/10.1183/09031936.00128008.

7. Ghoorah K, De Soyza A, Kunadian V. Increased cardiovascular risk in patients with chronic obstructive pulmonary disease and the potential mechanisms linking the two conditions: a review. Cardiol Rev 2013;21:196–202.

8. Agarwal SK, Heiss G, Barr RG, et al. Airflow obstruction, lung function, and risk of incident heart failure: the Atherosclerosis Risk in Communities (ARIC) study. Eur J Heart Fail 2012;14(4):414–22. http://dx.doi.org/10.1093/eurjhf/hfs016.

9. Mapel DW, Dedrick D, Davis K. Trends and cardiovascular co-morbidities of COPD patients in the Veterans Administration Medical System, 1991-1999. COPD 2005;2(1):35–41.

10. Anthonisen NR, Connett JE, Enright PL, et al, Lung Health Study Research Group. Hospitalizations and mortality in the Lung Health Study. Am J Respir Crit Care Med 2002;166(3):333–9.

11. Divo M, Cote C, de Torres JP, et al. Comorbidities and risk of mortality in patients with chronic obstructive pulmonary disease. Am J Respir Crit Care Med 2012;186(2):155–61. http://dx.doi.org/10.1164/rccm.201201-0034OC.

12. Holguin F, Folch E, Redd SC, et al. Comorbidity and mortality in COPD-related hospitalizations in the United States, 1979 to 2001. Chest 2005;128:2005–11.

13. Bang KM, Gergen PJ, Kramer R, et al. The effect of pulmonary impairment on all-cause mortality in a national cohort. Chest 1993;103(2):536–40.

14. Campo G, Guastaroba P, Marzocchi A, et al. Impact of chronic obstructive pulmonary disease on long-term outcome after ST-segment elevation myocardial infarction receiving primary percutaneous coronary intervention. Chest 2013. http://dx.doi.org/10.1378/chest.12-2313.

15. Hole DJ, Watt GC, Davey-Smith G, et al. Impaired lung function and mortality risk in men and women: finding from the Renfrew and Paisley prospective population study. BMJ 1996;313:711–5 [discussion: 715–6].

16. Sin DD, Man SF. Why are patients with chronic obstructive pulmonary disease at increased risk of cardiovascular diseases? The potential role of systemic inflammation in chronic obstructive pulmonary disease. Circulation 2003;107(11):1514–9.

17. Iwamoto H, Yokoyama A, Kitahara Y, et al. Airflow limitation in smokers is associated with subclinical atherosclerosis. Am J Respir Crit Care Med 2009;179(1):35–40.

18. van Gestel YR, Flu WJ, van Kuijk JP, et al. Association of COPD with carotid wall intima-media thickness in vascular surgery patients. Respir Med 2010;104(5):712–6.

19. Ross R. The pathogenesis of atherosclerosis: a perspective for the 1990s. Nature 1993;362(6423):801–9.

20. Agusti A, Edwards LD, Rennard SI, et al, Evaluation of COPD Longitudinally to Identify Predictive Surrogate End-points (ECLIPSE) Investigators. Persistent systemic inflammation is associated with poor clinical outcomes in COPD: a novel phenotype. PLoS One 2012;7(5):e37483.

21. Celli BR, Locantore N, Yates J, et al, ECLIPSE Investigators. Inflammatory biomarkers improve clinical prediction of mortality in chronic obstructive pulmonary disease. Am J Respir Crit Care Med 2012;185(10):1065–72.

22. McAllister DA, Maclay JD, Mills NL, et al. Diagnosis of myocardial infarction following hospitalisation for exacerbation of COPD. Eur Respir J 2012;39:1097–103. http://dx.doi.org/10.1183/09031936.00124811.

23. Hurst JR, Donaldson GC, Perera WR, et al. Use of plasma biomarkers at exacerbation of chronic obstructive pulmonary disease. Am J Respir Crit Care Med 2006;174(8):867–74.

24. Maclay JD, MacNee W. Cardiovascular disease in COPD: mechanisms. Chest 2013;143(3):798–807. http://dx.doi.org/10.1378/chest.12-0938.

25. Libby P, Theroux P. Pathophysiology of coronary artery disease. Circulation 2005;111(25):3481–8.

26. Coulson JM, Rudd JH, Duckers JM, et al. Excessive aortic inflammation in chronic obstructive pulmonary disease: an 18 F-FDG PET pilot study. J Nucl Med 2010;51(9):1357–60.

27. Lattimore J, Wilcox I, Nakhla S, et al. Repetitive hypoxia increases lipid loading in human macrophages—a potentially atherogenic effect. Atherosclerosis 2005;179(2):255–9.

28. Ichikawa H, Flores S, Kvietys PR, et al. Molecular mechanisms of anoxia/reoxygenation-induced neutrophil adherence to cultured endothelial cells. Circ Res 1997;81(6):922–31.

29. Hartmann G, Tschöp M, Fischer R, et al. High altitude increases circulating interleukin-6, interleukin-1 receptor antagonist and C-reactive protein. Cytokine 2000;12(3):246–52.

30. Savransky V, Nanayakkara A, Li J, et al. Chronic intermittent hypoxia induces atherosclerosis. Am J Respir Crit Care Med 2007;175(12):1290–7.

31. Chen L, Einbinder E, Zhang Q, et al. Oxidative stress and left ventricular function with chronic intermittent hypoxia in rats. Am J Respir Crit Care Med 2005;172(7):915–20.

32. Thomson AJ, Drummond GB, Waring WS, et al. Effects of short-term isocapnic hyperoxia and hypoxia on cardiovascular function. J Appl Physiol 2006;101:809–16.

33. Skwarski KM, Morrison D, Barratt A, et al. Effects of hypoxia on renal hormonal balance in normal

subjects and in patients with COPD. Respir Med 1998;92(12):1331–6.

34. Heindl S, Lehnert M, Criée CP, et al. Marked sympathetic activation in patients with chronic respiratory failure. Am J Respir Crit Care Med 2001;164: 597–601.

35. Curtis BM, O'Keefe JH Jr. Autonomic tone as a cardiovascular risk factor: the dangers of chronic fight or flight. Mayo Clin Proc 2002;77:45–54.

36. Cordero A, Bertomeu-Martínez V, Mazón P, et al. Clinical features and hospital complications of patients with acute coronary syndromes according to smoking habits. Med Clin (Barc) 2012;138(10):422–8. http://dx.doi.org/10.1016/j.medcli.2011.01.016.

37. Bernhard D, Wang XL. Smoking, oxidative stress and cardiovascular diseases—do anti-oxidative therapies fail? Curr Med Chem 2007;14:1703–12.

38. Brook RD, Rajagopalan S. Particulate matter, air pollution, and blood pressure. J Am Soc Hypertens 2009;3:332–50.

39. Talukder MA, Johnson WM, Varadharaj S, et al. Chronic cigarette smoking causes hypertension, increased oxidative stress, impaired NO bioavailability, endothelial dysfunction, and cardiac remodeling in mice. Am J Physiol Heart Circ Physiol 2011; 300(1):H388–96.

40. Alessandri C, Basili S, Violi F, et al. Chronic Obstructive Bronchitis and Haemostasis Group. Hypercoagulability state in patients with chronic obstructive pulmonary disease. Thromb Haemost 1994;72(3):343–6.

41. Ashitani JI, Mukae H, Arimura Y, et al. Elevated plasma procoagulant and fibrinolytic markers in patients with chronic obstructive pulmonary disease. Intern Med 2002;41(3):181–5.

42. Libby P. Inflammation in atherosclerosis. Nature 2002;420(6917):868–74.

43. Cote C, Zilberberg MD, Mody SH, et al. Haemoglobin level and its clinical impact in a cohort of patients with COPD. Eur Respir J 2007;29:923–9.

44. Weber FP. The prognostic significance of secondary polycythaemia in cardio-pulmonary cases. Proc R Soc Med 1913;6:83–98.

45. Minet C, Vivodtzev I, Tamisier R, et al. Reduced six-minute walking distance, high fat-free-mass index and hypercapnia are associated with endothelial dysfunction in COPD. Respir Physiol Neurobiol 2012;183(2):128–34. http://dx.doi.org/10.1016/j.resp.2012.06.017.

46. Barr RG, Mesia-Vela S, Austin JH, et al. Impaired flow mediated dilation is associated with low pulmonary function and emphysema in ex-smokers: the Emphysema and Cancer Action Project (EMCAP) Study. Am J Respir Crit Care Med 2007; 176:1200–7.

47. Eickhoff P, Valipour A, Kiss D, et al. Determinants of systemic vascular function in patients with stable

chronic obstructive pulmonary disease. Am J Respir Crit Care Med 2008;178:1211–8.

48. Maclay JD, McAllister DA, Mills NL, et al. Vascular dysfunction in chronic obstructive pulmonary disease. Am J Respir Crit Care Med 2009;180:513–20.

49. Vlachopoulos C, Aznaouridis K, Stefanadis C. Prediction of cardiovascular events and all-cause mortality with arterial stiffness: a systematic review and meta-analysis. J Am Coll Cardiol 2010;55:1318–27.

50. Sabit R, Bolton CE, Edwards PH, et al. Arterial stiffness and osteoporosis in chronic obstructive pulmonary disease. Am J Respir Crit Care Med 2007;175(12):1259–65.

51. Mills NL, Miller JJ, Anand A, et al. Increased arterial stiffness in patients with chronic obstructive pulmonary disease: a mechanism for increased cardiovascular risk. Thorax 2008;63(4):306–11.

52. McAllister DA, Maclay JD, Mills NL, et al. Arterial stiffness is independently associated with emphysema severity in patients with chronic obstructive pulmonary disease. Am J Respir Crit Care Med 2007;176:1208–14.

53. Maclay JD, McAllister DA, Rabinovich R, et al. Systemic elastin degradation in chronic obstructive pulmonary disease. Thorax 2012;67:606–12.

54. Rutten FH, Cramer MJ, Grobbee DE, et al. Unrecognized heart failure in elderly patients with stable chronic obstructive pulmonary disease. Eur Heart J 2005;26(18):1887–94.

55. Boudestein LC, Rutten FH, Cramer MJ, et al. The impact of concurrent heart failure on prognosis in patients with chronic obstructive pulmonary disease. Eur J Heart Fail 2009;11(12):1182–8. http://dx.doi.org/10.1093/eurjhf/hfp148.

56. Mascarenhas J, Lourenco P, Lopes R, et al. Chronic obstructive pulmonary disease in heart failure. Prevalence, therapeutic and prognostic implications. Am Heart J 2008;155:521–5.

57. De Blois J, Simard S, Atar D, et al. COPD predicts mortality in heart failure: the Norwegian Heart Failure Registry. J Card Fail 2010;16:225–9.

58. Iversen KK, Kjaergaard J, Akkan D, et al. The prognostic importance of lung function in patients admitted with heart failure. Eur J Heart Fail 2010; 12(7):685–91. http://dx.doi.org/10.1093/eurjhf/hfq050.

59. Watz H, Waschki B, Meyer T, et al. Decreasing cardiac chamber sizes and associated heart dysfunction in COPD, role of hyperinflation. Chest 2010; 138(1):32–8.

60. Barr RG, Bluemke DA, Ahmed FS, et al. Percent emphysema, airflow obstruction, and impaired left ventricular filling. N Engl J Med 2010;362(3):217–27.

61. Shih H, Webb C, Conway W, et al. Frequency and significance of cardiac arrhythmias in chronic obstructive lung disease. Chest 1988;94:44–8.

62. Sekine Y, Kesler KA, Behnia M, et al. COPD may increase the incidence of refractory supraventricular arrhythmias following pulmonary resection for non-small cell lung cancer. Chest 2001;120:1783–90.

63. Mathew JP, Fontes ML, Tudor IC, et al. A multicenter risk index for atrial fibrillation after cardiac surgery. JAMA 2004;291:1720–9.

64. Ryynänen OP, Soini EJ, Lindqvist A, et al. Bayesian predictors of very poor health related quality of life and mortality in patients with COPD. BMC Med Inform Decis Mak 2013;13:34. http://dx.doi.org/10.1186/1472-6947-13-34.

65. Reed RM, Eberlein M, Girgis RE, et al. Coronary artery disease is under-diagnosed and under-treated in advanced lung disease. Am J Med 2012;125(12):1228.e13–22. http://dx.doi.org/10.1016/j.amjmed.2012.05.018.

66. Hawkins NM, Huang Z, Pieper KS, et al. Chronic obstructive pulmonary disease is an independent predictor of death but not atherosclerotic events in patients with myocardial infarction: analysis of the Valsartan in Acute Myocardial Infarction Trial (VALIANT). Eur J Heart Fail 2009;11(3):292–8. http://dx.doi.org/10.1093/eurjhf/hfp001.

67. Donaldson GC, Hurst JR, Smith CJ, et al. Increased risk of myocardial infarction and stroke following exacerbation of COPD. Chest 2010;137(5):1091–7.

68. Mackay DF, Irfan MO, Haw S, et al. Meta-analysis of the effect of comprehensive smoke-free legislation on acute coronary events. Heart 2010;96:1525–30.

69. Sin DD, Man SF, Marciniuk DD, et al. The effects of fluticasone with or without salmeterol on systemic biomarkers of inflammation in chronic obstructive pulmonary disease. Am J Respir Crit Care Med 2008;177(11):1207–14. http://dx.doi.org/10.1164/rccm.200709-1356OC.

70. Calverley PM, Anderson JA, Celli B, et al. Cardiovascular events in patients with COPD: TORCH study results. Thorax 2010;65(8):719–25. http://dx.doi.org/10.1136/thx.2010.136077.

71. Verhamme KM, Afonso A, Romio S, et al. Use of tiotropium Respimat(R) SMI vs. tiotropium Handihaler(R) and mortality in patients with COPD. Eur Respir J 2013;42:606–15.

72. Celli B, Decramer M, Leimer I, et al. Cardiovascular safety of tiotropium in patients with COPD. Chest 2010;137(1):20–30. http://dx.doi.org/10.1378/chest.09-0011.

73. Dransfield MT, Rowe SM, Johnson JE, et al. Use of beta blockers and the risk of death in hospitalised patients with acute exacerbations of COPD. Thorax 2008;63(4):301–5.

74. Dobler CC, Wong KK, Marks GB. Associations between statins and COPD: a systematic review. BMC Pulm Med 2009;9:32. http://dx.doi.org/10.1186/1471-2466-9-32.

75. Mancini GB, Etminan M, Zhang B, et al. Reduction of morbidity and mortality by statins, angiotensin-converting enzyme inhibitors, and angiotensin receptor blockers in patients with chronic obstructive pulmonary disease. J Am Coll Cardiol 2006;47:2554–60.

76. Gottlieb SS, McCarter RJ, Vogel RA. Effect of beta-blockade on mortality among high-risk and low-risk patients after myocardial infarction. N Engl J Med 1998;339(8):489–97.

77. Hunt SA, Abraham WT, Chin MH, et al. 2009 focused update incorporated into the ACC/AHA 2005 Guidelines for the Diagnosis and Management of Heart Failure in Adults: a report of the American College of Cardiology Foundation/American Heart Association Task Force on Practice Guidelines developed in collaboration with the International Society for Heart and Lung Transplantation. Circulation 2009;119:e391–479.

78. Poole-Wilson PA, Swedberg K, Cleland JG, et al. Comparison of carvedilol and metoprolol on clinical outcomes in patients with chronic heart failure in the Carvedilol Or Metoprolol European Trial (COMET): randomised controlled trial. Lancet 2003;362:7–13.

79. Heart Failure Society of America, Lindenfeld J, Albert NM, Boehmer JP, et al. HFSA 2010 comprehensive heart failure practice guideline. J Card Fail 2010;16:e1–194.

80. Andreas S, Anker SD, Scanlon PD, et al. Neurohumoral activation as a link to systemic manifestations of chronic lung disease. Chest 2005;128(5):3618–24.

81. Rutten FH, Zuithoff NP, Hak E, et al. Beta-blockers may reduce mortality and risk of exacerbations in patients with chronic obstructive pulmonary disease. Arch Intern Med 2010;170(10):880–7. http://dx.doi.org/10.1001/archinternmed.2010.112.

82. Hawkins NM, Jhund PS, Simpson CR, et al. Primary care burden and treatment of patients with heart failure and chronic obstructive pulmonary disease in Scotland. Eur J Heart Fail 2010;12(1):17–24. http://dx.doi.org/10.1093/eurjhf/hfp160.

83. Salpeter S, Ormiston T, Salpeter E. Cardioselective beta-blockers for chronic obstructive pulmonary disease. Cochrane Database Syst Rev 2005;(4):CD003566.

84. Stefan MS, Rothberg MB, Priya A, et al. Association between β-blocker therapy and outcomes in patients hospitalised with acute exacerbations of chronic obstructive lung disease with underlying ischaemic heart disease, heart failure or hypertension. Thorax 2012;67(11):977–84. http://dx.doi.org/10.1136/thoraxjnl-2012-201945.

85. Ekström MP, Hermansson AB, Ström KE. Effects of cardiovascular drugs on mortality in severe chronic obstructive pulmonary disease. Am J Respir Crit

Care Med 2013;187(7):715–20. http://dx.doi.org/10.1164/rccm.201208-1565OC.

86. Mortensen EM, Copeland LA, Pugh MJ, et al. Impact of statins and ACE inhibitors on mortality after COPD exacerbations. Respir Res 2009;10:45. http://dx.doi.org/10.1186/1465-9921-10-45.

87. Agusti AG, Noguera A, Sauleda J, et al. Systemic effects of chronic obstructive pulmonary disease. Eur Respir J 2003;21:347–60.

88. Gosselink R, Troosters T, Decramer M. Peripheral muscle weakness contributes to exercise limitation in COPD. Am J Respir Crit Care Med 1996;153:976–80.

89. Shrikrishna D, Hopkinson NS. Chronic obstructive pulmonary disease: consequences beyond the lung. Clin Med 2012;12:71–4.

90. Decramer M, Gosselink R, Troosters T, et al. Muscle weakness is related to utilization of health care resources in COPD patients. Eur Respir J 1997;10:417–23.

91. Swallow EB, Reyes D, Hopkinson NS, et al. Quadriceps strength predicts mortality in patients with moderate to severe chronic obstructive pulmonary disease. Thorax 2007;62:115–20.

92. Seymour JM, Spruit MA, Hopkinson NS, et al. The prevalence of quadriceps weakness in COPD and the relationship with disease severity. Eur Respir J 2010;36:81–8.

93. Shrikrishna D, Hopkinson NS. Skeletal muscle dysfunction in chronic obstructive pulmonary disease. Respir Med 2009;5:7–13 COPD Update.

94. Hopkinson NS, Polkey MI. Does physical inactivity cause chronic obstructive pulmonary disease? Clin Sci 2010;118:565–72.

95. Shrikrishna D, Patel M, Tanner RJ, et al. Quadriceps wasting and physical inactivity in patients with COPD. Eur Respir J 2012. http://dx.doi.org/10.1183/09031936.00170111.

96. Wust RC, Degens H. Factors contributing to muscle wasting and dysfunction in COPD patients. Int J Chron Obstruct Pulmon Dis 2007;2:289–300.

97. Schols AM, Soeters PB, Dingemans AM, et al. Prevalence and characteristics of nutritional depletion in patients with stable COPD eligible for pulmonary rehabilitation. Am Rev Respir Dis 1993;147:1151–6.

98. Bernard S, LeBlanc P, Whittom F, et al. Peripheral muscle weakness in patients with chronic obstructive pulmonary disease. Am J Respir Crit Care Med 1998;158:629–34.

99. Mostert R, Goris A, Weling-Scheepers C, et al. Tissue depletion and health related quality of life in patients with chronic obstructive pulmonary disease. Respir Med 2000;94:859–67.

100. Marquis K, Debigare R, Lacasse Y, et al. Midthigh muscle cross-sectional area is a better predictor of mortality than body mass index in patients with chronic obstructive pulmonary disease. Am J Respir Crit Care Med 2002;166:809–13.

101. Whittom F, Jobin J, Simard PM, et al. Histochemical and morphological characteristics of the vastus lateralis muscle in patients with chronic obstructive pulmonary disease. Med Sci Sports Exerc 1998;30:1467–74.

102. Gosker HR, Engelen MP, van Mameren H, et al. Muscle fiber type IIX atrophy is involved in the loss of fat-free mass in chronic obstructive pulmonary disease. Am J Clin Nutr 2002;76:113–9.

103. Sala E, Roca J, Marrades RM, et al. Effects of endurance training on skeletal muscle bioenergetics in chronic obstructive pulmonary disease. Am J Respir Crit Care Med 1999;159:1726–34.

104. Jobin J, Maltais F, Doyon JF, et al. Chronic obstructive pulmonary disease: capillarity and fiber characteristics of skeletal muscle. J Cardiopulm Rehabil 1998;18:432–7.

105. Allaire J, Maltais F, Doyon JF, et al. Peripheral muscle endurance and the oxidative profile of the quadriceps in patients with COPD. Thorax 2004;59:673–8.

106. Rabinovich RA, Bastos R, Ardite E, et al. Mitochondrial dysfunction in COPD patients with low body mass index. Eur Respir J 2007;29:643–50.

107. Engelen MP, Deutz NE, Wouters EF, et al. Enhanced levels of whole-body protein turnover in patients with chronic obstructive pulmonary disease. Am J Respir Crit Care Med 2000;162:1488–92.

108. Plant PJ, Brooks D, Faughnan M, et al. Cellular markers of muscle atrophy in chronic obstructive pulmonary disease (COPD). Am J Respir Cell Mol Biol 2010;42:461–71.

109. Rabinovich RA, Vilaro J. Structural and functional changes of peripheral muscles in chronic obstructive pulmonary disease patients. Curr Opin Pulm Med 2010;16:123–33.

110. Dekhuijzen PN, Decramer M. Steroid-induced myopathy and its significance to respiratory disease: a known disease rediscovered. Eur Respir J 1992;5:997–1003.

111. Decramer M, de Bock V, Dom R. Functional and histologic picture of steroid-induced myopathy in chronic obstructive pulmonary disease. Am J Respir Crit Care Med 1996;153:1958–64.

112. Hopkinson NS, Man WD, Dayer MJ, et al. Acute effect of oral steroids on muscle function in chronic obstructive pulmonary disease. Eur Respir J 2004;24(1):137–42.

113. Takabatake N, Nakamura H, Abe S, et al. The relationship between chronic hypoxemia and activation of the tumor necrosis factor-α system in patients with chronic obstructive pulmonary disease. Am J Respir Crit Care Med 2000;161:1179–84.

114. Preedy VR, Smith DM, Sugden PH. The effects of 6 hours of hypoxia on protein synthesis in rat tissues in vivo and in vitro. Biochem J 1985;228:179–85.

115. Vohwinkel CU, Lecuona E, Sun H, et al. Elevated CO_2 levels cause mitochondrial dysfunction and impair cell proliferation. J Biol Chem 2011;286: 37067–76.

116. Yende S, Waterer GW, Tolley EA, et al. Inflammatory markers are associated with ventilatory limitation and muscle dysfunction in obstructive lung disease in well functioning elderly subjects. Thorax 2006; 61:10–6.

117. Remels AH, Gosker HR, Schrauwen P, et al. TNF-α impairs regulation of muscle oxidative phenotype: implications for cachexia? FASEB J 2010;24: 5052–62.

118. Pinto-Plata VM, Müllerova H, Toso JF, et al. C-Reactive protein in patients with COPD, control smokers and non-smokers. Thorax 2006;61:23–8.

119. Ries AL, Bauldoff GS, Carlin BW, et al. Pulmonary rehabilitation: joint ACCP/AACVPR evidence-based clinical practice guidelines. Chest 2007; 131:4S–42S.

120. Meyer A, Zoll J, Charles AL, et al. Skeletal muscle mitochondrial dysfunction during chronic obstructive pulmonary disease: central actor and therapeutic target. Exp Physiol 2013;98:1063–78.

121. MacIntyre NR. Oxygen therapy and exercise response in lung disease. Respir Care 2000;45: 194–200.

122. Cardellach F, Alonso JR, López S, et al. Effect of smoking cessation on mitochondrial respiratory chain function. J Toxicol Clin Toxicol 2003;41(3): 223–8.

123. Koechlin C, Couillard A, Simar D, et al. Does oxidative stress alter quadriceps endurance in chronic obstructive pulmonary disease? Am J Respir Crit Care Med 2004;169:1022–7.

124. Broekhuizen R, Wouters EF, Creutzberg EC, et al. Polyunsaturated fatty acids improve exercise capacity in chronic obstructive pulmonary disease. Thorax 2005;60:376–82.

125. Ettinger MP. Aging bone and osteoporosis: strategies for preventing fractures in the elderly. Arch Intern Med 2003;163(18):2237–46.

126. Lehouck A, Boonen S, Decramer M, et al. COPD, bone metabolism, and osteoporosis. Chest 2011;139(3): 648–57. http://dx.doi.org/10.1378/chest.10-1427.

127. Kanis JA. WHO Study Group Assessment of fracture risk and its application to screening for postmenopausal osteoporosis: synopsis of a WHO report. Osteoporos Int 1994;46:368–81.

128. Graat-Verboom L, Wouters EF, Smeenk FW, et al. Current status of research on osteoporosis in COPD: a systematic review. Eur Respir J 2009; 341:209–18.

129. Calverley PM, Anderson JA, Celli B, et al. Salmeterol and fluticasone propionate and survival in chronic obstructive pulmonary disease. N Engl J Med 2007;356:775–89.

130. Vrieze A, de Greef MH, Wijkstra PJ, et al. Low bone mineral density in COPD patients related to worse lung function, low weight and decreased fat-free mass. Osteoporos Int 2007;18:1197–202.

131. Jorgensen NR, Schwarz P, Holme I, et al. The prevalence of osteoporosis in patients with chronic obstructive pulmonary disease: across sectional study. Respir Med 2007;101:177–85.

132. Romme EA, Murchison JT, Edwards LD, et al. CT measured bone attenuation in patients with chronic obstructive pulmonary disease: relation to clinical features and outcomes. J Bone Miner Res 2013. http://dx.doi.org/10.1002/jbmr.1873.

133. Kjensli A, Falch JA, Ryg M, et al. High prevalence of vertebral deformities in COPD patients: relationship to disease severity. Eur Respir J 2009;33: 1018–24.

134. Mazokopakis EE, Starakis IK. Recommendations for diagnosis and management of osteoporosis in COPD men. ISRN Rheumatol 2011;2011:901416.

135. Weinstein RS, Wan C, Liu Q, et al. Endogenous glucocorticoids decrease skeletal angiogenesis, vascularity, hydration, and strength in aged mice. Aging Cell 2010;9:147–61.

136. Langhammer A, Forsmo S, Syversen U. Long-term therapy in COPD: any evidence of adverse effect on bone? Int J Chron Obstruct Pulmon Dis 2009; 4:365–80.

137. Manolagas SC, Weinstein RS. New developments in the pathogenesis and treatment of steroid-induced osteoporosis. J Bone Miner Res 1999; 14(7):1061–6.

138. Mathioudakis AG, Amanetopoulou SG, Gialmanidis IP, et al. Impact of long-term treatment with low-dose inhaled corticosteroids on the bone mineral density of chronic obstructive pulmonary disease patients: aggravating or beneficial? Respirology 2013;18(1):147–53. http://dx.doi.org/10. 1111/j.1440-1843.2012.02265.

139. Liang B, Feng Y. The association of low bone mineral density with systemic inflammation in clinically stable COPD. Endocrine 2012;42(1):190–5. http:// dx.doi.org/10.1007/s12020-011-9583-x.

140. Hardy R, Cooper MS. Bone loss in inflammatory disorders. J Endocrinol 2009;201(3):309–20.

141. Ritchlin CT, Haas-Smith SA, Li P, et al. Mechanisms of TNF-alpha- and RANKL-mediated osteoclastogenesis and bone resorption in psoriatic arthritis. J Clin Invest 2003;111(6):821–31.

142. Kovacic JC, Lee P, Baber U, et al. Inverse relationship between body mass index and coronary artery calcification in patients with clinically significant coronary lesions. Atherosclerosis 2012;221(1):176–82. http://dx.doi.org/10.1016/j. atherosclerosis.2011.11.020.

143. Ebeling PR. Osteoporosis in men. N Engl J Med 2008;358(14):1474–82.

144. Gennari L, Bilezikian JP. Osteoporosis in men. Endocrinol Metab Clin North Am 2007;36(2):399–419.

145. Plotkin LI, Aguirre JI, Kousteni S, et al. Bisphosphonates and estrogens inhibit osteocyte apoptosis via distinct molecular mechanisms downstream of extracellular signal-regulated kinase activation. J Biol Chem 2005;280(8):7317–25.

146. Ringe JD, Faber H, Farahmand P, et al. Efficacy of risedronate in men with primary and secondary osteoporosis: results of a 1-year study. Rheumatol Int 2006;26(5):427–31.

147. Misiorowski W. Parathyroid hormone and its analogues—molecular mechanisms of action and efficacy in osteoporosis therapy. Endokrynol Pol 2011;62(1):73–8.

148. Patel AR, Hurst JR. Extrapulmonary comorbidities in chronic obstructive pulmonary disease: state of the art [review]. Expert Rev Respir Med 2011; 5(5):647–62. http://dx.doi.org/10.1586/ers.11.62.

149. Kanis JA, McCloskey EV, Johansson H, et al, National Osteoporosis Guideline Group. Case finding for the management of osteoporosis with FRAX—assessment and intervention thresholds for the UK. Osteoporos Int 2008;19(10):1395–408.

150. Schols AM, Broekhuizen R, Weling-Scheepers CA, et al. Body composition and mortality in chronic obstructive pulmonary disease. Am J Clin Nutr 2005;82(1):53–9.

151. Collins PF, Elia M, Stratton RJ. Nutritional support and functional capacity in chronic obstructive pulmonary disease: a systematic review and meta-analysis. Respirology 2013. http://dx.doi.org/10.1111/resp.12070.

152. Ferreira IM, Brooks D, White J, et al. Nutritional supplementation for stable chronic obstructive pulmonary disease. Cochrane Database Syst Rev 2012;(12):CD000998. http://dx.doi.org/10.1002/14651858.CD000998.pub3.

153. Schols AM, Gosker HR. The pathophysiology of cachexia in chronic obstructive pulmonary disease. Curr Opin Support Palliat Care 2009; 3(4):282–7. http://dx.doi.org/10.1097/SPC.0b013e328331e91c.

154. Cano NJ, Roth H, Court-Ortuné I, et al. Nutritional depletion in patients on long-term oxygen therapy and/or home mechanical ventilation. Eur Respir J 2002;20:30–7.

155. Vermeeren MA, Creutzberg EC, Schols AM, et al, COSMIC Study Group. Prevalence of nutritional depletion in a large out-patient population of patients with COPD. Respir Med 2006;100:1349–55.

156. Landbo C, Prescott E, Lange P, et al. Prognostic value of nutritional status in chronic obstructive pulmonary disease. Am J Respir Crit Care Med 1999;160:1856–61.

157. Fuenzalida CE, Petty TL, Jones ML. The immune response to short nutritional intervention in advanced COPD. Am Rev Respir Dis 1990; 142(1):49–56.

158. DeBellis HF, Fetterman JW Jr. Enteral nutrition in the chronic obstructive pulmonary disease (COPD) patient. J Pharm Pract 2012;25(6):583–5. http://dx.doi.org/10.1177/0897190012460827.

159. Malone A. Enteral formula selection: a review of selected product categories. Pract Gastroenterol 2005;28:56–8.

160. de Batlle J, Sauleda J, Balcells E, et al. Association between Ω3 and Ω6 fatty acid intakes and serum inflammatory markers in COPD. J Nutr Biochem 2011;23(7):817–21.

161. World Health Organization. Overweight and obesity: a new nutrition emergency? Monitoring the rapidly emerging public health problem of overweight and obesity: the WHO global database on body mass index. SCN News 2004;5–12.

162. Poulain M, Doucet M, Major GC, et al. The effect of obesity on chronic respiratory diseases: pathophysiology and therapeutic strategies. CMAJ 2006;174:1293–9.

163. Pitta F, Troosters T, Spruit MA, et al. Characteristics of physical activities in daily life in chronic obstructive pulmonary disease. Am J Respir Crit Care Med 2005;171:972–7.

164. Dallman MF, la Fleur SE, Pecoraro NC, et al. Minireview: glucocorticoids—food intake, abdominal obesity, and wealthy nations in 2004. Endocrinology 2004;145:2633–8.

165. Franssen FM, O'Donnell DE, Goossens GH, et al. Obesity and the lung: 5. Obesity and COPD. Thorax 2008;63:1110–7. http://dx.doi.org/10.1136/thx.2007.086827.

166. Bastard JP, Maachi M, Lagathu C, et al. Recent advances in the relationship between obesity, inflammation, and insulin resistance. Eur Cytokine Netw 2006;17:4–12.

167. Yudkin JS. Adipose tissue, insulin action and vascular disease: inflammatory signals. Int J Obes Relat Metab Disord 2003;27(Suppl 3):S25–8.

168. Young T, Palta M, Dempsey J, et al. The occurrence of sleep disordered breathing among middle-aged adults. N. Engl. J Med 1993;328:1230–5.

169. Young T, Peppard PE, Gottlieb DJ. Epidemiology of obstructive sleep apnea: a population health perspective. Am J Respir Crit Care Med 2002; 165:1217–39.

170. McNicholas WT. Chronic obstructive pulmonary disease and obstructive sleep apnea: overlaps in pathophysiology, systemic inflammation, and cardiovascular disease. Am J Respir Crit Care Med 2009;180:692–700.

171. Fletcher EC. Chronic lung disease in the sleep apnea syndrome. Lung 1990;168(Suppl):751–61.

172. Ioachimescu OC, Teodorescu M. Integrating the overlap of obstructive lung disease and obstructive

sleep apnoea: OLDOSA syndrome. Respirology 2013;18(3):421–31. http://dx.doi.org/10.1111/resp.12062.

173. Clini E, Sturani C, Rossi A, et al. The Italian multicentre study on noninvasive ventilation in chronic obstructive pulmonary disease patients. Eur Respir J 2002;20:529–38.

174. Butterworth CE, Fielding JF, Finch CA, et al. Nutritional anaemias. Report of a WHO scientific group. World Health Organ Tech Rep Ser 1968;405:5–37.

175. John M, Hoernig S, Doehner W, et al. Anemia and inflammation in COPD. Chest 2005;127(3):825–9.

176. Chambellan A, Chailleux E, Similowski T, et al. Prognostic value of the hematocrit in patients with severe COPD receiving long-term oxygen therapy. Chest 2005;128:1201–8.

177. Rutten EP, Franssen FM, Spruit MA, et al. Anemia is associated with bone mineral density in chronic obstructive pulmonary disease. COPD 2013;10:286–92.

178. Weiss G. Pathogenesis and treatment of anaemia of chronic disease. Blood Rev 2002;16:87–96.

179. Schönhofer B, Wenzel M, Geibel M, et al. Blood transfusion and lung function in chronically anemic patients with severe chronic obstructive pulmonary disease. Crit Care Med 1998;26:1824–8.

180. Barnes PJ. Neural control of human airways in health and disease. Am Rev Respir Dis 1986;134:1289–314.

181. van Gestel AJ, Steier J. Autonomic dysfunction in patients with chronic obstructive pulmonary disease (COPD). J Thorac Dis 2010;2(4):215–22.

182. Buda AJ, Pinsky MR, Ingles NB, et al. Effect of intrathoracic pressure on left ventricular performance. N Engl J Med 1979;301:453–9.

183. Undem BJ, Kollarik M. The role of vagal afferent nerves in chronic obstructive pulmonary disease. Proc Am Thorac Soc 2005;2:355–60.

184. Dempsey JA, Sheel AW, St Croix CM. Respiratory influences on sympathetic vasomotor outflow in humans. Respir Physiol Neurobiol 2002;130:3–20.

185. Tug T, Terzi SM, Yoldas TK. Relationship between the frequency of autonomic dysfunction and the severity of chronic obstructive pulmonary disease. Acta Neurol Scand 2005;112(3):183–8.

186. Purdue MP, Gold L, Jarvholm B, et al. Impaired lung function and lung cancer incidence in a cohort of Swedish construction workers. Thorax 2007;62(1):51–6.

187. Punturieri A, Szabo E, Croxton TL. Lung cancer and chronic obstructive pulmonary disease: needs and opportunities for integrated research. J Natl Cancer Inst 2009;101(8):554–9.

188. Mannino DM, Aguayo SM, Petty TL, et al. Low lung function and incident lung cancer in the United States: data from the First National Health and Nutrition Examination Survey follow-up. Arch Intern Med 2003;163:1475–80.

189. Tockman MS, Anthonisen NR, Wright EC, et al. Airways obstruction and the risk for lung cancer. Ann Intern Med 1987;106(4):512–8.

190. Skillrud DM, Offord KP, Miller RD. Higher risk of lung cancer in chronic obstructive pulmonary disease. A prospective, matched, controlled study. Ann Intern Med 1986;105(4):503–7.

191. Anthonisen NR, Skeans MA, Wise RA, et al. The effects of a smoking cessation intervention on 14.5-year mortality: a randomized clinical trial. Ann Intern Med 2005;142:233–9.

192. Wilson DO, Weissfeld JL, Balkan A, et al. Association of radiographic emphysema and airflow obstruction with lung cancer. Am J Respir Crit Care Med 2008;178:738–44.

193. Young RP, Hopkins RJ, Christmas T, et al. COPD prevalence is increased in lung cancer independence of age, gender and smoking history. Eur Respir J 2009;34:380–6.

194. Papi A, Casoni G, Caramori G, et al. COPD increases the risk of squamous histological subtype in smokers who develop non-small cell lung carcinoma. Thorax 2004;59(8):679–81.

195. Jacobson BA, Alter MD, Kratzke MG, et al. Repression of cap-dependent translation attenuates the transformed phenotype in non-small cell lung cancer both in vitro and in vivo. Cancer Res 2006;66(8):4256–62.

196. Krysan K, Lee JM, Dohadwala M, et al. Inflammation, epithelial to mesenchymal transition, and epidermal growth factor receptor tyrosine kinase inhibitor resistance. J Thorac Oncol 2008;3(2):107–10.

197. Brody JS, Spira A. Chronic obstructive pulmonary disease, inflammation and lung cancer. Proc Am Thorac Soc 2006;3:535–8.

198. Yao HW, Rahman I. Current concepts on the role of inflammation in COPD and lung cancer. Curr Opin Pharmacol 2009;9:375–83.

199. Lin WW, Karin M. A cytokine-mediated link between innate immunity, inflammation, and cancer. J Clin Invest 2007;117:1175–83.

200. Wright JG, Christman JW. The role of nuclear factor kappa B in the pathogenesis of pulmonary diseases: implications for therapy. Am J Respir Med 2003;2:211–9.

201. Teramoto S, Kume H. The role of nuclear factor-kappa B activation in airway inflammation following adenovirus infection and COPD. Chest 2001;119:1294–5.

202. O'Byrne KJ, Dalgleish AG. Chronic immune activation and inflammation as the cause of malignancy. Br J Cancer 2001;85:473–83.

203. Parimon T, Chien JW, Bryson CL, et al. Inhaled corticosteroids and risk of lung cancer among patients

with chronic obstructive pulmonary disease. Am J Respir Crit Care Med 2007;175:712–9.

204. van Gestel YR, Hoeks SE, Sin DD, et al. COPD and cancer mortality: the influence of statins. Thorax 2009;64:963–7.

205. Young RP, Hopkins RJ. How the genetics of lung cancer may overlap with COPD. Respirology 2011;16(7):1047–55. http://dx.doi.org/10.1111/j.1440-1843.2011.02019.x.

206. Schwartz AG, Ruckdeschel JC. Familial lung cancer: genetic susceptibility and relationship to chronic obstructive pulmonary disease. Am J Respir Crit Care Med 2006;173:16–22.

207. Malhotra D, Thimmulappa R, Navas-Acien A, et al. Decline in Nrf2 regulated antioxidants in COPD lungs due to loss of its positive regulator DJ-1. Am J Respir Crit Care Med 2008;178:592–604.

208. Cho HY, Reddy SP, Kleeberger SR. Nrf2 defends the lung from oxidative stress. Antioxid Redox Signal 2006;8:76–87.

209. Krieken JH, Hiemstra PS. Expression of epidermal growth factors and their receptors in the bronchial epithelium of subjects with chronic obstructive pulmonary disease. Am J Clin Pathol 2006;125:184–92.

210. Hill K, Geist R, Goldstein RS, et al. Anxiety and depression in end-stage COPD. Eur Respir J 2008;31(3):667–77. http://dx.doi.org/10.1183/09031936.00125707.

211. Engstrom CP, Persson LO, Larsson S, et al. Functional status and well being in chronic obstructive pulmonary disease with regard to clinical parameters and smoking: a descriptive and comparative study. Thorax 1996;51:825–30.

212. Dowson C, Laing R, Barraclough R, et al. The use of the Hospital Anxiety and Depression Scale (HADS) in patients with chronic obstructive pulmonary disease: a pilot study. N Z Med J 2001;114:447–9.

213. van Manen JG, Bindels PJ, Dekker FW, et al. Risk of depression in patients with chronic obstructive pulmonary disease and its determinants. Thorax 2002;57:412–6.

214. van Ede L, Yzermans CJ, Brouwer HJ. Prevalence of depression in patients with chronic obstructive pulmonary disease: a systematic review. Thorax 1999;54:688–92.

215. Kunik ME, Roundy K, Veazey C, et al. Surprisingly high prevalence of anxiety and depression in chronic breathing disorders. Chest 2005;127:1205–11.

216. Hanania NA, Müllerova H, Locantore NW, et al. Evaluation of COPD Longitudinally to Identify Predictive Surrogate Endpoints (ECLIPSE) study investigators. Determinants of depression in the ECLIPSE chronic obstructive pulmonary disease cohort. Am J Respir Crit Care Med 2011;183(5):604–11. http://dx.doi.org/10.1164/rccm.201003-0472OC.

217. Anisman H, Merali Z, Hayley S. Neurotransmitter, peptide and cytokine processes in relation to depressive disorder: comorbidity between depression and neurodegenerative disorders. Prog Neurobiol 2008;85(1):1–74.

218. Almagro P, Calbo E, Ochoa-de-Echaguen A, et al. Mortality after hospitalization for COPD. Chest 2002;121:1441–8.

219. Ng TP, Niti M, Tan WC, et al. Depressive symptoms and chronic obstructive pulmonary disease: effect on mortality, hospital readmission, symptom burden, functional status, and quality of life. Arch Intern Med 2007;167:60–7.

220. Fan VS, Ramsey SD, Giardino ND, et al. Sex, depression, and risk of hospitalization and mortality in chronic obstructive pulmonary disease. Arch Intern Med 2007;167:2345–53.

221. de Voogd JN, Wempe JB, Köeter GH, et al. Depressive symptoms as predictors of mortality in patients with COPD. Chest 2009;135:619–25. http://dx.doi.org/10.1378/chest.08-0078. Prepublished online November 24, 2008.

222. Mannino DM, Thorn D, Swensen A, et al. Prevalence and outcomes of diabetes, hypertension and cardiovascular disease in COPD. Eur Respir J 2008;32(4):962–9.

223. Rabinovich RA, MacNee W. Chronic obstructive pulmonary disease and its comorbidities. Br J Hosp Med (Lond) 2011;72(3):137–45.

224. Rana JS, Mittleman MA, Sheikh J, et al. Chronic obstructive pulmonary disease, asthma, and risk of type 2 diabetes in women. Diabetes Care 2004;27:2478–84.

225. Poulain M, Doucet M, Drapeau V, et al. Metabolic and inflammatory profile in obese patients with chronic obstructive pulmonary disease. Chron Respir Dis 2008;5(1):35–41.

226. Chakrabarti B, Angus RM, Agarwal S, et al. Hyperglycaemia as a predictor of outcome during non-invasive ventilation in decompensated COPD. Thorax 2009;64(10):857–62.

227. Baker EH, Janaway CH, Philips BJ, et al. Hyperglycaemia is associated with poor outcomes in patients admitted to hospital with acute exacerbations of chronic obstructive pulmonary disease. Thorax 2006;61(4):284–9.

228. Marquis K, Maltais F, Duguay V, et al. The metabolic syndrome in patients with chronic obstructive pulmonary disease. J Cardiopulm Rehabil 2005;25:226–32.

229. Fabbri LM, Luppi F, Beghe B, et al. Complex chronic comorbidities of COPD. Eur Respir J 2008;31:204–12. http://dx.doi.org/10.1183/09031936.00114307.

230. Clini E, Crisafulli E, Radaeli A, et al. COPD and the metabolic syndrome: an intriguing association. Intern Emerg Med 2013;8(4):283–9.

231. Agusti A. Systemic effects of chronic obstructive pulmonary disease: what we know and what we don't know (but should). Proc Am Thorac Soc 2007;4:522–5.

232. van Eeden SF, Sin DD. Chronic obstructive pulmonary disease: a chronic systemic inflammatory disease. Respiration 2008;75:224–38.

233. Garcia-Rio F, Miravitlles M, Soriano JB, et al. Systemic inflammation in chronic obstructive pulmonary disease: a population-based study. Respir Res 2010;11:63.

234. Sin DD, Anthonisen NR, Soriano JB, et al. Mortality in COPD: role of comorbidities. Eur Respir J 2006; 28(6):1245–57.

235. Gan WQ, Man SF, Sin DD. Association between chronic obstructive pulmonary disease and systemic inflammation: a systematic review and a meta-analysis. Thorax 2004;59:574–80.

236. Fabbri LM, Rabe KF. From COPD to chronic systemic inflammatory syndrome? Lancet 2007;370: 797–9.

237. Gea J, Barreiro E, Orozco-Levi M. Systemic inflammation in COPD. Clin Pulm Med 2009;16:233–42.

238. Luppi F, Franco F, Beghe B, et al. Treatment of chronic obstructive pulmonary disease and its comorbidities. Proc Am Thorac Soc 2008;5:848–56.

239. Rennard SI. Inflammation in COPD: a link to systemic comorbidities. Eur Respir Rev 2007;16:91–7.

240. Yanbaeva DG, Dentener MA, Creutzberg EC, et al. Systemic effects of smoking. Chest 2007;131: 1557–66.

241. Gan WQ, Man SF, Sin DD. The interactions between cigarette smoking and reduced lung function on systemic inflammation. Chest 2005;127:558–64.

242. Maclay JD, McAllister DA, Macnee W. Cardiovascular risk in chronic obstructive pulmonary disease. Respirology 2007;12:634–41.

243. Sevenoaks MJ, Stockley RA. Chronic obstructive pulmonary disease, inflammation and comorbidity—a common inflammatory phenotype? Respir Res 2006;7:70.

244. Donaldson GC, Seemungal TA, Patel IS, et al. Airway and systemic inflammation and decline in lung function in patients with COPD. Chest 2005; 128:1995–2004.

245. Eagan TM, Ueland T, Wagner PD, et al. Systemic inflammatory markers in COPD: results from the Bergen COPD Cohort Study. Eur Respir J 2010; 35:540–8.

246. Walter RE, Wilk JB, Larson MG, et al. Systemic inflammation and COPD: the Framingham Heart Study. Chest 2008;133:19–25.

247. Pinto-Plata V, Toso J, Lee K, et al. Use of proteomic patterns of serum biomarkers in patients with chronic obstructive pulmonary disease: correlation with clinical parameters. Proc Am Thorac Soc 2006;3:465–6.

248. Sin DD, Leung R, Gan WQ, et al. Circulating surfactant protein D as a potential lung-specific biomarker of health outcomes in COPD: a pilot study. BMC Pulm Med 2007;7:13.

249. Bozinovski S, Hutchinson A, Thompson M, et al. Serum amyloid A is a biomarker of acute exacerbations of chronic obstructive pulmonary disease. Am J Respir Crit Care Med 2008;177:269–78.

250. Sparrow D, Glynn RJ, Cohen M, et al. The relationship of the peripheral leukocyte count and cigarette smoking to pulmonary function among adult men. Chest 1984;86:383–6.

251. Burnett D, Chamba A, Hill SL, et al. Neutrophils from subjects with chronic obstructive lung disease show enhanced chemotaxis and extracellular proteolysis. Lancet 1987;2:1043–6.

252. Aldonyte R, Jansson L, Piitulainen E, et al. Circulating monocytes from healthy individuals and COPD patients. Respir Res 2003;4:11.

253. Hodge SJ, Hodge GL, Reynolds PN, et al. Increased production of TGF-beta and apoptosis of T lymphocytes isolated from peripheral blood in COPD. Am J Physiol Lung Cell Mol Physiol 2003;285:L492–9.

254. Domagala-Kulawik J, Hoser G, Dabrowska M, et al. Increased proportion of Fas positive CD8+ cells in peripheral blood of patients with COPD. Respir Med 2007;101:1338–43.

255. Fairclough L, Urbanowicz RA, Corne J, et al. Killer cells in chronic obstructive pulmonary disease. Clin Sci (Lond) 2008;114:533–41.

256. Sin DD, Vestbo J. Biomarkers in chronic obstructive pulmonary disease. Proc Am Thorac Soc 2009;6:543–5.

257. Agusti A, Calverley P, Celli B, et al. Characterisation of COPD heterogeneity in the ECLIPSE cohort. Respir Res 2010;11:122–36.

258. Dickens JA, Miller B, Edwards L, et al. For the Evaluation of COPD Longitudinally to Identify Surrogate Endpoints (ECLIPSE) study investigators. Respir Res 2011;12:146.

259. Vanfleteren LE, Spruit MA, Groenen M, et al. Clusters of comorbidities based on validated objective measurements and systemic inflammation in patients with chronic obstructive pulmonary disease. Am J Respir Crit Care Med 2013;187(7):728–35. http://dx.doi.org/10.1164/rccm.201209-1665OC.

Biomarkers in COPD

Alvar Agusti, MD, PhD[a],*, Don D. Sin, MD, PhD[b]

KEYWORDS

- Chronic bronchitis • Emphysema • Outcomes • Smoking • Treatment

KEY POINTS

- Chronic obstructive pulmonary disease (COPD) is a complex and heterogeneous disease that affects 200 million patients worldwide.
- Over the past decade or so, there has been a great deal of interest in the identification and validation of biomarkers of potential clinical use in COPD.
- Adequately validated biomarkers can contribute to improved patient care.
- The recognition of the plasma inflammome in COPD is a major conceptual breakthrough, which may enable the discovery of plasma (inflammatory) biomarkers for clinical and research use for certain COPD phenotypes.

INTRODUCTION

Chronic obstructive pulmonary disease (COPD) is a complex and heterogeneous disease.[1] The severity of airflow limitation (assessed by forced expiratory volume in the first second of expiration [FEV_1]) has been traditionally used to diagnose, assess, and guide the therapy for patients with COPD.[2] Yet, FEV_1 is poorly related to other clinically relevant characteristics of the disease, such as symptoms, health status, exercise capacity, frequency of exacerbations, prevalence of comorbidities, or causes of death (**Fig. 1**).[3] FEV_1 alone, therefore, does not describe the complexity of the disease; other measures are needed in clinical practice to assess patients, predict their risk, guide their treatment, and assess their response to it (ie, their outcomes).[4]

Because of this limitation, over the past decade or so, there has been a great deal of interest in the identification and validation of biomarkers of potential clinical use in COPD. Here, the authors (1) review some general concepts in the field, (2) discuss currently validated biomarkers in COPD, and (3) speculate on potential future developments.

MARKERS AND OUTCOMES: GENERAL CONCEPTS

A marker is "a measurement that is associated with, and believed to be related patho-physiologically to, a relevant clinical outcome"[5]; clinical outcome is defined as "a consequence of the disease experienced by the patient,"[5] such as death, symptoms, exacerbations, weight loss, exercise limitation, and use of health care resources, among others.[5] The relationship between markers and outcomes is neither unique nor simple[5] because of the following: (1) A given outcome (ie, mortality) may associate with multiple markers (FEV_1, Pao_2, body mass index, and/or the Body mass index-Obstruction-Dyspnea-Exercise [BODE] index). (2) Their relationship can have different shapes (linear, parabolic, U or J); in fact, specific shapes can be more appropriate for different markers. Hence, a marker intended to diagnose the presence or absence of a given disease should ideally have a nonlinear relationship with the outcome of interest (existence of the disease), whereas a marker used to assess the clinical effect of a given therapeutic intervention

---

[a] Thorax Institute, Hospital Clinic, IDIBAPS, Universitat de Barcelona and CIBER Enfermedades Respiratorias (CIBERES), Villarroel 170, 08036 Barcelona, Spain; [b] Division of Respirology, Department of Medicine, The Institute for Heart and Lung Health, James Hogg Research Center, St Paul's Hospital, University of British Columbia, 1081 Burrard Street, Vancouver, BC, V6Z 1Y6, Canada

* Corresponding author. Institut del Tòrax, Hospital Clínic, Villarroel 170, Barcelona 08036, Spain.
E-mail address: Alvar.Agusti@clinic.ub.es

Clin Chest Med 35 (2014) 131–141
http://dx.doi.org/10.1016/j.ccm.2013.09.006
0272-5231/14/$ – see front matter © 2014 Elsevier Inc. All rights reserved.

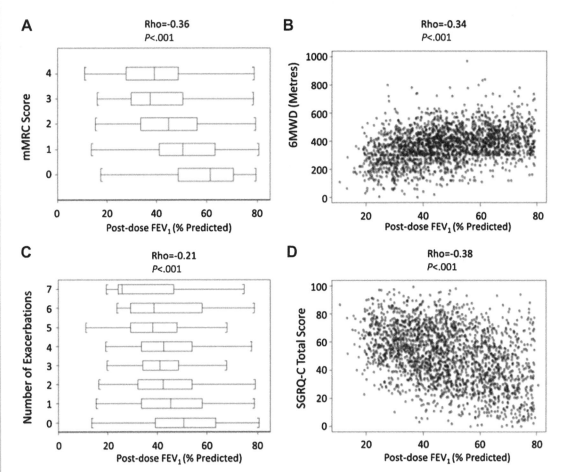

Fig. 1. Poor relationship between the severity of airflow limitation (FEV₁) and several clinically relevant domains of COPD, including breathlessness (mMRC [modified Medical Research Council] scale) (*A*), exercise capacity (6-minute walking distance [6MWD]) (*B*), frequency of exacerbations (*C*), and health status (Saint George Respiratory Questionnaire [SGRQ-C]) (*D*). For further explanations see text. (*Adapted from* Agusti A, Calverley P, Celli B, et al. Characterisation of COPD heterogeneity in the ECLIPSE cohort. Respir Res 2010;11:131; with permission.)

should preferentially have a linear relationship with it. (3) Their relationship can be modified by internal factors (eg, presence/absence of comorbidity) and/or external factors (eg, access to health care). (4) When very well characterized, markers can effectively substitute outcomes (for instance, high blood pressure is such a good marker of cardiovascular disease that it is, in fact, considered a disease in itself).

Depending on their use in clinical practice, several types of markers can be identified[5]: (1) *Diagnostic markers* can have the form of a dichotomous variable (present/absent) or can be measured on a continuous scale. In this latter case, however, a threshold value is needed, as it is the case of patients with α_1 antitrypsin deficiency or the use of the FEV₁/forced vital capacity ratio for the diagnosis of COPD.[6] (2) *Markers of disease severity* can have more than 2 levels (ie, mild/moderate/severe/very severe), and chosen ranges

may or may not be evidence based (ie, GOLD [Global Strategy for the Diagnosis, Management and Prevention of Chronic Obstructive Pulmonary Disease] grades of airflow limitation severity).[6] (3) *Markers of disease progression* can be either a continuous variable (ie, rate of decline of FEV₁)[7] or a categorical variable (ie, presence/absence: respiratory failure). (4) There are *markers of treatment effect,* such as changes in FEV₁ or exercise capacity. Other terms often used in this field are *surrogate markers* and *composite markers. Surrogate marker* is a term that is used when a given marker is actually a substitute of the marker of primary interest (ie, carbon monoxide lung diffusing capacity [DL$_{CO}$] and emphysema). Because COPD is a complex and multicomponent condition, a single marker may not adequately describe this complexity (or the results of therapeutic interventions); thus, *composite markers* are used (ie, the BODE index).[8]

BIOMARKERS: DEFINITION AND REQUIREMENTS

A biomarker is a special type of marker that has been defined as "a measurement of any *molecule or material (eg, cells, tissue) that reflects the dis-ease process.*"[9] This more restrictive definition excludes functional (or imaging) measurements from the more general concept of a marker discussed earlier and is used in the text later.

Adequately validated biomarkers can contribute to improve patient care by (1) allowing early detection of subclinical disease, (2) improving the diagnosis of acute or chronic syndromes, (3) stratifying patients' risk, (4) selecting the most appropriate therapy for a given patient, and/or (5) monitoring disease progression and response to therapy.[10]

To achieve these goals, a biomarker should ideally fulfill the following attributes[5,11]: (1) *relevance* (related to a specific disease); (2) *sensitivity* (able to detect clinically relevant differences); (3) *specificity* (not influenced by confounding variables); (4) *reliability* (the capacity to perform consistently in different settings); (5) *consistency* (similar instruments produce similar results); (6) *repeatability* (it only changes when disease changes); (7) *interpretability* (it is clinically meaningful); (8) *simplicity* (feasible in routine clinical practice); and, finally, (9) *cost-effective* (its cost is lower that the savings it produces). However, as shown in **Table 1**, not all of these attributes are essential for different stakeholders.[5] **Fig. 2** summarizes the criteria recommended for the assessment of novel biomarkers for clinical use.[10]

Statements in bold font are given the highest priority.

BIOMARKERS IN COPD: WHERE ARE WE NOW?

Over the past few years, several biomarkers have been intensively studied in COPD and are relatively close to use in clinical practice. The better-validated ones are discussed below. Of note, however, the authors focus on biomarkers that can be measured in the systemic circulation because of their easy accessibility. Others of potential relevance, such as those in sputum or exhaled air, are not discussed here.

Fibrinogen: the Most Promising Biomarker

The most evolved and promising blood biomarker in COPD is fibrinogen, which is currently being evaluated by the US Food and Drug Administration (FDA) for qualification.[12] Plasma fibrinogen has been variably associated with the risk of COPD, disease progression, and mortality (both total and disease specific), independent of other well-established risk factors, such as age, cigarette smoking, and lung function.[12] The relationship with mortality is particularly notable and strong in both COPD specifically as well as general population cohorts. For instance, in the largest meta-analysis of its kind that included 154 211 participants across 31 prospective studies with 1.38 million person-years of follow-up, Danesh and colleagues[13] showed that

---

Table 1
Different biomarker requirements for different stakeholders

Requirement	GPs	Hospital Specialist	Payers	Pharmaceutical Industry	Regulatory Authorities	Scientists	Patients
Clinical utility	—	X	—	—	X	—	—
Sensitivity	—	X	—	X	X	X	—
Specificity	X	X	—	—	X	X	—
Reliability	X	X	—	X	X	X	X
Simplicity	X	—	—	—	—	—	—
Clarity	X	—	X	—	X	—	—
Practicality	—	—	—	X	—	—	—
Generalizability	—	—	—	X	X	—	—
Simplicity	—	—	—	X	—	—	X
Biologic credibility	—	—	—	—	—	X	—
Cost-effective	—	—	X	—	—	—	—

Abbreviation: GP, general practitioner.
Data from Jones PW, Agusti AGN. Outcomes and markers in the assessment of chronic obstructive pulmonary disease. Eur Respir J 2006;27:823.

1) Can the clinician measure the biomarker?

    a)   **Accurate and reproducible analytical method(s)**
    b)   **Pre-analytical issues (including stability) evaluated and manageable**
    c)   **Assay is accessible**
    d)   Available assays provide high through-put and rapid turn-around
    e)   Reasonable cost

2) Does the biomarker add new information?

    a)   **Strong and consistent association between the biomarker and the outcome or disease of interest in multiple studies**
    b)   **Information adds to or improves upon existing tests**
    c)   Decision-limits are validated in more than one study
    d)   Evaluation includes data from community-based populations

3) Will the biomarker help the clinician to manage patients?

    a)   **Superior performance to existing diagnostic tests, or**
    b)   **Evidence that associated risk is modifiable with specific therapy, or**
    c)   **Evidence that biomarker-guided triage or monitoring enhances care**
    d)   Consider each of multiple potential uses (SEE PANEL B)

Fig. 2. Criteria for assessment of novel biomarkers for clinical use. Statements in bold font are given the highest priority. (*Adapted from* Morrow DA, de Lemos JA. Benchmarks for the assessment of novel cardiovascular biomarkers. Circulation 2007;115:950; with permission.)

a 1-g/L plasma increase in fibrinogen was associated with a 3.7-fold increase in the risk of COPD-specific mortality. In this meta-analysis, the relationship between plasma fibrinogen levels and COPD mortality was stronger among lifetime never smokers than in current or ex-smokers (hazard ratio of 5.5 vs 3.7 for all participants). Similar (though less striking) data have been noted in several population-based cohorts, including the National Health and Nutrition Examination survey 3, Atherosclerosis Risk in Communities, and the Cardiovascular Health Studies, comprising more than 30 000 participants.[14] In the Evaluation of COPD Longitudinally to Identify Predictive Surrogate Endpoints (ECLIPSE) study, one of the largest prospective COPD-specific cohort studies to date, plasma fibrinogen was only weakly associated with total mortality over 3 years and was outperformed by serum interleukin (IL)-6[15] However, one limitation of the ECLIPSE study was that only 9.1% of the cohort died during these 3 years of follow-up, which may have reduced the power to detect significant changes.

Some have suggested the possibility of using plasma fibrinogen for predicting exacerbations. In the ECLIPSE study, elevated plasma fibrinogen levels were associated with an increased risk of exacerbations in patients with moderate to severe COPD. A 1 SD increase in plasma fibrinogen level was associated with a 35% increase in the risk of exacerbations (defined as the use of antibiotics and/or systemic corticosteroids for acute worsening of symptoms) ($P<.0001$).[16] Plasma fibrinogen was particularly useful in discriminating

frequent exacerbators (defined as those with 2 or more exacerbations per year) from those without any exacerbations (relative risk [RR] of 2.0, $P<.0002$). Its ability to discriminate frequent exacerbators from infrequent exacerbators (defined as 1 exacerbation per year) was less, with an RR of 1.60 ($P<.04$). Similar findings were noted in the COPD and Seretide: A Multi-Center Intervention and Characterization study whereby a 1-g/L increase in the plasma fibrinogen level was associated with a 77% increase in the risk of severe exacerbation as defined by a COPD-related hospitalization.[17] An increased risk of COPD hospitalization related to elevated plasma fibrinogen levels has also been noted in the Copenhagen City Heart Study.[18] Together, these studies strongly suggest that elevated plasma fibrinogen is a very promising biomarker for selecting patients at high risk of exacerbations and mortality (**Table 2**).

Plasma fibrinogen may also prognosticate disease progression. However, the data for this outcome are less abundant and less stable. Although the older studies have reported increased risk of disease progression with elevated plasma fibrinogen levels,[18] the more recent ECLIPSE study failed to show a significant relationship between plasma fibrinogen levels and the rate of decline in FEV_1.[7] The reason for the discordance is unclear. On average, patients with more severe COPD have higher plasma fibrinogen levels than those with mild to moderate disease. However, because the variation around these mean values is high, plasma fibrinogen is probably

Table 2
Promising blood biomarker for predicting mortality in large-scale COPD studies

Biomarker	Approximate Relationship	References
Fibrinogen	1-g/L increase in levels is associated with a 3.5-fold increase in COPD mortality and 2.2-fold increase in total mortality	Danesh et al[13]
CRP	1-SD increase in levels is associated with 67% increase in the risk of deaths from respiratory failure and 2.32-fold increase in deaths from lung cancer	Kaptoge et al[49]
IL-6	In a head-to-head study, serum IL-6 levels outperformed CRP and fibrinogen in predicting 3-y mortality in the ECLIPSE study	Celli et al[15]
Total bilirubin	1-mg/dL reduction in levels is associated with 36% increase in total mortality and 86% increase in COPD-specific mortality	Horsfall et al[34]

Abbreviation: CRP, C-reactive protein.

not a clinically useful tool in diagnosing COPD or prognosticating disease progression.

The data on plasma fibrinogen levels as a diagnostic biomarker for exacerbation have also been variable and mixed. Some studies have suggested that plasma fibrinogen levels increase during acute exacerbations, whereas others[19,20] have shown no significant difference in plasma levels between periods of exacerbations and stability.[21] Most of these studies (whether positive or negative) have been plagued by relatively small sample sizes and confounded by the use of therapeutic interventions, such as antibiotics and systemic corticosteroids. Additional studies will be needed in the future to confirm (or refute) fibrinogen as a diagnostic biomarker for exacerbation.

Other Acute Phase Reactants Regulated by IL-6

Other promising plasma biomarkers include C-reactive protein (CRP) and serum amyloid protein (SAA) (see **Table 2**). Bozinovski and colleagues[22] identified SAA in a nontargeted proteomics experiment involving serum collected in patients who were acutely experiencing exacerbations versus serum collected in the same patients during periods of clinical stability. They found that during acute exacerbations, SAA levels increased by 6.5 fold compared with levels observed during clinical stability (7.7 mg/L vs 57.6 mg/L, P<.01). In contrast, serum levels of CRP increased by only 1.7 fold in the same samples (4.6 mg/L vs 12.4 mg/L, P<.01). SAA was particularly notable in discriminating exacerbations that led to hospitalizations or respiratory failure with an area under the curve of 0.88. In contrast, it had only a modest effect in discriminating ambulatory exacerbations from no exacerbations with an area under the curve of 0.71. Importantly, by the 10th day of exacerbation (and with acute exacerbation

treatment consisting of bronchodilators, antibiotics, and systemic corticosteroids), SAA recovered to near baseline levels.[20] Indeed, in this study, with treatment, the patients' SAA levels decreased by more than 92% from its peak levels before treatment initiation (1.8 mg/L vs 25.5 mg/L, P<.05). In contrast, serum CRP levels decreased by 83%, IL-6 levels decreased by 61%, and tumor necrosis factor (TNF)-α decreased by 36%.[20] Together, these data suggest that SAA is a promising diagnostic biomarker for exacerbation.

CRP is the prototypical acute-phase reactant that has been evaluated in various settings as a biomarker. Although its primary use is in detecting acute inflammatory or infectious events, it is increasingly being used to guide statin therapy for the primary prevention of cardiovascular events.[23] On average, patients with COPD have elevated CRP levels.[24] However, there is a lot of variation in data across the mean. Thus, CRP levels cannot be used as a diagnostic clinical tool. Although CRP levels are associated with an increased risk of mortality in COPD,[25,26] the signal is less robust and less consistent than that for fibrinogen. Moreover, unlike plasma fibrinogen, CRP levels have not been consistently associated with increased frequency of COPD exacerbations.[17,26] Similar to SAA, CRP levels have been shown to increase during acute exacerbations and decrease with recovery.[27] However, the variation around the mean is very large, suggesting a relatively small signal-to-noise ratio. Moreover, as previously pointed out, in head-to-head comparisons, SAA seems to be a more robust biomarker of exacerbation compared with CRP.[20,22] CRP may have a role in elucidating cardiovascular comorbidities in patients with COPD and may provide guidance regarding the use of statins in patients with COPD.[28,29]

Fibrinogen, SAA, and CRP are variably controlled by IL-6. Serum IL-6 levels have been assessed as a possible biomarker in COPD. In the ECLIPSE study, serum IL-6 levels were significantly related to total mortality. Indeed, it outperformed plasma fibrinogen, CRP, IL-8, and pneumoproteins (see later discussion), such as surfactant protein D (SP-D) and club cell secretory protein 16 (CCSP-16). However, the net incremental benefit in predicting mortality beyond nonbiomarker risk factors, such as age and BODE score, was small, increasing the area under the curve from 0.686 to only 0.708.[15] One major issue with IL-6 is that it is relatively non-repeatable over time. In the ECLIPSE study, among stable patients (ie, free of exacerbations), only 37% of patients with COPD had a 3-month IL-6 measurement that was within 25% of the baseline measurement. In contrast, 89% of patients had a 3-month plasma fibrinogen level that was within 25% of the baseline measurement.[30] CRP is one of the least robust measurements, with only 21% of patients having a 3-month measurement within 25% of the baseline level.

Emerging Biomarkers

There are several promising biomarkers in the pipeline. Receptor for advanced glycation end products (RAGE) and its ligand, advanced glycation end products (AGE), are subjects of great interest in COPD. AGEs are formed in a series of chemical reactions that variably glycate proteins or lipids (ie, addition of a simple sugar moiety). Once glycated, these lipid or protein molecules bind nonspecifically to normal tissue, such as endothelium or epithelium, altering its structure and function. Cells contain innate receptors called RAGE that bind with AGEs and mediate cellular responses that upregulate proinflammatory promoters, such as nuclear factor kappa B.[31] Wu and colleagues[31] have shown, using immunohistochemistry of lung tissue specimens, that COPD lungs have increased protein expression of AGE and RAGE in the airways. Miniati and colleagues[32] have shown that soluble AGE levels, which are decoy receptors for AGEs and, thus, attenuate tissue inflammation, are reduced in patients with COPD and are related directly to the severity of the airflow limitation.[33] Whether sRAGE or any components of the glycation pathways are associated with clinical end points, such as disease progression or mortality, in COPD is unknown.

Bilirubin is a well-known breakdown product of heme in red blood cells. It is widely used as one of the parameters of liver function, though its clinical use extends to diagnosing hemolysis and congenital disorders, such as Gilbert syndrome. One important property of bilirubin is its antioxidant capacity. Using data from more than 500 000 adults without any overt signs of hepatobiliary disease

from a UK primary care research database (the Health Improvement Network), Horsfall and colleagues[34] showed that the risk of COPD mortality was inversely related to serum bilirubin levels. In this study, a 1-mg/dL decrease in serum bilirubin was associated with an 86% increase in the risk of COPD mortality, a 2.9-fold increase in the risk of lung cancer mortality, and 36% increase in total mortality, after adjustments for age, body mass index, smoking status, and other factors.[34] The major limitation of this study, however, was that participants' lung function was not assessed using spirometry. Thus, the validity of the COPD definition is not certain. Nevertheless, these data raise the possibility of using a widely available and relatively inexpensive blood test for risk stratifying patients for future COPD-related morbidity and mortality.

Pneumoproteins

Because all of the abovementioned proteins and molecules are not predominantly produced by lung tissues, they lack specificity for COPD and their use may be confounded by comorbidities or other factors. To address this limitation, some have focused on proteins that are largely (though not exclusively) synthesized or modified in the lungs. These proteins are sometimes referred to as *pneumoproteins*. The best-studied pneumoproteins to date in this category are SP-D and CCSP-16 (previously known as Clara cell secretory protein-16). Although serum SP-D levels do not relate to disease severity or disease progression, they are increased in patients with COPD and are associated with an increased risk of exacerbation (though very weakly so).[35] Importantly, short-term use of either systemic or inhaled corticosteroids is associated with a reduction in serum SP-D levels, which in turn is associated with improved health status.[35,36] Because glucocorticosteroids are known to increase surfactant protein expression in lungs, it is widely thought that the reduction in serum levels associated with corticosteroid therapy is related to the decreased transfer of SP-D from lungs into the systemic circulation (ie, decreased leakage). Plasma SP-D levels have also been associated with an increased risk of total and cardiovascular mortality[37]; similar to fibrinogen, SP-D levels have a high repeatability index over 3 months,[30] suggesting robustness in the circulation.

In the ECLIPSE study, the best biomarker of disease progression was CCSP-16.[7] There are 2 major reasons why this may be the case. First, CCSP-16 is a very stable and robust biomarker in plasma. Over 3 months, 90% of patients with COPD have similar CCSP-16 levels (defined as 2 values within 25% of each other).[30] Second, CCSP-16 is produced largely by club cells and nonciliated bronchiolar cells in the airways. Thus, plasma levels are modified directly by the health and functional performance of these cells in the lungs. In the ECLIPSE study, 1-SD increase in serum CCSP-16 levels was associated with a 33-mL increase in baseline FEV_1 and 4 mL/y in the rate of decline in FEV_1 over 3 years. Although the overall contribution of CCSP-16 to disease progression was small, it still outperformed CRP, IL-6, and fibrinogen as a plasma biomarker of COPD progression.[7] Dissimilar to SP-D, CCSP-16 levels in plasma are not particularly responsive to systemic or inhaled corticosteroids.[38]

Pulmonary and activation-regulated chemokine (PARC/CCL-18) is another lung-predominant inflammatory protein that is found in serum. In both the ECLIPSE study and the Lung Health Study (LHS), serum PARC/CCL-18 levels were associated with an increased risk of mortality and, in LHS, were also associated with reduced lung function. However, dissimilar to CCSP-16 or SP-D, it is not a particularly robust biomarker in serum with a relatively low repeatability index. Only approximately 40% of patients with COPD have a 3-month value that is within 25% of the baseline value.[30] This finding may explain some of the discordant FEV_1 and disease progression data between the ECLIPSE study and LHS. PARC/CCL-18 levels are responsive to systemic but not inhaled corticosteroids.

Other Biomarkers

Serum adiponectin is an intriguing biomarker in COPD. In humans, adiponectin is almost exclusively produced in adipose tissue and is thought to be the main regulator of proinflammatory adipokines, such as TNF-α and IL-6. Although it is mainly synthesized by adipose tissue, blood levels decrease with the increasing body mass and fat content of individuals. In plasma, adiponectin molecules self-aggregate and form homotrimers and even higher-order structures, which are thought to be the most biologically active forms. In COPD, as in the general population, high serum adiponectin levels are associated with a reduced risk of cardiovascular morbidity and mortality. However, high serum levels are associated with an increased risk of disease progression and COPD-related mortality. Thus, serum adiponectin levels have a neutral effect on total mortality in COPD.[39]

Biomarkers of Therapeutic Responses

One of the main uses of biomarkers in clinical medicine is to guide therapeutic interventions. In COPD, the use of corticosteroids for acute exacerbations is well accepted, though there is large between-subject variability in response. Bafadhel and colleagues[40] conducted a randomized controlled trial to test the hypothesis that only patients who demonstrate peripheral eosinophilia (defined as an eosinophil count of 2% or greater in the peripheral circulation) would benefit from systemic corticosteroids. They showed that biomarker-directed therapy (which targeted systemic corticosteroids only to those with significant peripheral eosinophilia) was noninferior to the standard therapy of providing systemic corticosteroid therapy to all patients during exacerbations.[40] By using the biomarker-targeted approach, systemic corticosteroids could be safely avoided in patients who failed to demonstrate a significant peripheral eosinophilia during exacerbations. These data have been complemented by another independent clinical trial conducted by Aaron and colleagues.[41] They showed that patients who demonstrated significant peripheral eosinophilia (defined by >2% eosinophil count) during acute exacerbations derived significant benefits from systemic corticosteroids. In contrast, among patients without significant eosinophilia, there was a trend toward improved outcomes among those given etanercept, a TNF-α antagonist (vs those given systemic corticosteroids[41]).

As mentioned previously, SP-D and PARC/CCL-18 are responsive to short-term corticosteroids. However, it is unclear whether these biomarkers can identify patients who are most likely to benefit from these drugs.

A Network Approach to Inflammation: the Systemic Inflammome

Many of the studies reviewed earlier focused on a single biomarker that was most often measured once at baseline and then related to the outcome of interest. This approach has 2 important limitations. First, the inflammatory response is extremely complex and involves the participation of numerous cell types and a myriad of inflammatory signals.[42] It is, therefore, unlikely that the measurement of a single biomarker can describe such complexity accurately. Second, the inflammatory response is a physiologic response without which all of us would succumb quickly from sepsis. Yet, it is designed to be a quick response that also resolves quickly,[42] as soon as the initiating trigger (infection or injury) is eliminated/repaired. Inflammation becomes pathologic when it does not resolve and persist through time. It is now clear that this is the case in COPD because inflammation persists despite quitting smoking a decade ago[43] for reasons that are still unclear.[44,45] Having these two caveats in mind, investigators in ECLIPSE measured 6 inflammatory biomarkers in peripheral blood (white blood cells count, CRP, IL-6, IL-8, fibrinogen, and TNFα) in 1755 patients with moderate to severe COPD, 297 smokers with normal spirometry, and 202 nonsmoker controls who were followed for 3 years.[46] Measurements were repeated twice (at baseline and 1 year later), and a network approach (**Fig. 3**) was used to describe the pattern of systemic inflammation (ie, the systemic inflammome) in these 3 groups of individuals. The main results showed the following[46]: (1) The inflammome induced by smoking was different from that associated with COPD (see **Fig. 3**). (2) Thirty percent of the patients with COPD did not show any evidence of systemic inflammation (neither at baseline or during the 1-year follow-up), whereas 16% of patients with COPD had persistent systemic inflammation (defined by the presence of 2 or more abnormal biomarkers both at baseline and 1 year later). (3) Most importantly, despite the fact that pulmonary abnormalities were similar in never-inflamed and persistently inflamed patients, the latter was associated with a much higher all-cause mortality (13% vs 2%, P<.001) and exacerbation frequency (1.5 [1.5] versus 0.9 [1.1] per year, P<.001) during 3 years of follow-up.[46]

Overall, these results identify a novel systemic inflammatory COPD phenotype that may be the target of specific research and treatment.

HOW CAN WE PROGRESS IN THE FIELD?

Biomarker discovery is moving rapidly in COPD; several biomarkers are poised to garner clinical uptake, with fibrinogen being the closest to FDA approval and qualification. Despite the rapid gains in knowledge in the pathogenesis of COPD, there remain substantial gaps. The emergence of non-targeted proteomics is a very attractive platform for interrogating novel biomarkers without the need of any a priori hypothesis. However, the current technology limits the number of proteins and peptides that can be detected to about 300 to 400 (representing fewer than 0.5% of suspected proteins/peptides in the human proteome). On the other hand, the entire human genome can be interrogated using microarray or, more recently, using sequencing technology. The main limits of this technology are the lack of standardization of data acquisition and processing and the lack of reproducibility of findings across studies. Moreover, COPD is a heterogeneous disorder with multiple phenotypes. It is essential that future studies carefully characterize their cohorts using sophisticated phenotyping tools, such as thoracic

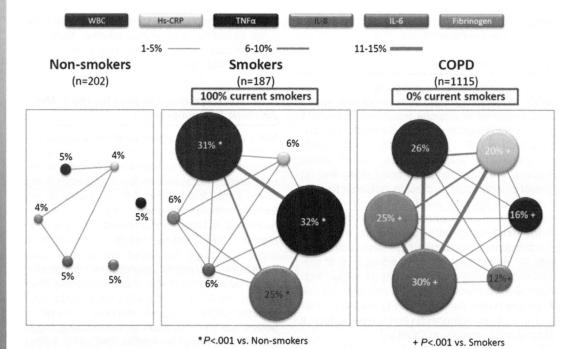

Fig. 3. Systemic inflammome as described in the ECLIPSE study. For further explanations see text. WBC, white blood cells. Hs-CRP, High-sensitivity-C reactive protein. (*Adapted from* Agusti A, Edwards LD, Rennard SI, et al. Persistent systemic inflammation is associated with poor clinical outcomes in COPD: a novel phenotype. PLoS ONE 2012;7:e37483.)

computed tomography and lung function measurements, and that the studies be large enough to evaluate biomarkers across different phenotypes. To this end, data and information sharing across large studies, such as ECLIPSE, SPIROMICS (Subpopulations and Intermediate Outcomes in COPD Study), COPDGene (Genetic Epidemiology of COPD), and CanCOLD (Canadian Cohort Obstructive Lung Disease) studies, should be encouraged to ensure that the data are collected in a similar fashion and analyzed using similar protocols. Moreover, when possible, data should be pooled across studies to ascertain hidden but robust biomarkers that may have been missed in a single study. This strategy has been proven particularly useful in genome association studies in asthma. This strategy should also work in COPD. In this vein, all studies (whether positive or negative) should be encouraged to deposit their data into a public repository for full data transparency and to encourage collaborations. Finally, complex diseases like COPD reflect the perturbations of the complex intracellular and intercellular network that links tissue and organ systems.[3] The emerging tools of network medicine offer a platform to systematically explore the molecular complexity of a particular disease as well as the molecular relationships among apparently distinct comorbid diseases,[47] like is frequently the case in COPD,[48] which is essential to identify and validate new biomarkers and drug targets.

SUMMARY

COPD is a complex disease that affects 200 million patients worldwide. The development of novel therapeutics has been slow owing in part to a lack of simple, sensitive, specific, and repeatable biomarker that can predict disease progression and other clinical outcomes. The recognition of the plasma inflammome in COPD is a major conceptual breakthrough, which may enable the discovery plasma (inflammatory) biomarkers for clinical and research use for certain COPD phenotypes. The pace of biomarker discovery will be further accelerated by the completion of several large (biomarker) cohort studies and with refinement of nontargeted and multiplex proteomic and genomic platforms.

REFERENCES

1. Agusti A, Calverley P, Celli B, et al. Characterisation of COPD heterogeneity in the ECLIPSE cohort. Respir Res 2010;11:122–36.
2. Rabe KF, Hurd S, Anzueto A, et al. Global strategy for the diagnosis, management, and prevention of chronic obstructive pulmonary disease: GOLD executive summary. Am J Respir Crit Care Med 2007;176:532–55.
3. Agusti A, Sobradillo P, Celli B. Addressing the complexity of chronic obstructive pulmonary disease: from phenotypes and biomarkers to scale-free networks, systems biology, and P4 medicine. Am J Respir Crit Care Med 2011;183:1129–37.
4. Vestbo J, Hurd SS, Agusti AG, et al. Global strategy for the diagnosis, management and prevention of chronic obstructive pulmonary disease, GOLD Executive Summary. Am J Respir Crit Care Med 2013;187(4):347–65.
5. Jones PW, Agusti AGN. Outcomes and markers in the assessment of chronic obstructive pulmonary disease. Eur Respir J 2006;27:822–32.
6. Vestbo J, Hurd SS, Agusti AG, et al. Global strategy for the diagnosis, management and prevention of chronic obstructive pulmonary disease, gold executive summary. Am J Respir Crit Care Med 2013;187: 347–65.
7. Vestbo J, Edwards LD, Scanlon PD, et al. Changes in forced expiratory volume in 1 second over time in COPD. N Engl J Med 2011;365:1184–92.
8. Celli BR, Cote CG, Marin JM, et al. The body-mass index, airflow obstruction, dyspnea, and exercise capacity index in chronic obstructive pulmonary disease. N Engl J Med 2004;350:1005–12.
9. Cazzola M, MacNee W, Martinez FJ, et al. Outcomes for COPD pharmacological trials: from lung function to biomarkers. Eur Respir J 2008;31:416–69.
10. Morrow DA, de Lemos JA. Benchmarks for the assessment of novel cardiovascular biomarkers. Circulation 2007;115:949–52.
11. Stockley RA. Biomarkers in COPD: time for a deep breath. Thorax 2007;62:657–60.
12. Duvoix A, Dickens J, Haq I, et al. Blood fibrinogen as a biomarker of chronic obstructive pulmonary disease. Thorax 2013;68:670–6.
13. Danesh J, Lewington S, Thompson SG, et al. Plasma fibrinogen level and the risk of major cardiovascular diseases and nonvascular mortality: an individual participant meta-analysis. JAMA 2005;294:1799–809.
14. Valvi D, Mannino DM, Mullerova H, et al. Fibrinogen, chronic obstructive pulmonary disease (COPD) and outcomes in two United States cohorts. Int J Chron Obstruct Pulmon Dis 2012;7:173–82.
15. Celli BR, Locantore N, Yates J, et al. Inflammatory biomarkers improve clinical prediction of mortality in chronic obstructive pulmonary disease. Am J Respir Crit Care Med 2012;185:1065–72.
16. Hurst JR, Vestbo J, Anzueto A, et al. Susceptibility to exacerbation in chronic obstructive pulmonary disease. N Engl J Med 2010;363:1128–38.
17. Groenewegen KH, Postma DS, Hop WC, et al. Increased systemic inflammation is a risk factor for COPD exacerbations. Chest 2008;133:350–7.

18. Dahl M, Tybjaerg-Hansen A, Vestbo J, et al. Elevated plasma fibrinogen associated with reduced pulmonary function and increased risk of chronic obstructive pulmonary disease. Am J Respir Crit Care Med 2001;164:1008–11.

19. Polatli M, Cakir A, Cildag O, et al. Microalbuminuria, von Willebrand factor and fibrinogen levels as markers of the severity in COPD exacerbation. J Thromb Thrombolysis 2008;26:97–102.

20. Koutsokera A, Kiropoulos TS, Nikoulis DJ, et al. Clinical, functional and biochemical changes during recovery from COPD exacerbations. Respir Med 2009;103:919–26.

21. Valipour A, Schreder M, Wolzt M, et al. Circulating vascular endothelial growth factor and systemic inflammatory markers in patients with stable and exacerbated chronic obstructive pulmonary disease. Clin Sci (Lond) 2008;115:225–32.

22. Bozinovski S, Hutchinson A, Thompson M, et al. Serum amyloid as a biomarker of acute exacerbations of chronic obstructive pulmonary disease. Am J Respir Crit Care Med 2008;177:269–78.

23. Ridker PM. C-reactive protein and the prediction of cardiovascular events among those at intermediate risk: moving an inflammatory hypothesis toward consensus. J Am Coll Cardiol 2007;49:2129–38.

24. Gan WQ, Man SF, Senthilselvan A, et al. Association between chronic obstructive pulmonary disease and systemic inflammation: a systematic review and a meta-analysis. Thorax 2004;59:574–80.

25. Man SF, Connett JE, Anthonisen NR, et al. C-reactive protein and mortality in mild to moderate chronic obstructive pulmonary disease. Thorax 2006;61: 849–53.

26. Dahl M, Vestbo J, Lange P, et al. C-reactive protein as a predictor of prognosis in chronic obstructive pulmonary disease. Am J Respir Crit Care Med 2007;175:250–5.

27. Hurst JR, Donaldson GC, Perera WR, et al. Use of plasma biomarkers at exacerbation of chronic obstructive pulmonary disease. Am J Respir Crit Care Med 2006;174:867–74.

28. Thomsen M, Dahl M, Lange P, et al. Inflammatory biomarkers and comorbidities in chronic obstructive pulmonary disease. Am J Respir Crit Care Med 2012;186:982–8.

29. Sin DD, Man SF. Why are patients with chronic obstructive pulmonary disease at increased risk of cardiovascular diseases? the potential role of systemic inflammation in chronic obstructive pulmonary disease. Circulation 2003;107:1514–9.

30. Dickens JA, Miller BE, Edwards LD, et al. COPD association and repeatability of blood biomarkers in the ECLIPSE cohort. Respir Res 2011;12:146.

31. Wu L, Ma L, Nicholson LF, et al. Advanced glycation end products and its receptor (RAGE) are increased in patients with COPD. Respir Med 2011;105:329–36.

32. Miniati M, Monti S, Basta G, et al. Soluble receptor for advanced glycation end products in COPD: relationship with emphysema and chronic cor pulmonale: a case-control study. Respir Res 2011;12:37.

33. Smith DJ, Yerkovich ST, Towers MA, et al. Reduced soluble receptor for advanced glycation end products in chronic obstructive pulmonary disease. Eur Respir J 2011;37:516–22.

34. Horsfall LJ, Rait G, Walters K, et al. Serum bilirubin and risk of respiratory disease and death. JAMA 2011;305:691–7.

35. Lomas DA, Silverman EK, Edwards LD, et al, Tal-Singer, and on behalf of the Evaluation of COPD Longitudinally to Identify Predictive Surrogate Endpoints study investigators. Serum surfactant protein D is steroid sensitive and associated with exacerbations of COPD. Eur Respir J 2009;34:95–102.

36. Sin DD, Man SFP, Marciniuk DD, et al. The effects of fluticasone with or without salmeterol on systemic biomarkers of inflammation in chronic obstructive pulmonary disease. Am J Respir Crit Care Med 2008;177:1207–14.

37. Hill J, Heslop C, Man SF, et al. Circulating surfactant protein-D and the risk of cardiovascular morbidity and mortality. Eur Heart J 2011;32:1918–25.

38. Lomas DA, Silverman EK, Edwards LD, et al. Evaluation of serum CC-16 as a biomarker for COPD in the ECLIPSE cohort. Thorax 2008;63:1058–63.

39. Yoon HI, Li Y, Man SF, et al. The complex relationship of serum adiponectin to COPD outcomes COPD and adiponectin. Chest 2012;142:893–9.

40. Bafadhel M, McKenna S, Terry S, et al. Blood eosinophils to direct corticosteroid treatment of exacerbations of chronic obstructive pulmonary disease. Am J Respir Crit Care Med 2012;186:48–55.

41. Aaron SD, Vandemheen KL, Maltais F, et al. TNFa antagonists for acute exacerbations of COPD: a randomised double-blind controlled trial. Thorax 2013;68:142–8.

42. Serhan CN, Brain SD, Buckley CD, et al. Resolution of inflammation: state of the art, definitions and terms. FASEB J 2007;21:325–32.

43. Hogg JC, Chu F, Utokaparch S, et al. The nature of small-airway obstruction in chronic obstructive pulmonary disease. N Engl J Med 2004;350:2645–53.

44. Cosio M, Saetta M, Agusti A. Immunological aspects of COPD. N Engl J Med 2009;360:2445–54.

45. Noguera A, Gomez C, Faner R, et al. An investigation of the resolution of inflammation (catabasis) in COPD. Respir Res 2012;13:101.

46. Agusti A, Edwards LD, Rennard SI, et al. Persistent systemic inflammation is associated with poor clinical outcomes in COPD: a novel phenotype. PLoS ONE 2012;7:e37483.

47. Barabasi AL, Gulbahce N, Loscalzo J. Network medicine: a network-based approach to human disease. Nat Rev Genet 2011;12:56–68.

48. Divo M, Cote C, de Torres JP, et al. Comorbidities and risk of mortality in patients with chronic obstructive pulmonary disease. Am J Respir Crit Care Med 2012;186:155–61.

49. Kaptoge S, Di AE, Lowe G, et al. C-reactive protein concentration and risk of coronary heart disease, stroke, and mortality: an individual participant meta-analysis. Lancet 2010;375:132–40.

Asthma and Chronic Obstructive Pulmonary Disease
Similarities and Differences

Dirkje S. Postma, MD, PhD[a],*, Helen K. Reddel, MD, PhD[b],
Nick H.T. ten Hacken, MD, PhD[a],
Maarten van den Berge, MD, PhD[a]

KEYWORDS

- Asthma • COPD • Inflammation • Remodeling • Overlap phenotype

KEY POINTS

- Asthma in childhood and chronic obstructive pulmonary disease (COPD) in smokers are easily distinguishable disease entities.
- There exist overlap phenotypes of asthma and COPD, such as asthma with neutrophilia and/or without bronchodilator response, and COPD with eosinophilia and/or some bronchodilator response.
- Differences in physiology, symptoms, inflammation, and remodeling between asthma and COPD are obscured by smoking. Hence asthma in a smoker and COPD appear similar (ie, they show phenotypic mimicry).
- A key component of overlap between asthma and COPD is the effect of aging.
- Some of the mechanisms driving airway obstruction and hyperresponsiveness are similar in asthma and COPD, and some are different.
- There is an unmet need to assess optimal treatment effects and safety in subphenotypes of asthma and COPD; phenotypes that have so far been excluded from pharmacologic studies.

INTRODUCTION

Asthma and chronic obstructive pulmonary disease (COPD) are both highly prevalent diseases worldwide. This issue of *Clinics in Chest Medicine* discusses different aspects of COPD, but in addition, the present article on overlap and differential signs and symptoms with asthma has been included. This is appropriate because it is often difficult to differentiate asthma from COPD, particularly at older ages. At that time in life, patients with asthma may have developed persistent airway obstruction, a characteristic that is a prerequisite for diagnosis of COPD according to the GOLD (Global Initiative for Chronic Obstructive Lung Disease) criteria.[1] This feature would not be a problem if asthma and COPD had the same clinical prognosis and response to pharmacologic treatment, and required similar management of the disease in clinical practice. However, this is often not the case.[2]

Asthma and COPD have been defined over the years in many different ways, and the heterogeneity in definitions in the literature contributes to the difficulty of evaluating evidence about the extent to which they overlap. The problem is confounded by the necessary reliance in many epidemiologic studies on self-reported diagnosis of asthma and COPD, and because, in clinical practice, these diagnoses are often assigned without lung function testing having been performed.

[a] University of Groningen, Department of Pulmonology, GRIAC research institute, University Medical Center Groningen, Hanzeplein 1, 9713 GZ Groningen, The Netherlands; [b] Department of Medicine, Woolcock Institute of Medical Research, University of Sydney, 431 Gleve Point Road, Gleve NSW 2037, Australia
* Corresponding author.
E-mail address: d.s.postma@umcg.nl

Clin Chest Med 35 (2014) 143–156
http://dx.doi.org/10.1016/j.ccm.2013.09.010
0272-5231/14/$ – see front matter © 2014 Elsevier Inc. All rights reserved.

Research on the clinical characterization, patho-physiology, prognosis, and management of asthma and COPD commenced with investigation of the extremes of the two conditions, namely:

1. Atopic individuals with asthma, never smokers or ex-smokers with less than 10 pack-year exposure, with significant bronchodilator reversibility at the time of study. These populations usually had an average age around 35 years.
2. Current or ex-smokers with fixed airway obstruction, generally with an age greater than 55 years.

This approach in research gave new insights into how best to treat the extreme phenotypes of asthma and COPD. However, many patients with asthma were excluded from these studies, particularly when they were smokers and showed no bronchodilator response at screening. Also excluded were many patients with COPD, especially when they showed an important reduction in airway obstruction after inhaling a bronchodilator.[3] As a result, such studies have not provided good insight into the management of asthma and COPD in daily practice, because it has been recognized that many patients do not fulfill the criteria of either asthma or COPD and show a mixture of both: the so-called overlap phenotype.[2] In the past, this concept was dismissed as representing the Dutch hypothesis,[4] but in more recent years the presence of overlap phenotypes has been widely accepted.[5–7]

When comparing asthma with COPD, it is important to realize that age has to be taken into account in every setting, because age induces changes in inflammation, immunologic responses, and mechanical properties of the lung.[8] Likewise, current smoking must be taken into account, because smoking induces inflammatory and remodeling changes in the lung and affects treatment response.[9,10] Hence it is not useful to compare young nonsmoking individuals with asthma and older smoking patients with COPD in their (dis)similarities in inflammatory cells and cytokines and in treatment response, because this is driven in both situations by differences in age and smoking status. Many studies in the past have overlooked the effects of both age and smoking and are therefore hampered in their interpretation as to whether asthma and COPD have comparable or distinct underlying mechanisms and treatment approaches.

This article discusses current knowledge on clinical features, inflammation and remodeling, genetics, and therapeutic response in asthma and COPD and discusses the overlap phenotypes.

DEFINITIONS

Asthma is currently defined as a chronic inflammatory disorder of the airways in which many cells and cellular elements play a role. The chronic inflammation is associated with airway hyperresponsiveness that leads to recurrent episodes of wheezing, breathlessness, chest tightness, and coughing, particularly at night or in the early morning. These episodes are usually associated with widespread, but variable, airflow obstruction within the lung that is often reversible either spontaneously or with treatment.[11,12] In contrast, COPD has for decades been defined as a preventable and treatable disease characterized by persistent airflow limitation that is usually progressive and associated with an enhanced chronic inflammatory response in the airways and the lung to noxious particles or gases. The following was added to this definition: "Exacerbations and comorbidities contribute to the overall severity in individual patients."[1] This definition of COPD is so vague that it fits many types of patients with distinct clinical characteristics, prognosis, and treatment response.[12] One of the important aspects here is that the airway obstruction in asthma, although often reversible, may be progressive in nature in a subset of patients with asthma,[13] leading to an overlap phenotype with COPD.

The definitions of asthma and COPD have been made to have a high sensitivity, but apparently their specificity is low. The problem is well acknowledged nowadays and recent studies suggest that 13% to 20% of patients with COPD have an overlap phenotype with asthma.[14] These patients have respiratory symptoms, have persistent airway obstruction, but some reversibility is still present after inhaling a bronchodilator and inflammatory markers are similar to those in asthma. Conversely, even 20% of patients with asthma at older ages have been given a diagnosis of COPD.[15]

CLINICAL FEATURES
Symptoms

It is difficult to differentiate asthma and COPD based on respiratory symptoms.[16] In the extremes with a sudden attack of wheeze and dyspnea after allergen exposure, it is clear that this is compatible with asthma. However, in the chronic forms, symptoms are many times more diffuse and patients with asthma may have symptoms of chronic cough and/or sputum production[17,18] formerly thought to imply COPD, especially when irreversible airway obstruction has developed.[19] In contrast, patients with COPD may have wheeze, a symptom formerly attributed solely to asthma.[20]

Moreover, an increase in the number of cigarettes smoked is associated with development of wheeze in COPD.[20] Thus, symptoms alone cannot rule out one or the other condition. Chronic cough and sputum production are associated with worse outcome in COPD,[21] but how this affects asthma has not been evaluated yet. Interestingly, atopic patients with COPD more frequently develop symptoms of cough and sputum production over time than nonatopic patients.[22]

Airway Obstruction and Reversibility

Bronchodilator response has been assumed to be a key differential parameter between asthma and COPD. However, bronchodilator response is frequently observed in patients with COPD in clinical practice, as well as in more recently designed clinical trials and in observational studies in patients with COPD.[23] Up to 50% of patients with COPD in the Understanding Potential Long-term Impacts on Function with TIOTropium (UPLIFT) study showed some bronchodilator response.[24] In another study, patients with COPD without a history of asthma showed a prevalence of bronchodilator response of 44%, with bronchodilator response being more frequently present in more severe disease.[25] This pattern is compatible with findings in the Evaluation of COPD longitudinally to Identify Surrogate Endpoints (ECLIPSE) cohort investigating 1831 patients with COPD tested before and after salbutamol inhalation.[26] In this study, it was concluded that the magnitude of postsalbutamol forced expiratory volume in 1 second (FEV_1) change is comparable between patients with COPD and smoking controls, but is lower with more severe airway obstruction and in the presence of emphysema.[26] Bronchodilator response status varied temporally in the latter study, but patients with consistent bronchodilator response (n = 227) did not differ in mortality, hospitalization, or exacerbation frequency from those with a lack of bronchodilator response, after adjustment for differences in baseline FEV_1.[26] One study suggested that the bronchodilator response in COPD is associated with eosinophilia, whereas absence of this response is associated with neutrophilia, possibly also explaining why some studies suggest a better inhaled corticosteroid (ICS) response in patients with reversible COPD.[27] In addition, it is debatable whether significant airway obstruction needs to be a prerequisite to define COPD, because emphysema may exist even without the presence of airway obstruction.[28]

When investigating a group of 228 patients with asthma followed for 26 years, it was shown that asthmatic patients may develop irreversible airway obstruction.[19] Although all of this cohort had reversible airway obstruction at baseline, at follow-up, 16% had developed irreversible airway obstruction, 23% had reduced carbon monoxide transfer coefficient, and 5% had both. Persistent airway obstruction was predicted by lower lung function, lower bronchodilator response, and milder hyperresponsiveness at baseline and was accompanied by the development of symptoms of chronic cough and sputum production. Patients with asthma with low transfer factor at follow-up had a higher total lung capacity and residual volume at baseline, but in multiple regression analysis this was no longer significant when pack-years of smoking were entered; higher pack-years significantly contributed to a lower transfer factor, but smoking was not independently associated with persistent airway obstruction. These observations may suggest that subtle signs of future features of COPD may already be present in early asthma. Another important message of this study is that persistent airway obstruction and reduced transfer factor are both signs of COPD, but they are distinct entities in asthma in terms of symptoms and causes. This message may have consequences for treatment approaches in asthma and the overlap phenotypes.

Small airway obstruction has long been recognized as one of the underlying mechanisms of COPD. In the last decades, it has become evident that small airway obstruction also contributes to the clinical presentation of asthma, although it is not clear yet whether this is only present in severe asthma or in mild asthma as well.[29–31] This gap in knowledge is predominantly caused by the lack of accurate and reproducible measures of small airway function suitable for general use. Signs of small airway dysfunction can already be present even 1 month after birth and they constitute a predictor of subsequent development of asthma.[32] However, it remains to be seen whether small airway changes in asthma and COPD originate from similar underlying mechanisms. The difference between inspiratory and expiratory X5, a measure of small airway obstruction, is larger in patients with COPD than in patients with asthma despite similar degrees of large airway obstruction as assessed with FEV_1.[33] Moreover, patients with COPD have greater ventilation heterogeneity than patients with asthma, as measured with slope, acinar component of ventilation heterogeneity (S_{acin}), a measure of the smallest airways where gas exchange takes place. In contrast, people with asthma predominantly have abnormalities in S_{cond}, a measure of the more proximal small conducting airways that are located before the acinus.[34] An additional contrast is that treatment with a bronchodilator induces an improvement in S_{cond} in patients with asthma, whereas it improves S_{acin} in patients with COPD[35,36] Galban and colleagues[37] identified functional small airway disease from computed tomography (CT) imaging across the spectrum of COPD severity and provided suggestive evidence that small airway narrowing and obliteration precede the onset of emphysema in COPD. Together these findings may suggest that the most peripherally located small airway disease contributes to COPD, and that the more proximally located contributes to asthma.

Atopy

Most children with asthma, and a large proportion of adult patients with asthma, are atopic.[38] It has long been overlooked that patients with COPD can be atopic as well but it is unclear whether this has clinical implications. A European study on severe asthma identified features of severe asthma that were distinct from milder forms of asthma.[39] It showed that patients with severe asthma were less frequently atopic and more frequently lacked a bronchodilator response than patients with milder disease.[39] In addition, patients with asthma with atopy respond better to ICS treatment than those without atopy.[39] Therefore, recommendations for the treatment of allergy are also included in the treatment guidelines of asthma. Recent studies showed that atopy can be present in patients with COPD as well and that the presence of allergy is a risk factor for future development of COPD.[40,41] Around 18% of patients with COPD were shown to be atopic in the European Respiratory Society study on Chronic Obstructive Pulmonary Disease (EUROSCOP) study,[22] and logistic regression provided evidence that atopic patients were more likely male, younger, and with a higher body mass index. Of importance, the presence of atopy was not associated with more severe airway obstruction.[22] Atopic patients with COPD more frequently develop symptoms of cough and sputum production when not using ICS treatment.[22] These symptoms were more likely to improve after ICS treatment of 2 years in atopic than in nonatopic patients with COPD. This finding is compatible with data from 1978 showing that atopic patients with COPD are the ones who benefit most from corticosteroid treatment.[42]

Airway Hyperresponsiveness

Airway hyperresponsiveness is a risk factor for development both of asthma and of COPD, as well as for a more rapid decline in lung function.[43]

In general, most patients with asthma express hyperresponsiveness, in contrast with about 60% of patients with COPD, even with mild disease in which the level of FEV_1 does not impinge on the severity of hyperresponsiveness.[44] However, the drivers of hyperresponsiveness in asthma and COPD, and whether different mechanisms are responsible for this phenomenon, have not been elucidated. There are many physiologic changes that may contribute to hyperresponsiveness: airway luminal diameter, airway wall thickness, smooth muscle mass, vascular engorgement, elastic recoil, airway inflammation, epithelial injury, and neural activity. Short-term treatment with ICS improves hyperresponsiveness in asthma, in conjunction with improvement of eosinophilic inflammation. After long-term ICS treatment, hyperresponsiveness may even disappear in a subset of patients with asthma.[45,46] In contrast, hyperresponsiveness improves to a smaller extent in COPD, in which it almost never disappears. One study investigating patients with asthma and COPD showed that a higher level of total serum immunoglobulin E predicted improvement in hyperresponsiveness with ICS.[47] This finding has not been investigated in other studies, but remains an interesting observation because this was present both in asthma and in COPD.[47] Although a common characteristic, this may be caused by different underlying mechanisms, which have only been studied to a limited extent in COPD. Chanez and colleagues[48] found that patients with COPD with asthmalike features (ie, eosinophilia and airway hyperresponsiveness) had thicker basement membranes than those without these features. Finkelstein and colleagues[49] investigated hyperresponsiveness in patients with COPD and showed that the airway wall internal to the smooth muscle layer of the small airways was thickened. A thicker airway wall was associated with more severe hyperresponsiveness. However, smooth muscle mass contributed more to hyperresponsiveness than adventitial or submucosal thickening.[50,51] This finding is similar with asthma, in which an increase in smooth muscle mass has also been shown to contribute to the presence and severity of hyperresponsiveness.[52,53] Even within asthma, different mechanisms contribute to severity of hyperresponsiveness. In older patients, this is predicted by air trapping and ventilation heterogeneity in the most distal small airways (S_{acin}), whereas ventilation heterogeneity in the more proximal small airways (S_{cond}) and inflammation predicts the severity of hyperresponsiveness in younger individuals with asthma.[54] Of interest, exhaled bronchial nitric oxide (NO), a parameter of large airway inflammation (usually related to eosinophilia) improved by ICS treatment in younger patients with asthma in conjunction with S_{cond}. However, the severity of hyperresponsiveness remaining after 3-month ICS treatment was best predicted by S_{cond} levels only.[55] It has yet to be established how small airway obstruction affects the severity of hyperresponsiveness in COPD. A recent cross-sectional and longitudinal study in COPD did not assess small airway function directly, but showed that a more severe hyperresponsiveness was associated with higher residual volume, a measure of air trapping related to small airway function, and with airway inflammation reflected by a higher number of neutrophils, macrophages, and lymphocytes in sputum and bronchial biopsies.[56] Severity of hyperresponsiveness was not associated with eosinophilic inflammation as suggested by Chanez and colleagues,[48] again suggesting that the mechanisms underlying hyperresponsiveness in asthma and COPD are at least partially different.

The Overlap Phenotype

There is no extensive literature available comparing the overlap phenotype with asthma on one hand and COPD on the other hand.[6,7,14,57,58] Some reviews have tried to give an overview[2,59,60] or to develop consensus on how best to define the overlap phenotype.[61] In epidemiologic studies in the United States and United Kingdom, 17% to 19% of patients with obstructive airway disease reported having both asthma and COPD, and these patients accounted for as many as 50% of patients with obstructive airway disease more than 50 years of age.[7] Thus, patients reporting to have been diagnosed with both asthma and COPD are generally older. However, as indicated earlier, diagnoses in population studies are often not based on lung function testing. When analyzing 175 individuals from a random population sample with objective measures, Weatherall and colleagues[58] performed a cluster analysis and showed 5 clusters: (1) severe and markedly variable airway obstruction with features of atopic asthma, chronic bronchitis, and emphysema; (2) features of emphysema alone; (3) atopic asthma with eosinophilic airway inflammation; (4) mild airway obstruction without other dominant phenotypic features; and (5) chronic bronchitis in nonsmokers. These findings make the situation even more complex. These investigators identified clusters 2 and 3 as clear emphysema and clear asthma respectively, whereas clusters 1, 4, and 5 represented various other overlapping phenotypes in asthma and COPD. However, Weatherall and colleagues[58] did not

examine the extent to which patients in these clusters differed with respect to other clinical or physiologic characteristics. In addition, these 5 clusters remain to be confirmed in other studies. Kauppi and colleagues[62] based an asthma and COPD diagnosis on UK guidelines and American Thoracic Society/European Respiratory Society criteria respectively. In this large group of patients with clinical disease, 1084 had asthma only, 237 COPD only, and 225 the overlap phenotype.[62] As expected, patients with asthma were younger, more frequently female, and less frequently had a history of smoking.[62] In addition, 26% of patients with asthma had been smoking for more than 10 years, compared with 72% and 76% of patients with COPD and the overlap phenotype respectively. The overlap group was between the asthma and COPD groups in other characteristics like gender, disease duration, pack-years smoking, lung function parameters, and comorbidities. These findings are compatible with those reported by Gibson and Simpson[2] in their review (ie, it was present in 64% of patients with the overlap syndrome, intermediate between a prevalence of 100% of patients with asthma and 25% of patients with COPD). Hypertension was highly prevalent as comorbidity with 32% in asthma, 41% in the overlap group, and 45% in patients with COPD, ages being on average 53, 61, and 64 years. However, it is also clear that the prevalence of comorbidities is higher in COPD than in asthma (**Table 1**), either as a result of long-standing smoking in COPD or because of the systemic inflammation present in COPD. In addition, patients with the overlap syndrome are more likely frequent exacerbators (ie, >2 exacerbations per year), have more gas trapping on CT, worse quality of life, more respiratory symptoms, more hospitalizations, and

---

Table 1
Proportion of patients with comorbidities

	Asthma (n = 1084)	Overlap (n = 225)	COPD (n = 237)
Hypertension	32.3	41.3	44.7
Coronary disease	7.7	19.1	25.3
Diabetes	6.8	12.9	19.8
Cerebrovascular disease	3.2	7.1	10.1
Peripheral vascular disease	0.6	3.6	7.2

Data from Kauppi P, Kupiainen H, Lindqvist A, et al. Overlap syndrome of asthma and COPD predicts low quality of life. J Asthma 2011;48(3):279–85.

consume much more health care resources than pure asthmatics.[6,7,14,57–62] Moreover, patients with the overlap phenotype are reported to have higher mortalities,[63] especially when peripheral blood eosinophilia is present.[64] Hardin and colleagues[14] additionally found that subjects with both COPD and asthma combined frequently have rhinitis, although it still remains to be established whether or not this reflects underlying atopy. Overall, data show that the overlap syndrome has characteristics between those of asthma and COPD, and is frequently present, irrespective of whether reported by patients or doctors, or objectively characterized.

GENETICS AND ENVIRONMENT

Genetic factors contribute to the development of both asthma and COPD, in conjunction with environmental factors. Many environmental factors contribute to both asthma and COPD and some only to either asthma or COPD alone. **Table 2** shows an overview of these factors as published in a recent review.[65] More severe airway hyperresponsiveness, lower lung function, maternal smoking during pregnancy, air pollution, and personal cigarette smoking are risk factors for development of both asthma and COPD. One of the features that drive several of these risk factors may be abnormal lung development in utero. It may be that this abnormal lung development, for

instance caused by maternal smoking, drives one of the underlying mechanisms of the abnormal lung response that patients with asthma and COPD express after inhalation of noxious stimuli that all individuals encounter, which then results in abnormal lung function measures, caused by airway inflammation and remodeling superimposed on this abnormal lung development. This mechanism would also explain, at least partially, the overlap syndrome if abnormal lung development in utero is the underlying mechanism of asthma and COPD.

There are additional differences in asthma and COPD caused by differences in the underlying genetic makeup of these two diseases. Genome-wide association studies (GWAS) have shown differential genes to be associated with COPD and asthma.[65,66] Recent GWAS have identified loci that harbor susceptibility genes for asthma and other pulmonary conditions. Many of the genes at these loci have unknown functions and have not previously been considered biologically plausible candidates for disease pathogenesis. Genes found by GWAS in asthma are *ORMDL3*, *GSMDB*, *IL18R1*, *IL1RL1*, *IL33*, *SMAD3*, *IL2RB*, *DENND1B*, *HLA-Dr/DQ* region, *PDE4D2*, *RAD50-IL13*, *WDR36*, *TLE4*, and *MYB*.[67] Studies have recently started to investigate the genome for subphenotypes of asthma. Thus, Himes and colleagues[68] found that the presence of a bronchodilator response is associated with *SPATS2*.

Table 2
Risk factors for asthma and COPD

Host factors	Male sex in childhood, female sex in adulthood	Family history of COPD
	(Family) history of asthma	Family history asthma/atopy
	Genetic constitution	Genetic constitution
	Airway hyperresponsiveness	Airway hyperresponsiveness
	Atopy	—
	Low lung function	Low lung function
	Overweight	
Perinatal factors	Maternal smoking	Maternal smoking
	Maternal diet	—
	Mode of delivery	—
Childhood exposures	Viral respiratory infections	Respiratory tract infections
	No breastfeeding	—
	Microbial deprivation	Maternal smoking
	Environmental tobacco smoke exposure	Indoor air pollution
	Air pollution	—
Adult exposures	Occupational exposures	Occupational exposures
	Cigarette smoking	Cigarette smoking
	Outdoor air pollution	Outdoor air pollution
	—	Indoor air pollution

From Postma DS, Kerkhof M, Boezen HM, et al. Asthma and chronic obstructive pulmonary disease: common genes, common environments? Am J Respir Crit Care Med 2011;183(12):1588–94; with permission.

However, this has not been tested in COPD so far. In addition, the level of lung function and its accelerated decline were investigated specifically in asthma.[69] Unfortunately, the numbers of individuals investigated were too small to find significant genome-wide associations. Nevertheless, this is the way forward to assess whether similar genes are associated with development of a fixed airflow obstruction in asthma and a more severe disease with a higher level of lung function decline in COPD. This research may determine whether similar and/or differential mechanisms are underlying the fixed airflow obstruction in asthma and COPD.

Several genes have been associated with COPD (defined usually by low FEV_1 and FEV_1/forced vital capacity <70%) in GWAS (ie, CHRNA3, CHRNB3/4, HHIP, and FAM13A). Furthermore, several genes have been associated with a lower lung function in the general population, like AGER, GPR126, GSTCD, HTR4, THSD4, and TSN1. However, a low lung function, in the general population without further testing, may reflect asthma, COPD, or both, especially at older age, which hampers the interpretation of genetics of COPD to a large extent. Therefore, the genes published so far might not be specific to asthma or COPD, but it could be hypothesized that they reflect abnormal lung development in utero, which by itself has not been tested so far. Moreover, because COPD encompasses several phenotypes such as chronic bronchitis, airway obstruction, and emphysema, and asthma may encompass individuals with persistent airway obstruction, it is not possible to tell which genes are associated with which phenotype of COPD if not tested formally.

Overlap of Asthma and COPD

Many candidate genes and genes found by GWAS have been associated on multiple occasions with asthma, and sometimes with COPD as well.[65] Bosse[66] recently published an overview of COPD genes found by GWAS and frequently replicated candidate genes. **Table 3** combines the data on the number of publications with association of genes with asthma and with COPD as reviewed in these two articles.[65,66] The common genes identified for both asthma and COPD are ADRB2, GSTM1, GSTP1, IL13, TGFB1, and TNF.[65] We reported that this, so far limited, list of candidate genes underlying both asthma and COPD might be extended in the near future, because some genes identified in COPD have not been studied yet in asthma or too few studies have been performed that have tried to replicate genes associated with asthma in COPD. In

Table 3
Number of reports showing genes that are replicated in asthma more than 10 times, and their positive reports in COPD, and the converse number of reports with more than 10 times replication of association with COPD and their reports in asthma

	Number of Reports in Asthma	Number of Reports in COPD
Genes >10 Times in Asthma and also Reported in COPD		
ADAM33	23	6
ADRB2	46	12
CCL5	12	1
CD14	34	2
GSTM1	6	16
GSTP1	17	16
HLA	15	2
IL4	23	3
IL10	18	7
IL13	38	9
IL1B	12	6
IL4R	43	2
LTA4	12	5
STAT6	15	1
TGFB1	12	13
TNF	28	20
Genes >10 Times in Asthma but not in COPD		
HLADRB1	32	Not reported
FCERB1	22	Not reported
FLG	18	Not reported
NPSR1	12	Not reported
ORMDL3	12	0
Genes >10 Times in COPD, but not in Asthma		
EPHX	Not tested	25
SERPINA1	0	19

From Postma DS, Kerkhof M, Boezen HM, et al. Asthma and chronic obstructive pulmonary disease: common genes, common environments? Am J Respir Crit Care Med 2011;183(12):1588–94, with permission; and Bosse Y. Updates on the COPD gene list. Int J Chron Obstruct Pulmon Dis 2012;7:607–31, with permission.

addition, it is likely that genes that affect lung development in utero and lung growth in early childhood in interaction with environmental detrimental stimuli, such as smoking and air pollution, are contributing to asthma in childhood, progression of asthma to a phenotype with persistent airway obstruction, as well as development of COPD (**Fig. 1**).[65] Additional genes and environmental factors drive specific immunologic

Common and distinct genes for asthma and COPD

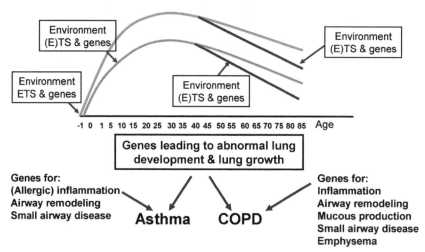

Fig. 1. Lung development, growth, and decline in interaction with genetic and environmental factors. Green line represents normal lung development, growth, and decline. Orange line represents abnormal prenatal lung development and growth. Red line represents abnormal lung decline caused by exposure to tobacco smoke. (E)TS, (environmental) tobacco smoke. (*From* Postma DS, Kerkhof M, Boezen HM, et al. Asthma and chronic obstructive pulmonary disease: common genes, common environments? Am J Respir Crit Care Med 2011;183(12):1588–94, copyright © 2011, American Thoracic Society; with permission.)

mechanisms that underlie asthma (like the Th2/Th1 (Thelper2/Thelper1) balance) and these may also contribute to the overlap phenotype of asthma and COPD (**Fig. 2**).

One approach to studying shared genes may be to compare the top hits of GWAS in distinct asthma and COPD populations. However, to unravel whether there exists an overlap phenotype that is genetically driven, a more fruitful method might be to search for shared genetics of asthma and COPD by performing a GWAS in one cohort including patients across the spectrum of chronic airways disease, and then examining whether the overlap phenotype has shared or distinct genes

with asthma and with COPD. Such a study would require a large number of well-characterized patients, but it seems the way forward.

INFLAMMATION AND REMODELING

Inflammation and remodeling are present in COPD throughout the bronchial tree and lung tissue. There are 3 distinct processes present, and in different combinations in COPD: (1) chronic sputum production and cough, so called chronic bronchitis; (2) small airway disease; and (3) emphysema, which is the loss of elastic tissue in the peripheral lung.[70] Respiratory bronchioles of young smokers are already inflamed,[70] likely reflecting early signs of COPD. This inflammation has been shown to predominantly comprise mononuclear cells in the airway wall and macrophages in the small airway lumen. In the peripheral airways of patients with established COPD, there is also an inflammatory infiltrate, in which neutrophils and predominantly CD8-positive lymphocytes as well as mast cells predominate (mast cells particularly in patients with centrilobular emphysema).[71,72] In addition, squamous cell metaplasia, fibrosis, and increased smooth muscle mass, associated with hypertrophy and hyperplasia of smooth muscle cells, are present.[73] Each of these components may contribute to airway narrowing, with consequences for severity of the disease and of respiratory symptoms. Moreover,

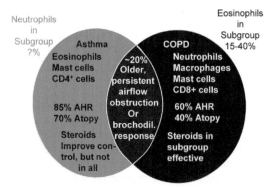

Fig. 2. The characteristics of patients with asthma, COPD, and the overlap phenotype. AHR, airway hyperresponsiveness.

goblet cell hyperplasia is frequently present and may contribute to chronic cough and phlegm in COPD, next to the contribution of increased mucus tenacity resulting from changes in soluble factors in the mucus, components that are different in asthma and COPD.[5] These types of inflammation and remodeling processes are also present in asthma (ie, increased numbers of eosinophils, CD4-positive lymphocytes and mast cells have been shown in both diseases).[5] Fabbri and colleagues[74] showed that patients with a history of asthma or a history of COPD with a similar level of airway obstruction and hyperresponsiveness have different inflammatory patterns (eosinophils in asthma and neutrophils in COPD), suggesting that there is no overlap in inflammatory pattern between asthma and COPD. However, in this case patients with COPD were all ex-smokers and current smokers and, as mentioned earlier, this may have skewed findings in the inflammatory pattern toward neutrophils, particularly because inflammation persists after smoking cessation in COPD.[75,76] Furthermore, although there was a significant difference in airway inflammation at a group level, there was also considerable overlap between asthma and COPD. Thus, these findings do not exclude an overlap phenotype of asthma and COPD.

Smoking induces inflammation in the lung with increased numbers of CD8 cells, neutrophils, mast cells, and macrophages in COPD.[77] It is not surprising that smoking in asthma induces comparable changes in inflammation (ie, more mast cells and fewer eosinophils in airway wall biopsies).[9] In addition, there is more remodeling in smokers with asthma, as reflected by more goblet cells and mucus-positive epithelium, increased epithelial thickness, and a higher proliferation rate of intact and basal epithelium in smokers with asthma.[9,22] Although asthma outside the context of smoking does not generally lead to neutrophilia, severe asthma is accompanied by a more neutrophilic inflammation compared with milder forms of asthma,[5,78] and some investigators have reported neutrophilic inflammation in patients with milder disease.[79] In contrast, severe asthma has a distinctive inflammatory phenotype as well: Benayoun and colleagues[80] showed that particularly high numbers of fibroblasts and airway smooth muscle hypertrophy in the proximal airways differentiates severe persistent asthma from milder asthma and COPD. Whether this is also the case in the smaller airways remains to be established. Next to neutrophilic asthma, there also exists a subset of patients with COPD with eosinophilia. The prevalence of eosinophilic COPD has been reported to range between 12% and 25% or even higher (up to 50% of stable patients with COPD).[81] This type of inflammatory cell in particular increases during exacerbations of COPD.[82] Bafadhel and colleagues[83] showed that the presence of blood eosinophilia (>2%) during an exacerbation of COPD may be a useful biomarker to direct corticosteroid therapy. In addition, it has been shown that stable patients with COPD and sputum eosinophilia can be effectively treated with inhaled steroids.[84]

Next to inflammation, remodeling plays a role in the clinical expression of asthma and COPD. It has been postulated that airway remodeling underlies the phenotypic overlap in asthma and COPD.[22] Airways are thickened in both asthma and COPD. However, Kuwano and colleagues[85] showed that the small airways in asthma are thicker than in COPD and healthy controls. Moreover, despite thickening of the airway wall in asthma, the airway lumen is larger[86] than in COPD, suggesting differential effects of airway wall thickening in asthma and COPD, possibly reflecting different underlying remodeling processes. This finding is underscored by the observation that patients with asthma generally do not develop emphysema. Parenchymal changes occur in asthma, in the sense of abnormal alveolar attachments and reduced numbers and changed geometry of elastic fibers.[87,88] These changes occur in the peribronchial region, whereas in emphysema there are widespread changes in lung tissue, not only in the peribronchiolar region, which differentiates people with asthma from patients with COPD with emphysema. However, there are also similarities with respect to remodeling in asthma and COPD, as recently pointed out in a review by Mauad and colleagues,[5] namely that structural changes occur in both diseases because of chronic inflammatory tissue injury, especially in the most severe cases. Because there are limited patterns of repair in the lungs, similar structural abnormalities may exist in some patients, possibly contributing to the clinical overlap. The latter review by Mauad and colleagues[5] and the studies discussed earlier show that some changes are characteristic of each disease (emphysema in COPD, epithelial desquamation and prominent increases in airway smooth muscle mass in the central airways in asthma), but in the overlap phenotype changes of both asthma and COPD may be present.

PHARMACOLOGIC RESPONSES

One of the difficulties in discussing treatment response in asthma and COPD is that patients with overlap phenotypes of asthma and COPD have been systematically excluded from drug trials, which are designed to include patients with pure COPD and pure asthma. This exclusion represents a problem for evidence-based guidelines on obstructive airway disease. Travers and colleagues[89] showed that only 5 of 100 individuals identified with COPD in a general population survey would fulfill inclusion criteria for major randomized controlled trials and reported comparable findings for asthma.[90] Thus, it is difficult to predict in an evidence-based way what the response to antiinflammatory and/or bronchodilator treatment would be in the full spectrum of COPD and the full spectrum of asthma.

Treatment of asthma and COPD is based on targeting inflammation and remodeling as well as counteracting contraction of the smooth muscles around the airways. Treatment is driven by the manifestations of disease both in asthma and COPD and aims to reduce symptoms, exacerbation frequency, and to improve health status, and, with severe disease, to improve exercise tolerance.[11] A proportion of patients with asthma or COPD does not achieve an acceptable level of control despite combination treatment with ICSs and long-acting bronchodilators, and has a more rapid loss of FEV_1 over time. This finding has been attributed to unresponsiveness of the underlying inflammatory and remodeling processes in the airways in the case of COPD. However, as mentioned earlier, it may also represent an overlap syndrome with neutrophilia in severe or persistent asthma, or clinicians may be treating patients with large-particle drugs, so the small airways are not being reached and inflammation and remodeling are not being adequately treated in either asthma or COPD.[30]

In general, lung function does not improve to a large extent in COPD and randomized studies have shown that the accelerated lung function decline, a major clinical characteristic of COPD, is not affected to a large extent by pharmacotherapy. However, 2 recent studies suggested that the decline in lung function can be significantly attenuated with ICS treatment, at least in a subset of patients with COPD, irrespective whether long acting beta agonists (LABAs) were added.[91,92] A recent meta-analysis showed that ICSs have immune-modulating effects in COPD,[93] hence this may be plausible. However, most studies do not show effects on lung function decline and the parameters that can predict a favorable ICS response in COPD remain to be determined.[94] Siva and colleagues[94] recently showed that patients with COPD with sputum eosinophilia (>3%) may respond better to ICS with respect to reduction in exacerbations, whereas the Groningen Leiden Universities Corticosteroids in Obstructive Lung Disease (GLUCOLD) study suggested that the presence of hyperinflation (a sign of small airway involvement) may predict a better response to ICS with respect to lung function decline, whereas disturbed diffusion capacity, a marker of emphysema, predicts a worse response.[95] Here, eosinophilia in sputum did not predict a better or worse response, suggesting that some markers associate with exacerbation frequency and others with lung function loss. The observation that signs of emphysema predict worse ICS response is plausible because regeneration of destroyed alveoli has never been shown in COPD, or in any other lung disease.

In eosinophilic asthma, ICS doses can be downtitrated based on sputum eosinophilia. Whether this is also the case in COPD, in which ICS doses have typically been much higher than in asthma, needs to be firmly established in future studies, but a pilot study suggested that this may be a good approach,[84] particularly given the concern about pneumonia with ICS in COPD (although not in asthma). However, in clinical practice it is difficult to perform sputum induction on regular basis, and, at least in asthma, the inflammatory profile can vary from visit to visit[96]; thus new inflammatory markers have to be found for optimal initiation and downtitration of ICS.

If a diagnosis of asthma or COPD is not reached, it could be worth establishing in all patients with airway obstruction, either asthma or COPD or overlap phenotypes, whether sputum eosinophilia is present, and, if so, initiating ICS treatment.[61] In addition, it could be worth starting long-acting bronchodilators if symptoms persist, because this improves clinical stability further. Welte and colleagues[97] showed that triple therapy (ICS with LABA and long-acting muscarinic anticholinergic) has great benefit in COPD, with many patients showing considerable bronchodilator responses (up to 50%). From this, it could be inferred that the overlap phenotype, in more severe disease, could benefit from triple therapy as well, which is also consistent with the observations of Magnussen and colleagues[98] showing that patients with COPD and concomitant asthma improve considerably with tiotropium bromide with respect to lung function and need for rescue medication.

SUMMARY

It is easy to differentiate pure asthma from pure COPD, because they reflect the extremes of a spectrum. However, in many, especially older, patients, features of both asthma and COPD can be present, leading to an overlap phenotype. There is no extensive literature available on the overlap phenotype, and interpretation of studies thus far has been hampered by differential age and smoking status in asthma and COPD. The balance of evidence so far suggests that the severity of airway obstruction and hyperresponsiveness in asthma, COPD, and the overlap phenotypes is driven by some similar and some different mechanisms. In addition, there is an unmet need to assess treatment effects in individuals with the overlap phenotype of asthma and COPD, because they have been consistently excluded from pharmacologic studies.

REFERENCES

1. Global initiative for chronic obstructive lung disease (GOLD). 2013. Available at: www.goldcopd.org.
2. Gibson PG, Simpson JL. The overlap syndrome of asthma and COPD: what are its features and how important is it? Thorax 2009;64(8):728–35.
3. Hanania NA, Celli BR, Donohue JF, et al. Bronchodilator reversibility in COPD. Chest 2011;140(4): 1055–63.
4. Postma DS, Boezen HM. Rationale for the Dutch hypothesis. Allergy and airway hyperresponsiveness as genetic factors and their interaction with environment in the development of asthma and COPD. Chest 2004;126(Suppl 2):96S–104S.
5. Mauad T, Dolhnikoff M. Pathologic similarities and differences between asthma and chronic obstructive pulmonary disease. Curr Opin Pulm Med 2008;14(1):31–8.
6. Contoli M, Baraldo S, Marku B, et al. Fixed airflow obstruction due to asthma or chronic obstructive pulmonary disease: 5-year follow-up. J Allergy Clin Immunol 2010;125(4):830–7.
7. Soriano JB, Davis KJ, Coleman B, et al. The proportional Venn diagram of obstructive lung disease: two approximations from the United States and the United Kingdom. Chest 2003;124(2):474–81.
8. Knudson RJ, Clark DF, Kennedy TC, et al. Effect of aging alone on mechanical properties of the normal adult human lung. J Appl Physiol 1977; 43(6):1054–62.
9. Broekema M, ten Hacken NH, Volbeda F, et al. Airway epithelial changes in smokers but not in ex-smokers with asthma. Am J Respir Crit Care Med 2009;180(12):1170–8.
10. Tomlinson JE, McMahon AD, Chaudhuri R, et al. Efficacy of low and high dose inhaled corticosteroid in smokers versus non-smokers with mild asthma. Thorax 2005;60(4):282–7.
11. Global INitiative for Asthma (GINA) guidelines. 2012. Available at: www.ginasthma.org.
12. Postma DS, Brusselle G, Bush A, et al. I have taken my umbrella, so of course it does not rain. Thorax 2012;67(1):88–9.
13. Broekema M, Volbeda F, Timens W, et al. Airway eosinophilia in remission and progression of asthma: accumulation with a fast decline of FEV(1). Respir Med 2010;104(9):1254–62.
14. Hardin M, Silverman EK, Barr RG, et al. The clinical features of the overlap between COPD and asthma. Respir Res 2011;12:127.
15. Akgun KM, Crothers K, Pisani M. Epidemiology and management of common pulmonary diseases in older persons. J Gerontol A Biol Sci Med Sci 2012;67(3):276–91.
16. Levy ML, Fletcher M, Price DB, et al. International Primary Care Respiratory Group (IPCRG) Guidelines: diagnosis of respiratory diseases in primary care. Prim Care Respir J 2006;15(1):20–34.
17. Rogers DF. Airway mucus hypersecretion in asthma: an undervalued pathology? Curr Opin Pharmacol 2004;4(3):241–50.
18. Thiadens HA, de Bock GH, Dekker FW, et al. Identifying asthma and chronic obstructive pulmonary disease in patients with persistent cough presenting to general practitioners: descriptive study. BMJ 1998;316(7140):1286–90.
19. Vonk JM, Jongepier H, Panhuysen CI, et al. Risk factors associated with the presence of irreversible airflow limitation and reduced transfer coefficient in patients with asthma after 26 years of follow up. Thorax 2003;58(4):322–7.
20. Watson L, Schouten JP, Lofdahl CG, et al. Predictors of COPD symptoms: does the sex of the patient matter? Eur Respir J 2006;28(2):311–8.
21. Prescott E, Lange P, Vestbo J. Chronic mucus hypersecretion in COPD and death from pulmonary infection. Eur Respir J 1995;8(8):1333–8.
22. Fattahi F, ten Hacken NH, Lofdahl CG, et al. Atopy is a risk factor for respiratory symptoms in COPD patients: results from the EUROSCOP study. Respir Res 2013;14(1):10.
23. Tashkin DP, Celli B, Decramer M, et al. Bronchodilator responsiveness in patients with COPD. Eur Respir J 2008;31(4):742–50.
24. Tashkin DP, Celli B, Senn S, et al. A 4-year trial of tiotropium in chronic obstructive pulmonary disease. N Engl J Med 2008;359(15):1543–54.
25. Bleecker ER, Emmett A, Crater G, et al. Lung function and symptom improvement with fluticasone propionate/salmeterol and ipratropium bromide/albuterol in COPD: response by beta-agonist reversibility. Pulm Pharmacol Ther 2008; 21(4):682–8.
26. Albert P, Agusti A, Edwards L, et al. Bronchodilator responsiveness as a phenotypic characteristic of established chronic obstructive pulmonary disease. Thorax 2012;67(8):701–8.
27. Papi A, Romagnoli M, Baraldo S, et al. Partial reversibility of airflow limitation and increased exhaled NO and sputum eosinophilia in chronic

obstructive pulmonary disease. Am J Respir Crit Care Med 2000;162(5):1773–7.

28. Mohamed Hoesein FA, de HB, Zanen P, et al. CT-quantified emphysema in male heavy smokers: association with lung function decline. Thorax 2011; 66(9):782–7.

29. Van den Berge M, ten Hacken NH, Cohen J, et al. Small airway disease in asthma and COPD: clinical implications. Chest 2011;139(2):412–23.

30. Van den Berge M, ten Hacken NH, Van der Wiel E, et al. Treatment of the bronchial tree from beginning to end: targeting small airway inflammation in asthma. Allergy 2013;68(1):16–26.

31. Van der Wiel E, ten Hacken NH, Postma DS, et al. Small-airways dysfunction associates with respiratory symptoms and clinical features of asthma: a systematic review. J Allergy Clin Immunol 2013; 131(3):646–57.

32. Turner SW, Palmer LJ, Rye PJ, et al. Infants with flow limitation at 4 weeks: outcome at 6 and 11 years. Am J Respir Crit Care Med 2002;165(9): 1294–8.

33. Paredi P, Goldman M, Alamen A, et al. Comparison of inspiratory and expiratory resistance and reactance in patients with asthma and chronic obstructive pulmonary disease. Thorax 2010; 65(3):263–7.

34. Verbanck S, Schuermans D, Paiva M, et al. Nonreversible conductive airway ventilation heterogeneity in mild asthma. J Appl Physiol 2003;94(4): 1380–6.

35. Verbanck S, Schuermans D, Noppen M, et al. Evidence of acinar airway involvement in asthma. Am J Respir Crit Care Med 1999;159(5 Pt 1):1545–50.

36. Verbanck S, Schuermans D, Van MA, et al. Conductive and acinar lung-zone contributions to ventilation inhomogeneity in COPD. Am J Respir Crit Care Med 1998;157(5 Pt 1):1573–7.

37. Galban CJ, Han MK, Boes JL, et al. Computed tomography-based biomarker provides unique signature for diagnosis of COPD phenotypes and disease progression. Nat Med 2012;18(11): 1711–5.

38. Kay AB. Overview of 'allergy and allergic diseases: with a view to the future. Br Med Bull 2000;56(4): 843–64.

39. The ENFUMOSA cross-sectional European multicentre study of the clinical phenotype of chronic severe asthma. European Network for Understanding Mechanisms of Severe Asthma. Eur Respir J 2003;22(3):470–7.

40. Sparrow D, O'Connor G, Weiss ST. The relation of airways responsiveness and atopy to the development of chronic obstructive lung disease. Epidemiol Rev 1988;10:29–47.

41. Weiss ST. Atopy as a risk factor for chronic obstructive pulmonary disease: epidemiological

evidence. Am J Respir Crit Care Med 2000; 162(3 Pt 2):S134–6.

42. Sahn SA. Corticosteroids in chronic bronchitis and pulmonary emphysema. Chest 1978;73(3): 389–96.

43. Postma DS, Kerstjens HA. Characteristics of airway hyperresponsiveness in asthma and chronic obstructive pulmonary disease. Am J Respir Crit Care Med 1998;158(5 Pt 3):S187–92.

44. Tashkin DP, Altose MD, Bleecker ER, et al. The lung health study: airway responsiveness to inhaled methacholine in smokers with mild to moderate airflow limitation. The Lung Health Study Research Group. Am Rev Respir Dis 1992;145(2 Pt 1):301–10.

45. Kerstjens HA, Brand PL, Hughes MD, et al. A comparison of bronchodilator therapy with or without inhaled corticosteroid therapy for obstructive airways disease. Dutch Chronic Non-Specific Lung Disease Study Group. N Engl J Med 1992; 327(20):1413–9.

46. Reddel HK, Jenkins CR, Marks GB, et al. Optimal asthma control, starting with high doses of inhaled budesonide. Eur Respir J 2000;16(2):226–35.

47. Kerstjens HA, Schouten JP, Brand PL, et al. Importance of total serum IgE for improvement in airways hyperresponsiveness with inhaled corticosteroids in asthma and chronic obstructive pulmonary disease. The Dutch CNSLD Study Group. Am J Respir Crit Care Med 1995;151(2 Pt 1):360–8.

48. Chanez P, Vignola AM, O'Shaugnessy T, et al. Corticosteroid reversibility in COPD is related to features of asthma. Am J Respir Crit Care Med 1997;155(5):1529–34.

49. Finkelstein R, Ma HD, Ghezzo H, et al. Morphometry of small airways in smokers and its relationship to emphysema type and hyperresponsiveness. Am J Respir Crit Care Med 1995;152(1):267–76.

50. Wiggs BR, Bosken C, Pare PD, et al. A model of airway narrowing in asthma and in chronic obstructive pulmonary disease. Am Rev Respir Dis 1992; 145(6):1251–8.

51. Rutgers SR, Timens W, Kauffman HF, et al. Markers of active airway inflammation and remodelling in chronic obstructive pulmonary disease. Clin Exp Allergy 2001;31(2):193–205.

52. Blacquiere MJ, Timens W, Melgert BN, et al. Maternal smoking during pregnancy induces airway remodelling in mice offspring. Eur Respir J 2009;33(5):1133–40.

53. Black JL, Panettieri RA Jr, Banerjee A, et al. Airway smooth muscle in asthma: just a target for bronchodilation? Clin Chest Med 2012;33(3):543–58.

54. Hardaker KM, Downie SR, Kermode JA, et al. Predictors of airway hyperresponsiveness differ between old and young patients with asthma. Chest 2011;139(6):1395–401.

55. Downie SR, Salome CM, Verbanck S, et al. Ventilation heterogeneity is a major determinant of airway hyperresponsiveness in asthma, independent of airway inflammation. Thorax 2007;62(8):684–9.

56. Van den Berge M, Vonk JM, Gosman M, et al. Clinical and inflammatory determinants of bronchial hyperresponsiveness in COPD. Eur Respir J 2012; 40(5):1098–105.

57. Shaya FT, Dongyi D, Akazawa MO, et al. Burden of concomitant asthma and COPD in a Medicaid population. Chest 2008;134(1):14–9.

58. Weatherall M, Travers J, Shirtcliffe PM, et al. Distinct clinical phenotypes of airways disease defined by cluster analysis. Eur Respir J 2009; 34(4):812–8.

59. Guerra S. Overlap of asthma and chronic obstructive pulmonary disease. Curr Opin Pulm Med 2005; 11(1):7–13.

60. Buist AS. Similarities and differences between asthma and chronic obstructive pulmonary disease: treatment and early outcomes. Eur Respir J Suppl 2003;39:30s–5s.

61. Soler-Cataluna JJ, Cosio B, Izquierdo JL, et al. Consensus document on the overlap phenotype COPD-asthma in COPD. Arch Bronconeumol 2012;48(9):331–7.

62. Kauppi P, Kupiainen H, Lindqvist A, et al. Overlap syndrome of asthma and COPD predicts low quality of life. J Asthma 2011;48(3):279–85.

63. Meyer PA, Mannino DM, Redd SC, et al. Characteristics of adults dying with COPD. Chest 2002; 122(6):2003–8.

64. Hospers JJ, Schouten JP, Weiss ST, et al. Asthma attacks with eosinophilia predict mortality from chronic obstructive pulmonary disease in a general population sample. Am J Respir Crit Care Med 1999;160(6):1869–74.

65. Postma DS, Kerkhof M, Boezen HM, et al. Asthma and chronic obstructive pulmonary disease: common genes, common environments? Am J Respir Crit Care Med 2011;183(12):1588–94.

66. Bosse Y. Updates on the COPD gene list. Int J Chron Obstruct Pulmon Dis 2012;7:607–31.

67. Hao K, Bosse Y, Nickle DC, et al. Lung eQTLs to help reveal the molecular underpinnings of asthma. PLoS Genet 2012;8(11):e1003029.

68. Himes BE, Jiang X, Hu R, et al. Genome-wide association analysis in asthma subjects identifies SPATS2L as a novel bronchodilator response gene. PLoS Genet 2012;8(7):e1002824.

69. Imboden M, Bouzigon E, Curjuric I, et al. Genome-wide association study of lung function decline in adults with and without asthma. J Allergy Clin Immunol 2012;129(5):1218–28.

70. Niewoehner DE, Kleinerman J, Rice DB. Pathologic changes in the peripheral airways of young cigarette smokers. N Engl J Med 1974;291(15):755–8.

71. Battaglia S, Mauad T, van Schadewijk AM, et al. Differential distribution of inflammatory cells in large and small airways in smokers. J Clin Pathol 2007;60(8):907–11.

72. Ballarin A, Bazzan E, Zenteno RH, et al. Mast cell infiltration discriminates between histopathological phenotypes of chronic obstructive pulmonary disease. Am J Respir Crit Care Med 2012;186(3): 233–9.

73. Baraldo S, Turato G, Saetta M. Pathophysiology of the small airways in chronic obstructive pulmonary disease. Respiration 2012;84(2):89–97.

74. Fabbri LM, Romagnoli M, Corbetta L, et al. Differences in airway inflammation in patients with fixed airflow obstruction due to asthma or chronic obstructive pulmonary disease. Am J Respir Crit Care Med 2003;167(3):418–24.

75. Rutgers SR, Postma DS, ten Hacken NH, et al. Ongoing airway inflammation in patients with COPD who do not currently smoke. Thorax 2000; 55(1):12–8.

76. Willemse BW, ten Hacken NH, Rutgers B, et al. Effect of 1-year smoking cessation on airway inflammation in COPD and asymptomatic smokers. Eur Respir J 2005;26(5):835–45.

77. Hogg JC, Chu F, Utokaparch S, et al. The nature of small-airway obstruction in chronic obstructive pulmonary disease. N Engl J Med 2004;350(26): 2645–53.

78. Shaw DE, Berry MA, Hargadon B, et al. Association between neutrophilic airway inflammation and airflow limitation in adults with asthma. Chest 2007;132(6):1871–5.

79. McGrath KW, Icitovic N, Boushey HA, et al. A large subgroup of mild-to-moderate asthma is persistently noneosinophilic. Am J Respir Crit Care Med 2012;185(6):612–9.

80. Benayoun L, Druilhe A, Dombret MC, et al. Airway structural alterations selectively associated with severe asthma. Am J Respir Crit Care Med 2003; 167(10):1360–8.

81. Saha S, Brightling CE. Eosinophilic airway inflammation in COPD. Int J Chron Obstruct Pulmon Dis 2006;1(1):39–47.

82. Bathoorn E, Liesker JJ, Postma DS, et al. Change in inflammation in out-patient COPD patients from stable phase to a subsequent exacerbation. Int J Chron Obstruct Pulmon Dis 2009;4:101–9.

83. Bafadhel M, McKenna S, Terry S, et al. Blood eosinophils to direct corticosteroid treatment of exacerbations of chronic obstructive pulmonary disease: a randomized placebo-controlled trial. Am J Respir Crit Care Med 2012;186(1):48–55.

84. Brightling CE, McKenna S, Hargadon B, et al. Sputum eosinophilia and the short term response to inhaled mometasone in chronic obstructive pulmonary disease. Thorax 2005;60(3):193–8.

85. Kuwano K, Bosken CH, Pare PD, et al. Small airways dimensions in asthma and in chronic obstructive pulmonary disease. Am Rev Respir Dis 1993; 148(5):1220–5.

86. Carroll N, Elliot J, Morton A, et al. The structure of large and small airways in nonfatal and fatal asthma. Am Rev Respir Dis 1993;147(2):405–10.

87. Carroll NG, Perry S, Karkhanis A, et al. The airway longitudinal elastic fiber network and mucosal folding in patients with asthma. Am J Respir Crit Care Med 2000;161(1):244–8.

88. Mauad T, Silva LF, Santos MA, et al. Abnormal alveolar attachments with decreased elastic fiber content in distal lung in fatal asthma. Am J Respir Crit Care Med 2004;170(8):857–62.

89. Travers J, Marsh S, Caldwell B, et al. External validity of randomized controlled trials in COPD. Respir Med 2007;101(6):1313–20.

90. Travers J, Marsh S, Williams M, et al. External validity of randomised controlled trials in asthma: to whom do the results of the trials apply? Thorax 2007;62(3):219–23.

91. Lapperre TS, Snoeck-Stroband JB, Gosman MM, et al. Effect of fluticasone with and without salmeterol on pulmonary outcomes in chronic obstructive pulmonary disease: a randomized trial. Ann Intern Med 2009;151(8):517–27.

92. Celli BR, Thomas NE, Anderson JA, et al. Effect of pharmacotherapy on rate of decline of lung function in chronic obstructive pulmonary disease: results from the TORCH study. Am J Respir Crit Care Med 2008;178(4):332–8.

93. Jen R, Rennard SI, Sin DD. Effects of inhaled corticosteroids on airway inflammation in chronic obstructive pulmonary disease: a systematic review and meta-analysis. Int J Chron Obstruct Pulmon Dis 2012;7:587–95.

94. Siva R, Green RH, Brightling CE, et al. Eosinophilic airway inflammation and exacerbations of COPD: a randomised controlled trial. Eur Respir J 2007; 29(5):906–13.

95. Snoeck-Stroband JB, Lapperre TS, Sterk PJ, et al. Fewer packyears smoking and less signs of emphysema predict long-term inhaled corticosteroid response in moderate to severe COPD: analysis of a randomized trial cohort. Abstract ATS. 2012.

96. Hancox RJ, Cowan DC, Aldridge RE, et al. Asthma phenotypes: consistency of classification using induced sputum. Respirology 2012;17(3):461–6.

97. Welte T, Miravitlles M, Hernandez P, et al. Efficacy and tolerability of budesonide/formoterol added to tiotropium in patients with chronic obstructive pulmonary disease. Am J Respir Crit Care Med 2009;180(8):741–50.

98. Magnussen H, Bugnas B, van NJ, et al. Improvements with tiotropium in COPD patients with concomitant asthma. Respir Med 2008;102(1):50–6.

Acute COPD Exacerbations

Jadwiga A. Wedzicha, MD, FRCP*, Richa Singh, MRCP,
Alex J. Mackay, MRCP

KEYWORDS

- COPD • Exacerbations • Respiratory viral infections • Bacterial infections

KEY POINTS

- Chronic obstructive pulmonary disease (COPD) exacerbations are important events in COPD and are major determinants of health status in COPD.
- The natural course of COPD is interrupted by episodes of respiratory symptom worsening, termed *exacerbations*.
- Optimal management of acute exacerbations not only increases the rate of exacerbation recovery but also affects exacerbation rates and prevents hospital admissions.
- There is a need for the development of novel antiinflammatory agents that are effective at COPD exacerbations.

IMPACT OF COPD EXACERBATIONS

The natural course of COPD is interrupted by episodes of respiratory symptom worsening, termed exacerbations.[1] COPD exacerbations are important events in COPD and are major determinants of health status in COPD. COPD exacerbations are also independent predictors of mortality in COPD and also drive disease progression, with approximately 25% of the lung function decline attributed to exacerbations.[2]

COPD is the second largest cause of emergency admissions in the United Kingdom, with 1 in 8 hospital emergency admissions resulting from COPD, accounting for more than £800 million ($1.3 billion) in direct health care costs.[3] COPD exacerbations are also associated with cardiovascular events, especially myocardial infarction,[4,5] and patients hospitalized with exacerbations of COPD are a particularly vulnerable group for ischemic events. Every new severe exacerbation requiring hospitalization increases the risk of a subsequent exacerbation, and every new severe exacerbation increases the risk of death, up to 5 times after

the 10th compared with after a first COPD hospitalization.[6] COPD exacerbations are also more common and more severe in the winter months, when there are already pressures on numbers of admissions in hospitals.

Thus, the COPD strategy document developed by the Global Initiative for Chronic Obstructive Lung Disease (GOLD) highlights the importance of avoiding future risk in COPD by preventing exacerbations.[7] In view of the wide impact of COPD exacerbations, any therapy that prevents exacerbations will also improve health status and prevent forced expiratory volume in the first second of expiration (FEV_1) decline.

DEFINITION OF EXACERBATIONS

The common symptoms of a COPD exacerbation are increase in dyspnea, sputum purulence, and cough, but other symptoms may include increased wheezing, chest discomfort, and symptoms of an upper airway cold. Physiologic changes at COPD exacerbations (eg, falls in peak flow or FEV_1) are

Conflicts of Interest: J.A. Wedzicha has received honoraria for lectures and/or advisory boards from GSK, Novartis, Boehringer, Pfizer, Bayer, Takeda, and Vifor Pharma. She has received research grants from Novartis, Johnson and Johnson, Takeda, and Chiesi.
Centre for Respiratory Medicine, Royal Free Campus, University College London, Rowland Hill Street, London NW3 2PF, UK
* Corresponding author.
E-mail address: w.wedzicha@ucl.ac.uk

chestmed.theclinics.com

generally small and not useful in predicting or monitoring exacerbations.[1]

An exacerbation of COPD is defined in the GOLD strategy in terms of health care utilization as "an acute event characterised by a worsening of the patient's respiratory symptoms that is beyond normal day-to-day variations and leads to a change in medication." There is considerable evidence, however, that approximately half of all COPD exacerbations identified by symptom worsening are not reported to health care professionals for treatment.[8] Furthermore, these unreported exacerbations, although generally of lesser severity than reported or treated exacerbations, also have an impact on health status.[8]

For this reason, considerable interest exists in the potential of patient-reported outcomes in studies of exacerbation, and one of these is an instrument specifically designed for exacerbations, the Exacerbations of Chronic Pulmonary Disease Tool (EXACT). Although it may be useful in assessing the severity of exacerbations and the response to acute exacerbation therapy,[9] detection of an exacerbation probably still depends on patient report. Recently, a study in the London COPD cohort has shown that EXACT scores at the peak of the exacerbation were higher in treated than untreated events (**Fig. 1**), suggesting that the symptomatic burden of the exacerbation drives a patient's need for therapy. Further data from this study showed that the change in EXACT score to detect an exacerbation is smaller in severe COPD than in milder patients and highlights the difficulty in assigning scores to changes in exacerbations that occur across the disease spectrum. The scores on the COPD assessment test (CAT) also rise on exacerbation and reflect severity of the exacerbation, but the CAT has not been developed or validated for use at exacerbation.[10]

CAUSES AND PATHOGENESIS OF EXACERBATION

A majority of COPD exacerbations are triggered by respiratory viral infections, especially rhinovirus, the cause of the common cold. Using molecular techniques, respiratory viruses can be identified in up to 60% of exacerbations.[11] Exacerbations associated with viruses tend to have greater airway and systemic inflammatory effects than those without any evidence of viral infection and are more common in the winter months, with more chance of hospital admission. Airway pollutants may also be associated with precipitating exacerbations, especially by interacting with respiratory viruses, although significant effects of pollution are seen only in global areas of high urban pollution.[12]

Bacteria are present in the lower airway and are known to be present in the stable state and colonize the airway. Although airway bacterial load increases at exacerbation, it is now considered that bacteria are not often the primary infective cause of the exacerbation but are secondary invaders after a viral trigger. The effect of the infective triggers is to increase inflammation further in a chronically inflamed airway, leading to an

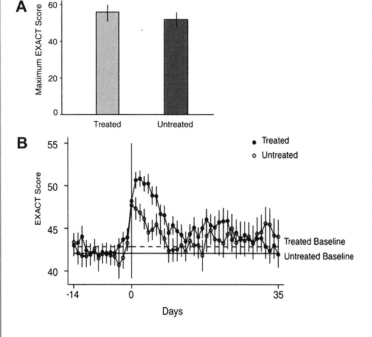

Fig. 1. (*A*) Maximum exacerbations of chronic pulmonary disease tool (EXACT) scores in chronic obstructive pulmonary disease patients treated and not treated with increased systemic therapy at exacerbation. Vertical lines represent standard errors. (*B*) Time course of EXACT scores during treated and untreated exacerbations. Vertical lines represent standard errors. (*From* Mackay AJ, Donaldson GC, Patel AR, et al. Detection and severity grading of COPD exacerbations using the exacerbations of Chronic Obstructive Pulmonary Disease Tool (EXACT). Eur Respir J 2013 Aug 29. [Epub ahead of print]).

increase in bronchoconstriction, edema, and mucus production, resulting in an increase in dynamic hyperinflation and symptoms of increased dyspnea characteristic of an exacerbation **Fig. 2.**[1] Thus, any intervention that reduces inflammation in COPD reduces the number and severity of exacerbation, whereas bronchodilators have an impact on exacerbation by their effects on reducing dynamic hyperinflation.

THE FREQUENT EXACERBATOR PHENOTYPE

Exacerbations become more frequent and severe as COPD severity increases. One distinct group of patients seems susceptible to exacerbations, irrespective of disease severity. This COPD phenotype of frequent exacerbations is stable over time and the major determinant of developing frequent exacerbations is a history of prior exacerbations.[13] This phenomenon is seen across all GOLD stages, including patients with stage 2 disease, of whom 22% had frequent exacerbations in the first year of the Evaluation of COPD Longitudinally to Identify Predictive Surrogate Endpoints (ECLIPSE) study.[14]

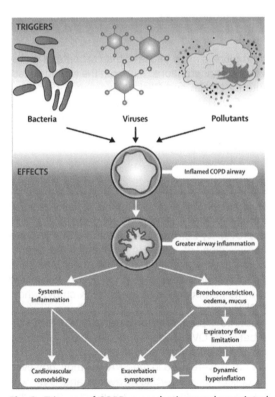

Fig. 2. Triggers of COPD exacerbations and associated pathophysiologic changes leading to increased exacerbation symptoms. (*From* Wedzicha JA, Seemungal TA. COPD exacerbations: defining their cause and prevention. Lancet 2007;370:787; with permission.)

Patients with a history of frequent exacerbations are at particular future risk of further events and death **Fig. 3.**[15] Studies have shown that this group of patients has worse quality of life, increased risk of hospitalization, and a greater chance of recurrent exacerbations. Frequent exacerbators also exhibit faster decline in lung function and may have worse functional status. Thus, it is vital to identify patients at risk of frequent exacerbations and target this group for therapy (**Table 1**).

EXACERBATION PREVENTION
Vaccines

In retrospective cohort studies of community-dwelling elderly patients, influenza vaccination is associated with a 27% reduction in the risk of hospitalization for pneumonia or influenza and a 48% reduction in the risk of death.[16] Thus, influenza vaccines are recommended in a majority of patients with COPD. There is less evidence for the role of pneumococcal polysaccharide vaccine in preventing exacerbations and hospital admissions in COPD, but large studies are currently under way with vaccines with improved immunogenicity. Nevertheless, pneumococcal vaccines are commonly administered to COPD patients.

Inhaled Corticosteroids and Long-acting Bronchodilators

Both inhaled corticosteroids (ICSs) and long-acting β-agonists (LABAs) reduce exacerbation frequency. In the Towards a Revolution in COPD Health (TORCH) study, where patients were followed over 3 years, both inhaled fluticasone and salmeterol reduced exacerbation frequency when administered separately in comparison with placebo.[17] The combination of fluticasone and salmeterol reduced exacerbation frequency further, in addition to improving health status and lung function in comparison with placebo. The combination of ICSs and LABAs also resulted in fewer hospital admissions over the study period. Reduction in exacerbation frequency has been also found with other LABA/ICS combinations, such as formoterol and budesonide. Guidelines indicate a LABA/ICS combination for patients with an FEV_1 below 50% predicted (groups C and D) and where there is a history of 2 or more exacerbations.

Long-acting *muscarinic antagonists* (LAMAs) also reduce exacerbation frequency. In the Understanding Potential Long-Term Impacts on Function with Tiotropium (UPLIFT) trial, patients were randomized to tiotropium or placebo for 4 years, with concomitant therapy allowed.[18] Although the primary endpoint of the trial (reduction in rate of decline in FEV_1) was negative, tiotropium was

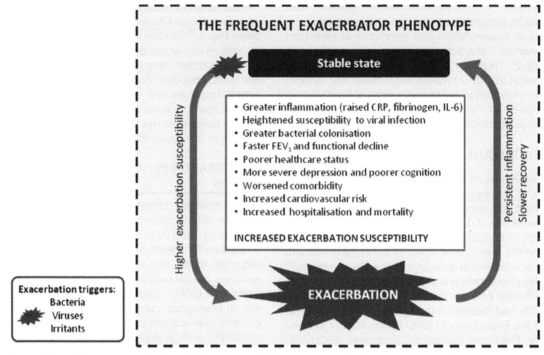

Fig. 3. Effect of COPD exacerbations in the group with frequent exacerbations. CRP, C-reactive protein; IL, interleukin. (*Adapted from* Wedzicha JA, Brill SE, Allinson JP, et al. Mechanisms and impact of the frequent exacerbator phenotype in chronic obstructive pulmonary disease. BMC Medicine 2013;11:181; with permission.)

associated with a reduction in exacerbation risk, related hospitalizations, and respiratory failure. The Prevention of Exacerbations with Tiotropium in COPD (POET-COPD) trial showed that, in patients with moderate to very severe COPD, tiotropium is more effective than salmeterol in preventing exacerbations.[19] In both the National Institute for Health and Clinical Excellence guidelines and GOLD strategy document, LAMAs can be used as an alternative to LABA/ICS to reduce exacerbations or in addition to the LABA/ICS combination as a triple therapy.[3]

Dual Bronchodilators

Dual inhaled long-acting bronchodilators contained in one inhaler are being introduced and the first one, approved by European regulators, is QVA that is a combination of a LABA (indacaterol) and a LAMA (glycopyrronium). QVA has been shown to produce increased bronchodilation compared with its components. In the SPARK study, where COPD patients were included with an FEV_1 of below 50% predicted and a history of COPD exacerbations, QVA reduced health care utilization exacerbation compared with glycopyrronium.[20] Diary cards were used in the SPARK study, however, to collect all exacerbation events and QVA was superior to both glycopyrronium and open-label tiotropium in the reduction of all exacerbations, that is, mild, moderate, and severe combined. Thus, future studies of dual bronchodilators must be designed to collect data on all exacerbation

---

Table 1
Strategies to prevent exacerbations

Pharmacologic Therapies for Exacerbation Prevention	Nonpharmacologic Therapies

• Antiviral therapy
• Vaccines
• Long-acting bronchodilators (LABAs/LAMAs)
• Combinations of LABA and ICS
• Dual bronchodilators (LABA + LAMA)
  ○ Phosphodiesterase-4 inhibitors
  ○ Mucolytics
  ○ Macrolide therapy
• Long-acting antibiotic therapy
	• Smoking cessation
	• Pollution control
	  ○ Pulmonary rehabilitation
	  ○ Home oxygen therapy
	  ○ Home ventilatory support

events as in the SPARK study. Availability of the new dual bronchodilators will change treatment algorithms because these therapies reduce both symptoms and prevent exacerbations.

Phosphodiesterase Inhibitors

Phosphodiesterase-4 inhibitors have broad antiinflammatory activity, inhibiting the airway inflammation associated with COPD, especially by reducing airway neutrophils that are key cells in COPD. Evidence from a pooled analysis of 2 large placebo-controlled, double-blind multicenter trials revealed a significant reduction of 17% in the frequency of moderate (glucocorticoid-treated) or severe (hospitalization/death) exacerbations with Roflumilast.[21] Only patients with an FEV_1 less than 50% (GOLD stages 3 and 4), presence of bronchitic symptoms, and a history of exacerbations, however, were enrolled. There currently are no comparator studies with ICSs. Weight loss was also noted in the roflumilast group, with a mean reduction of 2.1 kg after 1 year, and was highest in obese patients. Therefore, after treatment with roflumilast, weight needs to be monitored carefully. Recent evidence also suggests that roflumilast may reduce the number of patients in the frequent exacerbator group after 12 months of therapy.[22]

Long-term Antibiotics

At present there is insufficient evidence to recommend routine prophylactic antibiotic therapy in the management of stable COPD, but some studies have shown promise. Erythromycin reduced the frequency of moderate and/or severe exacerbations (treated with systemic steroids, treated with antibiotics, or hospitalized) and shortened exacerbation length when taken twice daily over 12 months by patients with moderate to severe COPD.[23] The macrolide azithromycin has been used as prophylaxis in patients with cystic fibrosis and when added to usual treatment azithromycin has also been shown to decrease exacerbation frequency and improve quality of life in COPD patients.[24] The benefits were most significant, however, in treatment-naive patients with mild disease (GOLD stage 2), and significant rates of hearing decrement (as measured by audiometry) and antibiotic resistance were found. Also, a recent large epidemiologic study has suggested a small increase in cardiovascular deaths in patients receiving azithromycin, particularly in those with a high baseline risk of cardiovascular disease.

Furthermore, intermittent pulsed moxifloxacin when given to stable patients has been shown to significantly reduce exacerbation frequency in a per protocol population and in a post hoc subgroup of patients with bronchitis at baseline.[25] This reduction did not meet statistical significance, however, in the intention-to-treat analysis, and further studies are required on nonmacrolide antibiotics, including assessment of safety.

Thus, before prescription of long-term antibiotics in COPD, patients should be treated with an optimum combination inhaled therapy, show evidence of ongoing frequent exacerbations, and be carefully assessed for risk of potential cardiovascular and auditory side effects.

Pulmonary Rehabilitation, Home Oxygen, and Ventilatory Support

There is some evidence from clinical trials that pulmonary rehabilitation programs reduce hospital stay. There is some evidence from epidemiologic studies in COPD patients that long-term oxygen therapy and noninvasive ventilatory support may reduce hospital admissions and prevent exacerbations,[26] but controlled trials have not yet addressed these issues. Although it is difficult to perform controlled trials of long-term oxygen therapy, there are ongoing studies of the role of home noninvasive ventilation in COPD patients who are hypercapnic and at risk of further events.

MANAGEMENT OF THE ACUTE EXACERBATION

After the earlier studies of Anthonisen and colleagues,[27] the standard management of an acute exacerbation consists of oral antibiotics, such as amoxicillin or doxycycline, if there is evidence of increased sputum purulence or increased sputum volume. Oral corticosteroids in short courses are also added depending on individual exacerbation severity, and there is recent evidence suggesting that shorter courses (5 days) may be as beneficial as longer ones, such as more conventional 14-day courses.[28] There is evidence that the earlier therapy is started at onset of exacerbation, the shorter the recovery of the event and less chance of hospital admission.[8] COPD exacerbations may show early recurrence, especially in patients who are frequent exacerbators. There is evidence that exacerbation therapy may prolong the time to subsequent events.[29] Thus, prompt and appropriate management of an exacerbation event not only will have an effect on optimizing recovery but also delay the time to the next event.

The use of oral corticosteroids at exacerbations is currently essential but it is possible that steroids may exacerbate bacterial infection at exacerbation in patients whose airways are colonized with bacteria, such as *Haemophilus influenzae* and

Streptococcus pneumoniae. There is a high risk of recurrent exacerbations in COPD patients and this may be due to secondary infection.[30] Thus, there is a need for the development of novel anti-inflammatory agents that are effective at COPD exacerbations. Optimal management of acute exacerbations not only will increase the rate of exacerbation recovery but also affect exacerbation rates and prevent hospital admissions.

REFERENCES

1. Wedzicha JA, Seemungal TA. COPD exacerbations: defining their cause and prevention. Lancet 2007; 370:786–96.
2. Donaldson GC, Seemungal TA, Bhowmik A, et al. The relationship between exacerbation frequency and lung function decline in chronic obstructive pulmonary disease. Thorax 2002;57:847–52.
3. National Institute for Health and Clinical Excellence (NICE). Chronic obstructive pulmonary disease: management of chronic obstructive pulmonary disease in adults in primary and secondary care. Update 2010. Available at: http://guidance.nice.org.uk/CG101/Guidance/pdf/English. Accessed December 18, 2013.
4. Donaldson GC, Hurst JR, Smith CJ, et al. Increased risk of myocardial infarction and stroke following exacerbation of COPD. Chest 2010;137:1091–7.
5. McAllister DA, Maclay JD, Mills NL. Diagnosis of myocardial infarction following hospitalisation for exacerbation of COPD. Eur Respir J 2012;39: 1097–103.
6. Suissa S, Dell'Aniello S, Ernst P. Long-term natural history of chronic obstructive pulmonary disease: severe exacerbations and mortality. Thorax 2012; 67(11):957–63.
7. Global Initiative for Chronic Obstructive Lung Disease (GOLD). Global strategy for the diagnosis, management and prevention of COPD. GOLD. Am J Respir Crit Care Med 2013. Available at: www.goldcopd.org. Accessed December 18, 2013.
8. Wilkinson TM, Donaldson GC, Hurst JR, et al. Early therapy improves outcomes of exacerbations of chronic obstructive pulmonary disease. Am J Respir Crit Care Med 2004;169:1298–303.
9. Mackay AJ, Donaldson GC, Patel AR, et al. Detection and severity grading of COPD exacerbations using the exacerbations of Chronic Obstructive Pulmonary Disease Tool (EXACT). Eur Respir J 2013. http://dx.doi.org/10.1183/09031936.00110913.
10. Mackay AJ, Donaldson GC, Patel AR, et al. Usefulness of the Chronic Obstructive Pulmonary Disease assessment test to evaluate severity of COPD exacerbations. Am J Respir Crit Care Med 2012;185:1218–24.
11. Seemungal TA, Harper-Owen R, Bhowmik A, et al. Respiratory viruses, symptoms and inflammatory markers in acute exacerbations and stable chronic obstructive pulmonary disease. Am J Respir Crit Care Med 2001;164:1618–23.
12. Peacock JL, Anderson HR, Bremner SA, et al. Outdoor air pollution and respiratory health in patients with COPD. Thorax 2011;66:591–6.
13. Seemungal TA, Donaldson GC, Paul EA, et al. Effect of exacerbation on quality of life in patients with chronic obstructive pulmonary disease. Am J Respir Crit Care Med 1998;157:1418–22.
14. Hurst JR, Vestbo J, Anzueto A, et al. Susceptibility to exacerbation in chronic obstructive pulmonary disease. N Engl J Med 2010;63:1128–38.
15. Wedzicha JA, Brill SE, Allinson JP, et al. Mechanisms and impact of the frequent exacerbator phenotype in chronic obstructive pulmonary disease. BMC Medicine 2013;11:181.
16. Nichol KL, Nordin JD, Nelson DB, et al. Effectiveness of influenza vaccine in the community-dwelling elderly. N Engl J Med 2007;357:1373–81.
17. Calverley PM, Anderson JA, Celli B, et al. Salmeterol and fluticasone propionate and survival in chronic obstructive pulmonary disease. N Engl J Med 2007;356:775–89.
18. Tashkin DP, Celli B, Senn S, et al. A 4-year trial of tiotropium in chronic obstructive pulmonary disease. N Engl J Med 2008;359:1543–54.
19. Vogelmeier C, Hederer B, Glaab T, et al. Tiotorpium versus salmeterol for the prevention of COPD exacerbations. N Engl J Med 2011;364(12): 1093–103.
20. Wedzicha JA, Decramer M, Fucker JH, et al. Analysis of COPD exacerbations with the dual bronchodilator QVA149 compared with glycopyrronium and tiotropium (SPARK): a randomized, double-blind, parallel-group study. Lancet Respir Med 2013;1: 199–209.
21. Calverley PM, Rabe KF, Goehring UM, et al. M2-124 and M2-125 study groups. Roflumilast in symptomatic chronic obstructive pulmonary disease: two randomised clinical trials. Lancet 2009;374(9691): 685–94 [Erratum appears in Lancet 2010; 376(9747):1146].
22. Wedzicha JA, Rabe KF, Martinez FJ, et al. Efficacy of roflumilast in the COPD frequent exacerbator phenotype. Chest 2013;143:1302–11.
23. Seemungal TA, Wilkinson T, Hurst JR, et al. Effect of erythromycin on exacerbations in COPD. Am J Respir Crit Care Med 2008;178:1139–47.
24. Albert RK, Connett J, Bailey WC, et al. Azithromycin for prevention of exacerbations of COPD. N Engl J Med 2011;365:689–98.
25. Sethi S, Jones PW, Theron MS, et al, PULSE Study group. Pulsed moxifloxacin for the prevention of exacerbations of chronic obstructive pulmonary disease: a randomized controlled trial. Respir Res 2010;11:10.

26. McEvoy RD, Pierce RJ, Hillman D, et al. Nocturnal non-invasive nasal ventilation in stable hypercapnic COPD: a randomised controlled trial. Thorax 2009; 64:561–6.

27. Anthonisen NR, Manfreda J, Warren CP, et al. Antibiotic therapy in exacerbations of chronic obstructive pulmonary disease. Ann Intern Med 1987;106: 196–204.

28. Leuppi JD, Schuetz P, Bingisser R. Short-term vs conventional glucocorticoid therapy in acute exacerbations of chronic obstructive pulmonary disease

the REDUCE randomized clinical trial. JAMA 2013; 309(21):2223–31.

29. Roede BM, Bresser P, Bindels PJ, et al. Antibiotic treatment is associated with a reduced risk of a subsequent exacerbation in obstructive lung disease: a historical population-based cohort. Thorax 2008; 63(11):968–73.

30. Hurst JR, Donaldson GC, Quint JK, et al. Temporal clustering of exacerbations in chronic obstructive pulmonary disease. Am J Respir Crit Care Med 2009;179:369–74.

Smoking Cessation

Stephen I. Rennard, MD*, David M. Daughton, MS

KEYWORDS

- Smoking • Cessation • Treatment • Pharmacotherapy

KEY POINTS

- Smoking is the major risk factor for lung cancer and contributes to risk for heart disease and many other conditions.
- Although the risks of smoking and the benefits of cessation are well recognized, for both generalist and specialist physicians, smoking cessation is often not a priority.
- Cigarette smoking should be regarded as a chronic relapsing disease.
- Optimal treatment requires a long-term approach, combining pharmacologic and nonpharmacologic interventions and close interactions between patient and clinician.

INTRODUCTION

Cigarette smoking is one of the major preventable causes of morbidity and mortality worldwide. It is the major risk factor for the development of chronic obstructive pulmonary disease (COPD) in the developed world and follows only indoor air pollution in the developing world. Smoking is the major risk factor for lung cancer and contributes to risk for heart disease and many other conditions. The adverse effects of smoking have been recognized at least since 1604,[1] and the overwhelming evidence linking smoking to disease was first reviewed in a Surgeon General's report in 1964.[2] The benefits of cessation are also well established and were the subject of a Surgeon General's report in 1990[3] and of a new report due in 2014.

Although the risks of smoking and the benefits of cessation are well recognized, for both generalist and specialist physicians, smoking cessation is often not a priority. This situation is unfortunate because more than 70% of adult smokers want to quit and interventions can help. Most have tried many times in the past. This situation often leads to a sense of futility, both for the smoker and the clinician. Undertreatment helps sustain this unhappy scenario. However, first-line smoking cessation interventions are not difficult, and all clinicians should be able to offer them to their patients.

The approach to cigarette smoking is to regard it as a chronic relapsing disease.[4] The role of the clinician is to help smokers achieve abstinence (remission), recognizing that relapses may occur. The proper model might be lymphoma, in which remissions are always regarded as successes and relapses are not failures but rather occasions that should lead to aggressive retreatment. In this article, the physiologic basis for smoking is reviewed and then both pharmacologic and nonpharmacologic approaches to treatment are addressed, with a discussion of practical issues.

PHYSIOLOGY OF SMOKING

There is a traditional view that regards smoking as a lifestyle choice and a habit. The decision to begin smoking is a choice, and in that context, it is a lifestyle choice. However, almost all smokers

Disclosures: Since 2010, S.I. Rennard has consulted with Pfizer on the topic of smoking cessation and conducted clinical trials sponsored by Pfizer. He has also consulted on other topics for GlaxoSmithKline which has smoking cessation products.

Division of Pulmonary, Critical Care, Sleep and Allergy, University of Nebraska Medical Center, 985910 Nebraska Medical Center, Omaha, Nebraska 68198-5910, USA

* Corresponding author.
E-mail address: srennard@unmc.edu

Clin Chest Med 35 (2014) 165–176
http://dx.doi.org/10.1016/j.ccm.2013.11.002

begin smoking in adolescence.[5] The choice to begin smoking is influenced by numerous social factors, which include not only the behaviors of family and friends but the promotion of smoking through advertising and public image. Smoking behavior is also strongly influenced by other social factors, including accessibility and cost.[6–8] Thus, although smoking is (in part) a lifestyle choice, it is clearly more than that. An alternative description is that it is a dangerous behavior, for which a susceptible population is at risk. Public health initiatives that are designed to influence smoking initiation among youth were initiated in the United States in the mid-1990s. These initiatives have had major impact on smoking prevalence.[9] Although public health initiatives are not reviewed here, they should be a part of any tobacco control program.

Nicotine is the most important psychologically active drug in tobacco, although there are others that are less well understood. Nicotine is a cholinergic agonist that acts specifically on a subset of cholinergic receptors, which have been classified as nicotinic receptors.[10,11] Nicotinic receptors are ion channels that are homopentamers or heteropentamers, which bind 2 ligand molecules.[12] The other major class of cholinergic receptors is muscarinic receptors, which are 7 membrane spanning G-protein coupled receptors that bind a single ligand molecule. Humans have 17 genes that code for distinct nicotinic receptor component chains, resulting in many potential pentamers. However, only a few play biological roles. Nine α and 3 β receptors are expressed in the brain. However, the $(\alpha4)(\beta2)$ complex, which can incorporate other subunits, including $\alpha5$, $\alpha6$, or $\beta3$, is believed to be a modulator of the effects of nicotine, and the $(\alpha4)_3(\beta2)_2$ subunit is believed to be particularly important in nicotine addiction. In support of the concept, deleting the β_2 receptor in mice eliminates behavioral responses to nicotine, whereas mutations in the gene can result in markedly increased sensitivity to nicotine[12] and the $(\alpha4)_3(\beta2)_2$ subunit is believed to be particularly important in nicotine addiction. In support of the concept, deleting the β_2 receptor in mice eliminates behavioral responses to nicotine, whereas mutations in the gene can result in markedly increased sensitivity to nicotine.[13]

By binding to the $(\alpha4)_3(\beta2)_2$ receptor, nicotine modulates the release of dopamine, which is a key mediator of pleasure and reward and plays a central role in the physiology of drug self-administration.[14] In particular, the release of dopamine is believed to mediate the euphoria associated with nicotine and many other addicting drugs. Nicotine also modulates the release of neurotransmitters in addition to dopamine and initiates both positive and negative feedback pathways, which may involve both changes in receptor expression and formation of neural connections. The overall effect in most individuals is an increase in nicotine self-administration together with a change in behavior (ie, addiction). These alterations can be long lasting. In rats, in utero exposures persist to adult life.[15] Adolescents may be particularly at risk for long-term alterations induced by nicotine.[16] These long-term effects may account for the persistent risk of relapse, which may be lifelong, which characterizes many addictions, including cigarette smoking. For this reason, an abstinent smoker is correctly regarded as in remission and at risk for relapse.

Some individuals, estimated at about 15% in the United States, are not addicted. Sometimes termed chippers, these individuals may smoke episodically and seem to not be fully addicted but may not be entirely normal either.[17,18] The physiologic basis for chippers is unclear, but may be related to genetic factors. It is an important point for the clinician, because this kind of behavior is well known to the general public and frequently confounds understanding of addiction.

Consistent with smoking being an addiction to nicotine, smokers adjust nicotine intake. If supplemental nicotine is provided, consumption is generally reduced.[19] Alternatively, if a smoker is obliged to reduce the number of cigarettes smoked, most maintain nicotine intake by altering the way in which individual cigarettes are smoked.[20] However, smoking is more than just an addiction to nicotine. Many cigarettes are smoked in social settings or habitually in association with other behaviors. In this regard, nicotine can augment the acquisition and persistence of conditioned behavior.[21] A smoker wishing to quit, therefore, must deal with both the biological effects caused directly by nicotine as well as with conditioned behaviors that likely have been potentiated by nicotine.

Nicotine is volatile. As a result, when air is sucked through the tip of a cigarette, the heated air causes nicotine in the unburned tobacco to volatilize. As the air passes through the cigarette, it cools, and the nicotine condenses on smoke particles, resulting in an aerosol that is about 1 μm in size, ideally suited to reach the alveolar space. Because nicotine is also lipid soluble in its neutral form, it can rapidly cross the alveolar space into the pulmonary capillary blood, reaching the brain in 15 to 20 seconds after a puff. The euphoric effects of nicotine depend in part on the kinetics: a rapid increase in levels at the receptors in the brain is associated with a greater hit. After absorption, nicotine redistributes into other body spaces, which leads to rapid decreases in arterial levels after smoking a cigarette is completed.[22] Nicotine is then metabolized, primarily in the liver by CYP450 enzymes, which lead to the formation of cotinine.[23] The nicotine half-life in the blood is 2 to 4 hours, so with continuing smoking throughout the day, nicotine levels increase. They are lowest in the early morning, and consistently, most addicted smokers report that the most potent cigarette is the first one smoked in the morning. Individuals who do not smoke within an hour of arising may not be heavily addicted. In contrast, heavily addicted smokers smoke within minutes of arising. This clinical observation forms a key part of the Fagerstrom Index, which is a widely used measure that assesses nicotine addition (**Table 1**).[24] The importance of nicotine kinetics in mediating its psychoactive effects is the basis for nicotine replacement as an aid for smoking cessation (see later discussion).

Table 1
Items and scoring for Fagerstrom test for nicotine dependence

Questions	Answers	Points
1. How soon after you wake up do you smoke your first cigarette?	Within 5 min	3
	6–30 min	2
	31–60 min	1
	After 60 min	0
2. Do you find it difficult to refrain from smoking in places where it is forbidden; eg, in church, at the library, in the cinema, etc?	Yes	1
	No	0
3. Which cigarette would you hate most to give up?	The first one in the morning	1
	All others	0
4. How many cigarettes/day do you smoke?	10 or less	0
	11–20	1
	21–30	2
	31 or more	3
5. Do you smoke more frequently during the first hours after waking than during the rest of the day?	Yes	1
	No	0
6. Do you smoke if you are so ill that you are in bed most of the day?	Yes	1
	No	0

From Heatherton TF, Kozlowski LT, Frecker RC, et al. The Fagerström test for nicotine dependence: a revision of the Fagerström Tolerance Questionnaire. Br J Addict 1991;86:1119–27. Copyright © 1991 KO Fagerstrom.

APPROACH TO A QUIT ATTEMPT

As noted earlier, smoking should be regarded as a primary addictive disorder.[4] Seventy-five percent of Americans wish to quit, but only 3% achieve prolonged abstinence in any year, indicating both the involuntary nature of the established addiction and the substantial need for treatment.[25] It is recommended that smoking status and willingness to quit be assessed at every health care visit.[4,26,27] However, individual readiness to quit (**Table 2**) is likely variable and may be related to acute health care events that may have no direct relationship to smoking.[28] Clinicians, therefore, must be prepared to exploit these windows of opportunity during which cessation attempts are made and may have greater success. To find these opportunities, the clinician must assess smoking status, hence the rationale for the recommendation for assessment at each visit.

The National Cancer Institute recommends using a 5-part approach, termed the 5As,[4,26,27] which follow the stages of change model. These stages are to ask patients about their smoking status, to assess their willingness to make a quit attempt, to advise smokers to stop, to assist them in their stop smoking efforts, and to arrange for follow-up visits to support the patient's efforts.

Routine inquiry about smoking may also favorably affect achievement of abstinence. In this regard, self-efficacy, the self-judged likelihood of success, seems to be a strong predictor of both success in a quit attempt[29] and the likelihood of subsequent relapse.[30] Failure to inquire about smoking is believed to send messages to the patient: that the physician does not care if the patient smokes; that the physician does not have an effective intervention; and that the physician does not

Table 2
Stages of change model for smoking cessation

Precontemplation	Not interested in quitting, likely unresponsive to direct intervention
Contemplation	Considering quitting, likely receptive to physician advice
Preparation	Actively preparing to make a quit attempt
Action	Quit attempt in progress
Maintenance	Avoidance of relapse (after a 6-mo remission)

Data from Prochaska JO, DiClemente CC. Stages of change in the modification of problem behaviors. Prog Behav Modification 1992;28:183–218.

think that the patient can quit, all of which can compromise self-efficacy. In support of the approach for routine assessment using the 5 As strategy, meta-analysis suggests that simple advice to quit from a clinician has a small but significant effect at boosting quit attempts and cessation.[27]

Quit attempts should be approached with the same strategy as inducing remission from lymphoma. Each treatment attempt should be given an optimal chance of success. In general, this strategy requires a combination of both pharmacotherapy, which can address some of the physiologic aspects of addiction, and nonpharmacologic approaches which can address the conditioned responses and other behavioral aspects of smoking. A staged approach, in which a person tries to quit on their own and, if unsuccessful, interventions of gradually increasing intensity are tried, is a misguided approach. Pharmacoeconomic analyses suggest that more intense programs are more cost-effective, because the less intense programs, which cost less, have less benefit.[31]

Whether smokers should quit with gradual reduction or tapering or with a sudden stop (eg. cold turkey) remains controversial. For most smokers, gradual cutting down can have initial success. First, a smoker can eliminate discretionary cigarettes that are smoked out of habit rather than to derive nicotine. As reduction proceeds, smokers can alter smoking behavior to maintain nicotine intake. However, as reduction continues, the smoker may begin to experience tobacco withdrawal symptoms. Rather than suffer prolonged discomfort, many taperers gradually return to their customary cigarette levels and do not succeed in quitting. In contrast, abrupt abstinence is often acutely stressful and leads to tobacco withdrawal symptoms. However, within a few weeks of total abstinence, complete abstainers experience less frequent cigarette cravings than taperers and are less prone to relapse. Nevertheless, some smokers may benefit from a tapering program,[32–34] and this can be used for selected individuals.

Most smokers are aware, at least in general, about the health hazards of smoking. In general, educational programs have proved disappointing as a means to achieve smoking abstinence.[4,26,27] Nevertheless, education about smoking is still regarded as useful, particularly when the information addresses specific patient concerns.

Group counseling programs to aid smoking cessation are available from several commercial and voluntary health organizations. Content generally includes lectures, group interactions, exercises on self-recognition of one's habit, some form of tapering method (leading to a quit day),

development of coping skills, and suggestions for relapse prevention. Programs sponsored by voluntary health organizations are generally the best cost value,[4,26,27] but are generally available only in large metropolitan areas and often on a sporadic basis. One-year success rates associated with group counseling programs are in the 15% to 35% range,[4,26,27] although the success rates likely reflect selection bias (ie, participants may be more motivated to quit).

Smoking cessation strategies are generally the same for special populations, including patients with COPD. In this regard, all 3 approved medications (nicotine replacement therapy [NRT], bupropion and varenicline) have been assessed in COPD and efficacy has been shown.[35–37] The hospital setting is an appropriate venue to begin treatment. Withdrawal symptoms are uncommon in the hospital, perhaps because of the enforced abstinence and unavailability of cigarettes. Follow-up after discharge seems to be particularly important for quit attempts initiated in the hospital.[38] Psychiatric comorbidities are not a contraindication to smoking cessation intervention. The cessation attempt does not compromise treatment of psychiatric disease, and successful abstinence can be achieved in that setting.[4,26,27]

STRATEGY FOR THE QUIT ATTEMPT

The greatest quit rates are achieved when nonpharmacologic support is combined with pharmacotherapy. The more extensive the support, the greater the success. However, many smokers do not accept referral to a group program. Limited counseling in the office can be provided to these individuals. In addition, telephone quit lines, which have shown efficacy,[39] are available toll-free and at no cost in many countries, including the United States and Canada. In the United States, the phone number is 1-800-Quit Now. Support can be found via the internet using smokefree.gov. Clinicians should encourage their patients to make use of these resources.

Several agents are available for pharmacotherapy. Selection of an agent should be based on past experience and individual patient issues. Nicotine Replacement Therapy (NRT) is often used as a first-line agent, because many clinicians have more experience with it and it has fewer adverse effects. The patch-plus regimen is often used, because of its increased efficacy, particularly for individuals who are more heavily addicted (Fagerstrom scores $\geq$7).[4,26,27,40] In contrast, an individual with a history of depression may be best treated with bupropion.[41] Individuals who achieved abstinence with an agent, but later relapsed, can be retreated with the same agent, but with specific attention to prevention of relapse. The details of specific agents are discussed later. NRT is generally started on the target quit date. Bupropion and varenicline are started 1 week before the quit date. Success has also been reported with varenicline started 1 to 5 weeks before the quit date.

A follow-up visit should be scheduled 10 days to 2 weeks after the quit date. This strategy allows assessment of adverse effects. However, the major reason for the visit is that it improves success rates, allowing the clinician to provide support to prevent relapse.

There are 4 specific issues that the clinician should anticipate with each quit attempt: withdrawal symptoms, cravings, depression, and weight gain. The clinician should prepare an action plan for each of these issues for each patient undergoing a quit attempt.

Withdrawal symptoms (**Box 1**) are experienced to a variable degree by most smokers undergoing a quit attempt. The symptoms generally peak within 72 hours then decrease gradually over the next 3 to 4 weeks. Common strategies that may help with withdrawal symptoms include increased levels of activity, deep breathing exercises, avoidance of high-risk situations, and use of other oral products (eg, cinnamon gum or chewable candies). Urges to smoke and withdrawal symptoms are greater when there is ready availability of cigarettes. As a result, it is important to remove all the cigarettes and smoking paraphernalia from the environment and to avoid situations in which cigarettes are provided by others.

Cravings to smoke are a feature of withdrawal. However, unlike the other symptoms, cravings can persist for years and are often precipitated by behaviors previously associated with smoking.

Generally, they decrease markedly in frequency but can still be intense. Cravings are times at which there is risk for relapse. Use of alcohol, which is often associated with smoking, can both precipitate craving and increase the risk of relapse.

Depression is experienced by many smokers during the first 3 months after cessation and is associated with a higher rate of relapse.[42] For most, the depression is mild and transient. For others, it may require treatment. Smoking has increased prevalence among individuals with depression, and both nicotine and other components of cigarette smoke have modest antidepressant effects. Some of the depression associated with cessation, therefore, may be an uncovering of a preexisting depression and may require counseling or pharmacotherapy.

Weight gain is a particularly difficult problem associated with smoking cessation.[4,26,27] Rapid weight gain for 6 to 8 weeks after cessation is common. A more gradual gain may follow. On average, 10 years after cessation, weight is increased 4.4 kg and 5.0 kg for men and women, respectively. Although the health risks associated with postcessation weight gain are unknown, they are likely surpassed by the health benefits of stopping smoking.

PHARMACOTHERAPY

Three classes of medication are approved as aids to smoking cessation (nicotine replacement, bupropion [Zyban, also sold under the trade name Wellbutrin to treat depression], and varenicline [Chantix]) and 2 others are available off-label (nortryptiline and clonidine), which have documented efficacy and are recommended as alternative therapies in current guidelines.[4,26,27,40]

NRT

There are 5 NRTs: lozenges, polacrilex (gum) and transdermal systems, which are available over the counter (OTC), and nasal spray and a nicotine inhaler, which are available with a prescription. Other nicotine preparations, including nicotine toothpicks and e-cigarettes, have been developed and marketed as consumer products. Their efficacy and safety in smoking cessation remain undetermined, and their use, particularly that of e-cigarettes, is controversial (see later discussion under harm reduction). There were initial reports of cardiac events when NRT products were used with concurrent smoking, which led the US Food and Drug Administration (FDA) to recommend against this practice. However, the FDA recently (April, 2013) removed this warning from the OTC

Box 1
Nicotine withdrawal symptoms (*Diagnostic and Statistical Manual of Mental Disorders, Fourth Edition*)

Dysphoric or depressed mood

Insomnia

Irritability, frustration, or anger

Anxiety

Difficulty concentrating

Restlessness

Decreased heart rate

Increased appetite or weight gain

formulations. These initial concerns are widely known by the general public, often inaccurately, and the current recommendations should be provided before the quit attempt.

NRT is usually started on a scheduled quit day, after which the smoker should be completely abstinent. If a smoker has some lapses, but is still interested in quitting, the quit attempt should continue. The concept is to replace nicotine to reduce the intensity of withdrawal. However, smokers' experience withdrawal symptoms, albeit with less intensity (see **Box 1**). The 5 approved formulations have similar 2-fold increases in quit rates over placebo when used alone.[4,26,27,43] They differ pharmacokinetically.[44] The transdermal systems provide the slowest delivery of nicotine but maintain steady state levels throughout the day. The other formulations, which can be administered ad lib, allow episodic dosing.

Nicotine polacrilex gum

Nicotine polacrilex gum is now commercially available OTC in 2-mg and 4-mg forms. The nicotine is bound to a resin and is released with chewing. Consequently, the rate of chewing influences nicotine delivery. At low pH nicotine is ionized, which prevents its absorption across the buccal mucosa. Thus, acidic foods or beverages can impair delivery of nicotine from the gum. The nicotine-containing saliva must be retained in the mouth as long as possible, because the nicotine must be absorbed across the buccal mucosa. If swallowed, the nicotine can cause local irritation of the stomach and can be absorbed. However, high first-pass metabolism in the liver limits blood nicotine levels. If chewed properly, blood levels peak after about 30 minutes[44] and achieve blood nicotine levels at less than 40% of customary smoking. A fixed dosage regimen rather than ad lib usage may have better success,[45] perhaps because it can produce higher blood nicotine levels. Some recommend that a smoker use 1 piece of gum every 1 to 2 hours for the first 6 weeks, followed by gradual reduction over 6 weeks. The long-term use of gum at times of craving to prevent relapse is also recommended. Some smokers can use sufficient gums to sustain nicotine addiction without smoking. Although this practice is not an approved use of NRT, it is recommended by some clinicians (see later discussion under harm reduction).

Nicotine gum is generally less effective in general practice and unsupervised settings than in clinical trials. This situation may be because of improper use of the gum, because chewing is important to its efficacy. Adverse effects of nicotine polacrilex gum include local effects (temporomandibular joint [TMJ] disease, trauma to dental appliances, sore jaw, oral irritation or ulcers, and excess salivation), effects from swallowed nicotine (hiccups), and effects from systemic absorption of nicotine (nausea, vomiting, abdominal pain, constipation, diarrhea, palpitations, and headache). Nicotine polacrilex gum is not recommended for those with poor dentition or who have dental appliances.[40]

Nicotine polacrilex lozenge

A nicotine polacrilex lozenge is also available OTC. Chewing is not required, but acid food or beverages impair absorption, as with gum. The lozenge is similar to the gum with regard to dosing, absorption, and duration of therapy.[46] Because it is not chewed, the lozenge does not share the problems related to TMJ disease or dental appliances. Other side effects are similar to those of gum.

Transdermal nicotine

Several transdermal patch delivery systems are available OTC. They are easy to use and maintain steady nicotine levels for 12 to 24 hours, achieving nicotine blood levels roughly 40% to 50% of a smoker of 30 cigarettes/d.[44] Perhaps because of the ease of use, transdermal nicotine systems have shown efficacy in the primary care setting.[28,47] The recommended duration of patches varies by product, but a minimum of 4 weeks of therapy is probably required to help achieve long-term abstinence.

Most commonly, patches are worn at night. This strategy provides a level of nicotine when a smoker awakes. This is a time when relapse is particularly likely, both because the low nicotine levels are associated with withdrawal and because smokers are familiar with the increased effect of a cigarette smoked on awakening. Both are likely reduced by maintaining nicotine levels during the night. However, nocturnal nicotine may disturb sleep, causing either vivid dreams or insomnia. Long-term use of the patch has not been observed, which suggests that the slow kinetics of nicotine delivery with transdermal systems is insufficient to sustain addiction.[48] As previously noted, early concerns about increased cardiac risk among individuals who smoked while wearing the patch have not been substantiated. In contrast, because patches lead to reduced smoking, they may decrease cardiac events.[49–51]

Nicotine inhaler

The nicotine inhaler is a plastic nicotine-containing cartridge that fits on a mouthpiece. Nicotine is not effectively delivered to the lungs, because the particle size is too large, but it is deposited and absorbed through the buccal mucosa. This situation results in pharmacokinetics that resemble nicotine polacrilex. Blood levels can be about one-third of conventional smoking but depend on frequency of use. Usual dosing is 6 to 16 cartridges per day for 6 to 12 weeks, followed by gradual reduction over 6 to 12 weeks. The inhaler recapitulates many actions associated with smoking: preparation of the device, oral stimulation, inhalation, and so forth. Thus, it may be effective for smokers in whom these behaviors are particularly strongly conditioned. The inhaler may cause irritation of the throat and mouth and may precipitate bronchospasm in individuals with reactive airways as well as cause the adverse effects associated with the lozenge.

Nicotine nasal spray

The nasal spray delivers nicotine to the nasal mucosal, through which it is absorbed. It has the most rapid pharmacokinetics of the currently available nicotine replacement formulations, but nicotine delivery is still slower than that of a cigarette.[44] Nasal irritation is common, particularly when initiating therapy. Recommended dosing is 1 to 2 sprays per hour, with a maximum of 80 sprays per day for the first 3 months. Because the spray delivers large amounts of nicotine rapidly, it may be particularly useful for heavily addicted smokers. It may also have a greater risk of nicotine overdose and may have a greater potential to sustain a long-term addiction.

Combinations of NRT

The patch-plus regimen,[52,53] which combines a transdermal system with an ad lib NRT, has become common practice, although its use is off-label. This approach provides a baseline of nicotine replacement but also increases nicotine dosing at times of urges. Because combination of a transdermal system with an ad lib modality has been shown to increase quit rates,[4,26,27,47,54] it is recommended by some as initial therapy.[40]

Bupropion

Bupropion is used both as an antidepressant (trade name, Wellbutrin). It is also effective as an aid for smoking cessation (trade name, Zyban).[4,26,27,55] It is thought to act by potentiating dopaminergic and noradrenergic signaling. It is important not to prescribe bupropion under both names to an individual, because overdosage can result.

Bupropion approximately doubles quit rates compared with placebo. In 1 trial, individuals with a history of depression seemed to benefit from bupropion but did not with nicotine replacement, suggesting that bupropion may be a superior initial choice in these individuals.[41] Combination of

nicotine replacement with bupropion seems to be more effective than either agent alone.

Recommended dosing is 150 mg daily for 3 days, followed by 150 mg twice daily. Steady state levels are achieved after 6 to 7 days, and thus, the target quit date should be approximately a week after the start of therapy. The 150-mg once-daily dose was nearly as effective as 150-mg twice daily.[56,57] As a consequence, many practitioners use the lower dose routinely. The appropriate duration of therapy has not been established. A 7-week course was the basis for regulatory approval, although a 12-week course is now commonly recommended. With prolonged therapy, secondary quits increase. Thus, therapy for 1 year results in more quits than therapy for 7 weeks.

The most common adverse effects are dry mouth, insomnia, agitation, and headache. An increase in blood pressure may occur, particularly when used in combination with NRT. Bupropion reduces seizure threshold, and a seizure risk of 0.1% has been reported. Because of its effects on seizure threshold, buproprion is contraindicated among those predisposed to seizures, or with anorexia nervosa or bulimia.

In 2008, concerns were raised for both bupropion and varenicline (see later discussion) with regard to a "possible association [with] suicidal events."[58] Because the benefits of smoking cessation were believed to outweigh any potential risks, the medicines were not withdrawn from the market, but a black box warning related to potential neuropsychiatric effects was added to the label. This warning states that patients and their caregivers should be alerted to the possibility of neuropsychiatric symptoms, and patients should be monitored for changes in behavior, hostility, agitation, depressed mood, suicidal ideation, and suicide attempts. Common practice is reassessing patients 3 to 7 days after the quit day. This strategy allows for both monitoring of adverse effects and the provision of additional support for the quit attempt. In this context, a second visit has been shown to greatly improve success.[4,26,27]

Varenicline

Varenicline is a partial agonist at the $(\alpha 4)(\beta 2)$ nicotinic receptor.[59] As a result, it partially activates the receptor, thereby reducing withdrawal symptoms. It also prevents nicotine from acting, thus reducing the rewarding and reinforcement effects associated with nicotine. This effect may help prevent a lapse from becoming a full relapse. Both reduction in withdrawal symptoms and reduction in the rewarding effects of smoking a cigarette have been reported in clinical trials.[60–63] Varenicline consistently improves success in quitting compared with placebo by an effect of 2-fold to 4-fold.[4,63]

Dosing is started at 0.5 mg orally once daily for 3 days, followed by 0.5 mg twice daily for 4 days and then 1 mg twice daily for 3 months. Treatment of a total of 6 months was associated with reduced relapse. A quit date is usually recommended for 1 week after starting medication. However, using a quitting window from 1 to 5 weeks had success that was comparable with a fixed quit rate.[64,65] The increased flexibility of this regimen may be helpful in exploiting windows of opportunity when patients are seen for another problem, and when motivation to make a quit attempt may be high.

The most common adverse reactions associated with varenicline are nausea, insomnia, visual disturbances, syncope, and skin reactions. The dose titration described earlier reduces nausea.[66] Varenicline has the same boxed warning as bupropion, indicating that patients and their caregivers should be alerted to the possibility of neuropsychiatric symptoms, and patients should be monitored for changes in behavior, hostility, agitation, depressed mood, suicidal ideation, and suicide attempts.[58] Clinical trials have failed to confirm psychiatric adverse effects, although they cannot be fully excluded.[67] One meta-analysis[68] reported a significant increase in cardiovascular events with varenicline. However, this analysis excluded studies with no events, a methodological flaw.[69] A subsequent meta-analysis,[69] which included all available studies, found no difference between varenicline and placebo. Current recommendations are that patients taking varenicline should be alert for development of new or worsening symptoms of cardiovascular disease.[70] Accidental injuries from falls and vehicular accidents have also been associated with varenicline.[71] As a result, the FDA has issued an advisory regarding operating heavy machinery while using varenicline.[72]

Off-label agents

Two off-label medications have documented efficacy for smoking cessation. Nortriptyline is a tricyclic antidepressant. Its efficacy in aiding smoking cessation is supported by both individual studies and meta-analyses.[55,73] The US Department of Health and Human Services (DHHS) guidelines recommend nortriptyline as a possible second-line agent for clinicians familiar with its use.[4,26,27] Major adverse effects of nortriptyline include drowsiness and dry mouth. As with other tricyclics, central nervous system and cardiovascular effects, including arrhythmias, may occur.

Clonidine is an α_2-adrenergic agonist used to treat hypertension. Several clinical trials have shown trends toward efficacy as an aid to smoking cessation, which is supported by a meta-analysis.[74] DHHS guidelines suggest that it can be considered by practitioners familiar with its use.[4,26,27] The most common important adverse effects are drowsiness, fatigue, dry mouth, and postural hypotension.

Smoking cessation has some associated risks. Depression may occur, as was discussed earlier. Exacerbations of ulcerative colitis have been reported to be increased after cessation.[75] Less well established are anecdotal reports that asthma may worsen after cessation, although smoking generally makes asthma worse.[76] Smoking leads to glucocorticoid resistance in asthma, and smoking cessation is generally associated with improvement in asthma.[77] Similarly, some individuals report worse cough and sputum with cessation. However, clinical studies have reported dramatic reductions in cough and sputum after cessation.[78,79]

HARM REDUCTION

Cigarette smoke contains up to 6000 components, which are generated by the complex chemical processes associated with curing and pyrolysis of the tobacco.[80] Nicotine is not among the most important toxic compounds in smoke. This factor has led to the concept that nicotine addiction could be addressed by nicotine replacement using a preparation that does not include the health-compromising toxins. This approach, termed harm reduction, is inherently controversial, because it involves supporting an addiction and, potentially, the use of less toxic tobacco products.[81,82]

As noted earlier, many smokers sustain an addiction to nicotine with NRT, most commonly nicotine polacrilex. Most clinicians view pharmacologic grade nicotine as less hazardous than smoking and, if smoking is the alternative, find this acceptable. The e-cigarette is more controversial. There are many e-cigarettes available. Their nicotine delivery is unregulated. In addition, the various products also contain many flavorants and other additives, the toxicity of which is unknown. Thus, the potential benefits of using e-cigarettes compared with conventional cigarettes is unknown, although it is likely that the e-cigarette delivers considerably less of most toxins. However, e-cigarettes may have other health issues. Because they are seen as a safer alternative to smoking, there are concerns that many smokers who would have quit opt to use e-cigarettes. Worse, some individuals may start using e-cigarettes because of their perceived lack of harm. After becoming addicted, these individuals may be at an increased risk for smoking conventional cigarettes.

Harm reduction with tobacco products is even more controversial. Several cigarette-like tobacco products that do not burn or burn very little tobacco have been developed. The personal and public health effects of these products are unknown. Snus is an unfermented tobacco product that is used orally and is not burned. It is widely used in Scandinavia, where it has been associated with dramatic reductions in risk of many cigarette-associated diseases.[83–86]

Because snus is a tobacco product produced and marketed as a consumer product, there is no experience with its use in a treatment setting.

SUMMARY

Cigarette smoking should be regarded as a chronic relapsing disease. However, it is a disease that can be effectively treated in many cases. Optimal treatment requires a long-term approach combining pharmacologic and nonpharmacologic interventions and close interactions between patient and clinician.

REFERENCES

1. King James I of England. A counterblaste to tobacco. 1604. Available at: http://www.laits.utexas.edu/poltheory/james/blaste/. Accessed September 2013.
2. US Department of Health, Education, and Welfare. Smoking and health. Report of the Advisory Committee to the Surgeon General of the Public Health Service. 1964.
3. US Department of Health and Human Services. The health benefits of smoking cessation. A report of the Surgeon General. Washington, DC: Department of Health and Human Services (US); 1990. p. 90–8416 Publication No. (CDC).
4. Fiore MC, Jaén CR, Baker TB, et al. Treating tobacco use and dependence: 2008 update. Clinical practice guideline. US Department of Health and Human Services, Public Health Service; 2008.
5. Escobedo LG, Anda RF, Smith PF, et al. Sociodemographic characteristics of cigarette smoking initiation in the United States. JAMA 1990;264: 1550–5.
6. Pierce JP, White VM, Emery SL. What public health strategies are needed to reduce smoking initiation? Tob Control 2012;21:258–64.
7. Headen SW, Bauman KE, Deane GD, et al. Are the correlates of cigarette smoking initiation different for black and white adolescents? Am J Public Health 1991;81:854–8.
8. In: Preventing tobacco use among youth and young adults: a report of the Surgeon General. Atlanta (GA): 2012.
9. Johnston LD, O'Malley PM, Bachman JG, et al. Monitoring the future national survey results on drug use, 1975–2012. Ann Arbor: University of Michigan; 2013.
10. Gotti C, Clementi F. Neuronal nicotinic receptors: from structure to pathology. Prog Neurobiol 2004; 74:363–96.
11. Drenan RM, Lester HA. Insights into the neurobiology of the nicotinic cholinergic system and nicotine addiction from mice expressing nicotinic receptors harboring gain-of-function mutations. Pharmacol Rev 2012;64:869–79.
12. Gotti C, Clementi F, Fornari A, et al. Structural and functional diversity of native brain neuronal nicotinic receptors. Biochem Pharmacol 2009;78: 703–11.
13. Changeux JP. Nicotine addiction and nicotinic receptors: lessons from genetically modified mice. Nat Rev Neurosci 2010;11:389–401.
14. Leslie FM, Mojica CY, Reynaga DD. Nicotinic receptors in addiction pathways. Mol pharmacol 2013;83:753–8.
15. Slotkin TA, Ryde IT, Seidler FJ. Additive and synergistic effects of fetal nicotine and dexamethasone exposure on cholinergic synaptic function in adolescence and adulthood: implications for the adverse consequences of maternal smoking and pharmacotherapy of preterm delivery. Brain Res Bull 2010;81:552–60.
16. Goriounova NA, Mansvelder HD. Short- and long-term consequences of nicotine exposure during adolescence for prefrontal cortex neuronal network function. Cold Spring Harb Perspect Med 2012;2: a012120.
17. Shiffman S. Tobacco "chippers"–individual differences in tobacco dependence. Psychopharmacology 1989;97:539–47.
18. Shiffman S, Paty JA, Gnys M, et al. Nicotine withdrawal in chippers and regular smokers: subjective and cognitive effects. Health Psychol 1995;14:301–9.
19. Benowitz NL, Jacob P. Intravenous nicotine replacement suppresses nicotine intake from cigarette smoking. J Pharmacol Exp Ther 1990;254: 1000–5.
20. Benowitz NL, Jacob P 3rd, Kozlowski LT, et al. Influence of smoking fewer cigarettes on exposure to tar, nicotine, and carbon monoxide. N Engl J Med 1986;315:1310–3.
21. Olausson P, Jentsch JD, Taylor JR. Repeated nicotine exposure enhances reward-related learning in the rat. Neuropsychopharmacology 2003;28: 1264–71.
22. Henningfield JE, London ED, Benowitz NL. Arterial-venous differences in plasma concentrations of

nicotine after cigarette smoking. JAMA 1990;263: 2049–50.

23. Hukkanen J, Jacob P 3rd, Benowitz NL. Metabolism and disposition kinetics of nicotine. Pharmacol Rev 2005;57:79–115.

24. Heatherton TF, Kozlowski LT, Frecker RC, et al. The Fagerstrom Test for nicotine dependence: a revision of the Fagerstrom Tolerance Questionnaire. Br J Addict 1991;86:1119–27.

25. Centers for Disease Control and Prevention (CDC). Cigarette smoking among adults and trends in smoking cessation–United States, 2008. MMWR Morb Mortal Wkly Rep 2009;58:1227–32.

26. Fiore MC, Bailey WC, Cohen SJ. Smoking cessation. Guideline technical report no. 18. Rockville (MD): US Department of Health and Human Services, Public Health Service, Agency for Health Care Policy and Research; 1997. Publication no. AHCPR 97-Noo4.

27. Fiore M, Bailey W, Cohen S, et al. Treating tobacco use and dependence. Rockville (MD): US Department Of Health and Human Services; 2000.

28. Daughton DM, Susman J, Sitorius M, et al. Transdermal nicotine therapy and primary care: importance of counseling, demographic and patient selection factors on one-year quit rates. Arch Fam Med 1998;7:425–30.

29. Gwaltney CJ, Metrik J, Kahler CW, et al. Self-efficacy and smoking cessation: a meta-analysis. Psychol Addict Behav 2009;23:56–66.

30. Gulliver SB, Hughes JR, Solomon LJ, et al. An investigation of self-efficacy, partner support and daily stresses as predictors of relapse to smoking in self-quitters. Addiction 1995;90:767–72.

31. Cromwell J, Bartosch WJ, Fiore MC, et al. Cost-effectiveness of the clinical practice recommendations in the AHCPR guideline for smoking cessation. JAMA 1997;278(21):1759–66.

32. Cinciripini PM, Wetter DW, McClure JB. Scheduled reduced smoking: effects on smoking abstinence and potential mechanisms of action. Addict Behav 1997;22:759–67.

33. Hughes JR, Solomon LJ, Livingston AE, et al. A randomized, controlled trial of NRT-aided gradual vs. abrupt cessation in smokers actively trying to quit. Drug Alcohol Depend 2010;111:105–13.

34. Lindson-Hawley N, Aveyard P, Hughes JR. Reduction versus abrupt cessation in smokers who want to quit. Cochrane Database Syst Rev 2012;(11):CD008033.

35. Anthonisen NR, Connett JE, Kiley JP, et al. Effects of smoking intervention and the use of an inhaled anticholinergic bronchodilator on the rate of decline of FEV1. JAMA 1994;272:1497–505.

36. Tashkin D, Kanner R, Bailey W, et al. Smoking cessation in patients with chronic obstructive pulmonary disease: a double-blind, placebo-controlled, randomised trial. Lancet 2001;357:1571–5.

37. Tashkin DP, Rennard S, Hays JT, et al. Effects of varenicline on smoking cessation in patients with mild to moderate COPD: a randomized controlled trial. Chest 2011;139:591–9.

38. Rigotti NA, Clair C, Munafo MR, et al. Interventions for smoking cessation in hospitalised patients. Cochrane Database Syst Rev 2012;(5):CD001837.

39. Stead LF, Perera R, Lancaster T. A systematic review of interventions for smokers who contact quitlines. Tob Control 2007;16(Suppl 1):i3–8.

40. Rennard SI, Rigotti NA, Daughton DM. Pharmacotherapy for smoking cessation in adults. In: UpToDate. 2013.

41. Jorenby DE, Leischow SJ, Nides MA, et al. A controlled trial of sustained-release bupropion, a nicotine patch, or both for smoking cessation. N Engl J Med 1999;340:685–91.

42. Allen SS, Hatsukami DK, Christianson D. Nicotine withdrawal and depressive symptomatology during short-term smoking abstinence: a comparison of postmenopausal women using and not using hormone replacement therapy. Nicotine Tob Res 2003;5:49–59.

43. Hajek P, West R, Foulds J, et al. Randomized comparative trial of nicotine polacrilex, a transdermal patch, nasal spray, and an inhaler. Arch Intern Med 1999;159:2033–8.

44. Rigotti NA. Clinical practice. Treatment of tobacco use and dependence. N Engl J Med 2002;346: 506–12.

45. Killen JD, Fortmann SP, Newman B, et al. Evaluation of a treatment approach combining nicotine gum with self-guided behavioral treatments for smoking relapse prevention. J Consult Clin Psychol 1990;58:85–92.

46. Dautzenberg B, Nides M, Kienzler JL, et al. Pharmacokinetics, safety and efficacy from randomized controlled trials of 1 and 2 mg nicotine bitartrate lozenges (Nicotinell). BMC Clin Pharmacol 2007; 7:11.

47. Smith SS, McCarthy DE, Japuntich SJ, et al. Comparative effectiveness of 5 smoking cessation pharmacotherapies in primary care clinics. Arch Intern Med 2009;169:2148–55.

48. Pickworth WB, Bunker EB, Henningfield JE. Transfermal nicotine: reduction of smoking with minimal abuse liability. Psychopharmacology (Berl) 1994; 115:9–14.

49. Nicotine replacement therapy for patients with coronary artery disease. Working Group for the Study of Transdermal Nicotine in Patients with Coronary artery disease. Arch Intern Med 1994; 154:989–95.

50. Mahmarian JJ, Moye LA, Nasser GA. Nicotine patch therapy in smoking cessation reduces the extent of exercise-induced myocardial ischemia. J Am Coll Cardiol 1997;30:125–30.

51. Joseph AM, Norma SM, Ferry LH. The safety of transdermal nicotine as an aid to smoking cessation in patients with cardiac disease. N Engl J Med 1996;335:1792–8.

52. Bohadana A, Nilsson F, Rasmussen T, et al. Nicotine inhaler and nicotine patch as a combination therapy for smoking cessation: a randomized, double-blind, placebo-controlled trial. Arch Intern Med 2000;160:3128–34.

53. Schneider NG, Cortner C, Gould JL, et al. Comparison of craving and withdrawal among four combination nicotine treatments. Hum Psychopharmacol 2008;23:513–7.

54. Piper ME, Smith SS, Schlam TR, et al. A randomized placebo-controlled clinical trial of 5 smoking cessation pharmacotherapies. Arch Gen Psychiatry 2009;66:1253–62.

55. Hughes JR, Stead LF, Lancaster T. Antidepressants for smoking cessation. Cochrane Database Syst Rev 2007;(1):CD000031.

56. Hurt RD, Sachs DP, Glover ED, et al. A comparison of sustained-release bupropion and placebo for smoking cessation. N Engl J Med 1997;337:1195–202.

57. Swan GE, McAfee T, Curry SJ, et al. Effectiveness of bupropion sustained release for smoking cessation in a health care setting: a randomized trial. Arch Intern Med 2003;163:2337–44.

58. The smoking cessation aids varenicline (marketed as Chantix) and bupropion (marketed as Zyban and generics): suicidal ideation and behavior. FDA Drug Safety Newsletter; 2009.

59. Coe JW, Brooks PR, Vetelino MG, et al. Varenicline: an alpha4beta2 nicotinic receptor partial agonist for smoking cessation. J Med Chem 2005;48:3474–7.

60. Gonzales D, Rennard SI, Nides M, et al. Varenicline, an alpha4beta2 nicotinic acetylcholine receptor partial agonist, vs sustained-release bupropion and placebo for smoking cessation: a randomized controlled trial. JAMA 2006;296:47–55.

61. Jorenby DE, Hays JT, Rigotti NA, et al. Efficacy of varenicline, an alpha4beta2 nicotinic acetylcholine receptor partial agonist, vs placebo or sustained-release bupropion for smoking cessation: a randomized controlled trial. JAMA 2006;296:56–63.

62. Tonstad S, Tonnesen P, Hajek P, et al. Effect of maintenance therapy with varenicline on smoking cessation: a randomized controlled trial. JAMA 2006;296:64–71.

63. Cahill K, Stead LF, Lancaster T. Nicotine receptor partial agonists for smoking cessation. Cochrane Database Syst Rev 2012;(4):CD006103.

64. Hughes JR, Russ CI, Arteaga CE, et al. Efficacy of a flexible quit date versus an a priori quit date approach to smoking cessation: a cross-study analysis. Addict Behav 2011;36:1288–91.

65. Rennard S, Hughes J, Cinciripini PM, et al. A randomized placebo-controlled trial of varenicline for smoking cessation allowing flexible quit dates. Nicotine Tob Res 2012;14:343–50.

66. Oncken C, Gonzales D, Nides M, et al. Efficacy and safety of the novel selective nicotinic acetylcholine receptor partial agonist, varenicline, for smoking cessation. Arch Intern Med 2006;166:1571–7.

67. Gunnell D, Irvine D, Wise L, et al. Varenicline and suicidal behaviour: a cohort study based on data from the General Practice Research Database. BMJ 2009;339:b3805.

68. Singh S, Loke YK, Spangler JG, et al. Risk of serious adverse cardiovascular events associated with varenicline: a systematic review and meta-analysis. CMAJ 2011;183:1359–66.

69. Prochaska JJ, Hilton JF. Risk of cardiovascular serious adverse events associated with varenicline use for tobacco cessation: systematic review and meta-analysis. BMJ 2012;344:e2856.

70. FDA. FDA Drug Safety Communication: Safety review update of Chantix (varenicline) and risk of cardiovascular adverse events. http://www.fda.gov/drugs/drugsafety/ucm330367.htm. Accessed April 1, 2013.

71. Moore TJ, Cohen MR, Furberg CD. Strong safety signal seen for new varenicline risks In: Institute for Safe Medicine Practices; 2008. www.ismp.org/docs/vareniclinestudy.asp. Accessed April 1, 2013.

72. FDA. Available at: http://www.fda.gov/Drugs/DrugSafety/DrugSafetyPodcasts/ccm077547.htm. 2008. Accessed April 1, 2013.

73. Stead LF, Lancaster T. Combined pharmacotherapy and behavioural interventions for smoking cessation. Cochrane Database Syst Rev 2012;(10):CD008286.

74. Gourlay SG, Stead LF, Benowitz NL. Clonidine for smoking cessation. Cochrane Database Syst Rev 2004;(3):CD000058.

75. Higuchi LM, Khalili H, Chan AT, et al. A prospective study of cigarette smoking and the risk of inflammatory bowel disease in women. Am J Gastroenterol 2012;107:1399–406.

76. Broekema M, ten Hacken NH, Volbeda F, et al. Airway epithelial changes in smokers but not in ex-smokers with asthma. Am J Respir Crit Care Med 2009;180:1170–8.

77. Polosa R, Thomson NC. Smoking and asthma: dangerous liaisons. Eur Respir J 2013;41:716–26.

78. Buist AS, Sexton GJ, Nagy JM, et al. The effect of smoking cessation and modification on lung function. Am Rev Respir Dis 1976;114:115–22.

79. Swan GE, Hodgkin JE, Roby T, et al. Reversibility of airways injury over a 12-month period following smoking cessation. Chest 1992;101:607–12.

80. Borgerding M, Klus H. Analysis of complex mixtures–cigarette smoke. Exp Toxicol Pathol 2005;57(Suppl 1):43–73.

81. Stratton K, Shetty P, Wallace R, et al. Clearing. Clearing the smoke: assessing the science base for tobacco harm reduction. Washington, DC: National Academy Press; 2001.

82. Rodu B. The scientific foundation for tobacco harm reduction, 2006–2011. Harm Reduct J 2011;8:19.

83. Hansson J, Galanti MR, Hergens MP, et al. Use of snus and acute myocardial infarction: pooled analysis of eight prospective observational studies. Eur J Epidemiol 2012;27:771–9.

84. Nordenvall C, Nilsson PJ, Ye W, et al. Tobacco use and cancer survival: a cohort study of 40,230 Swedish male construction workers with incident cancer. Int J Cancer 2013;132:155–61.

85. Arefalk G, Hergens MP, Ingelsson E, et al. Smokeless tobacco (snus) and risk of heart failure: results from two Swedish cohorts. Eur J Prev Cardiol 2012; 19:1120–7.

86. Lee PN. Summary of the epidemiological evidence relating snus to health. Regul Toxicol Pharmacol 2011;59:197–214.

Current Drug Treatment, Chronic and Acute

Peter Calverley, DSc, FMedSc

KEYWORDS

- Bronchodilators • Inhaled corticosteroids • COPD and exacerbations

KEY POINTS

- Increasing the dose or number of bronchodilators together with a short course of oral corticosteroids reduces the severity of chronic obstructive pulmonary disease (COPD) exacerbation.
- Supplementary methylxanthine treatment adds nothing to exacerbation management except risk for patients.
- Long-acting antimuscarinics should be given once daily as a first-line treatment of COPD, although new once daily long-acting beta-agonists may prove equally effective.
- Adding inhaled corticosteroids to a long-acting beta-agonist prevents exacerbations in severe disease and seems to be effective in some once daily combination treatments.
- Pneumonia is seen with all treatments containing fluticasone-related drugs, but appears to be less evident with budesonide. Once-daily tiotropium seems safe when given as a dry power, but there are concerns about its use when inhaled from a soft mist system.

INTRODUCTION

The appropriate management of chronic obstructive pulmonary disease (COPD) involves more than taking prescription medicines. The key components have been set out in detail in many treatment guidelines, both national and international.[1–3] They include the avoidance of identified risk factors, especially tobacco smoking, and the optimization of daily physical activity, topics covered elsewhere in this volume.

For a few patients with severe disease, noninvasive ventilation can be a lifesaving treatment in the acute episode,[4] although not all patients benefit.[5] There is a role for long-term domiciliary oxygen treatment, which is widely used in the United States and can reduce mortality and even improve exercise performance.[6,7] However, the effectiveness of ambulatory oxygen has been challenged[8]; the use of oxygen to relieve breathlessness after exercise having been shown to be ineffective when compared with room air.[9] These considerations do not seem to have dented the popularity of this treatment, with patients and their physicians indicating the limits of evidence-based clinical practice. However for many patients with COPD, a key part of their care remains the drugs their doctors prescribe and in recent years both the choice of treatment and the evidence for its effectiveness has improved.

This article reviews the key components of the pharmacologic treatment of COPD, both acute and chronic, with an emphasis on those recent studies, which are likely to change practice in the next few years.

DRUG TREATMENT IN ACUTE EXACERBATIONS

Acute exacerbations of COPD drive the morbidity and cost associated with this disease and the markers of an increased risk of dying, especially after the patients have been hospitalized.[10] In patients with more severe COPD and those attending

Respiratory Research, Clinical Sciences Department, Institute of Ageing & Chronic Diseases, University Hospital Aintree, Lower Lane, Liverpool L9 7AL, UK
E-mail address: pmacal@liverpool.ac.uk

Clin Chest Med 35 (2014) 177–189
http://dx.doi.org/10.1016/j.ccm.2013.09.009

the emergency department, breathlessness is the dominant symptom; there are good data showing that this results from a mixture of static and dynamic hyperinflation and consequent restriction on tidal volume.[11,12] Worsening lung mechanics leads to the deterioration in ventilation-perfusion matching and an increase in dead space, producing hypoxemia with or without hyperpnoea. Hence, the management of the acute episode focuses on reversing or limiting these physiologic abnormalities. The distress and ill health of the hospitalized patient makes the conduct of randomized control trials difficult or risky and so we have almost no clinical trial data to support the use of oxygen to either reduce breathlessness or improve outcomes in COPD. We do know that oxygen-induced hypercapnia can be dangerous,[13] but for physicians to take the opposite view and not prescribe oxygen to critically ill patients would seem to be perverse.

Similar considerations apply to drug treatment, but here there is at least some direct physiologic evidence of benefit resulting from studies conducted over the last decade.

Inhaled bronchodilators are the key components of management. For good practical reasons related to the speed of onset of action and the risk of adverse effects, the inhaled route is preferred for both acute and chronic treatment, and the main drug classes are beta-agonists (BA) and antimuscarinic (MA), which are also known as anticholinergic drugs.

There is little evidence for a dose-response effect with either BA or MA in COPD, although some data for unstable disease suggest a potential benefit of high doses of ipratropium.[14] However, many physicians prescribe nebulized BA, usually salbutamol in doses of 2.5 to 5.0 mg or MA such as ipratropium 250 to 500 mcg alone, or in combination with each other, to reduce symptoms in hospitalized patients with exacerbations. Adding ipratropium to salbutamol did not change the rate of recovery of forced expiratory volume in the first second of expiration (FEV_1) in one small UK study,[15] which did not examine other markers of lung mechanics or symptoms. However, there is evidence that even at high doses of BA, adding another drug of a different class can produce physiologically important reductions in end expiratory lung volumes,[16] changes similar to those observed after combination bronchodilators in acutely ill patients with COPD.[12]

There are no good studies to indicate when this high-dose treatment should be discontinued; this decision is usually an empiric one, made by the attending physician. Patients often think high-dose nebulized drugs during an exacerbation should be continued during their chronic care; but the evidence for this is lacking and is confused by the facial cooling effects of the nebulized mist, which can decrease acute breathlessness.[17] Other considerations related to the reimbursement of nebulized drugs may also be potent reasons why these agents are considered. The most common adverse events are tachycardia and palpitations with high doses of BA while hypokalemia is not a problem in normal clinical practice. MA drugs are well tolerated, although there is a risk of inducing glaucoma if mist from a facial mask enters the eyes of susceptible patients.

Intravenous aminophylline was used as the primary treatment of hospitalized acute COPD exacerbations long before safer inhaled bronchodilators were available, and it is still often added to the treatment of patients with severe breathlessness caused by acute COPD. However, xanthenes are weak bronchodilators and only effective at near-toxic doses.[18] Data from Rice and colleagues[19] suggested that it was ineffective when used acutely. This finding was confirmed in a large randomized controlled trial that showed that aminophylline reduced arterial carbon dioxide slightly but made no difference to the rate of recover, symptoms, lung function, or to the time spent in hospital.[20] Given the toxicity of this therapy, it should not be used in hospitalized patients with COPD. A trial of the acute effects of the phosphodiesterase IV inhibitor roflumilast in acute exacerbations of COPD is currently being conducted; but until these data are available, this drug is not recommended for acute use.

Acute exacerbations are characterized by an increase in inflammation,[21] triggered by infections and/or environmental insults, which produce the acute deterioration in lung mechanics noted earlier. Two therapies have been applied to reduce inflammation and shorten the acute episode.

High-dose enteral or parenteral corticosteroids have been tested in a limited number of studies. With one exception, patients were recruited from the emergency department (ED) or had been hospitalized; in these settings, corticosteroid treatment delayed the time to relapse (including relapses occurring within 30 days of an ED visit), reduced the number of treatment failures related to the primary event, and accelerated the rate at which lung function improved (**Fig. 1**), thereby reducing the hospital stay.[22–24] Lower doses of oral prednisolone (approximately 30 mg/d) were as effective as large doses of methylprednisolone. Although the large trials gave treatment for 10 to 14 days, most of the benefit accrues in the first week; one small study has shown that 10 days of treatment is better than 3 days.[25]

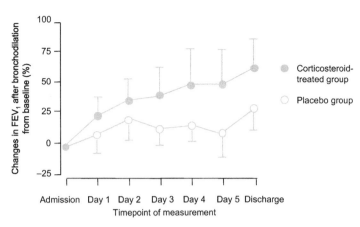

Fig. 1. Rate of recovery of FEV_1 in hospitalized patients with COPD treated with oral corticosteroids (*closed circles*) or placebo (*open circles*). (*Adapted from* Davies L, Angus RM, Calverley PM. Oral corticosteroids in patients admitted to hospital with exacerbations of chronic obstructive pulmonary disease: a prospective randomised controlled trial. Lancet 1999;354(9177):456–60; with permission.)

Data on ambulatory output patient events are very limited, but arterial oxygen tension improved more rapidly in those patients given prednisolone.[26] This treatment is widely prescribed for exacerbations of COPD in the community, particularly in Western Europe. Hyperglycemia is somewhat more common in corticosteroid-treated COPD exacerbations, but the degree is as likely to be a marker of the severity of the insult as the use of short courses of corticosteroids per see. The major risk of oral corticosteroid treatment is that it is sustained and converted into chronic oral therapy, which is hazardous to patients, producing a host of undesirable complications, including marked muscle weakness and immobility.[27]

The alternative and potentially complementary method of modifying exacerbation-related inflammation is the prescription of antibiotics with courses normally lasting 5 to 7 days. The choice of treatment is best determined by local sensitivity patterns to *Haemophilus influenzae* and *Streptococcus pneumoniae*, the dominant causes of these episodes.[28] In practice, coverage of other pathogens likely to cause pneumonia is also sensible, given the difficulties of distinguishing pneumonias from COPD exacerbations.[29] Only a few studies have compared antibiotics with placebo in COPD exacerbations, most trials having been comparator studies of microbiological cure rates. However, one community-based randomized controlled trial in Dutch patients all treated with oral prednisolone is instructive. This study showed that patients who had a history of cough, sputum production, and breathlessness recovered more rapidly when randomized to antibiotic treatment than with placebo,[30] a finding that confirmed the observations by Anthonisen and colleagues[31] some 25 years earlier.[32] There is database evidence that patients in intensive care unit (ICU) with COPD exacerbations who receive antibiotics have better outcomes,[32] and so the threshold for prescription in hospitalized patients should probably be lower than in the community at large.

Table 1 summarizes the current approaches to drug treatment and the management of acute exacerbations of COPD.

DRUG TREATMENT IN CHRONIC MANAGEMENT

Management approaches to stable COPD still rely heavily on drug treatment, but the way in which patients are evaluated and in which treatments are used have recently changed. **Box 1** summarizes the principal goals of medical treatment, whereas **Figs. 2** and **3** illustrate the preferred management approaches advocated by the Global Initiative in Obstructive Lung Disease (GOLD) and by the evidence-based UK National Institute of Health and Clinical Excellence's (NICE) guidelines.[33,34] Drug therapy is based on the use of long-acting inhaled bronchodilators, whereas shorter-acting inhaled treatments for rapid onset, usually salbutamol, are reserved for rescue treatment, when symptoms increase unexpectedly (eg, after exercise or during exacerbations). The efficacy of short-acting beta-agonists (SABA) treatment in reducing symptoms like this is not well established. Bronchodilators and phosphodiesterase 4 (PDE4) antagonists are considered in detail elsewhere; but before examining how these treatments are deployed, it is worth considering the current evidence for the use of inhaled corticosteroids (ICS) alone or in combination with other drugs.

ICS AND COPD

ICS have revolutionized the management of bronchial asthma for the first-line treatment of patients with persistent symptoms.[35] They decrease eosinophilic inflammation dramatically but have little, if

Table 1
Pharmacologic management of COPD exacerbations

Drug	Setting	Route	Dose	Comment
Bronchodilator (SABA/SAMA)	OP	Inhaled	2 puffs 3–4/h	Frequency of use should decrease over 48 h or seek help
	IP	Inhaled	Salbutamol 2.5 or 5 mg and Ipratropium 500 mcg 6/h	Nebulized till symptoms resolve
Corticosteroids	OP and IP	Oral	Prednisolone 30 mg	Give for 7–10 d and stop
Antibiotics	OP	Oral	Drug with appropriate sensitivity	Give for 5–7 d in patients with worse cough and sputum and dyspnea
	IP	Oral	Drug with appropriate sensitivity	Give for 5–7 d if one or more of the aforementioned; parenteral route seldom needed

To be used with appropriate supportive care and subsequent preventive management.
Abbreviations: IP, hospitalized in-patient or ED attendee; OP, outpatient; SABA, short-acting beta-agonist; SAMA, short-acting anti-muscarinic agents.

any, effect on inflammation and COPD, at least over 6 weeks to 3 months of treatment,[36,37] although some effects, in some patients, have been reported over longer periods.[38] Given the observed benefits of high-dose corticosteroids during exacerbations, it was reasonable to assess whether ICS had any effects in stable patients with COPD.

After 10 years, the general consensus can be summarized as follows:

- ICS have no effect on the rate of decline of lung function in lung disease in patients with GOLD grade 1 and 2 disease who smoke and in patients with severe COPD.[39–42] The different views derived from post hoc meta-analysis[43] and patient level meta-analysis[44] about whether these conclusions are correct, are likely to say more about the methodology than the effect of ICS.
- Small but consistent increases in FEV_1 are observed, the degree differing with the initial severity of airflow obstruction. This finding likely reflects the patients studied because improvement with short-acting bronchodilators is greater in patients with moderate severity disease than those with severe problems.[45] At any given GOLD grade, the change in postbronchodilator lung function with ICS is similar to that seen with roflumilast.[46,47]
- There is a reduction in the number of exacerbations defined by the need for medical treatment in patients treated with ICS.[42,48] This reduction seems to be especially true for episodes treated with oral corticosteroids, even though the doctor is blind to the background preventative medication.[49]
- ICS is not associated with any change in mortality as compared with placebo, but neither is mortality likely to be reduced.[50] This finding is contrary to the initial impression based on the result of the database analysis whereby confounding by disease severity may have played a role.[51] By contrast, combining a long-acting beta-agonist (LABA) with an ICS produced a trend to improvement mortality relative to placebo and a significantly better mortality than what was seen with ICS alone in the TORCH (TOwards a Revolution in COPD Health) trial.[50]
- ICS have not been conclusively shown to increase the risk of osteoporosis or cataracts, at least over a 3-year study in a randomized controlled trial. The background frequency with which these occur in patients with COPD makes it difficult to detect a small effect.[52] However, pneumonia, reported by physicians and subsequently confirmed radiologically, is more common in ICS-treated patients with COPD.[53] This effect is shown most clearly for fluticasone[49] and more

Box 1
Goals of COPD Management

- Improve lung function
- Prevent disease progression
- Relieve symptoms
- Improve exercise tolerance
- Improve health status
- Prevent and treat exacerbations
- Prevent and treat complications
- Reduce mortality
- Minimize side effects from treatment

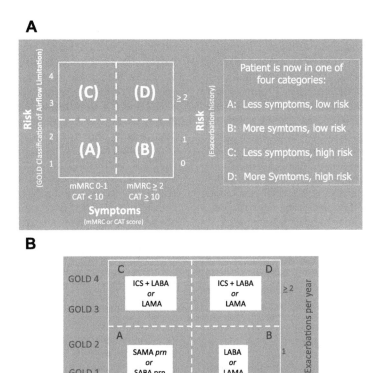

Fig. 2. Assessment by symptom severity and future risk as proposed by Vestbo and colleagues.[33] (*A*) Indicates groups in nonproportional quadrants, and (*B*) indicates the suggested initial treatment of patients in each quadrant. CAT, COPD Assessment Test; ICS, inhaled corticosteroids; LABA, long-acting beta-agonist; LAMA, long-acting anti-muscarinic agents; mMRC, modified Medical Research council breathlessness scale; prn, as needed; SABA, short-acting beta-agonist; SAMA, short-acting anti-muscarinic agents.

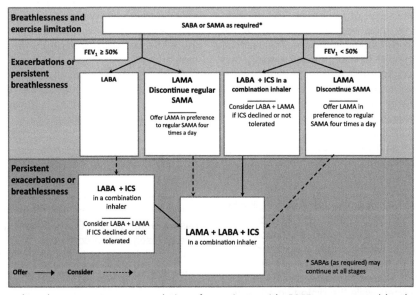

Fig. 3. Evidence-based treatment recommendations for patients with COPD as suggested by the UK National Institute for Clinical Excellence. ICS, inhaled corticosteroids; LABA, long-acting beta-agonist; LAMA, long-acting anti-muscarinic agents; SABA, short-acting beta-agonist; SAMA, short-acting anti-muscarinic agents. (*Adapted from* O'Reilly J, Jones MM, Parnham J, et al. Management of stable chronic obstructive pulmonary disease in primary and secondary care: summary of updated NICE guidance. BMJ 2010;340:c3134; with permission.)

recently for fluticasone furoate[54]; the signal with budesonide was smaller and did not reach statistical significance.[55] In the Investigating New Standards for Prophylaxis in Reduction of Exacerbations (INSPIRE) study, the excess of pneumonia events in patients treated with an ICS/LABA combination treatment was mainly caused by exacerbations that failed to resolve.[29] Patients treated with ICS have a higher airway bacterial load,[56] although whether this is a causal association and relates to the greater number of pneumonia events remains to be determined.

Based on these findings, there is consensus that ICS should not be used as the only regular treatment of COPD or combined with regular short-acting bronchodilators. Their role together with LABA is considered further later.

EVIDENCE-BASED THERAPY

The movement toward evidence-based therapy is both logical and desirable. Identifying areas where there is good evidence from randomized controlled trials (RCT) and other areas where practice is supported mainly by professional consensus is clinically helpful. However, some unintended consequences have arisen and effect the guidance in COPD care. Careful analysis of data, according to prespecified questions, with either systematic review or formal data pooling in a meta-analysis has become the preeminent way of determining the value of treatment. This method has reached its most sophisticated form in the GRADE (Grading Recommendations Assessment, Development and Evaluation) guideline methodology, which weighs data by the strength of the studies assessed on technical grounds and offers nuanced terms in support of an eventual recommendation for treatment.

There are limitations to this approach. Pooling underpowered studies to produce a conclusion can produce the disconcerting effect of a firm recommendation being overturned with a better-powered RCT report. Subtle differences in the a priori event rate of discontinuous variables, like exacerbations, can modify the conclusions drawn or at least the strength of the recommendations supporting them. Differential drop out in patients randomized to placebo treatment, a recurrent feature in recent COPD studies,[57,58] means that the study quality is penalized while the distorting effect and the loss of the sicker patients who drop out while using placebo decreases the chance of a positive outcome.[59] Most importantly, the questions answered by the guidelines are shrunk to ones for which sufficient RCT data are available; this often means that they focus on drug treatment and its use rather than considering the wider aspects relevant to the care of patients with COPD.

Two recent contrasting approaches illustrate these issues. The GOLD guidelines have, for the past decade, drawn on an expert panel of changing composition to review new data about COPD management, expanding the recommendations in its original report, by applying a standard methodology to consider important new data.[2] The 2011 version of the GOLD document changed its focus because the task of analyzing all of the recommendations using a grade approach has become prohibitively expensive.[33] Similar concerns have inhibited a full review of the previous American Thoracic Society/European Respiratory Society's (ATS/ERS) COPD guidelines. Instead, the new version of GOLD offers a management strategy with some preferred options for treatment. This version allows it to escape criticism as a guideline but means that its recommendations are less clearly evidenced based than in the past.

By contrast, the greater resources available to the American College of Physicians (ACP) (working jointly with the ERS and ATS) and to the UK government have allowed them to ask specific grade-based questions, producing focused recommendations.[34,60] The UK NICE updated a previous expert group approach and discovered a wider range of questions than did the ACP. Even so, many specific issues remain unanswered, particularly relating how long to continue with the specific treatment before it is changed, how best to assess the success of therapy, and how strong the evidence is in favor of one treatment rather than another.

As examples of these different approaches, the remainder of this review focuses on the similarities and differences brought up by these well-written, authoritative documents.

EVALUATING PATIENTS

For the last decade, there has been a strong emphasis on the need to monitor spirometry, preferably after a bronchodilator, to determine the disease severity in COPD. Treatment guidance has been closely anchored to this, by both the ATS/ERS' guidelines and in the NICE COPD revision. The current spirometric severity grades advocated by GOLD are as follows:

1. FEV_1 greater than 80% predicted: mild
2. FEV_1 79% to 50% predicted: moderate
3. FEV_1 49% to 30% predicted: severe
4. FEV_1 less than 30% predicted: very severe

Clinical trials have been aligned with these criteria and, hence, data on new drugs can be evaluated relative to their predecessors. However, patient well-being, expressed as either symptoms or health status, is only poorly related to FEV_1[61] and is significantly influenced by the number of COPD exacerbations.[62] To capture this component and make patient evaluation more clinically relevant, the 2011 GOLD revision separated patients into those with mild/moderate disease (GOLD grades 1 and 2) and severe/very severe disease (GOLD grades 3 and 4). In addition, the presence of symptoms evaluated by either an Medical Research Council (MRC) breathlessness score of 2 or greater or a COPD assessment test score of 10 or more was used to further subdivide patient groups.[63,64] FEV_1 was considered a marker of future risk, as was the number of exacerbations, with patients with a history of frequent exacerbations with 2 or more exacerbations forming a distinct phenotype[65] that predicted more future problems. The resulting matrix displayed in **Fig. 2** gives rise to 4 possible groups, A to D, each with a potentially different treatment approach.

The NICE approach also stratified patients with a cutoff point of an FEV_1 of 50% predicted and based initial treatment recommendations on the responses of patient groups defined spirometrically. However, they did consider the possibility that symptoms might be persistent or associated with recurrent exacerbations, despite treatment; therefore, they offered a follow-up treatment option for patients who had already received the first-line therapy but continued to have problems. This approach is somewhat closer to the one that operates in outpatient clinics and is helpful when spirometry is readily available. For many clinicians, the GOLD approach is attractive because it stresses not only spirometry but also the importance of symptoms and exacerbations.

The exact size of the patient population contained within each of the GOLD quadrants is open to debate and seems to depend on whether hospital-based or population-based cohorts are studied.[66] Impaired spirometry rather than simply high numbers of exacerbation seemed to determine the patients in groups C and D. There is some uncertainty about the equivalence of the MRC and the COPD Assessment Test (CAT) cut points, and it is hoped that this will be resolved.[67]

Ultimately, the GOLD proposal needs to be tested prospectively, both for its robustness and its clinical utility. Nonetheless, this new classification represents an important step forward in the way that patients with COPD are managed and treatment choices are evaluated.

INITIAL DRUG THERAPY

The preferred initial choices of drug treatment are shown in **Figs. 2**B and **3** and are remarkably similar in both the GOLD and NICE approaches. Patients with well-preserved lung function and relatively few symptoms, which would equate to a CAT score of less than 10, can be tried on short-acting bronchodilators, with no clear preference between SABA or short-acting anti-muscarinic agents (SAMA). How effective such an approach might be has never been studied, and this recommendation remains largely consensus based.

If patients have an FEV_1 of more than 50% predicted, are more symptomatic, but have no exacerbation history, then either a long-acting anti-muscarinic agents (LAMA) or a long-acting beta-agonists (LABA) should be tried. Since the NICE evidence review, Vogelmeier and colleagues[68] have published convincing evidence that using once-daily tiotropium is more effective than twice-daily salmeterol in preventing COPD exacerbations, regardless of the background use of ICS. Whether the same would be true for once-daily LABA, such as indacaterol, is still to be established. Several studies have suggested that these drugs are at least equivalent in terms of their lung function and health status changes[69,70]; but to date, a direct comparison based on exacerbation frequency has not been presented.

For patients with more severe disease spirometrically, the first-line options are either an LAMA or an LABA/ICS combination. There are clear data to show that LABA/ICS is more effective than its components in reducing exacerbations, improving health status and lung function, and in exercise capacity.[50] Patients who would be included in the GOLD C group because of increased exacerbations rather than poor lung function (a small number in secondary care practice) also benefit from LABA/ICS treatment.[71] However, most patients with more substantial reductions in FEV_1 will also be symptomatic and have an exacerbation history; here the NICE data review suggests that either LAMA or a combination can be given with a slight preference for the combination based on data about secondary end points, such as hospitalization, study drop out, and health status, described in the INSPIRE study.[49] However, the primary outcome of that study was to show equivalence between the treatments in terms of preventing exacerbations.

ALTERNATIVE THERAPIES

Unlike GOLD, NICE makes explicit evidence-based recommendations for treatment when exacerbations remain frequent and/or breathlessness cannot be reduced to acceptable levels. For patients in GOLD grades 1 and 2, the suggestion is to add another long-acting broncho-dilator of a different class to that used initially. Until recently, there has been only limited evidence of efficacy from this approach, with most of the data coming from the Canadian Optimal trial, with combination drugs performing disappoint-ingly, relative to tiotropium therapy.[72] However, a recent 6-month study comparing once-daily inda-caterol with the LAMA glycopyrronium in a combi-nation inhaler showed that the combination was superior to either component alone in terms of improving lung function over 3 months. The changes in health status were rather more equiv-ocal and no exacerbation data were presented.[73] However, the well-conducted SPARK study has shown in more severe disease a small but signifi-cant reduction in COPD exacerbation rates when these 2 bronchodilators are given compared with either agent alone, lending stronger support to the value of dual bronchodilator therapy.[74]

The next option for these patients with less se-vere spirometric impairment and the preferred second-line option for those with an FEV_1 of less than 50% predicted is to use the combination of LABA/LAMA and ICS. There are data to show that this triple therapy can reduce exacerba-tion and improve morning symptoms, at least then the budesonide-formoterol combination is used.[75] In practice, such a combined regimen has been widely adopted in patients with COPD or those at risk of hospitalization. This approach is supported by the GOLD guideline and may be a first-line choice for some patients.

The GOLD system also offers data about the PDE4 inhibitor roflumilast, which has been shown to prevent corticosteroid-treated exacerbations, in patients with a history of these events, who also have chronic bronchitis and an FEV_1 of less than 50% predicted.[76] It seems effective in pa-tients who use ICS (but not LABA)[77] or those who use either LABA or LAMA (but not ICS).[47] It is most effective when the background exacerba-tion rate is high[78] and converts frequent exacerba-tors to infrequent exacerbators. Further studies investigating the effect of roflumilast on top of either LABA/ICS or triple therapy are currently ongoing.[79] However, the most common side ef-fects seen with roflumilast are a pharmacologically predictable increase in nausea, diarrhea, and, more surprisingly, weight loss, which are likely to limit its use in some patients.

A range of other alternative treatments is sug-gested by GOLD, although not necessarily in any preferred order of use. Again, this represents expert preference because specific studies defining clinical effectiveness in comparable groups are lacking. GOLD also offers some op-tions for cheaper treatment for more cash-limited health care systems, although the comparability of studies conducted when there is almost no background therapy, even with short-acting bron-chodilators to trials whereby other effective agents were already deployed, is difficult to evaluate.[80]

EMERGING ISSUES

All of the aforementioned treatments have the po-tential for adverse effects as well as beneficial ones. As noted in the acute episodes, beta-agonists can produce troublesome tremor and palpitations, particularly in older patients, although the metabolic effects, including hypokalemia, are not troublesome. Patients with coexisting cardiac disease are common in COPD, although the evi-dence to date suggests that the use of beta-agonists alone or in combination with ICS is not associated with an increased mortality and may actually be beneficial.[81] LAMA drugs, such as tio-tropium, are absorbed somewhat more readily than ipratropium; the use of these agents seems to be associated with more cases of urinary reten-tion.[82,83] Dry mouth is not a major side effect and is reported less frequently with tiotropium than ipra-tropium. The twice-daily anticholinergic aclinidium does not seem to have this side effect.[84]

Initial concerns about an excess recurrence of cardiac deaths with LAMA treatments have been allayed by data from the follow-up of patients in the large randomized controlled Understanding the Potential Long term Improvement in Function with Tiotropium (UPLIFT) trial whereby overall fewer patients died if randomized to tiotropium treat-ment.[85] Recently, anxieties have been raised about the use of a soft-mist aerosol form of tiotropium, which is available in Western Europe. Greater numbers of deaths were reported on patients ran-domized to this treatment in the regulatory studies, which were not primarily designed to assess mor-tality risk.[86,87] This finding has led some to call for this delivery system to be discontinued and is un-likely to become available in the United States until these issues are resolved. Important information about this problem will come from the TIOtropium Safety and Performance in Respimat (TIOSPIR) study of more than 17,000 patients who are receiving either 2 different doses of tiotropium from the soft-mist inhaler or conventional tio-tropium from the dry power device.[88]

A range of new drugs belonging to the LABA and LAMA classes given once or twice daily alone or in combination with each other or inhaled corticosteroids are in the process of development and registration. One such combination of the LABA vilanterol and the inhaled corticosteroid fluticasone furoate has received a favorable assessment at a Food and Drug Administration advisory panel.

At present, no new twice-daily LABA drugs have been evaluated; but twice-daily aclidinium bromide has been licensed for use in the United States and Western Europe, and studies combining this with formoterol are ongoing. Once-daily inhaled indacaterol has been combined with glycopyrronium, as noted earlier,[73,74] and is also being studied together with mometasone furoate, an ICS that can prove effective when given once daily.[89]

A new LABA, olodaterol, is being combined with tiotropium; but these studies have used the soft-mist delivery system discussed earlier, and their outcome will be influenced by the results of TIO-SPIR. The vilanterol/fluticasone furoate combination has been investigated in several doses[90] and in replicate 1-year studies.[54] The inhaled steroid adds relatively little to the bronchodilator effect, but this is associated with fewer exacerbations than is seen with the LABA alone (**Fig. 4**). As with other fluticasone preparations, pneumonia was more common when the ICS was used; but overall, the combination of 25 mcg vilanterol and 200 mcg fluticasone furoate gave the most favorable benefit/risk profile.

Ultimately, the plethora of newer chemically and clinically similar entities will need a clear-sighted appraisal of the cost-effectiveness of treatment before these agents can be recommended in future treatment guidelines. The next generation of clinical trials will need to define not just whether the treatment works relative to a placebo comparator (an approach which seems to be increasingly unethical, given the established effects of treatment) but also how much benefit such treatment provides for the patients and payer. Defining when it is appropriate to add treatment to existing regimens or replace components of a current therapy will be our next challenge.

SUMMARY

Choosing the optimal drug therapy is a key component of the management of COPD. Acute exacerbation treatment, whether in the community or hospital, has changed little in recent years and involves increasing the frequency and/or dose of inhaled bronchodilators, giving a short (up to 10 days) course of oral prednisolone, having a low threshold for starting antibiotics of an appropriate spectrum to cover likely pathogens, and avoiding the use of methylxanthines.

Chronic treatment choices are influenced by baseline lung function, symptom intensity, and how often patients have exacerbated in the past. Short-acting reliever treatment with beta-agonists or antimuscarinics may be appropriate for patients with few symptoms and preserved lung function; but at present, long-acting antimuscarinic treatment is the first-line option when managing patients whose FEV_1 is more than 50% predicted. Those with more severe disease spirometrically and/or a history of 2 or more exacerbations per year gain benefits from either long-acting antimuscarinics but especially from combinations of LABA and ICS. These 3 treatment approaches can be combined if there are persistent problems, especially in patients who exacerbate often.

Other agents, such as PDE4 inhibitor roflumilast, can be considered as an alternative to ICS and may prove helpful in disease that is difficult to manage with triple treatment, although this has yet to be definitely established. Many other options exist, with once-daily combinations of bronchodilators and bronchodilator corticosteroids becoming available in the near future.

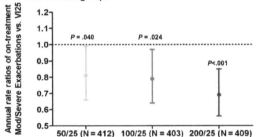

Fig. 4. Effect on exacerbation rate of adding the once-daily inhaled corticosteroid fluticasone furoate to the long-acting inhaled beta-agonist vilanterol (VI) in a 1-year clinical trial. Note the improvement in exacerbation rate with the corticosteroid in the absence of significant differences in FEV_1. Mod, moderate. (*Adapted from* Dransfield MT, Bourbeau J, Jones PW, et al. Once-daily inhaled fluticasone furoate and vilanterol vs vilanterol only for prevention of exacerbations of COPD: two replicate double-blind, parallel-group, randomised controlled trials. Lancet Respir Med 2013;1:210–23; with permission.)

REFERENCES

1. Celli BR, MacNee W. Standards for the diagnosis and treatment of patients with COPD: a summary of the ATS/ERS position paper. Eur Respir J 2004; 23(6):932–46.

2. Rabe KF, Hurd S, Anzueto A, et al. Global strategy for the diagnosis, management, and prevention of

chronic obstructive pulmonary disease: GOLD executive summary. Am J Respir Crit Care Med 2007;176(6):532–55.

3. National Collaborating Centre for Chronic Conditions. Chronic obstructive pulmonary disease. National clinical guideline on management of chronic obstructive pulmonary disease in adults in primary and secondary care. Thorax 2004; 59(Suppl 1):1–232.

4. Lightowler JV, Wedzicha JA, Elliott MW, et al. Non-invasive positive pressure ventilation to treat respiratory failure resulting from exacerbations of chronic obstructive pulmonary disease: cochrane systematic review and meta-analysis. BMJ 2003; 326(7382):185.

5. Chakrabarti B, Angus RM, Agarwal S, et al. Hyperglycaemia as a predictor of outcome during non invasive ventilation in decompensated COPD. Thorax 2009;64(10):857–62.

6. Albert P, Calverley PM. Drugs (including oxygen) in severe COPD. Eur Respir J 2008;31(5):1114–24.

7. O'Donnell DE, D'Arsigny C, Webb KA. Effects of hyperoxia on ventilatory limitation during exercise in advanced chronic obstructive pulmonary disease. Am J Respir Crit Care Med 2001;163(4): 892–8.

8. Lacasse Y, Lecours R, Pelletier C, et al. Randomised trial of ambulatory oxygen in oxygen-dependent COPD. Eur Respir J 2005;25(6):1032–8.

9. Stevenson NJ, Calverley PM. Effect of oxygen on recovery from maximal exercise in patients with chronic obstructive pulmonary disease. Thorax 2004;59(8):668–72.

10. Suissa S, Dell'Aniello S, Ernst P. Long-term natural history of chronic obstructive pulmonary disease: severe exacerbations and mortality. Thorax 2012; 67(11):957–63.

11. Parker CM, Voduc N, Aaron SD, et al. Physiological changes during symptom recovery from moderate exacerbations of COPD. Eur Respir J 2005;26(3): 420–8.

12. Stevenson NJ, Walker PP, Costello RW, et al. Lung mechanics and dyspnea during exacerbations of chronic obstructive pulmonary disease. Am J Respir Crit Care Med 2005;172(12):1510–6.

13. Austin MA, Wills KE, Blizzard L, et al. Effect of high flow oxygen on mortality in chronic obstructive pulmonary disease patients in prehospital setting: randomised controlled trial. BMJ 2010;341:c5462. http://dx.doi.org/10.1136/bmj.c5462.:c5462.

14. Gross NJ, Petty TL, Friedman M, et al. Dose response to ipratropium as a nebulized solution in patients with chronic obstructive pulmonary disease. A three-center study [see comments]. Am Rev Respir Dis 1989;139(5):1188–91.

15. Moayyedi P, Congleton J, Page RL, et al. Comparison of nebulised salbutamol and ipratropium bromide with salbutamol alone in the treatment of chronic obstructive pulmonary disease. Thorax 1995;50(8):834–7.

16. Hadcroft J, Calverley PM. Alternative methods for assessing bronchodilator reversibility in chronic obstructive pulmonary disease. Thorax 2001; 56(9):713–20.

17. Parshall MB, Schwartzstein RM, Adams L, et al. An official American Thoracic Society statement: update on the mechanisms, assessment, and management of dyspnea. Am J Respir Crit Care Med 2012;185(4):435–52.

18. McKay SE, Howie CA, Thomson AH, et al. Value of theophylline treatment in patients handicapped by chronic obstructive lung disease. Thorax 1993; 48(3):227–32.

19. Rice KL, Leatherman JW, Duane PG, et al. Aminophylline for acute exacerbations of chronic obstructive pulmonary disease. A controlled trial. Ann Intern Med 1987;107(3):305–9.

20. Duffy N, Walker P, Diamantea F, et al. Intravenous aminophylline in patients admitted to hospital with exacerbations of chronic obstructive pulmonary disease: a prospective randomised controlled trial. Thorax 2005;60(9):713–7.

21. Qiu Y, Zhu J, Bandi V, et al. Biopsy neutrophilia, neutrophil chemokine and receptor gene expression in severe exacerbations of chronic obstructive pulmonary disease. Am J Respir Crit Care Med 2003;168(8):968–75.

22. Niewoehner DE, Erbland ML, Deupree RH, et al. Effect of systemic glucocorticoids on exacerbations of chronic obstructive pulmonary disease. N Engl J Med 1999;340(25):1941–7.

23. Davies L, Angus RM, Calverley PM. Oral corticosteroids in patients admitted to hospital with exacerbations of chronic obstructive pulmonary disease: a prospective randomised controlled trial. Lancet 1999;354(9177):456–60.

24. Aaron SD, Vandemheen KL, Hebert P, et al. Outpatient oral prednisone after emergency treatment of chronic obstructive pulmonary disease. N Engl J Med 2003;348(26):2618–25.

25. Sayiner A, Aytemur ZA, Cirit M, et al. Systemic glucocorticoids in severe exacerbations of COPD [see comments]. Chest 2001;119(3):726–30.

26. Thompson WH, Nielson CP, Carvalho P, et al. Controlled trial of oral prednisone in outpatients with acute COPD exacerbation. Am J Respir Crit Care Med 1996;154(2 Pt 1):407–12.

27. Decramer M, de Bock V, Dom R. Functional and histologic picture of steroid-induced myopathy in chronic obstructive pulmonary disease. Am J Respir Crit Care Med 1996;153(6 Pt 1):1958–64.

28. Wedzicha JA, Seemungal TA. COPD exacerbations: defining their cause and prevention. Lancet 2007;370(9589):786–96.

29. Calverley PM, Stockley RA, Seemungal TA, et al. Reported pneumonia in patients with COPD: findings from the INSPIRE study. Chest 2011;139(3): 505–12.

30. Daniels JM, Snijders D, de Graaff CS, et al. Antibiotics in addition to systemic corticosteroids for acute exacerbations of chronic obstructive pulmonary disease. Am J Respir Crit Care Med 2010; 181(2):150–7.

31. Anthonisen NR, Manfreda J, Warren CP, et al. Antibiotic therapy in exacerbations of chronic obstructive pulmonary disease. Ann Intern Med 1987; 106(2):196–204.

32. Rothberg MB, Pekow PS, Lahti M, et al. Antibiotic therapy and treatment failure in patients hospitalized for acute exacerbations of chronic obstructive pulmonary disease. JAMA 2010;303(20):2035–42.

33. Vestbo J, Hurd SS, Agusti AG, et al. Global strategy for the diagnosis, management and prevention of chronic obstructive pulmonary disease, GOLD executive summary. Am J Respir Crit Care Med 2013;187(4):347–65.

34. O'Reilly J, Jones MM, Parnham J, et al. Management of stable chronic obstructive pulmonary disease in primary and secondary care: summary of updated NICE guidance. BMJ 2010;340:c3134. http://dx.doi.org/10.1136/bmj.c3134.:c3134.

35. Bateman ED, Hurd SS, Barnes PJ, et al. Global strategy for asthma management and prevention: GINA executive summary. Eur Respir J 2008; 31(1):143–78.

36. Hattotuwa KL, Gizycki MJ, Ansari TW, et al. The effects of inhaled fluticasone on airway inflammation in chronic obstructive pulmonary disease: a double-blind, placebo-controlled biopsy study. Am J Respir Crit Care Med 2002;165(12):1592–6.

37. Bourbeau J, Christodoulopoulos P, Maltais F, et al. Effect of salmeterol/fluticasone propionate on airway inflammation in COPD: a randomised controlled trial. Thorax 2007;62(11):938–43.

38. Lapperre TS, Snoeck-Stroband JB, Gosman MM, et al. Effect of fluticasone with and without salmeterol on pulmonary outcomes in chronic obstructive pulmonary disease: a randomized trial. Ann Intern Med 2009;151(8):517–27.

39. Vestbo J, Sorensen T, Lange P, et al. Long-term effect of inhaled budesonide in mild and moderate chronic obstructive pulmonary disease: a randomised controlled trial. Lancet 1999;353(9167): 1819–23.

40. Pauwels RA, Lofdahl CG, Laitinen LA, et al. Long-term treatment with inhaled budesonide in persons with mild chronic obstructive pulmonary disease who continue smoking. N Engl J Med 1999; 340(25):1948–53.

41. The Lung Health Study Research Group. Effect of inhaled triamcinolone on the decline in pulmonary function in chronic obstructive pulmonary disease. N Engl J Med 2000;343:1902–9.

42. Burge PS, Calverley PM, Jones PW, et al. Randomised, double blind, placebo controlled study of fluticasone propionate in patients with moderate to severe chronic obstructive pulmonary disease: the ISOLDE trial. BMJ 2000;320(7245):1297–303.

43. Sutherland ER, Allmers H, Ayas NT, et al. Inhaled corticosteroids reduce the progression of airflow limitation in chronic obstructive pulmonary disease: a meta-analysis. Thorax 2003;58(11):937–41.

44. Soriano JB, Sin DD, Zhang X, et al. A pooled analysis of FEV1 decline in COPD patients randomized to inhaled corticosteroids or placebo. Chest 2007; 131(3):682–9.

45. Albert P, Agusti A, Edwards L, et al. Bronchodilator responsiveness as a phenotypic characteristic of established chronic obstructive pulmonary disease. Thorax 2012;67(8):701–8.

46. Rabe KF, Bateman ED, O'donnell D, et al. Roflumilast–an oral anti-inflammatory treatment for chronic obstructive pulmonary disease: a randomised controlled trial. Lancet 2005;366(9485):563–71.

47. Fabbri LM, Calverley PM, Izquierdo-Alonso JL, et al. Roflumilast in moderate-to-severe chronic obstructive pulmonary disease treated with long acting bronchodilators: two randomised clinical trials. Lancet 2009;374(9691):695–703.

48. Kardos P, Wencker M, Glaab T, et al. Salmeterol/fluticasone propionate versus salmeterol on exacerbations in severe chronic obstructive pulmonary disease. Am J Respir Crit Care Med 2007;175(2): 144–9.

49. Wedzicha JA, Calverley PM, Seemungal TA, et al. The prevention of chronic obstructive pulmonary disease exacerbations by salmeterol/fluticasone propionate or tiotropium bromide. Am J Respir Crit Care Med 2008;177(1):19–26.

50. Calverley PM, Anderson JA, Celli B, et al. Salmeterol and fluticasone propionate and survival in chronic obstructive pulmonary disease. N Engl J Med 2007;356(8):775–89.

51. Kiri VA, Pride NB, Soriano JB, et al. Inhaled corticosteroids in chronic obstructive pulmonary disease: results from two observational designs free of immortal time bias. Am J Respir Crit Care Med 2005;172(4):460–4.

52. Ferguson GT, Calverley PM, Anderson JA, et al. Prevalence and progression of osteoporosis in patients with COPD. Results from TORCH. Chest 2009;136(6):1456–65.

53. Crim C, Calverley PM, Anderson JA, et al. Pneumonia risk in COPD patients receiving inhaled corticosteroids alone or in combination: TORCH study results. Eur Respir J 2009;34(3):641–7.

54. Dransfield MT, Bourbeau J, Jones PW, et al. Once-daily inhaled fluticasone furoate and vilanterol

versus vilanterol only for prevention of exacerbations of COPD: two replicate double-blind, parallel-group, randomised controlled trials. Lancet Respir Med 2013;1(30):210–23.

55. Sin DD, Tashkin D, Zhang X, et al. Budesonide and the risk of pneumonia: a meta-analysis of individual patient data. Lancet 2009;374(9691):712–9.

56. Garcha DS, Thurston SJ, Patel AR, et al. Changes in prevalence and load of airway bacteria using quantitative PCR in stable and exacerbated COPD. Thorax 2012;67(12):1075–80.

57. Vestbo J, Anderson JA, Calverley PM, et al. Bias due to withdrawal in long-term randomised trials in COPD: evidence from the TORCH study. Clin Respir J 2011;5(1):44–9.

58. Kesten S, Plautz M, Piquette CA, et al. Premature discontinuation of patients: a potential bias in COPD clinical trials. Eur Respir J 2007;30(5): 898–906.

59. Calverley PM, Rennard SI. What have we learned from large drug treatment trials in COPD? Lancet 2007;370(9589):774–85.

60. Qaseem A, Wilt TJ, Weinberger SE, et al. Diagnosis and management of stable chronic obstructive pulmonary disease: a clinical practice guideline update from the American College of Physicians, American College of Chest Physicians, American Thoracic Society, and European Respiratory Society. Ann Intern Med 2011;155(3):179–91.

61. Spencer S, Calverley PM, Burge PS, et al. Health status deterioration in patients with chronic obstructive pulmonary disease. Am J Respir Crit Care Med 2001;163(1):122–8.

62. Spencer S, Calverley PM, Burge PS, et al. Impact of preventing exacerbations on deterioration of health status in COPD. Eur Respir J 2004;23(5): 698–702.

63. Bestall JC, Paul EA, Garrod R, et al. Usefulness of the Medical Research Council (MRC) dyspnoea scale as a measure of disability in patients with chronic obstructive pulmonary disease. Thorax 1999;54(7):581–6.

64. Jones PW, Harding G, Berry P, et al. Development and first validation of the COPD assessment test. Eur Respir J 2009;34(3):648–54.

65. Hurst JR, Vestbo J, Anzueto A, et al. Susceptibility to exacerbation in chronic obstructive pulmonary disease. N Engl J Med 2010;363(12):1128–38.

66. Han MK, Muellerova H, Curran-Everett D, et al. GOLD 2011 disease severity classification in COPDGene: a prospective cohort study. Lancet Respir Med 2013;1:43–9.

67. Jones P, Adamek L, Nadeau G, et al. Comparisons of health status scores with MRC grades in a primary care COPD population: implications for the new GOLD 2011 classification. Eur Respir J 2013; 42(3):647–54.

68. Vogelmeier C, Hederer B, Glaab T, et al. Tiotropium versus salmeterol for the prevention of exacerbations of COPD. N Engl J Med 2011;364(12):1093–103.

69. Jones PW, Barnes N, Vogelmeier C, et al. Efficacy of indacaterol in the treatment of patients with COPD. Prim Care Respir J 2011;20(4):380–8.

70. Donohue JF, Fogarty C, Lotvall J, et al. Once-daily bronchodilators for chronic obstructive pulmonary disease: indacaterol versus tiotropium. Am J Respir Crit Care Med 2010;182(2):155–62.

71. Jenkins CR, Jones PW, Calverley PM, et al. Efficacy of salmeterol/fluticasone propionate by GOLD stage of chronic obstructive pulmonary disease: analysis from the randomised, placebo-controlled TORCH study. Respir Res 2009;10:59.

72. Aaron SD, Vandemheen KL, Fergusson D, et al. Tiotropium in combination with placebo, salmeterol, or fluticasone-salmeterol for treatment of chronic obstructive pulmonary disease: a randomized trial. Ann Intern Med 2007;146(8):545–55.

73. Vogelmeier C, Bateman ED, Pallante J, et al. Efficacy and safety of once-daily QVA149 compared with twice-daily salmeterol–fluticasone in patients with chronic obstructive pulmonary disease (ILLUMINATE): a randomised, double-blind, parallel group study. Lancet Respir Med 2013;1(1):51–60.

74. Wedzicha JA, Decramer M, Ficker JH, et al. Analysis of chronic obstructive pulmonary disease exacerbations with the dual bronchodilator QVA149 compared with glycopyrronium and tiotropium (SPARK): a randomised, double-blind, parallel-group study. Lancet Respir Med 2013;1(3):199–209.

75. Welte T, Miravitlles M, Hernandez P, et al. Efficacy and tolerability of budesonide/formoterol added to tiotropium in patients with chronic obstructive pulmonary disease. Am J Respir Crit Care Med 2009;180(8):741–50.

76. Calverley PM, Rabe KF, Goehring UM, et al. Roflumilast in symptomatic chronic obstructive pulmonary disease: two randomised clinical trials. Lancet 2009;374(9691):685–94.

77. Rennard SI, Calverley PM, Goehring UM, et al. Reduction of exacerbations by the PDE4 inhibitor roflumilast–the importance of defining different subsets of patients with COPD. Respir Res 2011; 12:18.

78. Bateman ED, Rabe KF, Calverley PM, et al. Roflumilast with long-acting beta2-agonists for COPD: influence of exacerbation history. Eur Respir J 2011;38(3):553–60.

79. Calverley PM, Martinez FJ, Fabbri LM, et al. Does roflumilast decrease exacerbations in severe COPD patients not controlled by inhaled combination therapy? The REACT study protocol. Int J Chron Obstruct Pulmon Dis 2012;7:375–82. http://dx.doi.org/10.2147/COPD.S31100.

80. Albert P, Calverley P. A PEACE-ful solution to COPD exacerbations? Lancet 2008;371(9629):1975–6.

81. Calverley PM, Anderson JA, Celli B, et al. Cardiovascular events in patients with COPD: TORCH study results. Thorax 2010;65(8):719–25.

82. Kesten S, Jara M, Wentworth C, et al. Pooled clinical trial analysis of tiotropium safety. Chest 2006; 130(6):1695–703.

83. Stephenson A, Seitz D, Bell CM, et al. Inhaled anticholinergic drug therapy and the risk of acute urinary retention in chronic obstructive pulmonary disease: a population-based study. Arch Intern Med 2011;171(10):914–20.

84. Jones PW, Singh D, Bateman ED, et al. Efficacy and safety of twice-daily aclidinium bromide in COPD patients: the ATTAIN study. Eur Respir J 2012;40(4):830–6.

85. Celli B, Decramer M, Kesten S, et al. Mortality in the 4 year trial of tiotropium (UPLIFT) in patients with COPD. Am J Respir Crit Care Med 2009;180(10): 948–55.

86. Singh S, Loke YK, Enright PL, et al. Mortality associated with tiotropium mist inhaler in patients with chronic obstructive pulmonary disease: systematic review and meta-analysis of randomised controlled trials. BMJ 2011;342:d3215. http://dx.doi.org/10.1136/bmj.d3215.:d3215.

87. Dong YH, Lin HH, Shau WY, et al. Comparative safety of inhaled medications in patients with chronic obstructive pulmonary disease: systematic review and mixed treatment comparison meta-analysis of randomised controlled trials. Thorax 2013;68(1):48–56.

88. Wise RA, Anzueto A, Calverley P, et al. The Tiotropium Safety and Performance in Respimat(R) Trial (TIOSPIR(R)), a large scale, randomized, controlled, parallel-group trial-design and rationale. Respir Res 2013;14:40. http://dx.doi.org/10.1186/1465-9921-14-40.

89. Calverley PM, Rennard S, Nelson HS, et al. One-year treatment with mometasone furoate in chronic obstructive pulmonary disease. Respir Res 2008;9:73.

90. Martinez FJ, Boscia J, Feldman G, et al. Fluticasone furoate/vilanterol (100/25; 200/25 mug) improves lung function in COPD: a randomised trial. Respir Med 2013;107(4):550–9.

Bronchodilators: Current and Future

Mario Cazzola, MD[a],*, Maria Gabriella Matera, MD, PhD[b]

KEYWORDS

- Chronic obstructive pulmonary disease • β_2-Agonists • Antimuscarinic agents • Methylxanthines
- Choice of bronchodilators • Emerging bronchodilators

KEY POINTS

- Bronchodilators are central in the symptomatic treatment of chronic obstructive pulmonary disease (COPD), although there is often limited reversibility of airflow obstruction.
- Three classes of bronchodilators (β_2-agonists, antimuscarinic agents, and methylxanthines) are currently available, which can be used individually, or in combination with each other or inhaled corticosteroids.
- It is still not known whether long-acting bronchodilators should be started in obstructed patients also in the absence of symptoms, whether it is better to start with a β-agonist or an antimuscarinic agent in patients with mild/moderate stable COPD, and whether once-daily or twice-daily dosing is preferable.
- Novel classes of bronchodilators have proved difficult to develop.
- It is likely that an approach using muscarinic antagonist β_2-agonist (MABA) molecules will provide the best opportunity to develop combinations that combine corticosteroids with 2 bronchodilator activities, and thus potentially achieve better efficacy than is apparent with the current combination products that dominate the treatment of COPD.

THE IMPORTANCE OF BRONCHODILATION IN COPD

The use of bronchodilators is one of the key elements in the treatment of chronic obstructive pulmonary disease (COPD), although there is often limited reversibility of airflow obstruction.[1] Bronchodilation aims at alleviating bronchial obstruction and airflow limitation, reducing hyperinflation, and improving emptying of the lung and exercise performance. Bronchodilators work by relaxing airway smooth muscle tone, leading to reduced respiratory muscle activity and improvements in ventilatory mechanics.[1] In particular, they reduce airway resistance and elastic loading of the inspiratory muscles during exercise at constant work rate.[2] Bronchodilators acting on peripheral airways

diminish air trapping, thereby reducing lung volumes. The lower operating lung volume allows patients to achieve the required alveolar ventilation during rest and exercise at a lower oxygen cost of breathing, improving symptoms and exercise capacity.[3]

The importance of bronchodilation explains why all guidelines highlight that inhaled bronchodilators are still the mainstay of the current management of COPD at all stages of the disease,[4–6] although the recent American College of Physicians (ACP)/American College of Chest Physicians (ACCP)/American Thoracic Society (ATS)/European Respiratory Society (ERS) guidelines conclude that no sufficient evidence exists to support bronchodilator treatment in asymptomatic COPD patients.[5]

[a] Unit of Respiratory Clinical Pharmacology, Department of System Medicine, University of Rome Tor Vergata, Via Montpellier 1, Rome 00133, Italy; [b] Unit of Pharmacology, Department of Experimental Medicine, Second University of Naples, Naples, Italy
* Corresponding author. Unità di Farmacologia Clinica Respiratoria, Dipartimento di Medicina dei Sistemi, Università di Roma Tor Vergata, Via Montpellier 1, Rome 00133, Italy.
E-mail address: mario.cazzola@uniroma2.it

Clin Chest Med 35 (2014) 191–201
http://dx.doi.org/10.1016/j.ccm.2013.10.005
0272-5231/14/$ – see front matter © 2014 Elsevier Inc. All rights reserved.

CLASSES OF BRONCHODILATORS

Three classes of bronchodilators, namely β_2-agonists, antimuscarinic agents, and methylxanthines, are currently available; these can be used individually, or in combination with each other or inhaled corticosteroids (ICSs). For both β_2-agonists and antimuscarinic agents, long-acting formulations are preferred over short-acting formulations.[6] Inhaled bronchodilators are preferred over oral bronchodilators and, in any case, because of relatively low efficacy and more side effects, treatment with theophylline is not recommended unless other long-term treatment bronchodilators are unavailable or unaffordable.[6] For patients whose COPD is not sufficiently controlled by monotherapy, guidelines recommend combining medications of different classes, in particular an inhaled antimuscarinic agent and a β_2-agonist, as a convenient way of delivering treatment and obtaining better lung function and improved symptoms.[6]

β_2-Agonists

β_2-Agonists act by mimicking some of the effects of epinephrine at several levels: (1) inhibitory action on airway smooth muscle; (2) stimulation of the heart, leading to increased heart rate, contraction, and conduction; (3) inhibition of the release of mediators from mast cells; (4) metabolic actions (eg, glycogenolysis in liver and skeletal muscle, resulting in an increase in glucose); (5) endocrine actions (increasing insulin and glucagon release); and (6) prejunctional action on parasympathetic ganglia, increasing or decreasing acetylcholine release.[1,7,8] In addition to their main bronchodilator effect, this class of drugs also protects against the actions of bronchoconstrictor stimuli.

Short-acting β_2-agonists (SABAs), such as salbutamol and terbutaline, have long been used as rescue medications for COPD. Their short half-life, however, limits their efficacy as maintenance medications. A volume of published evidence supports the role of long-acting β_2-agonists (LABAs) in the treatment of stable COPD.[1,7,8] There are currently 3 LABAs: formoterol and salmeterol, which are twice-daily LABAs, and indacaterol, a once-daily LABA. Physiologic studies have shown that β_2-agonists dilate the airways and reduce air trapping, leading to reduced dyspnea, improved lung function, and improved exercise tolerance for patients.[9] Moreover, they reduce the frequency of COPD exacerbations[10] and offer a potential survival advantage.[11] Of note, LABAs, rather than SABAs, also have the potential to improve the mucociliary component of COPD.[12]

All β_2-agonists can induce increased heart rate, palpitations, vasodilation, and reflex tachycardia.[1,7,8] These agents can also produce a transient decrease in the partial pressure of arterial oxygen despite concomitant bronchodilation, an effect that is of doubtful clinical significance.[1,7,8] β_2-Agonists induce glycogenolysis and raise blood sugar levels. In addition, they can cause hypokalemia because of stimulation in the skeletal muscle of the Na^+,K^+-ATPase–driven pump coupled to β_2-adrenoceptors.[1,7,8] Dose-related tremor is one of the most characteristic adverse effects after administration of β_2-agonists, as they can directly stimulate β_2-adrenoceptors on skeletal muscle.[13] Although prolonged or repeated use of β_2-agonists may lead to tolerance to rescue SABA, in patients with COPD the long-term use of β_2-agonists results in sustained improvements in bronchodilatory activity, with no indication of development of tolerance.[14]

Antimuscarinic Agents

Cholinergic parasympathetic nerves contribute to the elevated tone of airway smooth muscle in COPD, and this primary reversible component of airway limitation is sensitive to muscarinic receptor antagonists.[1,15] Acetylcholine (ACh) and other bronchoconstrictor mediators can also be released from nonneuronal cells to act on airway smooth muscle cells and other cells involved in the chronic inflammatory response in COPD and airway remodeling.[1,15] The effects of ACh are mediated by a family of 5 G-protein–coupled receptors (M_1–M_5). These receptors have distinct anatomic distribution and functions. Only subtypes M_1 to M_3 are expressed in airways.[15] The contraction of airway smooth muscle cells in response to ACh is predominantly mediated via M_3 receptors.[1,15]

There are currently 2 short-acting antimuscarinic agents (SAMAs) (ipratropium bromide and oxitropium bromide), 1 twice-daily long-acting antimuscarinic agent (LAMA) (aclidinium bromide), and 2 once-daily LAMAs (tiotropium bromide and glycopyrronium bromide) that have been licensed for use in the treatment of COPD.

Aclidinium bromide, 400 μg twice daily, shows clinically meaningful effects in lung function and other important supportive outcomes, such as health-related quality of life, dyspnea, and nighttime/early-morning symptoms, and is safe.[16] Tiotropium bromide is a once-daily treatment for COPD that provides 24-hour bronchodilation, and improves symptoms and health-related quality of life.[1,15] LAMAs offer distinct advantages over SAMAs in terms of maintaining 24-hour bronchodilation.[1,15] However, although tiotropium bromide provides 24-hour bronchodilation, it takes

2 to 8 days to achieve maximal bronchodilation and 2 to 3 weeks to reach steady-state plasma levels.[1,15] Glycopyrronium bromide, 50 μg once daily, provides clinically significant 24-hour bronchodilation but with a rapid onset of action that is faster than that of tiotropium, and a favorable safety and tolerability profile.[17]

Administration of antimuscarinic agents often results in a bad taste and dryness in the mouth.[1] These agents can cause urinary retention in older men.[1] Thus, these medications should be used with caution in patients with prostatic hypertrophy or bladder-outlet obstruction. Several ophthalmic side effects, including blurred vision, elevated intraocular pressure, acute or worsening narrow-angle glaucoma, and cataracts, have been reported with the use of inhaled antimuscarinic agents.[1] Concerns have been raised about possible associations of antimuscarinic agents with cardiovascular morbidity and mortality.[18,19] The cardiovascular adverse events include arrhythmias (including supraventricular tachycardia and atrial fibrillation), angina, nonspecific chest pain, and edema.[1]

Methylxanthines

Methylxanthines (eg, theophylline, aminophylline) may act as nonselective phosphodiesterase (PDE) inhibitors, but have been reported to have a range of nonbronchodilating actions that may be potentially beneficial.[1] Theophylline at low concentrations increases histone deacetylase (HDAC) activity in alveolar macrophages, and in vitro reverses the steroid resistance induced by oxidative stress.[20] The molecular mechanism of action of theophylline in restoring HDAC2 seems to be through selective inhibition of phosphoinositide 3-kinase δ, which is activated by oxidative stress in patients with COPD.[15] Moreover, it can interfere with certain intracellular kinases.[21] Patients receiving regimens that include theophylline seem to have slightly increased risks of mortality, COPD exacerbations, and COPD hospitalizations compared with patients receiving the same regimens without theophylline, although it offers minimal benefits in terms of lung function.[22] Because of its toxicity at levels close to the therapeutic range, theophylline is rarely used as a first-line COPD medication. It has been used as a modestly effective bronchodilator, but in low doses theophylline is still considered to be an add-on therapy in those with severe or very severe COPD.[1]

Theophylline has a narrow therapeutic index; serum levels slightly outside of the target range may lead to serious toxicity or lack of efficacy.[1] The most commonly reported adverse effects

associated with theophylline include anorexia, nausea, headache, and sleep disturbance. Theophylline was also found to worsen symptoms of gastroesophageal reflux disease and to cause cardiac arrhythmias. Given that most of these adverse effects can be avoided at lower plasma levels, monitoring of the therapeutic drug level plays a pivotal role.[1]

THE CHOICE OF BRONCHODILATORS IN STABLE COPD

It is noteworthy that in almost all guidelines no distinction is made as to which class of bronchodilators should be considered first, but they only recommend the use of long-acting broncholytic agents. Unfortunately, it is still not known whether long-acting bronchodilators should be started in obstructed patients also in absence of symptoms, whether it is better to start with a β-agonist or an antimuscarinic agent in patients with mild/moderate stable COPD, and whether once-daily or twice-daily dosing is preferable.[23] Moreover, there is no real guidance on when 2 bronchodilators with different mechanisms of action must be combined.[23]

When Starting Treatment with Bronchodilators

As already mentioned, there is insufficient evidence to support bronchodilator treatment in asymptomatic patients,[5] although some studies report that mild and even moderate airflow obstruction can occur without complaints or symptoms,[24] and several surveys revealed a cohort of COPD patients with silent obstruction who had no chronic cough, phlegm, and/or dyspnea, although they had airflow limitation in spirometry tests.[25–27] Early intervention might possibly avoid or delay the onset of symptoms and other clinical manifestations, such as exacerbations, and their long-term consequences. However, this hypothesis needs to be tested in appropriate prospective studies. In any case, a consensus initiative for optimizing therapeutic appropriateness among Italian specialists concluded that regular therapy with long-acting bronchodilators should be started in obstructed patients in both the presence and absence of symptoms.[28]

Choice of Treatment Based on Effectiveness

The National Institute for Health and Clinical Excellence of England and Wales, in its 2010 update of COPD treatment guidelines, reviewed all studies that compared LABAs and LAMAs, and conclude that there was no evidence to favor one treatment over another.[4] Therefore, the choice of agents to treat the diagnosed COPD condition depends mainly on individual response, cost, side effects, and availability,[29] and therapy often starts with an empiric choice and recording of clinical response to treatment.

Nonetheless, data from efficacy trials are providing valuable information on choosing between inhaled therapies. Data suggest that twice-daily LABAs (salmeterol and formoterol) are preferable to SABAs (ipratropium)[30,31]; a twice-daily antimuscarinic agent, aclidinium bromide, may be more effective than a LABA,[32] whereas once-daily tiotropium, a LAMA[33,34] and indacaterol, a once-daily LABA,[35] are superior to twice-daily LABAs. The Prevention of Exacerbations with Tiotropium in COPD (POET-COPD) trial showed that in patients with moderate to very severe COPD, tiotropium is more effective than salmeterol in preventing exacerbations.[34]

In any case, a blinded comparison in COPD of the once-daily LABA indacaterol and the once-daily LAMA tiotropium showed that both bronchodilators demonstrated spirometric efficacy; however, compared with tiotropium, indacaterol provided significantly greater improvements in clinical outcomes.[36] Moreover, a systematic review that explored the efficacy and safety of indacaterol in comparison with tiotropium showed that indacaterol induced statistically and clinically significant reductions in the use of rescue medication and dyspnea, and improvement in health status.[37] Since the updated 2011 Global Strategy for the Diagnosis, Management, and Prevention of Chronic Obstructive Pulmonary Disease (GOLD) for prescribing bronchodilators for patients with COPD based on the goals of reducing symptoms and reducing the risk of exacerbations,[6] a recent post hoc analysis compared the efficacy of available once-daily inhaled bronchodilators, indacaterol and tiotropium, according to baseline dyspnea severity using pooled data from 3 clinical studies.[38] The overall findings demonstrated that indacaterol was generally equivalent or superior to open-label tiotropium depending on the dyspnea category.[38] These data suggest that for patients with less dyspnea, indacaterol 150 μg is an appropriate initial choice if symptoms are not controlled with short-acting bronchodilators. The results also suggest that indacaterol 300 μg is the preferred indacaterol dose for patients with more dyspnea, and that tiotropium would be an appropriate alternative treatment.[38]

Choice of Treatment Based on Safety

Salpeter[39] pooled all the data from randomized placebo-controlled trials of at least 3 months' duration to evaluate the risk for COPD hospitalizations, respiratory mortality, and total mortality. The results suggested that antimuscarinic agents should be the bronchodilator of choice in COPD because their use was associated with a 30% reduction in COPD hospitalizations and a 70% reduction in respiratory mortality, without a significant effect on total mortality, whereas β_2-agonists were associated with poorer disease control.

Nonetheless, there has been uncertainty about whether antimuscarinic agents increase or decrease cardiovascular risk in the treatment of patients with COPD.[18,40] Recently, it caution in prescribing inhaled antimuscarinic agents has been suggested for patients with preexisting arrhythmias or cardiac disease.[41] In fact, these agents can cause progressively increasing tachycardia by blocking vagal effects of M_2 receptors on the sinoatrial nodal pacemaker.[42] For each patient, the benefit of dyspnea relief and reduction in COPD exacerbations should be weighed against the potential risks of serious cardiovascular adverse effects.[42]

Regrettably, even inhaled β_2-agonists may have adverse effects on the myocardium in COPD patients suffering from preexisting cardiac arrhythmias,[43] also because of the presence of β_2-adrenoreceptors in the heart.[44] Moreover, the adverse effects of β_2-agonists are likely to be exacerbated in COPD patients with coexistent chronic heart failure.[45]

All of these issues constitute a genuine problem when considering use of a bronchodilator for the treatment of patients suffering from COPD, because there is solid evidence that these patients are at increased risk of cardiovascular disease.[46]

When Combining Two Bronchodilators with Different Mechanisms of Action

In real life, COPD dyspneic patients who have only a single bronchodilator available often assume additional doses of their bronchodilator in the hope of relieving dyspnea when they are unable to perceive bronchodilation or must perform an exercise.[47] Unfortunately, only a proportion of patients with COPD require such additional doses, and in many patients an additional dose does not induce any substantial improvement in lung function.[48] Alternatively, the therapeutic option is to add a SABA, such as salbutamol, as rescue medication to achieve rapid relief of bronchospasm, even if patients are under regular treatment with a LABA or a LAMA.[14,49,50]

However, most specialists believe that patients not controlled by a single bronchodilator should be given 2 bronchodilators with different mechanisms of action.[28] Certainly this seems to be a good choice because using multiple drugs in combination may lower doses of individual agents, decrease adverse effects, simplify medication regimens, and improve compliance. The scientific rationale for combining a β-agonist with an antimuscarinic agent in COPD fully supports this opinion.[51] Complementary bronchodilation may be obtained either by directly relaxing the smooth muscle through stimulation of β_2-adrenoceptors or by inhibiting the action of ACh at muscarinic receptors with antimuscarinic agents, and indirectly by decreasing the release of ACh through the modulation of cholinergic neurotransmission by prejunctional β_2-adrenoceptors stimulated by the addition of a β_2-agonist, thereby amplifying the relaxation of bronchial smooth muscle induced by the antimuscarinic agent.[51]

In its last version, the GOLD Executive Summary[6] recommends that combination of bronchodilators may be considered if symptoms are not improved with single agents. However, it highlights that good long-term studies are lacking and also that combination treatment seems to be expensive in many countries.

Nonetheless, studies of LABA/LAMA combinations to date indicate that combining different classes of bronchodilator results in significantly greater improvements in lung function and other meaningful outcomes such as inspiratory capacity, dyspnea, symptom scores, rescue medication use, and health status in comparison with individual drugs.[52] A meta-analysis of 8 trials found significant increases in forced expiratory volume in 1 second (FEV_1) and forced vital capacity, and improved dyspnea score, when formoterol was added to tiotropium.[53] A recent 12-week study that investigated the approach of dual bronchodilation using indacaterol and tiotropium, showed that, compared with tiotropium monotherapy, indacaterol plus tiotropium provided greater bronchodilation and lung deflation.[54]

It must be highlighted that because of their pharmacologic action, LABAs and LAMAs may have the potential to increase heart rate and alter other cardiac events. Therefore, there is a concern about a possible increase in adverse events with combination therapy. However, although, as already mentioned, good long-term studies are still lacking, cardiac effects seem to be relatively rare. Of note, the aforementioned mentioned meta-analysis documented a trend toward a decrease rather than an increase in adverse events among patients treated with combination therapy, although the difference was not statistically significant.[53]

Although a dissertation on ICSs is beyond the scope of this review, it must be underlined that in patients with stable COPD, it is still unclear whether and when it is preferable to add a second bronchodilator with a different mechanism of action or if it is better to introduce an ICS as an alternative.[23] Moreover, it is imperative to establish whether LAMA/LABA combination therapy is preferred over LAMA plus LABA/ICS, and whether addition of an ICS to the LAMA/LABA combination provides additional clinical value.[23] Dual and triple therapy seem to be the most promising for patients with moderate to very severe COPD. However, data are still too scarce and studies too short to generate a strong recommendation.[55]

FUTURE DEVELOPMENTS
Novel Classes

Novel classes of bronchodilators have proved difficult to develop,[1] but the continued interest in generating new agents that act via emerging targets has identified at least 8 new classes: (1) selective PDE inhibitors; (2) potassium-channel openers; (3) vasoactive intestinal peptide (VIP) analogues; (4) Rho kinase inhibitors; (5) brain natriuretic peptide (BNP) and analogues; (6) nitric oxide (NO) donors; (7) E-prostanoid (EP) receptor 4 agonists; and (8) bitter-taste receptor agonists.[1]

PDE4 inhibitors have minimal direct effects of clinical relevance on airway smooth muscle. By contrast, it has long been appreciated that PDE3 is the prevalent isoenzyme in the airway smooth muscle that leads to smooth muscle relaxation. Consequently, dual PDE3/PDE4 inhibitors are under development. The mechanisms underlying the apparent synergistic effects of dual PDE3/PDE4 inhibition are unclear. However, it has been suggested that PDE3 (which is predominantly localized to the particulate cellular fraction) and PDE4 (which is predominantly cytosolic) can regulate different pools of cyclic adenosine monophosphate (cAMP).[56] A nonemetic mixed PDE3/PDE4 inhibitor, RPL554, which has been demonstrated to be both a bronchodilator and anti-inflammatory,[56] has already successfully undergone several phase 2 clinical trials in patients with COPD.[1]

Potassium-channel openers are not effective in treating COPD because their vasodilating activity limits the dose that can be administered.[1,57] Clinical application of VIP is limited by its vasodilating activity and, moreover, by its short plasma half-life.[1,57] VIP analogues do not seem to be longer lasting in their bronchodilatory effect. Rho kinase inhibitors are able to relax human isolated bronchial preparations, but information on their effect in humans is still lacking.[1,57] BNP is able to induce a time-dependent and concentration-dependent increase in levels of cyclic guanosine monophosphate in human airway smooth muscle cells, and induces a weak but intriguing relaxant effect on human airway smooth muscle through the activation of the natriuretic peptide receptor A.[58,59] However, there is no information on its broncholytic effects in humans. NO-donor compounds relax human airways in vitro,[1] and this has raised the possibility that such compounds may prove to be useful as novel bronchodilators. However, it is still difficult to carefully target NO release to lungs at an optimal concentration so as to achieve a beneficial action and limit possible adverse effects, particularly on the cardiovascular system.[1] In any case, there is evidence that the NO-releasing salbutamol, NCX-950, has greater relaxant and anti-inflammatory properties in the human bronchi and in mice when compared with salbutamol alone.[60] Stimulation of the EP_4 receptor with prostaglandin E_2 (PGE_2) leads to a direct stimulation of the adenylyl cyclase via the $G\alpha_s$ subunit, which converts adenosine triphosphate to cAMP. Thus, highly potent EP_4 subtype-selective receptor agonists have been suggested to have therapeutic potential without side effects.[61] In the respiratory system, stimulation of extraoral type 2 taste receptors (T2Rs) expressed in respiratory epithelia and smooth muscle has been implicated in protective airway reflexes, ciliary beating, and bronchodilation.[62] Agonists to these receptors may make up a new class of useful direct bronchodilators for treating obstructive lung disease, but because they are members of the G-protein–coupled receptor superfamily, they may undergo desensitization.[63]

New Traditional Bronchodilators

Several once-daily LABAs, olodaterol (BI1744 CL), vilanterol (GSK642444), and abediterol (LAS10097), are currently undergoing development.[7,8,64] These agents are single enantiomers of the (R)-configuration and have a near full-agonist profile at human β_2-adrenoreceptors. All produce a dose-dependent rapid bronchodilation, which is maintained over 24 hours, with a safety and tolerability profile similar to that of placebo.

Several LAMAs are also in clinical development.[1,15,64] Umeclidinium bromide is being developed as a once-daily treatment of COPD. It is a potent antagonist of ACh in vitro, with a longer duration of action than tiotropium bromide. Single and repeat doses of umeclidinium produced clinically relevant improvements in lung function over 24 hours in patients with COPD. It is well tolerated, but the incidence of drug-related adverse

events has been shown to be dose related. Glycopyrronium bromide, already on the market as a once-daily LAMA (NVA237), is also in clinical development in several different formulations and by several pharmaceutical companies. EP-101 is an inhalation solution formulation of glycopyrronium bromide optimized for administration via the investigational eFlow Nebulizer System. CHF-5259 is another inhaled formulation of glycopyrronium bromide that is delivered using a pressurized metered-dose inhaler (pMDI). PT001 is also delivered via a novel pMDI that uses a porous particle–based suspension technology, which allows better targeting of drugs to the airways and enables the development of products with improved physical stability and uniformity of dose content. Contrary to NVA237, all these new formulations are being developed as twice-daily bronchodilators. CHF-5407 is a potent antagonist with a dissociation half-life at M_3 receptors comparable with that of tiotropium bromide, with a more rapid dissociation from M_2 receptors. In vivo, the bronchodilator profile of CHF-5407 is comparable with that of tiotropium bromide. BEA2180 is a once-daily LAMA. In a 24-week trial of 2080 patients, both tiotropium and BEA2180 were effective at improving lung function and reducing the symptoms of COPD, and were generally well tolerated.[65] TD-4208, AZD8683, and V-0162 are other antimuscarinic agents in development for respiratory disease, but unfortunately there are still no relevant data available.

Several once-daily LABA/LAMA combinations, including QVA149 (combination of indacaterol and glycopyrronium bromide), vilanterol plus umeclidinium bromide, and olodaterol plus tiotropium bromide, are in clinical development as fixed-dose combinations.[1,7,8,15,64]

Once-daily QVA149 caused significant and clinically meaningful improvements in lung function in comparison with the component monotherapies indacaterol and glycopyrronium, as well as significant improvements versus tiotropium and placebo over 26 weeks in patients with COPD.[66] Moreover, QVA149 provided significant, sustained, and clinically meaningful improvements in lung function in comparison with a twice-daily salmeterol-fluticasone combination in patients with moderate to severe COPD, with significant symptomatic benefit.[67] Dual bronchodilation with QVA149 significantly reduced the rate of exacerbations compared with both glycopyrronium and tiotropium.[68] QVA149 at a supratherapeutic dose in healthy volunteers had no relevant impact on heart rate and QTcF (QT interval corrected for heart rate using Fridericia's formula) when compared with placebo.[69] There was no tachycardic or QTcF effect of QVA149 when compared with supratherapeutic doses of its monocomponents indacaterol and glycopyrronium alone. QVA149 also had less of an effect on heart rate and QTcF than salmeterol alone. Overall, QVA149 had a good tolerability profile.

Once-daily dosing with umeclidinium bromide in combination with vilanterol in patients with moderate to very severe COPD was well tolerated over 28 days.[70] A 24-week trial has documented that once-daily umeclidinium bromide/vilanterol 125/25 μg was well tolerated in subjects with COPD, and produced improvements in lung function, dyspnea, and health-related quality of life compared with placebo, umeclidinium 125 μg, and vilanterol 25 μg.[71] Another 24-week trial has shown that umeclidinium bromide/vilanterol 125/25 μg and umeclidinium bromide/vilanterol 62.5/25 μg are well tolerated and show increased efficacy in lung function in comparison with tiotropium 18 μg or vilanterol 25 μg for the once-daily treatment of COPD.[72] Of note, no evidence of an effect on QTcF was observed following 10 days of inhaled umeclidinium bromide/vilanterol 125/25 μg or umeclidinium 500 μg in comparison with placebo.[73] At a supratherapeutic dose, umeclidinium bromide/vilanterol 500/100 μg increased QTcF on average by 8.2 milliseconds (90% CI: 6.2, 10.2) at 30 minutes only compared with placebo.

Two dose-finding studies have been conducted to identify the optimal doses of olodaterol and tiotropium to be used in combination. An initial trial evaluated the bronchodilator efficacy of olodaterol (2, 5, or 10 μg) when added to tiotropium 5 μg, in a comparison with tiotropium 5 μg monotherapy, in 360 COPD patients. After once-daily treatment for 4 weeks, peak FEV_1 response from baseline was significantly increased for all doses of olodaterol plus tiotropium compared with tiotropium; trough FEV_1 response from baseline was significantly increased for olodaterol plus tiotropium (10/5 μg) when compared with tiotropium.[74] A second study involving 232 COPD patients tested various doses of tiotropium (1.25, 2.5, and 5 μg) in combination with olodaterol either 5 μg or 10 μg, and efficacy was measured against the respective doses of olodaterol as monotherapy.[75] The addition of tiotropium to olodaterol resulted in improvements in lung-function parameters in comparison with olodaterol monotherapy over 4 weeks. Incremental increases in FEV_1 were observed with increasing doses of tiotropium. Compared with olodaterol monotherapy, the combination of tiotropium and olodaterol further increased lung function. Treatment with combinations of tiotropium/olodaterol once daily was well

tolerated at all doses, and no safety concerns were identified. Taking into consideration data from this study, the long-term efficacy and safety of 2.5 and 5 μg tiotropium combined with 5 μg olodaterol as a fixed-dose combination is being investigated in the TOviTO phase 3 clinical trial program.

As there is a progressive attempt to shift attention toward controlling nocturnal symptoms and those present on awakening, which are indicated by epidemiologic studies to be the most troublesome for COPD patients,[76] the twice-daily dosing of bronchodilators is still considered a useful approach at least for the symptomatic treatment of COPD. Therefore, 2 twice-daily LABA/LAMA fixed-dose combinations, aclidinium/formoterol and glycopyrronium bromide/formoterol, are under development. The few clinical data available suggest that the addition of formoterol fumarate to aclidinium bromide results in greater bronchodilation than formoterol fumarate or aclidinium bromide alone. However, a large phase 3 program is involving a huge number of patients with moderate to severe COPD, and consists of large long-term (from 24 to 52 weeks) pivotal clinical trials.[77] PT003 is an inhaled combination of PT001 (glycopyrronium bromide) and formoterol fumarate, delivered via hydrofluoroalkane (HFA) metered-dose inhaler (MDI). Doses of PT003 from 2.4/9.6 μg to 18/9.6 μg demonstrated superior bronchodilation in comparison with glycopyrronium MDI 18 μg and formoterol fumarate MDI 9.6 μg ($P \leq .001$) for the primary end point FEV_1 area under the $curve_{0-12}$ on day 7, and were also statistically significantly superior to tiotropium ($P \leq .020$).[78] All treatments were well tolerated, and overall safety was comparable between PT003, its components, and tiotropium.

Bifunctional (or dual pharmacophore) muscarinic β_2-agonist molecules (MABA) constitute a novel approach to dual bronchodilator therapy by combining muscarinic antagonism (MA) and β_2-agonism (BA) in a single molecule.[79] This approach may offer several advantages over combination therapy of 2 separate drug entities,[1] which include the benefit of delivering a fixed ratio into every region of the lung, reducing the complexity of combination inhalers via a single pharmacokinetic profile, a uniform ratio of activities at the cellular level, and a simplified clinical development program. However, one limitation of MABA molecules is that the ratio of MA and BA activities cannot be adjusted as needed, which limits dosing flexibility.[79] GSK961081 will likely be the first MABA to be commercialized. It is able to elicit a bronchodilator effect that was significantly greater than that induced by salmeterol in moderate and severe COPD patients, with 400 µg/d as the best dosage,[80] and to induce sustained bronchodilation similar to that of tiotropium plus salmeterol, but with a more rapid onset of action.[81] AZD2115 and LAS190792 are another 2 MABAs under development.

A growing body of evidence suggests that triple therapy with LABAs, LAMAs, and ICS is efficacious in patients with more severe COPD, such as those with frequent exacerbations. The development of fixed triple-combination inhalers and novel molecules for once-daily treatment regimens are likely to improve patient adherence and facilitate the evaluation of treatment.[82] However, only Triohale pMDI has been marketed as the world's first triple-combination inhaler to be taken only once a day (tiotropium 9 µg, formoterol fumarate 6 µg, ciclesonide 200 µg).[83] This formulation is a suspension-based product and is the only pMDI to contain 3 therapeutics in one device. The 3 drugs are suspended in HFA 227, with apparently no other additives. The combination of glycopyrronium/beclomethasone dipropionate/formoterol is under clinical evaluation,[64] although it is likely that the MABA approach will provide the best opportunity to develop combinations that combine corticosteroids with 2 bronchodilator activities and, thus, potentially achieve better efficacy than is apparent with the current combination products that dominate the treatment of COPD.[84]

REFERENCES

1. Cazzola M, Page CP, Calzetta L, et al. Pharmacology and therapeutics of bronchodilators. Pharmacol Rev 2012;64:450–504.
2. Thomas M, Decramer M, O'Donnell DE. No room to breathe: the importance of lung hyperinflation in COPD. Prim Care Respir J 2013;22:101–11.
3. O'Donnell DE, Banzett RB, Carrieri-Kohlman V, et al. Pathophysiology of dyspnea in chronic obstructive pulmonary disease: a roundtable. Proc Am Thorac Soc 2007;4:145–68.
4. National Clinical Guideline Centre. Chronic obstructive pulmonary disease: management of chronic obstructive pulmonary disease in adults in primary and secondary care. London: National Clinical Guideline Centre; 2010. Available at: http://guidance.nice.org.uk/CG101/Guidance/pdf/English. Accessed March 20, 2013.
5. Qaseem A, Wilt TJ, Weinberger SE, et al. Diagnosis and management of stable chronic obstructive pulmonary disease: a clinical practice guideline update from the American College of Physicians, American College of Chest Physicians, American Thoracic Society, and European Respiratory Society. Ann Intern Med 2011;155:179–91.
6. Vestbo J, Hurd SS, Agustí AG, et al. Global strategy for the diagnosis, management, and prevention of chronic obstructive pulmonary disease: GOLD executive summary. Am J Respir Crit Care Med 2013;187:347–65.
7. Cazzola M, Calzetta L, Matera MG. β_2-Adrenoceptor agonists: current and future direction. Br J Pharmacol 2011;163:4–17.
8. Cazzola M, Page CP, Rogliani P, et al. β_2-Agonist therapy in lung disease. Am J Respir Crit Care Med 2013;187:690–6.
9. Decramer ML, Hanania NA, Lötvall JO, et al. The safety of long-acting β_2-agonists in the treatment of stable chronic obstructive pulmonary disease. Int J Chron Obstruct Pulmon Dis 2013;8:53–64.
10. Wang J, Nie B, Xiong W, et al. Effect of long-acting beta-agonists on the frequency of COPD exacerbations: a meta-analysis. J Clin Pharm Ther 2012;37:204–11.
11. Suissa S, Ernst P, Vandemheen KL, et al. Methodological issues in therapeutic trials of COPD. Eur Respir J 2008;31:927–33.
12. Rogers DF. Mucociliary dysfunction in COPD: effect of current pharmacotherapeutic options. Pulm Pharmacol Ther 2005;18:1–8.
13. Cazzola M, Matera MG. Tremor and β_2-adrenergic agents: is it a real clinical problem? Pulm Pharmacol Ther 2012;25:4–10.
14. Cazzola M, Rogliani P, Ruggeri P, et al. Chronic treatment with indacaterol and airway response to salbutamol in stable COPD. Respir Med 2013;107:848–53.
15. Cazzola M, Page C, Matera MG. Long-acting muscarinic receptor antagonists for the treatment of respiratory disease. Pulm Pharmacol Ther 2013;26:307–17.
16. Cazzola M, Page C, Matera MG. Aclidinium bromide for the treatment of chronic obstructive pulmonary disease. Expert Opin Pharmacother 2013;14:1205–14.
17. Buhl R, Banerji D. Profile of glycopyrronium for once-daily treatment of moderate-to-severe COPD. Int J Chron Obstruct Pulmon Dis 2012;7:729–41.
18. Lee TA, Pickard AS, Au DH, et al. Risk for death associated with medications for recently diagnosed chronic obstructive pulmonary disease. Ann Intern Med 2008;149:380–90.
19. Singh S, Loke YK, Enright PL, et al. Mortality associated with tiotropium mist inhaler in patients with chronic obstructive pulmonary disease: systematic review and meta-analysis of randomised controlled trials. BMJ 2011;342:d3215.
20. Ito K, Lim S, Caramori G, et al. A molecular mechanism of action of theophylline: induction of histone deacetylase activity to decrease inflammatory gene expression. Proc Natl Acad Sci U S A 2002;99:8921–6.

21. To Y, Ito K, Kizawa Y, et al. Targeting phosphoinositide-3-kinase-δ with theophylline reverses corticosteroids insensitivity in chronic obstructive pulmonary disease. Am J Respir Crit Care Med 2010;182:897–904.

22. Lee TA, Schumock GT, Bartle B, et al. Mortality risk in patients receiving drug regimens with theophylline for chronic obstructive pulmonary disease. Pharmacotherapy 2009;29:1039–53.

23. Cazzola M, Segreti A, Rogliani P. Comparative effectiveness of drugs for chronic obstructive pulmonary disease. Drugs Today (Barc) 2012;48:785–94.

24. van den Boom G, Rutten-van Mölken MP, Tirimanna PR, et al. Association between health-related quality of life and consultation for respiratory symptoms: results from the DIMCA programme. Eur Respir J 1998;11:67–72.

25. d'Andiran G, Schindler C, Leuenberger P. The absence of dyspnoea, cough and wheezing: a reason for undiagnosed airflow obstruction? Swiss Med Wkly 2006;136:425–33.

26. Shin C, Lee S, Abbott RD, et al. Respiratory symptoms and undiagnosed airflow obstruction in middle-aged adults: the Korean health and genome study. Chest 2004;126:1234–40.

27. Lu M, Yao WZ, Zhong NS, et al. Asymptomatic patients of chronic obstructive pulmonary disease in China. Chin Med J 2010;123:1494–9.

28. Cazzola M, Brusasco V, Centanni S, et al. Project PriMo: sharing principles and practices of bronchodilator therapy monitoring in COPD: a consensus initiative for optimizing therapeutic appropriateness among Italian specialists. Pulm Pharmacol Ther 2013;26:218–28.

29. Ohar JA, Donohue JF. Mono- and combination therapy of long-acting bronchodilators and inhaled corticosteroids in advanced COPD. Semin Respir Crit Care Med 2010;31:321–33.

30. Rennard SI, Anderson W, ZuWallack R, et al. Use of a long-acting inhaled β2-adrenergic agonist, salmeterol xinafoate, in patients with chronic obstructive pulmonary disease. Am J Respir Crit Care Med 2001;163:1087–92.

31. Dahl R, Greefhorst LA, Nowak D, et al. Inhaled formoterol dry powder versus ipratropium bromide in chronic obstructive pulmonary disease. Am J Respir Crit Care Med 2001;164:778–84.

32. Singh D, Magnussen H, Kirsten A, et al. A randomised, placebo- and active-controlled dose-finding study of aclidinium bromide administered twice a day in COPD patients. Pulm Pharmacol Ther 2012;25:248–53.

33. Donohue JF, van Noord JA, Bateman ED, et al. A 6- month, placebo-controlled study comparing lung function and health status changes in COPD patients treated with tiotropium or salmeterol. Chest 2002;122:47–55.

34. Vogelmeier C, Hederer B, Glaab T, et al. Tiotropium versus salmeterol for the prevention of exacerbations of COPD. N Engl J Med 2011; 364:1093–103.

35. Vogelmeier C, Magnussen H, LaForce C, et al. Profiling the bronchodilator effects of the novel ultra-long-acting β2-agonist indacaterol against established treatments in chronic obstructive pulmonary disease. Ther Adv Respir Dis 2011;5: 345–57.

36. Buhl R, Dunn LJ, Disdier C, et al. Blinded 12-week comparison of once-daily indacaterol and tiotropium in COPD. Eur Respir J 2011;38:797–803.

37. Rodrigo GJ, Neffen H. Comparison of indacaterol with tiotropium or twice-daily long-acting β-agonists for stable COPD: a systematic review. Chest 2012; 142:1104–10.

38. Mahler DA, Buhl R, Lawrence D, et al. Efficacy and safety of indacaterol and tiotropium in COPD patients according to dyspnoea severity. Pulm Pharmacol Ther 2013;26:348–55.

39. Salpeter SR. Bronchodilators in COPD: impact of β-agonists and anticholinergics on severe exacerbations and mortality. Int J Chron Obstruct Pulmon Dis 2007;2:11–8.

40. Singh S, Loke YK, Furberg CD. Inhaled anticholinergics and risk of major adverse cardiovascular events in patients with chronic obstructive pulmonary disease: a systematic review and meta-analysis. JAMA 2008;300:1439–50.

41. Singh S, Loke YK, Enright P, et al. Pro-arrhythmic and pro-ischaemic effects of inhaled anticholinergic medications. Thorax 2013;68:114–6.

42. Cazzola M, Calzetta L, Matera MG. The cardiovascular risk of tiotropium: is it real? Expert Opin Drug Saf 2010;9:783–92.

43. Cazzola M, Imperatore F, Salzillo A, et al. Cardiac effects of formoterol and salmeterol in patients suffering from COPD with preexisting cardiac arrhythmias and hypoxemia. Chest 1998;114:411–5.

44. Cazzola M, Matera MG, Donner CF. Inhaled β2-adrenoceptor agonists: cardiovascular safety in patients with obstructive lung disease. Drugs 2005;65:1595–610.

45. Matera MG, Martuscelli E, Cazzola M. Pharmacological modulation of β-adrenoceptor function in patients with coexisting chronic obstructive pulmonary disease and chronic heart failure. Pulm Pharmacol Ther 2010;23:1–8.

46. Cazzola M, Calzetta L, Bettoncelli G, et al. Cardiovascular disease in asthma and COPD: a population-based retrospective cross-sectional study. Respir Med 2012;106:249–56.

47. Cazzola M, Santus P, Castagna F, et al. Addition of an extra dose of salmeterol Diskus to conventional dose of salmeterol Diskus in patients with COPD. Respir Med 2002;96:439–43.

48. Cazzola M, Segreti A, Stirpe E, et al. Effect of an additional dose of indacaterol in COPD patients under regular treatment with indacaterol. Respir Med 2013;107:107–11.

49. Cazzola M, Di Perna F, Noschese P, et al. Effects of formoterol, salmeterol or oxitropium bromide on airway responses to salbutamol in COPD. Eur Respir J 1998;11:1337–41.

50. Cazzola M, Santus P, D'Adda A, et al. Acute effects of higher than standard doses of salbutamol and ipratropium on tiotropium-induced bronchodilation in patients with stable COPD. Pulm Pharmacol Ther 2009;22:177–82.

51. Cazzola M, Molimard M. The scientific rationale for combining long-acting β_2-agonists and muscarinic antagonists in COPD. Pulm Pharmacol Ther 2010; 23:257–67.

52. van der Molen T, Cazzola M. Beyond lung function in COPD management: effectiveness of LABA/LAMA combination therapy on patient-centred outcomes. Prim Care Respir J 2012;21:101–8.

53. Wang J, Jin D, Zuo P, et al. Comparison of tiotropium plus formoterol to tiotropium alone in stable chronic obstructive pulmonary disease: a meta-analysis. Respirology 2011;16:350–8.

54. Mahler DA, D'Urzo A, Bateman ED, et al. Concurrent use of indacaterol plus tiotropium in patients with COPD provides superior bronchodilation compared with tiotropium alone: a randomised, double-blind comparison. Thorax 2012;67:781–8.

55. Rodrigo GJ, Plaza V, Castro-Rodríguez JA. Comparison of three combined pharmacological approaches with tiotropium monotherapy in stable moderate to severe COPD: a systematic review. Pulm Pharmacol Ther 2012;25:40–7.

56. Boswell-Smith V, Cazzola M, Page CP. Are phosphodiesterase 4 inhibitors just more theophylline? J Allergy Clin Immunol 2006;117:1237–43.

57. Matera MG, Page CP, Cazzola M. Novel bronchodilators for the treatment of chronic obstructive pulmonary disease. Trends Pharmacol Sci 2011;32:495–506.

58. Matera MG, Calzetta L, Parascandolo V, et al. Relaxant effect of brain natriuretic peptide in non-sensitized and passively sensitized isolated human bronchi. Pulm Pharmacol Ther 2009;22:478–82.

59. Matera MG, Calzetta L, Passeri D, et al. Epithelium integrity is crucial for the relaxant activity of brain natriuretic peptide in human isolated bronchi. Br J Pharmacol 2011;163:1740–54.

60. Lagente V, Naline E, Guenon I, et al. A nitric oxide-releasing salbutamol elicits potent relaxant and anti-inflammatory activities. J Pharmacol Exp Ther 2004;310:367–75.

61. Buckley J, Birrell MA, Maher SA, et al. EP_4 receptor as a new target for bronchodilator therapy. Thorax 2011;66:1029–35.

62. Clark AA, Liggett SB, Munger SD. Extraoral bitter taste receptors as mediators of off-target drug effects. FASEB J 2012;26:4827–31.

63. Robinett KS, Deshpande DA, Malone MM, et al. Agonist-promoted homologous desensitization of human airway smooth muscle bitter taste receptors. Am J Respir Cell Mol Biol 2011;45:1069–74.

64. Cazzola M, Rogliani P, Segreti A, et al. An update on bronchodilators in Phase I and II clinical trials. Expert Opin Investig Drugs 2012;21:1489–501.

65. Abrahams R, Moroni-Zentgraf P, Ramsdell J, et al. Safety and efficacy of the once-daily anticholinergic BEA2180 compared with tiotropium in patients with COPD. Respir Med 2013;107:854–62.

66. Barnes N, Bateman E, Gallagher N, et al. QVA149 once daily provides superior bronchodilation versus indacaterol, glycopyrronium, tiotropium and placebo: the SHINE study [abstract]. Thorax 2012;67:A147–8.

67. Vogelmeier CF, Bateman ED, Pallante JM, et al. Efficacy and safety of once-daily QVA149 compared with twice-daily salmeterol-fluticasone in patients with chronic obstructive pulmonary disease (ILLUMINATE): a randomised, double-blind, parallel group study. Lancet Respir Med 2013;1:51–60.

68. Wedzicha JA, Decramer M, Ficker J, et al. Dual bronchodilation with QVA149 reduces COPD exacerbations: the SPARK study [abstract]. Am J Respir Crit Care Med 2013;187:A2428.

69. Drollmann A, Brown M, Sechaud R, et al. Effect of once-daily QVA149 on cardiac safety in healthy volunteers [abstract]. Am J Respir Crit Care Med 2013;187:A1480.

70. Feldman G, Walker RR, Brooks J, et al. 28-Day safety and tolerability of umeclidinium in combination with vilanterol in COPD: a randomized placebo-controlled trial. Pulm Pharmacol Ther 2012;25:465–71.

71. Celli BR, Crater G, Kilbride S, et al. A 24-week randomized, double-bind, placebo-controlled study of the efficacy and safety of once-daily umeclidinium/vilanterol 125/25 mcg in COPD [abstract]. Am J Respir Crit Care Med 2013;187:A2435.

72. Anzueto A, Decramer M, Kaelin T, et al. The efficacy and safety of umeclidinium/vilanterol compared with tiotropium or vilanterol over 24 weeks in subjects with COPD [abstract]. Am J Respir Crit Care Med 2013;187:A4268.

73. Kelleher D, Tombs L, Crater G, et al. A placebo- and moxifloxacin-controlled thorough QT study of umeclidinium monotherapy and umeclidinium/vilanterol combination in healthy subjects [abstract]. Am J Respir Crit Care Med 2013;187:A1487.

74. Maltais F, Beck E, Webster D, et al. Four weeks once daily treatment with tiotropium+olodaterol (BI 1744) fixed dose combination compared with

tiotropium in COPD patients [abstract]. Eur Respir J 2010;36:1014s.

75. Aalbers R, Maleki-Yazdi MR, Hamilton A, et al. Dose-finding study for tiotropium and olodaterol when administered in combination via the Respimat inhaler in patients with COPD [abstract]. Eur Respir J 2012;40:525–526s.

76. Kessler R, Partridge MR, Miravitlles M, et al. Symptom variability in patients with severe COPD: a pan-European cross-sectional study. Eur Respir J 2011; 37:264–72.

77. Cazzola M, Rogliani P, Matera MG. Aclidinium bromide/formoterol fumarate fixed-dose combination for the treatment of chronic obstructive pulmonary disease. Expert Opin Pharmacother 2013;14:775–81.

78. Reisner C, Gotfried M, Denenberg MB, et al. Low doses of pearl therapeutics' LAMA/LABA combination MDI (GFF MDI, PT003) provide superior bronchodilation compared to components and to open-label Spiriva Handihaler in a randomized, double-blind, placebo-controlled phase IIb study in patients with COPD [abstract]. Am J Respir Crit Care Med 2013;187:A2434.

79. Hughes AD, McNamara A, Steinfeld T. Multivalent dual pharmacology muscarinic antagonist and β_2 agonist (MABA) molecules for the treatment of COPD. Prog Med Chem 2012;51:71–95.

80. Wielders PL, Ludwig-Sengpiel A, Locantore N, et al. A new class of bronchodilator improves lung function in COPD: a trial with GSK961081. Eur Respir J 2013; 42:972–81.

81. Bateman ED, Kornmann O, Ambery C, et al. Pharmacodynamics of GSK961081, a bi-functional molecule, in patients with COPD. Pulm Pharmacol Ther 2013;26:581–7.

82. Bjerg A, Lundbäck B, Lötvall J. The future of combining inhaled drugs for COPD. Curr Opin Pharmacol 2012;12:252–5.

83. Salama RO, Young PM, Rogueda P, et al. Advances in drug delivery: is triple therapy the future for the treatment of chronic obstructive pulmonary disease? Expert Opin Pharmacother 2011;12: 1913–32.

84. Norman P. Novel dihydroquinoline-based MABAs; clues to the identity of LAS-190792: evaluation of WO20111411802. Expert Opin Ther Pat 2012;22: 185–92.

How Phosphodiesterase 4 Inhibitors Work in Patients with Chronic Obstructive Pulmonary Disease of the Severe, Bronchitic, Frequent Exacerbator Phenotype

Mark A. Giembycz, BSc, PhD[a],*, Robert Newton, BSc, PhD[b]

KEYWORDS

- Phosphodiesterase 4 inhibitors • Roflumilast • COPD phenotypes • Gene transactivation
- Combination therapies • Acute exacerbations

KEY POINTS

- The novel, antiinflammatory drug, roflumilast, is efficacious in patients with severe chronic obstructive pulmonary disease (COPD) who have chronic bronchitis and a history of frequent exacerbations.
- This COPD phenotype is associated with mucus hypersecretion, an increased risk of bacterial colonization and infection, and a high level of inflammation. Such patients are most likely to derive clinical benefit from antiinflammatory drugs, such as the phosphodiesterase 4 inhibitor, roflumilast.
- The antiinflammatory benefit of roflumilast alone and in the presence of an inhaled corticosteroid/long-acting β_2-adrenoceptor agonist combination therapy may be caused, in part, by the de novo expression of a variety of antiinflammatory genes.

INTRODUCTION

Chronic obstructive pulmonary disease (COPD) is an umbrella term that describes a heterogeneous collection of distinct, debilitating, pulmonary-related disorders that, in many individuals, coexist. COPD is defined clinically by a progressive and largely irreversible decrement in expiratory airflow[1] that is often associated with airway collapse, fibrosis, edema, mucus hypersecretion, airway and systemic inflammation, skeletal muscle wasting, pulmonary hypertension, right sided heart failure, and venous thromboembolism. The variable extent to which an individual presents with one or more of these clinical

Financial disclosures and conflicts of interest: Grant support for M.A. Giembycz is from the Canadian Institutes for Health Research (CIHR; MOP 93742), the Lung Association, Alberta and North West Territories, Takeda, Gilead Sciences, GlaxoSmithKline, and AstraZeneca. Grant support for R. Newton is from the CIHR (MOP 68828), the Lung Association, Alberta and North West Territories, Takeda, Gilead Sciences, GlaxoSmithKline, and AstraZeneca. The authors state no conflict of interest.
 [a] Department of Physiology & Pharmacology, Airways Inflammation Research Group, Snyder Institute for Chronic Diseases, University of Calgary, 3280 Hospital Drive Northwest, Calgary, Alberta T2N 4N1, Canada; [b] Department of Cell Biology & Anatomy, Airways Inflammation Research Group, Snyder Institute for Chronic Diseases, University of Calgary, 3280 Hospital Drive Northwest, Calgary, Alberta T2N 4N1, Canada
* Corresponding author.
E-mail address: giembycz@ucalgary.ca

Clin Chest Med 35 (2014) 203–217
http://dx.doi.org/10.1016/j.ccm.2013.09.007

entities accounts for the wide spectrum of disease seen in clinical practice. COPD typically affects middle-aged and elderly people, and it is a general perception that chronic cigarette smoking is the primary cause.[2,3] However, long-term exposure of individuals to biomass fuel combustion products, used largely in the process of indoor cooking, also is now recognized as a significant cause especially in developing countries.[4]

COPD heterogeneity is probably caused by a complex interplay between genetic factors, which remain largely indeterminate, and the environment, in which tobacco smoke and pollutants are primary players.[5–8] It is intuitive that phenotypic diversity of COPD precludes effective treatment. Because current pharmacotherapies were not rationally designed to target distinct phenotypes, the current one-size fits all approach to management is inherently flawed and poorly effective. Therefore, although COPD heterogeneity is problematic, it nevertheless creates potential opportunities for the design of therapies tailored to the phenotype of interest.[9] In 2012, 4 broad COPD clinical phenotypes (denoted A–D) were proposed based on prognostic and therapeutic relevance (**Fig. 1**A).[10,11] According to this taxonomy, which is distinct from the groups defined in the Global Initiative for Chronic Obstructive Lung Disease (GOLD) guidelines (see **Fig. 1**B; www.goldcopd.org/uploads/users/files/GOLD_Report_2013_Feb20.pdf), patients are categorized as having infrequent exacerbations (A), an asthma/COPD overlap (B), exacerbations with emphysema (C), or exacerbations

with chronic bronchitis (D). This article focuses on patients of the D phenotype. These patients have severe disease (GOLD stage 3–4), present with a history of productive cough or expectoration (>3 months per year and for more than 2 consecutive years) and respond to the novel, antiinflammatory drug, roflumilast (marketed variably as Daxas, Daliresp, and Libertek). Frequent exacerbations of COPD are associated, maybe causally, with mucus hypersecretion, an increased risk of bacterial colonization and infection, and a high level of inflammation.[12] Together, these characteristics suggest that patients of a severe, bronchitic phenotype are most likely to derive clinical benefit from antiinflammatory drugs, such as the phosphodiesterase (PDE) 4 inhibitor, roflumilast. A post hoc analysis of 2 phase III studies (AURA, M2-124; HERMES, M2-125[13]) found that roflumilast (500 µg daily for 1 year) transformed patients classified as frequent exacerbators at the outset of the trial into a more stable, infrequent exacerbator phenotype.[14]

PDE4 INHIBITORS AND COPD

PDEs represent a superfamily of enzymes that degrade the second messenger molecules cyclic adensosine-3′,5′-monophosphate (cAMP) and/or cyclic guanosine-3′,5′-monophophate to the catalytically inactive, corresponding 5′-nucleoside monophosphates. Following the first identification of a PDE activity more than 50 years ago,[15] 11 molecularly, biochemically, and immunologically distinct enzyme families have been clearly

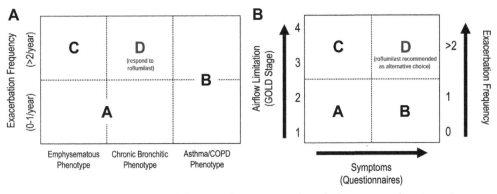

Fig. 1. Classification of COPD. (*A*) The subdivision of COPD into 4 broad phenotypes wherein patients are categorized as having infrequent exacerbations (A), an asthma/COPD overlap (B), exacerbations with emphysema (C), or exacerbations with chronic bronchitis (D). (*B*) The Global Initiative for Chronic Obstructive Lung Disease classification of COPD, which is based on airflow limitation, exacerbation history, and symptoms (determined by questionnaire). Patients are classified as low risk, fewer symptoms (A), low risk, more symptoms (B), high risk, fewer symptoms (C), or high risk, more symptoms (D). The phosphodiesterase (PDE) 4 inhibitor, roflumilast, is a recommended treatment option for group D patients in both classifications (shown in red). (*Adapted from* Miravitlles M, Jose Soler-Cataluna J, Calle M, et al. Treatment of COPD by clinical phenotypes. Putting old evidence into clinical practice. Eur Respir J 2013;41(6):1252–6.)

defined.[16] Since then, there has been considerable interest in the cAMP-specific PDE4 family as an intracellular target that could be exploited to therapeutic advantage for a multitude of diseases associated with chronic inflammation, including COPD. Despite compelling preclinical evidence of efficacy,[17–19] the PDE4 inhibitors that have progressed to phase II and phase III clinical evaluation have had a regrettable rate of attrition, in part, because of unfavorable adverse-effect profiles.[20–22] However, after almost 30 years of research and development, the European Medicines Agency, in April 2010, recommended approval of the first PDE4 inhibitor, roflumilast, for the "maintenance treatment of patients with severe COPD associated with chronic bronchitis who have a history of frequent exacerbations" (www.ema.europa.eu/docs/en_GB/ document_library/Summary_of_opinion_-_Initial_ authorisation/human/001179/WC500089626.pdf). Roflumilast was subsequently approved by Health Canada (www.hc-sc.gc.ca/dhp-mps/prodpharma/ applic-demande/regist/reg_innov_dr-eng.php), the United States Food and Drug Administration (www.fda.gov/NewsEvents/Newsroom/Press Announcements/ucm244989.htm), and other regulatory agencies globally. The approval of roflumilast for COPD is significant because it is thought to provide clinical benefit by suppressing inflammation.[18,23,24] Moreover, the recommendation that roflumilast be used in a defined population of chronic bronchitic patients in whom exacerbation frequency is high and inflammation severe represents the first example of a drug that targets (albeit not by design) a specific COPD phenotype.

A TRIPLE COMBINATION THERAPY?

GOLD recently updated its recommendations for the treatment of stable COPD to include roflumilast as a second-choice medication in high-risk patients with severe (stages 3–4) symptomatic disease (www.goldcopd.org/uploads/users/files/ GOLD_Report_2013_Feb20.pdf). This clinical positioning dictates that roflumilast should be prescribed to patients with severe disease (defined as group D patients in both of the classifications shown in **Fig. 1**) taking, minimally, an inhaled corticosteroid (ICS)/long-acting β_2-adrenoceptor agonist (LABA) combination therapy. Data accrued from the roflumilast clinical development program (reviewed in Refs.[23–27]) indicate that there may be a clinical rationale for combining a PDE4 inhibitor with an ICS or an ICS/LABA combination therapy. In a pooled post hoc analysis of 2 phase III studies (OPUS, M2-111; RATIO, M2-112), roflumilast reduced exacerbation frequency in a subgroup of patients with severe COPD who were

taking an ICS concomitantly, whereas patients not taking an ICS derived no such benefit.[28] Lung function was also improved in patients diagnosed with COPD associated with chronic bronchitis, with or without coexisting emphysema, which was greater if they had received concomitant ICS relative to placebo.[28] However, 2 additional phase III trials (AURA, M2-124; HERMES, M2-125), also in patients with severe COPD, found that roflumilast reduced exacerbation rates in the absence of an ICS,[13] indicating that PDE4 inhibition alone is sufficient for clinical benefit to be realized. Although the reason(s) for this discrepancy is debatable, the possibility that the efficacy of roflumilast and an ICS together may be superior to either drug alone is attractive from a therapeutics standpoint. A meta-analysis of several trials involving almost 12,000 patients with COPD confirmed the superiority of an ICS/LABA combination therapy rather than a LABA alone in reducing the rate of acute exacerbations.[29] Given that LABAs and PDE4 inhibitors, which can both mediate their effects by increasing cAMP, are predicted to interact additively or, in theory, synergistically at the molecular level, the possibility that further improvement could be achieved with an ICS/LABA/PDE4 inhibitor triple combination therapy should be considered. Frequent exacerbations of COPD are associated with a high level of inflammation[12] and may be more responsive to these drug interventions if they are given in combination rather than individually as monotherapies. In 2011, the REACT (Roflumilast in the prevention of COPD Exacerbations while taking Appropriate Combination Treatment) study was initiated to test such a hypothesis. This 1-year investigation will compare the effects of roflumilast and placebo on exacerbation rates in patients with severe to very severe airflow limitation, symptoms of chronic bronchitis, and at least 2 exacerbations in the previous year, who are treated with ICS/LABA combination therapy, with or without a long-acting, muscarinic receptor antagonist.[30]

SCIENTIFIC RATIONALE FOR ADDING ON A PDE4 INHIBITOR TO AN ICS/LABA COMBINATION THERAPY: A CASE FOR GENE TRANSACTIVATION

Glucocorticoids as a monotherapy are poorly effective in COPD (cf asthma) and are contraindicated[31] because of doubts about efficacy and potential adverse effects including pneumonia and tuberculosis.[32,33] Nevertheless, the results of a recent meta-analysis suggest that the potential benefit of an ICS/LABA combination therapy is a reduction in acute exacerbations.[29] From a clinical perspective, this suggests that ICS/LABA combination therapies should only be used in patients classified as frequent exacerbators. Given that inflammation is assumed to be more prevalent and/or severe in these patients, adding on a PDE4 inhibitor might impart additional benefit through the ability of each component of the combination to act individually, additively, or cooperatively to repress inflammation. Notwithstanding multiple nongenomic mechanisms, which have been reviewed extensively elsewhere (see Ref.[18] for review), the remainder of this article focuses on the concept that the clinical efficacy of roflumilast in COPD is derived, in part, from its ability either alone or in combination with an ICS and LABA to induce and/or enhance the expression of a variety of genes that collectively suppress inflammation and improve lung function.

In considering the potential for drug interactions, a mechanistic basis is required. It is thought that the primary mode of action of glucocorticoids, more commonly known as corticosteroids or simply steroids, is to repress the expression of proinflammatory genes, including those that encode cytokines, chemokines, and growth factors.[34] Two general mechanisms have been described in which the glucocorticoid receptor (GR) may act either to directly repress gene transcription (transrepression) or to activate gene transcription (transactivation). In terms of antiinflammatory actions, the most widely accepted of these mechanisms is transrepression, in which the agonist-bound GR, through ill-defined tethering interactions, prevents transcription factors such as nuclear factor kappa B (NF-κB) and activator protein 1 (AP-1) from inducing the expression of target proinflammatory genes. Transrepression may also occur via a direct interaction of the agonist-bound GR to negative glucocorticoid response elements (GREs) located in the promoter regions of target genes.[35] However, glucocorticoids are often only partial inhibitors of proinflammatory gene transcription, implying that processes in addition to transcriptional repression must contribute to their in vivo antiinflammatory activity.[34,36] In this respect, considerable evidence is available that transactivation of genes encoding proteins with antiinflammatory properties also constitutes a major mechanism of glucocorticoid action.[37] For example, glucocorticoids are able to transcriptionally induce the expression of the NF-κB inhibitor protein, IκBα, and this represents a mechanism of repression that involves transactivation by GR.[38,39] The expression of the antiinflammatory gene, GILZ (glucocorticoid-induced leucine zipper; HUGO gene name, transforming growth factor β-stimulated clone 22; domain family member 3 [TSC22D3]), similarly is significantly

upregulated in bronchial biopsies harvested from human asthmatic subjects given a high dose of budesonide by a mechanism thought to involve GR-mediated transactivation.[40]

The empirical demonstration that a glucocorticoid can promote gene transactivation in vivo in human subjects is of particular therapeutic relevance because cAMP can augment glucocorticoid-induced gene expression,[41] possibly by enhancing the binding of ligand-bound GRs to GREs on target genes.[42] This effect was initially reported in the early 1990s following overexpression of cAMP-dependent protein kinase (PKA) in cAMP response element binding protein (CREB)–deficient F9 embryonal carcinoma cells.[43] LABAs and other cAMP-increasing agents, including PDE4 inhibitors, produce the same effect by a mechanism that involves the activation of PKA.[41,44–47] Although this interaction was initially identified from experiments using artificial reporter constructs, it became clear that many bona fides glucocorticoid-inducible genes are regulated similarly.[41,44–47] In many cases, the cAMP-increasing agent alone is without effect, but interacts with glucocorticoid in a positive cooperative fashion. For example, LABAs and PDE4 inhibitors do not promote transcription of a simple GRE reporter. However, they markedly enhance the maximum response produced by the glucocorticoid without changing its potency,[41,46] which indicates that cAMP can boost the intrinsic efficacy (vide infra) of the GR agonist (Fig. 2A). In the presence of a LABA, or a PDE4 inhibitor, a glucocorticoid is therefore able to produce a given level of response but at a significantly lower concentration (see Fig. 2A). As an example, selective PDE4 inhibition with roflumilast potentiates the ability of formoterol to enhance the expression of luciferase from a GRE reporter stably transfected into the human BEAS-2B airway epithelial cell line (see Fig. 2A) as well as the expression of several putative, glucocorticoid-inducible antiinflammatory genes.[46] This effect is described pharmacologically by a sinistral displacement of the LABA concentration-response curve (see Fig. 2A), indicating that the cells are now more sensitive to the LABA. In the absence of evidence that cAMP can enhance GR-mediated transrepression, these results collectively add weight to the importance of transactivation as a mechanism of glucocorticoid action.[34] Moreover, the data also have potential clinical relevance because they provide a plausible explanation for the superior efficacy of ICS/LABA combination therapies in several respiratory diseases relative to an ICS alone as a monotherapy. Such positive interactions are clear for patients with moderate to severe asthma[48–51] and similar, albeit less impressive, data are available in

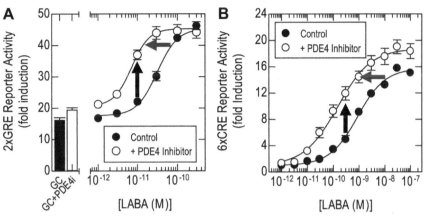

Fig. 2. PDE4 inhibition potentiates the ability of LABAs to promote cAMP response element (CRE)–dependent transcription and enhance GRE-dependent transcription. (*A*) The BEAS-2B human airway epithelial cell line was stably transfected with 2 copies of a GRE upstream of the luciferase gene and stimulated concurrently with the glucocorticoid (GC), fluticasone propionate (100 nM) and the LABA, formoterol, in the absence and presence of the PDE4 inhibitor (PDE4i), roflumilast. (*B*) The results of a similar study in which BEAS-2B cells were stably transfected with 6 copies of a CRE upstream of the same luciferase gene and exposed to the LABA, indacaterol, in the absence and presence of the PDE4 inhibitor, GSK 256066. In both cases, PDE4 inhibition produced a sinistral displacement of the LABA concentration-response curve (*red arrow*) and thereby augmented transcription, especially at low LABA concentrations (*blue arrow*).

COPD.[29] The treatment of acute bronchiolitis with a combination of dexamethasone and adrenaline (an endogenous agonist that activates the β_2-adrenoceptor) or salbutamol was recently reported to significantly reduce the frequency of acute hospitalizations relative to either treatment alone.[52,53] Although β_2-adrenoceptor agonists are not antiinflammatory as monotherapies, these data strongly suggest that they can interact with glucocorticoids to deliver enhanced clinical benefit that is superior to the effect of a glucocorticoid alone. On a molecular level, we suggest that these beneficial effects might derive, in part, from the ability of cAMP to enhance glucocorticoid-induced gene expression, which requires the activation of the canonical cAMP signaling cascade. Adding on a PDE4 inhibitor could therefore potentiate β_2-adrenoceptor–mediated cAMP formation and thereby further enhance antiinflammatory gene expression. This effect might be particularly relevant in cells in which β_2-adrenoceptor signaling is weak because of low receptor number and/or poor coupling efficiency. A PDE4 inhibitor might transform a proinflammatory or immune cell that is normally insensitive to a LABA into one that generates a cAMP signal of sufficient magnitude to enhance glucocorticoid-induced gene expression (vide infra).

PDE4 inhibitors and LABAs alone and in combination could also impart clinical benefit in COPD by promoting the transactivation of antiinflammatory genes that is independent of their ability to enhance the genomic effects of glucocorticoids. A prior microarray study in the BEAS-2B human bronchial epithelial cell line identified more than 200 genes that were upregulated more than 2-fold by the LABA, indacaterol, and the PDE4 inhibitor, GSK 256066 (authors' unpublished data). Many of these genes are glucocorticoid insensitive but, nevertheless, have documented antiinflammatory activity. Moreover, on some genes, the PDE4 inhibitor and LABA in combination could interact synergistically (see **Fig. 2**B). Thus, superior efficacy of a triple combination therapy can be envisaged by considering that each component can work in several distinct, and mutually cooperative, ways, Stated differently, the rationale for combining these drugs is based on the assumption that distinct subpopulations of genes exist that are induced by glucocorticoid alone, cAMP alone, and by both glucocorticoid and cAMP with potential for additivity and/or synergy. In this last group, it is conceivable that genes could respond to both glucocorticoid and cAMP in combination, but not necessarily to each individually. The possibility that LABAs and PDE4 inhibitors can also upregulate distinct subpopulations of cAMP-inducible genes is also worthy of consideration in view of the mounting evidence that distinct subcellular compartments of cyclic nucleotides can be generated in an agonists-dependent manner.

WHY ICS/LABA COMBINATION THERAPIES ARE NOT ENOUGH

Logic dictates that, for a glucocorticoid and a LABA to interact additively or synergistically, target tissues must express functional GR and β_2-adrenoceptors in sufficient numbers. Although GR is expressed ubiquitously, consistent with the pleiotropic effects produced by cortisol in humans, its density varies considerably across tissues.[54] In immune and proinflammatory cells, the rank order of GR expression (high to low) is estimated to be airway smooth muscle $\geq$ bronchial epithelium > alveolar macrophages > eosinophils $\geq$ peripheral blood mononuclear cells (lymphocytes and monocytes) > neutrophils.[55–58] Based on this ranking, it can be speculated that low GR number in neutrophils may explain, in part, why inflammation in COPD is insensitive to glucocorticoids as a monotherapy.[59] In these same cell types, β_2-adrenoceptor density is also low and/or coupling to downstream effectors inefficient. Compared with airway myocytes and epithelial cells, which express approximately 30,000 to 40,000 and 8000 to 9000 sites/cell respectively,[60–62] alveolar macrophages,[63] eosinophils,[64] neutrophils,[65] and T lymphocytes[66] express few β_2-adrenoceptors (~6000, ~4000, ~900, and ~750 sites/cell respectively). The ability of a LABA to enhance the expression of glucocorticoid-inducible antiinflammatory genes could therefore be minimal or not happen at all in cell types in which functional β_2-adrenoceptor number is limiting. This effect is compounded if functional GR number is also low. It is in these β_2-adrenoceptor–poor cells that the potential therapeutic benefit of adding on a PDE4 inhibitor could

be most realized. This concept is illustrated in **Fig. 3**, which shows responses in 2 hypothetical cells, A and B, that express the β_2-adrenoceptor in high and low copy number respectively. In each panel, the term system maximum (E_m) is indicated. E_m is the maximum achievable tissue (but not necessarily agonist) response and is both an agonist-dependent and tissue-dependent parameter. In a cell with high β_2-adrenoceptor density (eg, an airway myocyte; A), a LABA might produce a response that equates to E_m. As a result, the amplitude of that response is unaffected by a PDE4 inhibitor but, because of second messenger amplification, the concentration-response curve is displaced to the left (ie, the system is now more sensitive to the LABA). In contrast, the same LABA in a cell with low β_2-adrenoceptor density or poor coupling efficiency (eg, a neutrophil; B), might produce a response considerably less than the E_m. In this situation, PDE4 inhibition could enhance the maximal effect toward E_m. Although there may be little change in agonist potency (quantified as the half maximal effective concentration [EC_{50}]), the system has, nevertheless, been sensitized such that a given level of response in the presence of a PDE4 inhibitor can now be produced by a lower concentration of the LABA (see **Fig. 3**). For a PDE4 inhibitor to work optimally in cells in which β_2-adrenoceptor number is limiting, the intrinsic efficacy of the LABA is an important parameter and highly relevant for the design of new ICS/LABA combination therapies.

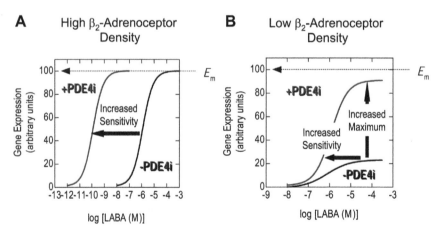

Fig. 3. Theoretical effects of PDE4 inhibition on LABA concentration-response curves constructed in cells expressing high and low β_2-adrenoceptor density. In each panel, the term system maximum (E_m) is indicated, which is the maximum achievable tissue response. In a cell with high β_2-adrenoceptor density (A) a LABA produces a response that equates to E_m (*red curve*). In the presence of a PDE4i, the amplitude of the LABA response is unaffected but the concentration-response curve is displaced to the left (*blue curve*). (B) A cell with low β_2-adrenoceptor density on which a LABA produces a response that is considerably less than the E_m. In this situation, PDE4 inhibition enhances the maximal effect of the LABA toward E_m, without changing its half maximal effective concentration [EC_{50}]. However, the cell is sensitized because a given level of response in the presence of a PDE4 inhibitor can now be produced by a lower concentration of the LABA.

The term intrinsic efficacy, as given by Furch-gott,[67] is defined as a quantal unit of stimulus given to a receptor and is solely an agonist-dependent parameter. Therefore, the ability of an agonist to produce response in a given tissue (ie, its efficacy) is the product of intrinsic efficacy (agonist dependent) and receptor number (tissue dependent). This pharmacodynamic concept is seen in eosinophils (low β_2-adrenoceptor density) in which salmeterol behaves as a β_2-adrenoceptor antagonist under conditions in which formoterol, which has a higher intrinsic efficacy, is an effective agonist.[68,69]

An additional theoretical advantage of a PDE4 inhibitor is its ability to potentiate the antiinflammatory activity of endogenous agonists that act through G-protein–coupled receptors (GPCRs) coupled to cAMP formation such as catecholamines, certain prostaglandins, and adenosine.

CANDIDATE ANTIINFLAMMATORY GENES

Several glucocorticoid and/or cAMP-inducible genes have recently been identified that, when expressed together, could collectively impart a clinically beneficial impact on those mechanisms that promote inflammation and predispose susceptible patients to acute exacerbations (vide infra). Moreover, their expression could contribute to the therapeutic benefit of roflumilast seen in patients with severe, bronchitic disease who have frequent, acute exacerbations. As transactivation becomes more accepted as a mechanism that contributes to the beneficial actions of glucocorticoids (rather than an entrenched and inaccurate view that it mediates only side effects)[70] it is likely that many more genes will be discovered that, when upregulated, would be advantageous in chronic inflammatory diseases such as COPD.

Mitogen-activated Protein Kinase Phosphatase 1

Mitogen-activated protein (MAP) kinases are central regulators of virtually all aspects of the inflammatory process, including proinflammatory gene expression.[71] The activity of these enzyme cascades is tightly controlled by reversible phosphorylation. Termination of MAP kinase signaling is mediated by a several phosphatases that dephosphorylate 2 critical amino acids that are targeted by upstream activating kinases. One of these phosphatases is MAP kinase phosphatase (MKP) 1 (HUGO gene name, dual-specificity phosphatase 1 [*DUSP1*]), for which extracellular-signal-regulated kinase, p38 MAP kinase and *c-jun*-N-terminal kinase (JNK), are substrates.[72] In humans and other species, *MKP-1* is profoundly induced

by glucocorticoids through the activation of a glucocorticoid-responsive region (located between −1380 and −1266bp of the *MKP-1* promoter)[73] and is implicated in the repression of several proinflammatory genes.[74–76] MKP-1 can prevent the activation of key proinflammatory transcription factors (eg, NF-κB, AP-1)[77,78] and also promote the destabilization of proinflammatory gene mRNAs.[74,79] In vivo, the ability of glucocorticoids to repress proinflammatory gene expression is impaired in *mkp-1*–deficient mice.[80] Acetylcholine-induced airways hyper-responsiveness in mice exposed to ozone is normalized by dexamethasone through the upregulation of *mkp-1*.[81]

In human bronchial epithelial cells and airway myocytes, *MKP-1* is also induced by cAMP-increasing agents, including LABAs and PDE4 inhibitors, by activating the canonical cAMP/PKA signaling cascade.[41,73,82] The human *MKP-1* promoter contains 2 *cis*-acting cAMP response elements[83] that can be activated by the transcription factor, CREB.[84] Moreover, a LABA and a glucocorticoid in combination have been shown to activate a human *MKP-1* promoter construct in an additive manner, indicating that these are transcriptionally regulated events.[73,82]

The mucus hypersecretion that can often occur in COPD is thought to be caused by overexpression of *MUC5AC*, which encodes a major gel-forming mucin.[85,86] Acute, bacteria-induced exacerbations of COPD are associated, maybe causally, with enhanced mucus production.[87] It has been shown recently that PDE4 inhibitors, by selectively targeting the PDE4B subtype, can attenuate *Streptococcus pneumoniae*–induced *MUC5AC* gene expression in human airway epithelial cells in vitro and in an in vivo murine model of otitis media by enhancing the expression of MKP-1.[75] This effect is thought to be transcriptional, because similar data were obtained with a MUC5AC luciferase reporter.[75] It is possible that some form of additional upregulation of MKP-1 could be produced when a PDE4 inhibitor is added on to a glucocorticoid alone or in combination with a LABA.

Glucocorticoid-induced Leucine Zipper

Glucocorticoid-induced leucine zipper (GILZ) is typically described as a very highly glucocorticoid-inducible gene.[88] Expression levels can increase dramatically in a range of cell types relevant to airways inflammatory disorders including bronchial epithelial cells, mast cells, airway myocytes, and T lymphocytes.[40,41,89,90] GILZ blocks the activity of certain key proinflammatory transcription factors including NF-κB and

AP-1.[89] There are 2 principal ways that inhibition may occur. One process involves the physical interaction of GILZ with NF-κB and AP-1 in the nucleus to inhibit their ability to promote transcription,[89,91,92] whereas other studies show that GILZ is localized to the cytoplasm[40] where it may suppress MAP kinase signaling.[93] Whichever mechanism applies, it is clear that GILZ can inhibit the expression of proinflammatory genes such as interleukin (IL)-8.[94]

Neither LABAs nor PDE4 inhibitors induce *GILZ* and their ability to enhance glucocorticoid-induced GILZ expression is modest compared with many of the other genes described here. However, in certain cells, such as human primary airway epithelia, synergy has been reported with formoterol and a high concentration of roflumilast.[46]

Regulator of G-protein Signaling 2

Regulators of G-protein signaling (RGS) represent a large group of GTPase-activating proteins that act as critical, negative modulators of GPCRs. By enhancing the intrinsic GTPase activity of active G proteins, RGSs promote guanosine 5′-monophosphate (GTP) hydrolysis and return the GPCR-G-protein complex to the resting state. RGS2 is selective for Gq[95] and inactivates receptors that typically mediate airway smooth muscle contraction. In mice lacking *rgs2*, the muscarinic M$_3$-receptor agonist, methacholine, produces exaggerated contractile responses of tracheal smooth muscle, whereas in vivo such animals display airways hyper-reactivity.[96] In human ASM cells, LABAs, including formoterol and salmeterol, induce *RGS2*. The magnitude of this effect is enhanced and the kinetics significantly protracted in the presence of a glucocorticoid, affording a long-lasting protection of the muscle against constrictor stimuli.[96] Similar data have been found in human airway epithelial cells in which RGS2 up-regulation could suppress proinflammatory responses mediated through Gq-linked GPCRs. RGS2 is reported to attenuate *MUC5AC* expression in human airway epithelial cells following activation of GPR68, a proton-sensing Gq-linked receptor that is more commonly known as ovarian cancer G-protein–coupled receptor-1.[97] Of particular interest is the finding that the PDE4 inhibitor, roflumilast, further enhanced the expression of RGS2 in these cells to a level greater than that produced by a combination of fluticasone propionate and formoterol.[46] If this also occurs in airways smooth muscle, the degree and/or duration of bronchoprotection afforded by ICS/LABA combination therapy could be extended further.

Cluster of Differentiation 200

Cluster of differentiation (CD) 200 is a transmembrane glycoprotein expressed on a variety of cells of both hematopoietic and nonhematopoietic origin (eg, neutrophils, airway epithelia, alveolar macrophages, mast cells, dendritic cells, lymphocytes). The receptor for CD200, CD200R, has a more restricted expression profile, being found primarily on myeloid and lymphoid cells. Together, CD200 and CD200R form an inhibitory ligand-receptor pair that results in a unidirectional, downregulation of proinflammatory responses in CD200R-bearing cells. In mice infected with influenza virus, the CD200/CD200R interaction blunts the activation of alveolar macrophages (which have high constitutive expression of CD200R compared with their systemic counterparts) as measured by proinflammatory cytokine generation.[98] Because acute exacerbations of COPD are triggered, primarily, by acute bouts of excessive inflammation in response to bacterial and viral infections, upregulation of *CD200* on epithelial and other airway cells could, by this mechanism, help reduce exacerbation frequency.[98] In this context, *CD200* is modestly induced on human airway epithelial cells by the glucocorticoid, fluticasone propionate. However, this effect is significantly enhanced by formoterol alone and, even more dramatically, in combination with roflumilast.[46]

Cysteine-rich Secretory Protein Limulus Clotting Factor C, Cochlin, Lgl1 Domain-containing 2

A similar function to CD200 may be attributed to CRISPLD2 (cysteine-rich secretory protein limulus clotting factor C, cochlin, Lgl1 domain-containing 2), which can function as a secreted lipopolysaccharide-binding protein in mice and humans.[99] The expression of this gene could also help reduce COPD exacerbations in response to infections with gram-negative bacteria by downregulating Toll-like receptor-4 (TLR4)–mediated proinflammatory responses. *CRISPLD2* was originally identified as a glucocorticoid-induced gene in rat lung[100] and, subsequently, shown to be upregulated in human airway epithelial cells by both fluticasone propionate and formoterol, which interact in a synergistic manner.[46] Moreover, although roflumilast at clinically relevant concentrations failed to increase *CRISPLD2* mRNA levels, it potentiated the induction produced by fluticasone propionate and formoterol in combination. CRISPLD2 also plays a critical role in branching morphogenesis in fetal lung and in the development of alveolae.[100] Whether these functions are pertinent in adults with emphysema is unclear.

p57[kip2]

An inhibitor of certain G1 cyclin/cyclin-dependent kinase complexes, p57[kip2] (kinase inhibitor protein 2 of 57 kDa; HUGO gene name, cyclin-dependent kinase inhibitor 1C [*CDKN1C*]), was originally reported to be involved in the antiproliferative actions of glucocorticoids in HeLa cells.[101] The findings that glucocorticoids induce *p57*[kip2] in airways smooth muscle and human bronchial epithelial cells[41] suggests that it may subserve a similar function in other tissues. In the context of COPD, the expression of *p57*[kip2] in airway structural cells could arrest mitogenesis and suppress airways remodeling, which is a characteristic feature of COPD.[102] In bovine airway myocytes, the combination of low concentrations of fluticasone propionate and formoterol inhibits the induction of a proliferative, hypocontractile phenotype produced by platelet-derived growth factor.[102] The findings that glucocorticoid-induced p57[kip2] expression is enhanced by formoterol alone, and more impressively by formoterol and roflumilast in combination, raises the possibility that an even greater effect could be produced with an ICS/LABA/PDE4 inhibitor triple combination therapy.[46,102] In addition, p57[kip2] may also block proinflammatory responses through its ability to inhibit JNK, one of the core MAP kinases.[103]

Suppressor of Cytokine Signaling 3

Suppressors of cytokine signaling (SOCS) are a family of 8 related proteins that terminate signals emanating from the interaction of proinflammatory mediators with IL-6Rα, IL-12Rβ2, and receptors for interferon-γ, granulocyte colony–stimulating factor, and leptin.[104] In vascular endothelial cells, *SOCS3* is a cAMP-inducible gene that is regulated independently of PKA by mechanisms that involve, minimally, cAMP-guanine nucleotide exchange factor-1 and downstream small GTPases, Rap1 and Ras.[105] The expression of *SOCS3* is also upregulated by cAMP-increasing agents in human airway epithelial cells[47,106] and synergy has been reported with a LABA (salmeterol) and a glucocorticoid (fluticasone propionate) in combination.[106] Moreover, in airway epithelial cells exposed to tobacco smoke, basal *SOCS3* expression was significantly downregulated and this was rescued by fluticasone propionate and salmeterol in combination.[106] Additivity or further synergy might be predicted in the presence of a PDE4 inhibitor. Given that IL-6 and leptin are increased in COPD and may correlate with disease severity,[107,108] the expression of SOCS3 by an ICS/LABA/PDE4 inhibitor triple combination therapy could help attenuate proinflammatory signals mediated by their cognate receptors.

Cylindromatosis

Polyubiquitination is an enzymatic process whereby ubiquitin molecules are added sequentially to susceptible protein substrates through the formation of covalent, intermolecular glycine-lysine (K) bonds.[109] Ubiquitin chains linked via K48 typically mark a given protein for proteosomal degradation. However, linkage via other lysines (eg, K63) facilitates several nondegradative processes[109] including the activation of the proinflammatory transcription factor, NF-κB,[110] and of JNK signaling cascades.[111] There is evidence that several upstream, K63-linked ubiquitinated proteins including tumor necrosis factor receptor-associated factor (TRAF) 6 and NF-κB essential modulator (NEMO) are required for an active NF-κB signaling complex to form.[112,113] Ubiquitination is a reversible process and the opposite reaction is catalyzed by a large group deubiquitinases that deconjugate protein-bound ubiquitin chains. A novel deubiquitinase, cylindromatosis (CYLD), was recently identified as an inducible, negative regulator of NF-κB through its ability to cleave ubiquitin molecules from several substrates including TRAF6 and NEMO and so prevent the formation of an active NF-κB signaling complex.[112,113] In the context of COPD exacerbations, several reports have documented that CYLD is upregulated by both gram-positive (eg, *S pneumoniae*) and gram-negative (eg, nontypeable *Haemophilus influenzae* [NTHi], *Escherichia coli*) bacteria to repress inflammation,[114] which may represent an autoinhibitory (protective) mechanism to oppose the deleterious effects of TLR4 activation.[115,116] Moreover, Komatsu and colleagues[117] reported in 2013 that inhibition of PDE4, specifically the PDE4B isoform, augments the induction of *CYLD* in human airway epithelial cells in response to NTHi and in the lungs of NTHi-infected mice. By using siRNA technology and *cyld*[−/−] mice, the same investigators showed that the PDE4 inhibitors, rolipram and roflumilast, suppressed proinflammatory cytokine generation in vitro and indices of pulmonary inflammation in vivo by a CYLD-dependent mechanism.[117] The sensitivity of *CYLD* to LABAs has not been investigated, but similar results in β2-adrenoceptor-expressing cells might be expected and for there to be some form of positive interaction with a PDE4 inhibitor. It is not known whether *CYLD* is a glucocorticoid-inducible gene.

Tristetraprolin

Posttranscriptional mechanisms are central to regulating gene expression. In this respect, the mRNA destabilizing protein, tristetraprolin

(TTP; HUGO gene name, zinc finger protein 36 homologue [*ZFP36*]), by binding to regulatory sequences in the 3'-untranslated regions of target mRNAs, provides feedback control of many inflammatory genes, including *TNF, IL1B, IL8,* and *CSF2*.[118] Thus, although *TTP* is primarily induced by inflammatory stimuli,[119] it is also upregulated by glucocorticoids to exert repression.[47,120,121] In addition, *TTP* is induced by β_2-adrenceptor agonists, PDE inhibitors (including inhibitors of PDE4), and other cAMP-increasing agents.[47,122] Such data support the beneficial effects of the cAMP and glucocorticoid pathways on TTP expression, but no obvious combinatorial effect was noted in BEAS-2B human bronchial epithelial cells treated with LABAs and glucocorticoid,[41] although additivity was reported when the same cells were exposed to glucocorticoid and the adenosine A_{2B}-receptor agonist, Bay 60–6583.[47]

GENE TRANSACTIVATION AND GLUCOCORTICOID RESISTANCE

The concept of gene transactivation as a mechanism of action of glucocorticoids also has relevance to the clinical phenomenon of reduced glucocorticoid responsiveness (variably reported as resistance, tolerance, insensitivity, or subsensitivity) such as that seen in COPD. Compelling evidence is available that the ability of glucocorticoids to induce transcriptional responses is impaired by a variety of proinflammatory stimuli including tobacco smoke extract, cytokines, growth factors, and viruses (both respiratory syncytial virus and human rhinovirus).[123–126] The expression of *GILZ, p57*^kip2, and *RGS2*, which may exert antiinflammatory, antiproliferative, and bronchoprotective effects respectively (vide supra), is inhibited by one or more of these proinflammatory insults.[123–127] The finding that LABAs can functionally rescue cells and tissues from this form of glucocorticoid subsensitivity[96,123] provides an attractive mechanism to explain the superior clinical benefit of ICS/LABA combination therapies. A PDE4 inhibitor, as part of a triple combination therapy, could further boost the transactivation potential of a glucocorticoid alone and in combination with a LABA in addition to any effect it might produce by itself.

A NOTE ON cAMP-INDUCED, ADVERSE-EFFECT GENES

A clinical concern of β_2-adrenoceptor agonists as monotherapies is their ability to upregulate the expression of a variety of proinflammatory signaling molecules including IL-6, IL-6R, IL-8,

IL-11, IL-15, and IL-20Rβ (authors' unpublished observations).[128] In asthmatic patients, this is an important issue because regular administration of β_2-adrenoceptor agonists is reported to promote pulmonary eosinophilia.[129,130] Whether this proinflammatory liability is also realized in patients with COPD is, currently, vague but should not be ignored. It is intuitive that the upregulation of adverse-effect genes could be replicated by a PDE4 inhibitor and be more pronounced if the PDE4 inhibitor is combined with a LABA because of their potential to synergize. Although this possibility needs to be carefully evaluated, it may not be problematic in the context of a triple combination therapy because a large number of these cAMP-inducible genes are repressed by glucocorticoids.[37,128] Unwanted actions of LABAs may also be mediated by Gsβγ heterodimers or through promiscuous coupling of the β_2-adrenoceptor to Gi.[131] At present, there is little evidence for such signal transduction in native systems (but see Refs.[132,133]) and, regardless, PDE4 inhibitors are not expected to potentiate responses mediated by these alternative signaling cascades.

SUMMARY AND FUTURE DIRECTIONS

Current international guidelines recommend that roflumilast be added on to an ICS/LABA combination therapy in high-risk patients with severe, bronchitic COPD who have frequent acute exacerbations. Evidence is presented here that a glucocorticoid, LABA, and PDE4 inhibitor in combination can interact in a complex manner to induce a panel of genes that could act collectively to suppress inflammation and improve lung function. Central to this concept is that this drug combination produces a unique gene induction fingerprint that is not reproduced by any components of the triple therapy alone. The clinical efficacy of roflumilast, when combined with an ICS and a LABA, is therefore attributable, in part, to the individual, additive, and often cooperative actions of these drugs on gene transcription.[134] In this respect, the results of the ongoing REACT study[30] are awaited with anticipation.

At present, side effects remain a continuing problem with PDE4 inhibitors, including roflumilast.[20,22] However, several strategies may result in the discovery of compounds with improved therapeutic ratios. These strategies include the selective targeting of certain PDE4 subtypes and the development of allosteric PDE4 inhibitors.[135,136] The possibility that multivalent (multifunctional) ligands, which feature 2 or more pharmacophores, may deliver superior efficacy is also an approach that is being explored. Single molecules that inhibit PDE4 and activate β_2-adrenoceptors at similar concentrations have been described.[137,138] These drugs would not have the potential disadvantage of an inhaled combination therapy in which unequal deposition of each component is always possible.

ACKNOWLEDGMENTS

We thank our colleague, Dr Richard Leigh, Department of Medicine, University of Calgary, for constructive comments on this article.

REFERENCES

1. Pauwels RA, Buist AS, Calverley PM, et al. Global strategy for the diagnosis, management, and prevention of chronic obstructive pulmonary disease. NHLBI/WHO Global Initiative for Chronic Obstructive Lung Disease (GOLD) workshop summary. Am J Respir Crit Care Med 2001;163:1256–76.
2. Hogg JC. Pathophysiology of airflow limitation in chronic obstructive pulmonary disease. Lancet 2004;364:709–21.
3. Hogg JC, Chu F, Utokaparch S, et al. The nature of small-airway obstruction in chronic obstructive pulmonary disease. N Engl J Med 2004;350:2645–53.
4. Laumbach RJ, Kipen HM. Respiratory health effects of air pollution: update on biomass smoke and traffic pollution. J Allergy Clin Immunol 2012;129:3–11.
5. Walter R, Gottlieb DJ, O'Connor GT. Environmental and genetic risk factors and gene-environment interactions in the pathogenesis of chronic obstructive lung disease. Environ Health Perspect 2000;108(Suppl 4):733–42.
6. Kleeberger SR, Cho HY. Gene-environment interactions in environmental lung diseases. Novartis Found Symp 2008;293:168–78.
7. Caramori G, Adcock I. Gene-environment interactions in the development of chronic obstructive pulmonary disease. Curr Opin Allergy Clin Immunol 2006;6:323–8.
8. Kleeberger SR, Peden D. Gene-environment interactions in asthma and other respiratory diseases. Annu Rev Med 2005;56:383–400.
9. Rennard SI, Vestbo J. The many "small COPDs": COPD should be an orphan disease. Chest 2008;134:623–7.
10. Miravitlles M, Soler-Cataluna JJ, Calle M, et al. A new approach to grading and treating COPD based on clinical phenotypes: summary of the Spanish COPD guidelines (GesEPOC). Prim Care Respir J 2013;22:117–21.
11. Miravitlles M, Jose Soler-Cataluna J, Calle M, et al. Treatment of COPD by clinical phenotypes. Putting old evidence into clinical practice. Eur Respir J 2013;41(6):1252–6.
12. Perera WR, Hurst JR, Wilkinson TM, et al. Inflammatory changes, recovery and recurrence at COPD exacerbation. Eur Respir J 2007;29:527–34.
13. Calverley PM, Rabe KF, Goehring UM, et al. Roflumilast in symptomatic chronic obstructive pulmonary disease: two randomised clinical trials. Lancet 2009;374:685–94.
14. Wedzicha1 JA, Rabe KF, Martinez FJ, et al. Efficacy of roflumilast in the chronic obstructive pulmonary disease frequent exacerbator phenotype. Chest 2012;143(5):1302–11.
15. Butcher RW, Sutherland EW. Adenosine 3',5'-phosphate in biological materials. I. Purification and properties of cyclic 3',5'-nucleotide phosphodiesterase and use of this enzyme to characterize adenosine 3',5'-phosphate in human urine. J Biol Chem 1962;237:1244–50.
16. Bender AT, Beavo JA. Cyclic nucleotide phosphodiesterases: molecular regulation to clinical use. Pharmacol Rev 2006;58:488–520.
17. Dastidar SG, Rajagopal D, Ray A. Therapeutic benefit of PDE4 inhibitors in inflammatory diseases. Curr Opin Investig Drugs 2007;8:364–72.
18. Hatzelmann A, Morcillo EJ, Lungarella G, et al. The preclinical pharmacology of roflumilast - a selective, oral phosphodiesterase 4 inhibitor in development for chronic obstructive pulmonary disease. Pulm Pharmacol Ther 2010;23:235–56.
19. Torphy TJ. Phosphodiesterase isozymes: molecular targets for novel antiasthma agents. Am J Respir Crit Care Med 1998;157:351–70.
20. Oba Y, Lone NA. Efficacy and safety of roflumilast in patients with chronic obstructive pulmonary disease: a systematic review and meta-analysis. Ther Adv Respir Dis 2013;7:13–24.
21. Giembycz MA. Life after PDE4: overcoming adverse events with dual-specificity phosphodiesterase inhibitors. Curr Opin Pharmacol 2005;5:238–44.
22. Giembycz MA. An update and appraisal of the cilomilast phase III clinical development programme for chronic obstructive pulmonary disease. Br J Clin Pharmacol 2006;62:138–52.
23. Giembycz MA, Field SK. Roflumilast: first phosphodiesterase 4 inhibitor approved for treatment of COPD. Drug Des Devel Ther 2010;4:147–58.
24. Gross NJ, Giembycz MA, Rennard SI. Treatment of chronic obstructive pulmonary disease with roflumilast - a new phosphodiesterase 4 inhibitor. COPD 2010;7:141–53.
25. Field SK. Roflumilast, a novel phosphodiesterase 4 inhibitor, for COPD patients with a history of exacerbations. Clin Med Insights Circ Respir Pulm Med 2011;5:57–70.
26. Cazzola M, Picciolo S, Matera MG. Roflumilast in chronic obstructive pulmonary disease: evidence from large trials. Expert Opin Pharmacother 2010;11:441–9.

27. Antoniu SA. New therapeutic options in the management of COPD - focus on roflumilast. Int J Chron Obstruct Pulmon Dis 2011;6:147–55.

28. Rennard SI, Calverley PM, Goehring UM, et al. Reduction of exacerbations by the PDE4 inhibitor roflumilast–the importance of defining different subsets of patients with COPD. Respir Res 2011; 12:18.

29. Nannini LJ, Lasserson TJ, Poole P. Combined corticosteroid and long-acting β_2-agonist in one inhaler versus long-acting β_2-agonists for chronic obstructive pulmonary disease. Cochrane Database Syst Rev 2012;(9):CD006829.

30. Calverley PM, Martinez FJ, Fabbri LM, et al. Does roflumilast decrease exacerbations in severe COPD patients not controlled by inhaled combination therapy? The REACT study protocol. Int J Chron Obstruct Pulmon Dis 2012;7:375–82.

31. O'Donnell DE, Aaron S, Bourbeau J, et al. Canadian Thoracic Society recommendations for management of chronic obstructive pulmonary disease - 2007 update. Can Respir J 2007; 14(Suppl B):5B–32B.

32. Brassard P, Suissa S, Kezouh A, et al. Inhaled corticosteroids and risk of tuberculosis in patients with respiratory diseases. Am J Respir Crit Care Med 2011;183:675–8.

33. Ernst P, Gonzalez AV, Brassard P, et al. Inhaled corticosteroid use in chronic obstructive pulmonary disease and the risk of hospitalization for pneumonia. Am J Respir Crit Care Med 2007;176:162–6.

34. Newton R, Leigh R, Giembycz MA. Pharmacological strategies for improving the efficacy and therapeutic ratio of glucocorticoids in inflammatory lung diseases. Pharmacol Ther 2010;125:286–327.

35. Surjit M, Ganti KP, Mukherji A, et al. Widespread negative response elements mediate direct repression by agonist-liganded glucocorticoid receptor. Cell 2011;145:224–41.

36. Clark AR. Anti-inflammatory functions of glucocorticoid-induced genes. Mol Cell Endocrinol 2007;275:79–97.

37. King EM, Chivers JE, Rider CF, et al. Glucocorticoid repression of inflammatory gene expression shows differential responsiveness by transactivation- and transrepression-dependent mechanisms. PLoS One 2013;8:e53936.

38. Scheinman RI, Cogswell PC, Lofquist AK, et al. Role of transcriptional activation of IκBα in mediation of immunosuppression by glucocorticoids. Science 1995;270:283–6.

39. Auphan N, DiDonato JA, Rosette C, et al. Immunosuppression by glucocorticoids: inhibition of NF-κB activity through induction of IκB synthesis. Science 1995;270:286–90.

40. Kelly MM, King EM, Rider CF, et al. Corticosteroid-induced gene expression in allergen-challenged asthmatic subjects taking inhaled budesonide. Br J Pharmacol 2012;165:1737–47.

41. Kaur M, Chivers JE, Giembycz MA, et al. Long-acting β_2-adrenoceptor agonists synergistically enhance glucocorticoid-dependent transcription in human airway epithelial and smooth muscle cells. Mol Pharmacol 2008;73:201–14.

42. Roth M, Johnson PR, Rudiger JJ, et al. Interaction between glucocorticoids and β_2 agonists on bronchial airway smooth muscle cells through synchronised cellular signalling. Lancet 2002;360:1293–9.

43. Rangarajan PN, Umesono K, Evans RM. Modulation of glucocorticoid receptor function by protein kinase A. Mol Endocrinol 1992;6:1451–7.

44. Miller AH, Vogt GJ, Pearce BD. The phosphodiesterase type 4 inhibitor, rolipram, enhances glucocorticoid receptor function. Neuropsychopharmacology 2002;27:939–48.

45. Wilson SM, Shen P, Rider CF, et al. Selective prostacyclin receptor agonism augments glucocorticoid-induced gene expression in human bronchial epithelial cells. J Immunol 2009;183: 6788–99.

46. Moodley T, Wilson SM, Joshi T, et al. Phosphodiesterase 4 inhibitors augment the ability of formoterol to enhance glucocorticoid-dependent gene transcription in human airway epithelial cells: a novel mechanism for the clinical efficacy of roflumilast in severe COPD. Mol Pharmacol 2013;83:894–906.

47. Greer S, Page CW, Joshi T, et al. Concurrent agonism of adenosine A$_{2B}$- and glucocorticoid receptors in human airway epithelial cells cooperatively induces genes with anti-inflammatory potential: a novel approach to treat COPD. J Pharmacol Exp Ther 2013;346(3):473–85.

48. Ducharme FM, Ni CM, Greenstone I, et al. Addition of long-acting β_2-agonists to inhaled corticosteroids versus same dose inhaled corticosteroids for chronic asthma in adults and children. Cochrane Database Syst Rev 2010;(5):CD005535.

49. Frois C, Wu EQ, Ray S, et al. Inhaled corticosteroids or long-acting β-agonists alone or in fixed-dose combinations in asthma treatment: a systematic review of fluticasone/budesonide and formoterol/salmeterol. Clin Ther 2009;31:2779–803.

50. Pauwels RA, Lofdahl CG, Postma DS, et al. Effect of inhaled formoterol and budesonide on exacerbations of asthma. Formoterol and Corticosteroids Establishing Therapy (FACET) International Study Group. N Engl J Med 1997;337:1405–11.

51. Shrewsbury S, Pyke S, Britton M. Meta-analysis of increased dose of inhaled steroid or addition of salmeterol in symptomatic asthma (MIASMA). BMJ 2000;320:1368–73.

52. Plint AC, Johnson DW, Patel H, et al. Epinephrine and dexamethasone in children with bronchiolitis. N Engl J Med 2009;360:2079–89.

53. Kuyucu S, Unal S, Kuyucu N, et al. Additive effects of dexamethasone in nebulized salbutamol or L-epinephrine treated infants with acute bronchiolitis. Pediatr Int 2004;46:539–44.

54. Su AI, Wiltshire T, Batalov S, et al. A gene atlas of the mouse and human protein-encoding transcriptomes. Proc Natl Acad Sci U S A 2004; 101:6062–7.

55. Pujols L, Mullol J, Roca-Ferrer J, et al. Expression of glucocorticoid receptor α- and β-isoforms in human cells and tissues. Am J Physiol Cell Physiol 2002;283:C1324–31.

56. Plumb J, Gaffey K, Kane B, et al. Reduced glucocorticoid receptor expression and function in airway neutrophils. Int Immunopharmacol 2012; 12:26–33.

57. Miller AH, Spencer RL, Pearce BD, et al. Glucocorticoid receptors are differentially expressed in the cells and tissues of the immune system. Cell Immunol 1998;186:45–54.

58. Adcock IM, Gilbey T, Gelder CM, et al. Glucocorticoid receptor localization in normal and asthmatic lung. Am J Respir Crit Care Med 1996;154:771–82.

59. Schleimer RP. Effects of glucocorticosteroids on inflammatory cells relevant to their therapeutic applications in asthma. Am Rev Respir Dis 1990;141: S59–69.

60. Johnson M. Effects of β2-agonists on resident and infiltrating inflammatory cells. J Allergy Clin Immunol 2002;110:S282–90.

61. Penn RB, Kelsen SG, Benovic JL. Regulation of β-agonist- and prostaglandin E2-mediated adenylyl cyclase activity in human airway epithelial cells. Am J Respir Cell Mol Biol 1994;11:496–505.

62. Kelsen SG, Higgins NC, Zhou S, et al. Expression and function of the β-adrenergic receptor coupled-adenylyl cyclase system on human airway epithelial cells. Am J Respir Crit Care Med 1995; 152:1774–83.

63. Liggett SB. Identification and characterization of a homogeneous population of β2-adrenergic receptors on human alveolar macrophages. Am Rev Respir Dis 1989;139:552–5.

64. Yukawa T, Ukena D, Kroegel C, et al. β2-Adrenergic receptors on eosinophils. Binding and functional studies. Am Rev Respir Dis 1990;141:1446–52.

65. Galant SP, Underwood S, Duriseti L, et al. Characterization of high-affinity β2-adrenergic receptor binding of (-)-[³H]-dihydroalprenolol to human polymorphonuclear cell particulates. J Lab Clin Med 1978;92:613–8.

66. Martinsson A, Larsson K, Hjemdahl P. Studies in vivo and in vitro of terbutaline-induced β-adrenoceptor desensitization in healthy subjects. Clin Sci (Lond) 1987;72:47–54.

67. Furchgott RF. The use of β-haloalkylamines in the differentiation of receptors and in the determination of dissociation constants of receptor-agonist complexes. Adv Drug Res 1966;3:21–55.

68. Rabe KF, Giembycz MA, Dent G, et al. Salmeterol is a competitive antagonist at β-adrenoceptors mediating inhibition of respiratory burst in guinea-pig eosinophils. Eur J Pharmacol 1993;231:305–8.

69. Munoz NM, Rabe KF, Vita AJ, et al. Paradoxical blockade of β-adrenergically-mediated inhibition of stimulated eosinophil secretion by salmeterol. J Pharmacol Exp Ther 1995;273:850–4.

70. Newton R. Molecular mechanisms of glucocorticoid action: what is important? Thorax 2000;55: 603–13.

71. Kyriakis JM, Avruch J. Mammalian mitogen-activated protein kinase signal transduction pathways activated by stress and inflammation. Physiol Rev 2001;81:807–69.

72. Clark AR, Martins JR, Tchen CR. Role of dual specificity phosphatases in biological responses to glucocorticoids. J Biol Chem 2008;283:25765–9.

73. Manetsch M, Ramsay EE, King EM, et al. Corticosteroids and β2-agonists upregulate mitogen-activated protein kinase phosphatase 1: in vitro mechanisms. Br J Pharmacol 2012;166:2049–59.

74. Quante T, Ng YC, Ramsay EE, et al. Corticosteroids reduce IL-6 in ASM cells via up-regulation of MKP-1. Am J Respir Cell Mol Biol 2008;39:208–17.

75. Lee J, Komatsu K, Lee BC, et al. Phosphodiesterase 4B mediates extracellular signal-regulated kinase-dependent up-regulation of mucin MUC5AC protein by Streptococcus pneumoniae by inhibiting cAMP-protein kinase A-dependent MKP-1 phosphatase pathway. J Biol Chem 2012; 287:22799–811.

76. Issa R, Xie S, Khorasani N, et al. Corticosteroid inhibition of growth-related oncogene protein-alpha via mitogen-activated kinase phosphatase-1 in airway smooth muscle cells. J Immunol 2007;178: 7366–75.

77. King EM, Holden NS, Gong W, et al. Inhibition of NF-κB-dependent transcription by MKP-1: transcriptional repression by glucocorticoids occurring via p38 MAPK. J Biol Chem 2009;284:26803–15.

78. Diefenbacher M, Sekula S, Heilbock C, et al. Restriction to Fos family members of Trip6-dependent coactivation and glucocorticoid receptor-dependent trans-repression of activator protein-1. Mol Endocrinol 2008;22:1767–80.

79. Lasa M, Abraham SM, Boucheron C, et al. Dexamethasone causes sustained expression of mitogen-activated protein kinase (MAPK) phosphatase 1 and phosphatase-mediated inhibition of MAPK p38. Mol Cell Biol 2002;22:7802–11.

80. Abraham SM, Lawrence T, Kleiman A, et al. Antiinflammatory effects of dexamethasone are partly dependent on induction of dual specificity phosphatase 1. J Exp Med 2006;203:1883–9.

81. Li F, Zhang M, Hussain F, et al. Inhibition of p38 MAPK-dependent bronchial contraction after ozone by corticosteroids. Eur Respir J 2011;37:933–42.

82. Manetsch M, Rahman MM, Patel BS, et al. Long-acting β_2-agonists increase fluticasone propionate-induced mitogen-activated protein kinase phosphatase 1 (MKP-1) in airway smooth muscle cells. PLoS One 2013;8:e59635.

83. Kwak SP, Hakes DJ, Martell KJ, et al. Isolation and characterization of a human dual specificity protein-tyrosine phosphatase gene. J Biol Chem 1994;269:3596–604.

84. Cho IJ, Woo NR, Shin IC, et al. H89, an inhibitor of PKA and MSK, inhibits cyclic-AMP response element binding protein-mediated MAPK phosphatase-1 induction by lipopolysaccharide. Inflamm Res 2009;58:863–72.

85. Innes AL, Woodruff PG, Ferrando RE, et al. Epithelial mucin stores are increased in the large airways of smokers with airflow obstruction. Chest 2006;130:1102–8.

86. Caramori G, Casolari P, Di Gregorio C, et al. MUC5AC expression is increased in bronchial submucosal glands of stable COPD patients. Histopathology 2009;55:321–31.

87. Dohrman A, Miyata S, Gallup M, et al. Mucin gene (MUC2 and MUC5AC) upregulation by Gram-positive and Gram-negative bacteria. Biochim Biophys Acta 1998;1406:251–9.

88. Ayroldi E, Riccardi C. Glucocorticoid-induced leucine zipper (GILZ): a new important mediator of glucocorticoid action. FASEB J 2009;23:3649–58.

89. Mittelstadt PR, Ashwell JD. Inhibition of AP-1 by the glucocorticoid-inducible protein GILZ. J Biol Chem 2001;276:29603–10.

90. Godot V, Garcia G, Capel F, et al. Dexamethasone and IL-10 stimulate glucocorticoid-induced leucine zipper synthesis by human mast cells. Allergy 2006;61:886–90.

91. Ayroldi E, Migliorati G, Bruscoli S, et al. Modulation of T-cell activation by the glucocorticoid-induced leucine zipper factor via inhibition of nuclear factor kappaB. Blood 2001;98:743–53.

92. Di Marco B, Massetti M, Bruscoli S, et al. Glucocorticoid-induced leucine zipper (GILZ)/NF-κB interaction: role of GILZ homo-dimerization and C-terminal domain. Nucleic Acids Res 2007;35:517–28.

93. Ayroldi E, Zollo O, Macchiarulo A, et al. Glucocorticoid-induced leucine zipper inhibits the Raf-extracellular signal-regulated kinase pathway by binding to Raf-1. Mol Cell Biol 2002;22:7929–41.

94. Eddleston J, Herschbach J, Wagelie-Steffen AL, et al. The anti-inflammatory effect of glucocorticoids is mediated by glucocorticoid-induced leucine zipper in epithelial cells. J Allergy Clin Immunol 2007;119:115–22.

95. Heximer SP, Watson N, Linder ME, et al. RGS2/G0S8 is a selective inhibitor of Gqα function. Proc Natl Acad Sci U S A 1997;94:14389–93.

96. Holden NS, Bell MJ, Rider CF, et al. β_2-Adrenoceptor agonist-induced RGS2 expression is a genomic mechanism of bronchoprotection that is enhanced by glucocorticoids. Proc Natl Acad Sci U S A 2011;108:19713–8.

97. Liu C, Li Q, Zhou X, et al. Regulator of G-protein signaling 2 inhibits acid-induced mucin5AC hypersecretion in human airway epithelial cells. Respir Physiol Neurobiol 2013;185:265–71.

98. Snelgrove RJ, Goulding J, Didierlaurent AM, et al. A critical function for CD200 in lung immune homeostasis and the severity of influenza infection. Nat Immunol 2008;9:1074–83.

99. Wang ZQ, Xing WM, Fan HH, et al. The novel lipopolysaccharide-binding protein CRISPLD2 is a critical serum protein to regulate endotoxin function. J Immunol 2009;183:6646–56.

100. Kaplan F, Ledoux P, Kassamali FQ, et al. A novel developmentally regulated gene in lung mesenchyme: homology to a tumor-derived trypsin inhibitor. Am J Physiol 1999;276:L1027–36.

101. Samuelsson MK, Pazirandeh A, Davani B, et al. p57^{kip2}, a glucocorticoid-induced inhibitor of cell cycle progression in HeLa cells. Mol Endocrinol 1999;13:1811–22.

102. Dekkers BG, Pehlic A, Mariani R, et al. Glucocorticosteroids and β_2-adrenoceptor agonists synergize to inhibit airway smooth muscle remodeling. J Pharmacol Exp Ther 2012;342:780–7.

103. Chang TS, Kim MJ, Ryoo K, et al. p57^{KIP2} modulates stress-activated signaling by inhibiting c-Jun NH$_2$-terminal kinase/stress-activated protein kinase. J Biol Chem 2003;278:48092–8.

104. Yoshimura A, Naka T, Kubo M. SOCS proteins, cytokine signalling and immune regulation. Nat Rev Immunol 2007;7:454–65.

105. Milne GR, Palmer TM, Yarwood SJ. Novel control of cAMP-regulated transcription in vascular endothelial cells. Biochem Soc Trans 2012;40:1–5.

106. Nasreen N, Khodayari N, Sukka-Ganesh B, et al. Fluticasone propionate and salmeterol combination induces SOCS-3 expression in airway epithelial cells. Int Immunopharmacol 2012;12:217–25.

107. Liang R, Zhang W, Song YM. Levels of leptin and IL-6 in lungs and blood are associated with the severity of chronic obstructive pulmonary disease in patients and rat models. Mol Med Rep 2013;7:1470–6.

108. Barnes PJ. The cytokine network in COPD. Am J Respir Cell Mol Biol 2009;41:631–8.

109. Hershko A, Ciechanover A. The ubiquitin system. Annu Rev Biochem 1998;67:425–79.

110. Jono H, Lim JH, Chen LF, et al. NF-kappaB is essential for induction of CYLD, the negative

regulator of NF-κB: evidence for a novel inducible autoregulatory feedback pathway. J Biol Chem 2004;279:36171–4.

111. Reiley W, Zhang M, Sun SC. Negative regulation of JNK signaling by the tumor suppressor CYLD. J Biol Chem 2004;279:55161–7.

112. Lim JH, Jono H, Komatsu K, et al. CYLD negatively regulates transforming growth factor-β-signalling via deubiquitinating Akt. Nat Commun 2012;3:771.

113. Sun SC. CYLD: a tumor suppressor deubiquitinase regulating NF-κB activation and diverse biological processes. Cell Death Differ 2010;17:25–34.

114. Lim JH, Ha UH, Woo CH, et al. CYLD is a crucial negative regulator of innate immune response in *Escherichia coli* pneumonia. Cell Microbiol 2008; 10:2247–56.

115. Lim JH, Jono H, Koga T, et al. Tumor suppressor CYLD acts as a negative regulator for non-typeable *Haemophilus influenza*-induced inflammation in the middle ear and lung of mice. PLoS One 2007;2:e1032.

116. Lim JH, Stirling B, Derry J, et al. Tumor suppressor CYLD regulates acute lung injury in lethal *Streptococcus pneumoniae* infections. Immunity 2007;27: 349–60.

117. Komatsu K, Lee JY, Miyata M, et al. Inhibition of PDE4B suppresses inflammation by increasing expression of the deubiquitinase CYLD. Nat Commun 2013;4:1684.

118. Anderson P. Post-transcriptional control of cytokine production. Nat Immunol 2008;9:353–9.

119. King EM, Kaur M, Gong W, et al. Regulation of tristetraprolin expression by interleukin-1β and dexamethasone in human pulmonary epithelial cells: roles for nuclear factor-κB and p38 mitogen-activated protein kinase. J Pharmacol Exp Ther 2009;330:575–85.

120. Smoak K, Cidlowski JA. Glucocorticoids regulate tristetraprolin synthesis and post-transcriptionally regulate tumor necrosis factor α inflammatory signaling. Mol Cell Biol 2006;26:9126–35.

121. Ishmael FT, Fang X, Galdiero MR, et al. Role of the RNA-binding protein tristetraprolin in glucocorticoid-mediated gene regulation. J Immunol 2008;180: 8342–53.

122. Jalonen U, Leppanen T, Kankaanranta H, et al. Salbutamol increases tristetraprolin expression in macrophages. Life Sci 2007;81:1651–8.

123. Rider CF, King EM, Holden NS, et al. Inflammatory stimuli inhibit glucocorticoid-dependent transactivation in human pulmonary epithelial cells: rescue by long-acting β2-adrenoceptor agonists. J Pharmacol Exp Ther 2011;338:860–9.

124. Salem S, Harris T, Mok JS, et al. Transforming growth factor-β impairs glucocorticoid activity in the A549 lung adenocarcinoma cell line. Br J Pharmacol 2012;166:2036–48.

125. Hinzey A, Alexander J, Corry J, et al. Respiratory syncytial virus represses glucocorticoid receptor-mediated gene activation. Endocrinology 2011; 152:483–94.

126. Rider CF, Miller-Larsson A, Proud D, et al. Modulation of transcriptional responses by poly(I:C) and human rhinovirus: effect of long-acting β2-adrenoceptor agonists. Eur J Pharmacol 2013;708:60–7.

127. Xie Y, Jiang H, Nguyen H, et al. Regulator of G protein signaling 2 is a key modulator of airway hyperresponsiveness. J Allergy Clin Immunol 2012;130:968–76.

128. Holden NS, Rider CF, Bell MJ, et al. Enhancement of inflammatory mediator release by β2-adrenoceptor agonists in airway epithelial cells is reversed by glucocorticoid action. Br J Pharmacol 2010;160: 410–20.

129. Manolitsas ND, Wang J, Devalia JL, et al. Regular albuterol, nedocromil sodium, and bronchial inflammation in asthma. Am J Respir Crit Care Med 1995;151:1925–30.

130. Gauvreau GM, Jordana M, Watson RM, et al. Effect of regular inhaled albuterol on allergen-induced late responses and sputum eosinophils in asthmatic subjects. Am J Respir Crit Care Med 1997;156:1738–45.

131. Giembycz MA, Newton R. Beyond the dogma: novel β2-adrenoceptor signalling in the airways. Eur Respir J 2006;27:1286–306.

132. Lecuona E, Ridge K, Pesce L, et al. The GTP-binding protein RhoA mediates Na, K-ATPase exocytosis in alveolar epithelial cells. Mol Biol Cell 2003;14:3888–97.

133. Wang WC, Schillinger RM, Malone MM, et al. Paradoxical attenuation of β2-AR function in airway smooth muscle by Gi-mediated counterregulation in transgenic mice over-expressing type 5 adenylyl cyclase. Am J Physiol Lung Cell Mol Physiol 2011;300:L472–8.

134. Giembycz MA, Newton R. Harnessing the clinical efficacy of phosphodiesterase 4 inhibitors in inflammatory lung diseases: dual-selective phosphodiesterase inhibitors and novel combination therapies. Handb Exp Pharmacol 2011;204:415–46.

135. Giembycz MA. Can the anti-inflammatory potential of PDE4 inhibitors be realized: guarded optimism or wishful thinking? Br J Pharmacol 2008;155:288–90.

136. Burgin AB, Magnusson OT, Singh J, et al. Design of phosphodiesterase 4D (PDE4D) allosteric modulators for enhancing cognition with improved safety. Nat Biotechnol 2010;28:63–70.

137. Shan WJ, Huang L, Zhou Q, et al. Dual β2-adrenoceptor agonists-PDE4 inhibitors for the treatment of asthma and COPD. Bioorg Med Chem Lett 2012; 22:1523–6.

138. Liu A, Huang L, Wang Z, et al. Hybrids consisting of the pharmacophores of salmeterol and roflumilast or phthalazinone: dual β2-adrenoceptor agonists-PDE4 inhibitors for the treatment of COPD. Bioorg Med Chem Lett 2013;23:1548–52.

New Drug Therapies for COPD

Clare L. Ross, MRCP, Trevor T. Hansel, FRCPath, PhD*

KEYWORDS

- COPD • Pharmacology • Bronchodilators • Antiinflammatory drugs • Antioxidants
- Protease inhibitors • Fibrosis • Lung regeneration

KEY POINTS

- It is proving a major challenge to produce new effective drugs for chronic obstructive pulmonary disease (COPD).
- Improved understanding of COPD pathophysiology, novel clinical trial designs, endpoints, imaging and biomarkers, noninvasive sampling, patient stratification, challenge models, and clinical trial designs is necessary to facilitate development of new drugs for COPD.
- Smoking cessation is fundamental and new approaches include antinicotine vaccines, cannabinoid receptor antagonists, and dopamine D3 receptor antagonists.
- Novel combinations of inhaled bronchodilators and corticosteroids are being introduced.
- Antiinfective drugs are important, with a recent focus on the viruses that commonly cause exacerbations.
- Antiinflammatory drugs are in development, including kinase inhibitors, chemokine receptor antagonists, inhibitors of innate immune mechanisms, and statins.
- Biologics used in rheumatoid diseases may also have a role; anti-IL-6 (tocilizumab) is promising.
- Antioxidants, mucolytics, antiproteases, and antifibrotics are all under active development.
- Aids to lung regeneration have potential to alter the natural history of COPD, including retinoids and mesenchymal stem cell therapy.

INTRODUCTION

New drugs for chronic obstructive pulmonary disease (COPD) have been largely based on existing classes of current therapies, involving new inhaled combinations of long-acting muscarinic antagonists (LAMAs), long-acting beta2-agonists (LABAs), and inhaled corticosteroids (ICS) (**Table 1**).[1] A useful reference source for new COPD medicines in development is the Pharmaceutical Research and Manufacturers of America (www.phrma.org). There is also an excellent series of topical articles on "The COPD Pipeline" provided by Nicholas J. Gross in the journal *COPD* (22 articles as of mid-2012). Although recent increases in knowledge of the inflammatory components contributing to COPD

have led to many new targets for COPD treatment,[2] very few new classes of drugs are being licensed, making this a controversial area for new drug development.[3]

Clinical studies with new drugs for COPD have been difficult for several reasons[4]:

- The immunopathology of COPD is complex and variable (**Fig. 1**). Cigarette smoke has widespread effects beyond the respiratory system, involving the large airways (bronchitis), small airways (bronchiolitis), lung interstitium (emphysema and interstitial lung disease), pulmonary vasculature (pulmonary artery hypertension), and systemic complications.[5–7] Pathologic features such as mucus

Imperial Clinical Respiratory Research Unit (ICRRU), Biomedical Research Centre (BMRC), Centre for Respiratory Infection (CRI), National Heart and Lung Institute (NHLI), St Mary's Hospital, Imperial College, Praed Street, Paddington, London W2 INY, UK
* Corresponding author.
E-mail address: t.hansel@imperial.ac.uk

Clin Chest Med 35 (2014) 219–239
http://dx.doi.org/10.1016/j.ccm.2013.10.003
0272-5231/14/$ – see front matter © 2014 Elsevier Inc. All rights reserved.

Table 1
Drugs to aid smoking cessation

Current treatments	First-line: • Nicotine replacement therapy • Bupropion • Varenicline (partial agonist for α4β2 nicotinic acetylcholine receptors) Second-line: • Nortriptyline • Clonidine
New approaches	• Antinicotine vaccines: NicVAX, SEL-068 • Electronic cigarettes • Novel nicotine formulations: eg, inhaled aerosolized nicotine (ARD-1600) • Nicotine partial agonist: cytisine • Cannabinoid receptor 1 antagonists: taranabant • Dopamine D3 receptor antagonists: GSK598809 • Monoamine oxidase inhibitors: selegiline

hypersecretion, small airway fibrosis, and lung destruction (emphysema) are notoriously difficult to reverse with drugs.

- COPD may be caused by the innate immune response to oxidants and microbes, with accelerated aging and autoimmune features. Bacteria and viruses may become more important in more severe COPD.[8]
- Preclinical models need to be improved for in vitro and in vivo (animal) studies.[9]
- COPD patients are often elderly, frail, and have multiple diseases associated with smoking. Cardiovascular diseases, metabolic syndrome, and malignancies may be present. Hence, these patients may be on a variety of medications. These factors may mean that it is difficult to recruit patients when there are strict entry criteria.
- A new therapy is more likely to be effective when used early in the natural history of COPD, before irreversible disease has occurred. However, delays in diagnosis are common and the disease is notoriously underdiagnosed.
- Small proof-of-concept studies in humans are poorly predictive of efficacy in clinical practice. Some clinical development plans for COPD have been discontinued after large-scale clinical trials, including Viozan, recombinant DNase (Pulmozyme), and cilomilast (Ariflo).

- Challenge models looking at the effects of cigarette smoke,[10] ozone, or lipopolysaccharide have been developed. On the other hand, smoking cessation is part of COPD patient care, providing an interesting situation of withdrawal of the stimulus.[10–12] As a model of COPD exacerbations, live experimental challenge can be performed with human rhinovirus (HRV) in patients with COPD.[13] Novel large scale clinical trial designs for COPD are also needed.[14]
- There is a need to identify and validate endpoints that can capture the considerable heterogeneity of pulmonary and systemic features. Forced expiratory volume in 1 second (FEV_1) is a commonly used endpoint in most clinical COPD trials. However, recently, the Evaluation of COPD Longitudinally to Identify Predictive Surrogate Endpoints (ECLIPSE) study has demonstrated that the annual rate of change in FEV_1 in COPD is highly variable in different subjects.[15] In addition, given that the FEV_1 declines very slowly during the natural history of COPD, an estimated 1000 subjects per sample group must be followed for a minimum of 3 years to have sufficient power to detect a 50% improvement in disease progression.[16]
- Phenotypes of COPD need to be defined and validated in order to tailor drugs to individual patients; it is becoming increasing clear that "one size does not fit all" in COPD.[17] This was demonstrated clearly by recent trials such as the National Emphysema Treatment Trial (NETT), which showed a mortality benefit in only a subgroup of patients undergoing lung volume reduction surgery.[18] Of special interest are approaches that use CT.[7,19]
- Samples of varying invasiveness and from different compartments are required. Sputum gene expression looks promising,[20] although exhaled breath condensate has been disappointing,[21] and there are few studies with exhaled nitric oxide.[22] However, assessment by proteomics of epithelial lining fluid from the airway of COPD patients is feasible,[23] and bronchial brushings can be carried out to assess gene expression.[24]
- There is a need to identify and validate biomarkers that may predict potential responders for specific therapy.[25–27] Gene expression or transcriptomics of the airway in COPD is of special interest.[20,24]
- Current therapy is merely palliative; it is becoming clear that there must be more focus on preventative and regenerative therapies. However, these are ambitious targets for new drugs.

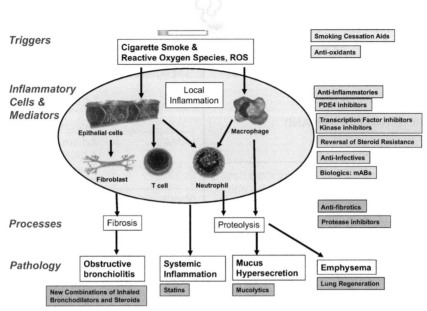

Fig. 1. Pathology, targets, and new drugs for COPD. An overview of some of the pathophysiologic processes involved in COPD, highlighting potential therapeutic targets for novel therapies. Cigarette smoke contains reactive oxygen species, particulates, and chemicals, which lead to a range of inflammatory effects: macrophage, epithelial cell, and CD8+ T cell activation. These cells in turn release neutrophil chemotactic factors. Numerous local inflammatory mediators are then released, along with proteases, which break down connective tissue in the lung, causing emphysema. Proteases are also important in stimulating mucus hypersecretion, which may manifest as chronic bronchitis. Profibrotic mediators are also released by epithelial cells, contributing to fibroblast proliferation and small airway fibrosis. Novel therapies include those aimed at local as well as systemic inflammation. The most ambitious target is to regenerate lung tissue in response to emphysema. mABs, monoclonal antibodies; PDE4, phosphodiesterase 4.

DRUGS TO AID SMOKING CESSATION

Smoking cessation is the first priority in the management of a COPD patient who smokes. To date, it is the only intervention shown to convincingly reduce the accelerated decline in pulmonary function and improve long-term prognosis (see **Fig. 1, Table 1**).[28,29] Success in quitting is increased by behavioral support in addition to a range of pharmacotherapies.[30] However, a recent systematic review has concluded that, in contrast to non-COPD smokers, neither the intensity of counseling nor the type of antismoking drug make a significant difference in smoking cessation results.[31]

The most widely used agents include nicotine replacement (in a variety of preparations), antidepressants such as bupropion and nortriptyline, and nicotine partial receptor agonists such as varenicline (which remains the most efficacious monotherapy for smoking cessation[32]). Cytisine, a partial agonist that binds with high affinity to the α4β2 subtype of the nicotine acetylcholine receptor is effective in sustaining abstinence at

12 months.[33] Other approaches currently under investigation include nicotine vaccines (with the associated benefits of infrequent dosing and prolonged effect); however, large trials of the current front-runners (NicVAx and NIC002) have been disappointing.[34,35] Both agents stimulate the production of antibodies that bind to nicotine and prevent it from crossing the blood-brain barrier. Novel nicotine products that can be given via the inhaled, topical (in the form of a spray) or orally dissolving film route are also under development, and detailed in a recent review.[36] Compounds are also being explored to target other neurotransmitters implicated in nicotine dependence such as dopamine, γ- aminobutyric acid (GABA), and glutamate.[37] These include trials of monoamine oxidase inhibitors such as selegiline.[36] The cannabinoid receptor system is thought to inhibit indirectly the dopamine-mediated rewarding properties of food and tobacco, and cannabinoid receptor 1 antagonists are undergoing evaluation, although trials have so far been disappointing.[36] There is increasing popularity of electronic cigarettes, which deliver nicotine via an electronic

battery-powered device resembling a cigarette, despite no formal demonstration of the efficacy and safety of such devices. These devices have the potential advantage of tackling the psychological and physical components of nicotine addiction; therefore, several large prospective studies are now underway.[38]

INHALED BRONCHODILATORS AND CORTICOSTEROIDS
Inhaled Bronchodilators

The development of improved bronchodilators has focused on finding better inhaled LABAs and LAMAs (**Table 2**).[39–41] Novel classes of bronchodilator have been difficult to develop because they often have additional unwanted effects on vascular smooth muscle, producing postural hypotension and headaches. Until recently, all LABAs required twice-daily dosing, but newer once-daily agents, ultra-LABAs (ULABAs), such as indacaterol, olodaterol, vilanterol, and carmoterol are proving to be effective.[39,42–44] Aclidinium bromide is a new LAMA that has an acute onset of action (compared with tiotropium's slower onset of action) but has disappointed in trials to date.[45,46] Other LAMAs with a more rapid onset of action are in development. Glycopyrronium bromide/NVA237 has been shown to provide comparable effects to tiotropium.[47–49] Another company is soon to start phase III trials with nebulized LAMA, EP-101, a glycopyrrolate solution. Two single-molecule, dual-action bronchodilators, muscarinic antagonist and beta2-agonists (MABAs), are in phase I and II trials, including GSK961081.

Studies looking at the benefits of dual LABA or LAMA (salmeterol or formoterol with tiotropium) therapy have demonstrated greater bronchodilation and fewer symptoms when the drugs are combined, than with either agent alone.[50–52] New ULABAs allow for once-daily administration of LABA-LAMA combination inhaler, and a recent study has demonstrated significant benefits in FEV_1 using QVA149 (a combination of glycopyrronium bromide and indacaterol) versus indacaterol alone or placebo.[53] Aclidinium has been combined with formoterol as a LAMA and LABA combination.[46]

Attempts to combine existing classes of drugs with additional agents have proved less successful, as demonstrated by the arrested development of the novel D2 dopamine receptor–β2 adrenoreceptor agonist sibenadet (Viozan). The rationale for this agent was based on observations that sensory afferent nerves were key mediators of COPD symptoms such as breathlessness, cough, and excess sputum production, and advocates of Viozan hypothesized that that activation of

Table 2 Inhaled bronchodilators and corticosteroids and corticosteroid-related approaches	
Ultralong-acting β2-agonists	Abadeterol AZD3199 Olodaterol (BI1744CL) Carmoterol Vilanterol (GSK642444) Indacaterol (QAB149)
LAMA	Aclidinium (LAS-34273) AZD8683 Umeclidinium (GSK573719) Glycopyrronium (NVA237)
Muscarinic antagonist and β2-agonist	AZD2115 GSK961081
LABA + LAMA	Formoterol + aclidinium Olodaterol + tiotropium Vilanterol + umeclidinium Indacaterol + glycopyrronium (QVA149)
ICS + Ultralong-acting β2-agonists	Beclomethasone + formoterol (Fostair) Fluticasone + vilanterol (Relovair) Mometasone + formoterol (Dulera) Fluticasone + formoterol (Flutiform) Mometasone + indacaterol (QMF149) Ciclesonide + formoterol
New corticosteroid-related approaches	Nonglucocorticoid steroids Selective glucocorticoid receptor agonists
Reversal of steroid resistance	Theophylline (histone deacetylase 2 activators) Phosphoinositide-3-kinase inhibitors LABAs and phosphodiesterase 4/LABAs (via phosphoinositide-3-kinase inhibition)

D2-receptors on such nerves would modulate their activity.[54] Although initial short-term studies were promising, the duration of the bronchodilator effect diminished as studies progressed and no sustained benefit was reported in a 1-year large-scale trial.[55]

ICS

Current United Kingdom and international guidance, despite little supporting evidence, recommend ICS for symptomatic patients with an FEV_1

lower than 50% and/or frequent exacerbations. These are usually prescribed in the form of a combination inhaler containing LABA. In reality ICS-LABA inhalers may be used inappropriately in an excessive number of COPD patients who do not meet the criteria outlined by the Global Initiative for Chronic Obstructive Lung Disease (GOLD) guidelines.[56] A Spanish study found a rate of inappropriate ICS use of 18.2%.[57]

A Cochrane review of the role of ICS included studies published up until July 2011.[58] This review concluded that long-term (>6 months) ICS use did not consistently reduce the rate of decline in FEV_1 in COPD patients. There was no statistically significant effect on mortality in COPD subjects, but long-term use of ICS did reduce the mean rate of exacerbations in those studies in which pooling of data was possible. In addition, there was slowing of the rate of decline in quality of life (measured by the St. George's Respiratory Questionnaire). There was an increased risk of oropharyngeal candidiasis and hoarseness with ICS use and, in the long-term studies, the rate of pneumonia was increased in the ICS group compared with the placebo group. Although ICS does seem to have some beneficial effects in COPD, when compared with long-acting bronchodilators, the latter agents seem to provide similar benefits to ICS or ICS-LABA combinations in exacerbation reduction without the side effects associated with ICS use.[59]

One alternative may be the use of nonglucocorticoid steroids. EPI-12323 is a once-daily, small molecule, inhaled nonglucocorticoid steroid and may not exhibit any of the classic side effects of glucocorticoid steroids. It may also be possible to avoid the unwanted side effects of glucocorticoids by selectively inducing transrepression genomic mechanisms (which are responsible for many desirable antiinflammatory and immunomodulating effects), whereas transactivation processes (associated with frequently occurring side effects) are simultaneously less affected.[60,61] An inhaled selective glucocorticoid receptor agonist is currently undergoing clinical trials.

For patients who remain symptomatic despite LABA-ICS combination, GOLD recommends triple therapy with LAMA, LABA, and ICS. The rationale behind this seems logical because all three agents work via different mechanisms on different targets, potentially allowing for lower doses of the individual agents to be used, accompanied by improved side-effect profiles. However, there has been a lack of sufficiently powered studies primarily addressing the benefits of triple therapy versus LABA-ICS therapy, or, indeed, versus dual LABA-LAMA therapy.[62,63] A single inhaler combining all three agents is currently in formational development, although

the ICS to be used has not been confirmed. Once-daily ICS are now in development to allow future trials with once-daily triple-therapy combined inhalers. These inhalers may well improve compliance, but titration of individual component drug doses may prove difficult, and disease severity seems to affect the drug dose-response curve.[64]

Steroid Resistance

Interestingly, ICS do not seem to suppress inflammation in COPD. One hypothesis attributes this to the marked reduction in histone deacetylase 2 (HDAC2), the nuclear enzyme that corticosteroids require to switch off activated inflammatory genes,[65] rendering these patients resistant to the effects of ICS. The reduction in HDAC2 is thought to be secondary to oxidative stress, both independent of and by way of activation of phosphoinositide-3-kinase-δ (PI3Kδ).[66] Inhibition of PI3Kδ has recently shown to restore corticosteroid sensitivity in mice[66] and may hold therapeutic promise.[67,68] One group has shown that formoterol reverses oxidative stress-induced corticosteroid insensitivity via PI3Kδ.[68] Low-dose theophylline has shown to enhance the antiinflammatory effects of steroids during exacerbations of COPD[69] and seems to have the capacity to restore the reduced HDAC2 activity in COPD macrophages.[70] More recently, roflumilast has shown to augment the ability of formoterol to enhance glucocorticoid-dependent gene transcription in human airway epithelial cells.[71]

ANTIINFECTIVE AND ANTIINFLAMMATORY AGENTS
Antibiotics

The Lung Health Study of North America revealed that lower respiratory tract illnesses promote FEV_1 decline in current smokers (**Table 3**).[72] There is growing evidence that exacerbations accelerate the progressive decline in lung function in COPD patients.[73] Several lines of evidence now implicate bacteria as an important cause of exacerbations[74] and bacterial colonization is frequently found in patients with COPD.[75] It is associated with the frequency of exacerbations.[76] There seems to be a correlation between bacterial colonization of lower airways and elevated levels of inflammatory mediators.[77] Finally, patients with severe COPD who receive inappropriate antibiotic treatment are vulnerable to multidrug-resistant infections.[78]

It has become increasingly difficult to develop new antibiotics, so that there is a need for novel types of therapy. Bacteriophages are bacterial

Table 3
Antiinfective and antiinflammatory agents

Antibacterials	Antibiotics, antimicrobial peptides, bacteriophages, vaccines
Antivirals	Antivirals (eg, neuraminidase inhibitors for influenza) Vaccines for influenza, HRV, and respiratory syncytial virus
Agents acting on pattern recognition by the innate immune system	Toll-like receptor inhibitors 2, 4, and 9 NLR agonists or antagonists RLR agonists or antagonists
Antagonists of cell surface receptors	CXCR2 antagonists (AZD5069); GSK1325756 CCR2 antagonists (CCR2b antagonist: AZD2423) Chemoattractant receptor-homologous molecule expressed on Th2 cells antagonists LTB_4 receptor antagonists Selectin antagonists
Phosphodiesterase (PDE)-4 inhibitors	PDE4i: roflumilast, tetomilast Inhaled selective PDE4B inhibitor: GSK25066 Dual selective PDE inhibitors Novel combinations: 　PDE4 +7A inhibition 　PDE3 + PDE4 inhibition (RPL554)
Kinase inhibition	p38 mitogen-activated protein kinase inhibitors (inhaled GSK610677) JNK inhibitors Syk inhibitors JAK/STAT inhibitors: tofacitinib
Transcription inhibition	NF-κB inhibitors: IKK2 inhibitors PI3K-γ/δ inhibitors Peroxisome proliferator-activated receptor-γ antagonists (rosiglitazone) Cyclosporine-A (inhaled)
Combating systemic inflammation	Statins

viruses that are approximately 10 times more numerous than bacteria in nature. Although they have been used in Russia for many decades as antibacterial agents, they have been used less in Western medicine.[79] Lytic phages are highly specific to particular bacteria and are well tolerated, with no risk of overgrowth of intestinal flora. They may be administered by inhalation, so may be effective in the treatment of respiratory bacterial infections.

Antimicrobial peptides, including α-defensins, β-defensins, and cathelicidins, are produced from epithelial and other cells in the respiratory tract and play a key role in innate immunity and stimulating adaptive immune responses.[80] These peptides may also be considered potential future therapies.

Although the molecular mechanisms for these effects are not fully clear, 14- and 15-membered ring macrolide antibiotics have several antiinflammatory effects in addition to their antibacterial actions.[81] It has been shown that these drugs decrease the production of cytokines in the lungs.[82] A recent large clinical trial, with more than 1142 volunteers, randomized subjects to daily administration of 250 mg of azithromycin or placebo for 1 year.[83] The median time to the first acute exacerbation in the azithromycin group was increased by 92 days, and the frequency of exacerbations in the azithromycin group was significantly reduced. However, deafness was observed in the treatment group as an adverse event. Another long-term, placebo-controlled clinical trial examining macrolides in the prevention of acute exacerbations used erythromycin at a dose of 250 mg twice daily for 1 year.[84] A nonantibiotic macrolide such as EM704, derived from the structure of erythromycin, has been shown to inhibit neutrophilic inflammation, the release of TGF-β, and fibrosis in a bleomycin model of pulmonary fibrosis.[85] Such nonantibiotic macrolides may be delivered by inhalation during an exacerbation and will not affect antibiotic resistance patterns.

Recently, pulsed antibiotic prophylaxis has been trialed. Moxifloxacin has shown to reduce the odds of exacerbation in stable COPD subjects when given once a day for 5 days every 8 weeks for 48 weeks.[86] New pneumococcal vaccines are also in development that may prove more effective than are their current counterparts.

Antivirals

With advances in diagnostic techniques for viruses, such as polymerase chain reaction, there is evidence that the most COPD exacerbations are associated with viral infections and that, of these, HRV is the most common cause[87] and can directly infect the lower respiratory tract.[88] Up-regulation of the HRV receptor, intercellular adhesion molecule 1, on epithelial cells occurs in COPD patients and this may cause predisposition to infection.[89] When infected, COPD primary bronchial epithelial cells elicit exaggerated antiviral therapies, especially in relation to HIV, development of resistance to proinflammatory response.[90] Although there have been remarkable strides in the development of antiviral therapies, especially in relation to HIV, development of resistance to viral therapy is a recurrent problem[91] and there are no effective antirhinoviral treatments to date. Recently, an important model of human RV16 challenge has been introduced as a model of exacerbations in patients with COPD.[13]

Respiratory syncytial virus (RSV) is increasingly recognized in adults with COPD[92] and it can persist in stable disease.[93] Treatment of RSV infection remains largely supportive, although a monoclonal antibody (MoAB) therapy against RSV F protein (palivizumab) is licensed for specialist use in restricted circumstances.[94]

Seasonal influenza is another important cause of exacerbations of COPD and there is the fear that an influenza pandemic could cause high mortality in patients with COPD.[95] It is important that all patients with COPD have adequate influenza immunization and that they be considered for early treatment in the event of an influenza-induced exacerbation of COPD. Apart from vaccines, there are two licensed antiviral agents against influenza: zanamivir and oseltamivir (Tamiflu).[96] Nevertheless, development of resistance is a major problem and new anti-influenza agents are being actively sought.[97]

Agents Acting on Innate Immunity

Cigarette smoke has long been known to increase the permeability of the respiratory epithelium, thus compromising the barrier function. Respiratory viruses have a particular predilection for respiratory epithelial cells and these can then initiate nonspecific inflammation. Once the respiratory physical barrier is penetrated, danger signals meet the next part of the immune system defense: the pattern recognition receptors (PRRs). Recently,

there has been recent dramatic progress in the understanding of the molecular and cellular details of how the innate nonspecific immune system is activated.[98] PRRs are thought to be central to the activation of the innate immune system and they have the capacity to drive chronic lung inflammation,[99] repair processes, fibrosis, and proteolysis. A unified theory can be made of how the development of mild-to-moderate COPD, as well as exacerbations of COPD, is mediated through interaction of reactive oxidant species (ROS), viruses, and bacteria with the innate immune system.[100] Molecular signatures on ROS, viruses, and bacteria, as well as from dead and damaged cells, cause rapid activation of the family of PRRs. Pathogen-associated molecular patterns (PAMPs) are found especially in the nucleic acid of the viruses that infect the respiratory epithelium and in various cell wall and cytoplasmic components of bacteria.[101] A variety of damage-associated molecular patterns (DAMPs) has been proposed, including high-mobility group box 1, S100 proteins, heat shock proteins (HSP), and extracellular matrix hyaluronans.

ROS activate Toll-like receptor (TLR) 2[102] and TLR4 using MyD88 signaling,[103,104] but they can also cause damage to membrane lipids and to DNA and thus activate DAMPs.[105,106] The cell wall of gram-negative bacteria contains lipopolysaccharide that activates cell surface TLR4, whereas various other bacterial components activate different cell surface TLRs. In contrast, viral nucleic acid motifs activate TLR3, 7, and 9, which are found on the inner surface of the endosomal membrane.

PRRs undergo extensive cross-talk with TLRs,[101] scavenger receptors,[107] and receptor for advanced glycation end-products (RAGE).[91,108] In addition, there are TLRs on endosomes that recognize viral nucleic acids and cytoplasmic PRRs that consist of retinoic acid-inducible gene-1 (RIG-1)-like receptors (RLRs), and NOD-like receptors (NLRs). Activation of PRRs takes place in COPD on epithelial cells, neutrophils, macrophages, smooth muscle[109] fibroblasts, and other cells of the airways. Acute cigarette smoke activates MyD88, a common adapter protein that is involved in the signaling of several TLRs (including TLR2, 4, 7, 8, and 9).[104]

Therefore, blocking PRRs, including TLRs that recognize and are activated by PAMPs on oxidants and infectious agents, may be a potential way of modulating disease activity in COPD. There are now intensive efforts to develop TLR-agonists and antagonists for treatment of diseases like COPD that involve inflammation and infection.[110] Eritoran, a synthetic TLR4 antagonist, has been shown to block influenza-induced lethality in mice, and may well provide a novel therapeutic approach for other infections.[111] PRRs activate a variety of signal transduction pathways, including NF-κB and mitogen-activated protein (MAP) kinase pathways, as well as type I interferon pathways in the case of viruses.[112] MyD88 offers another target for therapy.[104,113]

Chemokine Receptor Antagonists

CXC and CC chemokine receptors are thought to be involved in COPD inflammation due to their role in neutrophil recruitment. The concentrations of CXC chemokines, including CXCL5 and CXCL8, are increased during exacerbations and, because they all signal through a common receptor, CXCR2, specific antagonists of this receptor may be useful in treating exacerbations. A small molecule CXCR1/2 antagonist (AZD8309) shows promise in inhibiting sputum neutrophils, after inhaled endotoxin, by approximately 80%,[114] suggesting that this could be useful in exacerbations and has the advantage of oral administration. A proof-of-principle study revealed that SCH527123, a novel, selective CXCR2 antagonist, causes significant attenuation of ozone-induced airway neutrophilia in healthy subjects.[115] However, experimental inflammation by ozone challenge is chiefly CXCL8-dependent, transient, and fully reversible in contrast to the pathologic inflammation occurring in the airways of subjects with COPD, which depends on multiple mediators and is chronic and largely irreversible. This highlights the difficulty with current models. Interestingly, SCH527123 has now undergone phase 2 studies in subjects with moderate-to-severe COPD, during which there were beneficial effects on sputum neutrophil counts and FEV_1 (reported at the ERS in 2010).

Several other oral CXCR2 antagonists such as AZD5069 are currently in phase II trials and include secondary outcome measures of circulating blood neutrophil levels.

CX3CL1 binds exclusively to CX3C chemokine receptor 1 (CX3CR1), and is unregulated in the lung tissue of smokers with COPD, making this an attractive target.[38]

An inhaled CCR1 antagonist (AZD4818) failed to show benefit in COPD,[116] although a CCR2b antagonist (AZD2423) is currently in trials.

Chemoattractant Receptor-homologous Receptor Antagonism

Chemoattractant receptor-homologous molecule expressed on Th2 cells (CRTH2) is a G-protein coupled receptor expressed by Th2 lymphocytes,

eosinophils, and basophils. The receptor mediates the activation and chemotaxis of these cell types in response to prostaglandin D2 (PGD_2), the major prostanoid produced by mast cell degranulation typically in the initial phase of IgE-mediated reactions but also thought to occur at sites of inflammation, such as the bronchial mucosa. As such, selective PGD_2 receptor antagonists (CRTh2 antagonists) are mainly in development for asthma.[117]

LTB_4 Receptor Antagonists

Serum concentrations of LTB_4, a potent neutrophil chemoattractant, are increased in patients with COPD.[118] LTB_4 activates BLT_1-receptors, which are expressed on neutrophils and T lymphocytes. Although BLT_1-antagonists have a relatively small effect on neutrophil chemotaxis in response to COPD sputum[119] and they have not proved to be effective in treating stable COPD, it is possible that they would have greater efficacy if used acutely, due to observations that LTB_4 is especially elevated during COPD exacerbations.[7]

LTA4H has been proposed as another potential therapeutic target because it is the enzyme responsible for generation of LTB_4 from leukotriene A2. However, another role for LTA4H has been observed, whereby it degrades another neutrophil chemoattractant, namely proline-glycine-proline (PGP),[120] thus therapeutic strategies inhibiting LTA4H to prevent LTB_4 generation may not reduce neutrophil recruitment due to simultaneous elevation in PGP levels, once again demonstrating the complexity of manipulating inflammatory processes in COPD.

Selectin Antagonism

The selectin family is a group of adhesion molecules involved in the initial activation and adhesion of leukocytes on the vascular endothelium, which facilitates their migration into the surrounding tissue. In a phase II trial in 77 COPD subjects, 28 days of bimosiamose (an inhaled pan-selectin antagonist) led to a significant decrease in the sputum macrophage count, and decreased CXCL8 and matrix metalloprotease (MMP)-9, whereas most lung function parameters also showed a small numeric increase with no difference in adverse events.[121] Trials with longer treatment durations are now required and an anti-selectin MoAB (EL246) is currently under predevelopment.[122]

Phosphodiesterase Inhibitors

Theophylline has some PDE inhibitor activities and it as been used in the treatment of COPD for more than 75 years. However, its use is limited by its narrow therapeutic range, side-effect profile, and drug interactions. Newer selective PDE inhibitors are anticipated to exhibit the beneficial effects of theophylline with an improved side-effect profile. PDE4 inhibitors have a broad spectrum of antiinflammatory effects and are effective in animal models of COPD. However, in human studies their effectiveness has been limited by side effects, such as nausea, diarrhea, and headaches.[123,124]

Development of selective orally active PDE4 inhibitors has predominantly involved cilomilast (Ariflo), roflumilast, and tetomilast in inflammatory bowel disease.[125] Cilomilast has been studied in five phase III studies: involving 2088 subjects on cilomilast and 1408 on placebo for 24 weeks.[126] Although an initial study was very encouraging in 424 patients with COPD assessed for 6 weeks,[127] benefits were not as great in a larger study for 6 months,[128] and cilomilast failed to convince in other phase III studies. As a result, the entire cilomilast program was terminated, providing a cautionary example of the difficulties in developing new drugs for COPD.

In contrast, roflumilast has proved more effective in long-term studies,[129–132] especially in decreasing exacerbations, and is now the first in this new class of agents licensed for treatment of severe COPD with bronchitis.[133,134] Roflumilast is given once daily (500 µg), but gastrointestinal adverse effects and weight loss are common on starting therapy. The Roflumilast in the Prevention of COPD Exacerbations While Taking Appropriate Combination Treatment (REACT) study aims to assess whether or not roflumilast will provide additional benefit when added to dual or triple therapy.[135] This will also go some way to confirming the safety of the drug and it's future use, although it may be that newer inhaled PDE4 inhibitors will prove preferable in terms of reduced side effects. To date, inhaled PDE4 inhibitors have been found to be ineffective.

Avoidance of targeting certain isoforms should help limit side effects because mouse studies have suggested that emesis is the result of PDE4D inhibition,[136] whereas PDE4B is the predominant subtype present in monocytes and neutrophils and is implicated in the inflammatory process. This insight has led to the design of PDE4 inhibitor modulators, which have one to two orders of magnitude less affinity for the PDE4D isoform, while maintaining other PDE4 inhibitory activities. However, more work is needed to confirm whether targeting specific subtypes really is more beneficial. In addition, mixed PDE4/7 inhibitors are under development that may have synergistic benefits. TPI 1100, which comprises two antisense oligonucleotides targeting the mRNA for the PDE4B/4D and PDE7A isoforms, has been shown to reduce neutrophil influx and key cytokines in an established smoking mouse model.[137] A final approach may be use of a PDE4 inhibitor in combination with other antiinflammatory drugs such as glucocorticoids[138] based on recent findings that these drugs together may impart clinical benefit beyond that achievable by an ICS or a PDE4 alone.[71]

Kinase Inhibitors

After decades of research on oral kinase inhibitors, a JAK inhibitor has been licensed in 2012 for the treatment of rheumatoid arthritis.[139] There is also progress with orally active Syk inhibitors in autoimmune disease. p38 (p38 MAP kinase) is activated by bacteria and viruses, as well as other inflammatory signals and, therefore, is another target for inhibition.[140,141] These phosphorylases are involved in cell-signaling cascades, which often result in the activation of proinflammatory nuclear transcription factors such as NF-κB. Several p38 MAP kinase inhibitors are now in clinical development, and the results of a phase II trial with losmapimod (an oral p38 MAP kinase inhibitor) were published last year. Although losmapimod did not have an effect on sputum neutrophils or lung function, there was a significant reduction in plasma fibrinogen levels after 12 weeks, and improvements in lung hyperinflation were noted.[142]

Other broad-spectrum antiinflammatory drugs in development include inhibitors of NF-κB and PI3K. However, there is much interaction between signaling pathways and it may be that a multipronged approach is required.[125,143] NF-κB inhibition can be attempted through a variety of approaches; namely by inhibiting the degradation of the inhibitor of NF-κB family of proteins (IκB), gene transfer of IκB or IκB kinase (IKK) inhibition. Several IKK inhibitors are in development.[38] PI3K inhibitors also have therapeutic potential,[144,145] and selective inhibition may restore glucocorticoid sensitivity.[146] There are drugs directed against both the δ- and γ-isoforms of PI3K,[147,148] as well as an inhaled dual γ/δ inhibitor.[149] In addition, peroxisome proliferator-activated receptor gamma (PPAR-γ) antagonists such as rosiglitazone may treat airway mucus hypersecretion.[150] Finally, new formulations of cyclosporine A (inhaled) are being developed for asthma and COPD.[151]

Statins

COPD is associated with a complex list of systemic manifestations, including systemic inflammation associated with cachexia and skeletal muscle weakness.[152,153] COPD also has an extensive association with comorbidities, such as cardiovascular diseases,[154] and it is recognized that new drugs are required for COPD and these comorbidities.[155] This subset of patients with persistent systemic inflammation has been associated with poor clinical outcomes, irrespective of their lung impairment.[156] It is recognized that skeletal muscle weakness and wasting may also be amenable to therapy.[157,158]

This has encouraged the use of statins in COPD because they have a range of systemic antiinflammatory effects.[159] Statins increase survival in patients with peripheral arterial disease and COPD,[160] and may reduce COPD exacerbations.[161] Furthermore, retrospective studies have shown that statins reduce the risk of death in patients with COPD.[162–164] The benefit on all-cause mortality depends on the level of underlying systemic inflammation, as assessed using high-sensitivity C-reactive protein (hsCRP) measurements.[165] Various academic institutions are currently conducting studies looking at the effect of statins on the frequency of COPD exacerbations in patients with moderate-to-severe COPD who are prone to exacerbations, but may not have other indications for statin treatment. In addition, statins have been associated with a reduced risk of extrapulmonary cancers in patients with COPD.[166]

MISCELLANEOUS ADDITIONAL CLASSES OF NEW DRUGS
Antioxidants

Each inhalation of cigarette smoke contains a large burden of ROS,[167] as well as many different chemical components that cause lung toxicity (**Table 4**).[168] In addition, oxidants are generated endogenously from activated inflammatory cells. Manipulation of the oxidant–antioxidant balance, therefore, seems to be a logical therapeutic strategy and there is a range of novel targets.[169,170] Resveratrol is a cardioprotective antioxidant in red

Table 4
Miscellaneous additional classes of new drugs

Antioxidants	• Dietary antioxidants • N-acetyl-cysteine, N-acystelyn, N-isobutyryl-cysteine, erdosteine, procysteine, carbocysteine • Thiols, spin traps • Enzyme mimetics: superoxide dismutase, catalase and glutathione peroxidase • Polyphenols
Mucolytics	• N-acetyl-cysteine and carbocysteine • Epidermal growth factor receptor tyrosine kinase inhibitors
Protease inhibitors	• Neutrophil elastase inhibitors: sivelestat (ONO-5046), silanediol isosteres, AZD 9688 • MMP-9 & MMP-12 inhibitors • Broad-spectrum MMP inhibitors: ilomastat, marimastat
Antifibrotics	Agents used in idiopathic pulmonary fibrosis • Pirfenidone • Endothelin antagonists • PDE5 inhibitor: sildenafil • MoABs: anti-TGF-β, anti-FGF, anti-IL-13, anti-αvβ6 integrin (STX-100), anti-CCL2 (CNTO 888)
Drugs to combat cachexia and muscle wasting	Growth hormone releasing factor analogue (tesamorelin)
MoABs	• Anti-TNFα • Anti-IL-1β • Anti-IL-6 (tocilizumab) • Anti-CXCL8 (IL-8) • Anti-IL-17, anti-IL-13, anti-IgE • Anti-TGF-β
Drugs to slow aging	Sirtuin 1 activator (GSK2245840)
Lung regeneration	• Retinoids (γ-selective retinoid agonist, palovarotene) • Mesenchymal stem cell therapy • Gly-his-lys (GHK) tripeptide

wine, whereas stilbenes are dietary antioxidants from tomatoes, but may not achieve sufficient levels in established COPD. Interestingly, resveratrol is also a sirtuin (SIRT) activator and this property has been proposed to account for antiaging effects.[171] There are theories that COPD represents an accelerated form of lung aging,[172,173] and this concept suggests that antiaging molecules may have potential in COPD.[174] Other dietary components such as sulforaphanes and chalcones are potential therapeutic antioxidants in COPD.[175]

N-acetyl-cysteine (NAC) is a potent reducing agent capable of increasing intracellular glutathione levels. In addition, its mucolytic properties can improve sputum clearance in COPD. In preclinical studies, NAC attenuated elastase-induced emphysema in rats,[176] but later clinical studies have yielded mixed results. A Cochrane review reported the beneficial effects on exacerbation frequency of NAC in chronic bronchitis,[177] but this was later followed by a large multicenter trial in which NAC had no effect on exacerbation frequency or FEV_1 decline.[178] Carbocysteine may be more promising. The PEACE study revealed a significant decline in COPD exacerbations using 500 mg carbocysteine three times a day daily in Chinese patients with COPD.[179] Both of these agents are undergoing further studies in COPD.

Stable glutathione compounds, superoxide dismutase (SOD) analogues, and radical scavengers are in development. Enzyme mimetics are being developed that enhance the activity or expression of antioxidant enzymes such as SOD and glutathione peroxidase, which can neutralize cellular ROS. Nitrone spin-traps are potent antioxidants, which inhibit the formation of intracellular ROS by forming stable compounds, whereas thioredoxin is a redox sensor inhibitor. Hydrogen sulfide (H_2S) is a potent antioxidant and GYY4137 is a novel H_2S-releasing molecule that protects against endotoxic shock in the rat[180]; however, all these agents are still being assessed in animal models.

Mucoactive Drugs

Secretions can accumulate in airway lumens, exacerbating airflow obstruction and increasing susceptibility to infections in COPD. A variety of drugs has been developed to treat airway mucus hypersecretion, as well as mucoactive drugs,[181] in addition to NAC and carbocysteine mentioned above. These agents combat targets such as epidermal growth factor receptor, tyrosine kinase inhibitors, and human calcium-activated chloride channel (hCACL2). PPAR-γ is an exciting target for drugs to treat airway mucus hypersecretion.[150] Surfactant protein B has recently been found to be associated with COPD exacerbations.[182] It is important to stress that mucus can be both protective and harmful in different situations in COPD. In a study using inhaled recombinant DNAse to treat acute exacerbations of COPD, the study was terminated due to a trend toward increased mortality in the treatment arm.[183]

Proteases

α1-Antitrypsin deficiency is a genetic disease that illustrates the importance of proteases in causing a subtype of COPD.[134,135] There have been recent advances in provision of augmentation therapy for α1-antitrypsin deficiency.[184] Neutrophil elastase (NE),[136] MMP-9,[137] and MMP-12[185] have been implicated in the pathogenesis of COPD, and provide targets for novel therapies.[186]

A novel oral inhibitor of NE, AZD9668, underwent a 12-week dose-finding study in subjects with COPD treated with tiotropium, but failed to show benefit.[187,188] An inhibitory effect of heparin has been shown on neutrophil elastase release, which is independent of the anticoagulant activity of this molecule.[189] However, a phase II trial of O-desulfated heparin in subjects with exacerbations of COPD was terminated at the end of last year due to a lack of efficacy. Interestingly, heparin is also a known inhibitor of selectin-mediated interactions, but a phase II trial in COPD exacerbation patients with PGX-100 (2-O, 3-O desulfated heparin) also failed to demonstrate efficacy and was terminated early.[122]

Attempts to readdress the protease-antiprotease imbalance with synthetic MMP inhibitors have been attempted,[190] but the development of musculoskeletal syndrome with marimastat is a prominent adverse effect.[191] AZD1236, a novel more selective inhibitor of MMP-9 and MMP-12, has failed to demonstrate convincing clinical efficacy in two studies over 6 weeks.[192,193] The role of other proteases in COPD remains unclear, but inhibitors of cysteine proteases are under development.

Fibrosis and Remodeling

There have been dramatic advances in the understanding of lung injury and idiopathic pulmonary fibrosis (IPF).[194–196] This has resulted in a flurry of drug development, for which excellent reviews are available.[197,198] Inflammation and fibrosis are related processes, and COPD and IPF have some common features.[199,200] Airway inflammation, resulting in tissue injury can result in peribronchial fibrosis when lung injury exceeds the lung's ability to repair. The resulting airways become narrowed, leading to airway obstruction. However, although these processes, inflammation, and fibrosis, may be closely related, it has also been postulated that fibrosis may occur alone in COPD. For example, in IPF there can be very little inflammation.[201] The process of fibrosis is prominent in the small airways as obstructive bronchiolitis, but excessive fibrosis may also contribute to emphysema. It has been recently recognized that fibroblasts and myofibroblasts may be resident cells, derived from bone marrow stem cells and blood-borne fibrocytes, or may be derived by epithelial to mesenchymal transition (EMT).[202,203] Therefore, strategies used to treat IPF (eg, pirfenidone) may be of benefit in COPD, but more research is needed in this area.[194,204]

A recent study has demonstrated that cigarette smoke induces EMT in differentiated bronchial epithelial cells via release and autocrine action of transforming growth factor-β1 (TGF-β1) as well as by enhancing oxidative stress, thus suggesting that EMT could participate in the COPD remodeling process of small bronchi such as peribronchiolar fibrosis.[205] Small-molecule inhibitors of TGF-β1 receptor tyrosine kinase have been developed: SD-208, however, has been shown to inhibit airway fibrosis in a model of asthma.[206]

Biologics: MoABs

Tumor necrosis factor α (TNF-α) has been implicated in the pathogenesis of COPD and seems to be a good therapeutic target. Indeed, an observational study in rheumatoid arthritis patients demonstrated that etanercept (a TNF-receptor antagonist) led to a reduction of 50% in the rate of hospitalization due to COPD exacerbations.[207] Although blocking TNF-α was not effective in stable COPD patients,[208–210] it is possible that administration during an acute exacerbation might be effective in view of the acutely increased TNF-α concentrations. However, there are major concerns that the TNF antibody infliximab increased the incidence of respiratory cancers in a COPD study (although this was not statistically significant),[208] and increased other types of cancer as well as infections in a study in severe asthma.[211] Future efforts may consider a more tailored approach using these agents in a subset of patients defined by an increased TNF-α axis. In addition, cachectic patients were found to have a small improvement in exercise capacity in post hoc analysis.[208] Inhibition of TNF-α production by inhibition of TNF-α converting enzyme is an alternative strategy.[38] A prominent effect of NF-κB and p38 MAP kinase inhibitor is the downstream inhibition of TNF-α synthesis.

An anti-CXCL8 (IL-8) MoAB was tested in COPD, but no improvement in health status or lung function was seen, possibly because the active bound form of CXCL8 was not recognized by the MoAB.[38] There is now special interest in assessing MoABs directed against IL-6, IL-1β, IL-17, IL-18, IL-1R, TGF-β, and granulocyte-macrophage colony-stimulating factor for effects in COPD. A humanized antibody against IL-6 receptors (tocilizumab) is effective in several other inflammatory diseases,[212] but there are no studies in COPD. Canakinumab, a MoAB to IL-1β, is already used in rare autoimmune diseases and is now in trials in COPD.[213] Th17 cells have recently been identified as a separate cell population that produce IL-17, which causes neutrophilia[214,215] and induce loss of HDAC2 and steroid insensitivity,[216] thus implicating another potential target, and phase II trials in psoriasis have been encouraging.[217,218] Finally, omalizumab, the anti-IgE MoAB approved for severe allergic asthma, has also now entered a study in a subgroup of COPD patients with elevated IgE levels.

Aging and Autoimmunity

COPD may be considered a disease of accelerated aging and geroprotectors are a novel therapeutic strategy.[219] SIRT1 and SIRT6 are attractive targets[220,221] because they can possess HDAC2 activity, protect against oxidative stress, and permit stabilization and repair of DNA. Another insight is that autoimmunity may have a role in COPD[222] and the immune system may be targeted against elastin[223] or epithelial cells.[224]

Lung Regeneration

Approaches to aid lung regeneration aim to correct the defect of emphysema and to replace destroyed lung interstitium. Human lungs have regenerative capacity, as demonstrated in Nepalese children given maternal vitamin A supplements.[225] This is not exclusive to children as demonstrated in an adult patient after pneumonectomy.[226] Attempts have been made to exploit this potential with new drugs to cause lung regeneration in COPD.[227–229]

Retinoids are known to promote alveolar septation in the developing lung and to stimulate alveolar repair in some animal models of emphysema. However, despite abrogation of elastase-induced emphysema in rats using all-trans retinoic acid,[230] subsequent attempts with retinoids and γ-retinoic acid receptor agonists in humans have been less promising.[231,232] The REPAIR study evaluated the effects of palovarotene (an oral γ-selective retinoid agonist) on lung density in emphysema secondary to α1-antitrypsin deficiency. Although effects on the primary endpoint were not significant, there was a trend toward an improvement in most functional parameters in subjects taking palovarotene for a year. Another group conducted a 2-year trial with this agent and reported their findings at the ATS in 2011. There was no overall improvement in FEV_1 in COPD subjects on the drug; however, subgroup analysis revealed a significant reduction in the rate of decline in FEV_1 and TLCO in subjects with lower lobe emphysema.

Mesenchymal stem cells (MSCs) also offer exciting regenerative potential.[228,233] MSCs exhibit potent antiinflammatory and immunomodulatory activities both in vitro and in vivo. This finding has led to a trial assessing the safety and efficacy of an IV preparation of allogenic MSCs (Prochymal).[234] The therapy was well tolerated and, although there were no significant differences in lung function tests or quality of life indicators, an early significant decrease in levels of circulating C-reactive protein was observed in some subjects. Another approach taken with MSCs was to populate a biologic connective tissue scaffold (which has been stripped of HLA-antigen expressing cells), which can then be used to grow autologous tissue before surgical implantation.[235]

SUMMARY

For the future treatment of COPD, it should be possible to have improved current drugs, antiinfective and antioxidant therapy, coupled with novel approaches directed against the innate immune system. In terms of the processes involved in COPD, there is rapid advancement of knowledge of viral responses and fibrosis, steroid-insensitive inflammation, autoimmunity, aberrant repair, accelerated aging, and appreciation of systemic disease and comorbidities. There is the need to develop validated noninvasive biomarkers for COPD and to have novel challenge models in animals and humans.[71] More interest has recently focused on cigarette-challenge models in an attempt to understand the exact immunologic responses to an acute smoke exposure event, to understand better the chronic changes that result from smoking.[68] In terms of clinical trial designs, these are adapted for bronchodilation, the natural history, and the prevention and treatment of COPD exacerbations and comorbidities. As is the case with many diseases, combinations of therapies may be the key to effective COPD treatment and prevention, and they may need to be given early in the disease. To develop novel drugs for COPD, it is clear that long-term studies in specific phenotypic groups, giving targeted therapy based on companion biomarkers, are needed. This would ideally use inhaled agents delivered directly to the intended site of action, with minimal unwanted side effects.[35] Overall, there is need for extensive collaboration between scientists, clinicians, the pharmaceutical industry, and drug regulators to identify and provide better therapy for patients with COPD.

REFERENCES

1. Ngkelo A, Adcock IM. New treatments for COPD. Curr Opin Pharmacol 2013;13(3):362–9.
2. Gross NJ. Novel antiinflammatory therapies for COPD. Chest 2012;142(5):1300–7.
3. Rabe KF, Wedzicha JA. Controversies in treatment of chronic obstructive pulmonary disease. Lancet 2011;378(9795):1038–47.
4. Martinez FJ, Donohue JF, Rennard SI. The future of chronic obstructive pulmonary disease treatment–difficulties of and barriers to drug development. Lancet 2011;378(9795):1027–37.
5. Hogg JC, Chu F, Utokaparch S, et al. The nature of small-airway obstruction in chronic obstructive pulmonary disease. N Engl J Med 2004;350(26): 2645–53.
6. Hansel TT, Barnes PJ. New drugs for exacerbations of chronic obstructive pulmonary disease. Lancet 2009;374(9691):744–55.
7. McDonough JE, Yuan R, Suzuki M, et al. Small-airway obstruction and emphysema in chronic obstructive pulmonary disease. N Engl J Med 2011;365(17):1567–75.
8. Brusselle GG, Joos GF, Bracke KR. New insights into the immunology of chronic obstructive pulmonary disease. Lancet 2011;378(9795):1015–26.
9. Churg A, Wright JL. Testing drugs in animal models of cigarette smoke-induced chronic obstructive pulmonary disease. Proc Am Thorac Soc 2009; 6(6):550–2.
10. van der Vaart H, Postma DS, Timens W, et al. Acute effects of cigarette smoke on inflammation and oxidative stress: a review. Thorax 2004; 59(8):713–21.
11. Willemse BW, Postma DS, Timens W, et al. The impact of smoking cessation on respiratory symptoms, lung function, airway hyperresponsiveness and inflammation. Eur Respir J 2004; 23(3):464–76.
12. Willemse BW, ten Hacken NH, Rutgers B, et al. Effect of 1-year smoking cessation on airway inflammation in COPD and asymptomatic smokers. Eur Respir J 2005;26(5):835–45.
13. Papi A, Contoli M, Caramori G, et al. Models of infection and exacerbations in COPD. Curr Opin Pharmacol 2007;7(3):259–65.

14. Calverley PM, Rennard SI. What have we learned from large drug treatment trials in COPD? Lancet 2007;370(9589):774–85.
15. Vestbo J, Edwards LD, Scanlon PD, et al. Changes in forced expiratory volume in 1 second over time in COPD. N Engl J Med 2011;365(13):1184–92.
16. Anthonisen N, Connett J, Friedman B, et al. Design of a clinical trial to test a treatment of the underlying cause of emphysema. Ann N Y Acad Sci 1991; 624(Suppl):31–4.
17. Han MK, Agusti A, Calverley PM, et al. Chronic obstructive pulmonary disease phenotypes: the future of COPD. Am J Respir Crit Care Med 2010; 182(5):598–604.
18. National Emphysema Treatment Trial Research Group. Patients at high risk of death after lung-volume-reduction surgery. N Engl J Med 2001; 345(15):1075–83.
19. Agusti A, Calverley PM, Celli B, et al. Characterisation of COPD heterogeneity in the ECLIPSE cohort. Respir Res 2010;11:122.
20. Qiu W, Cho MH, Riley JH, et al. Genetics of sputum gene expression in chronic obstructive pulmonary disease. PLoS One 2011;6(9):e24395.
21. MacNee W, Rennard SI, Hunt JF, et al. Evaluation of exhaled breath condensate pH as a biomarker for COPD. Respir Med 2011;105(7):1037–45.
22. Gelb AF, Barnes PJ, George SC, et al. Review of exhaled nitric oxide in chronic obstructive pulmonary disease. J Breath Res 2012;6(4):047101.
23. Franciosi L, Govorukhina N, Fusetti F, et al. Proteomic analysis of human epithelial lining fluid by microfluidics-based nanoLC-MS/MS: a feasibility study. Electrophoresis 2013. [Epub ahead of print].
24. Steiling K, van den Berge M, Hijazi K, et al. A dynamic bronchial airway gene expression signature of chronic obstructive pulmonary disease and lung function impairment. Am J Respir Crit Care Med 2013;187(9):933–42.
25. Woodruff PG. Novel outcomes and end points: biomarkers in chronic obstructive pulmonary disease clinical trials. Proc Am Thorac Soc 2011; 8(4):350–5.
26. Verrills NM, Irwin JA, He XY, et al. Identification of novel diagnostic biomarkers for asthma and chronic obstructive pulmonary disease. Am J Respir Crit Care Med 2011;183(12):1633–43.
27. Rosenberg SR, Kalhan R. Biomarkers in chronic obstructive pulmonary disease. Transl Res 2012; 159(4):228–37.
28. Scanlon PD, Connett JE, Waller LA, et al. Smoking cessation and lung function in mild-to-moderate chronic obstructive pulmonary disease. The lung health study. Am J Respir Crit Care Med 2000; 161(2 Pt 1):381–90.
29. Tonnesen P, Carrozzi L, Fagerstrom KO, et al. Smoking cessation in patients with respiratory diseases: a high priority, integral component of therapy. Eur Respir J 2007;29(2):390–417.
30. Stead LF, Lancaster T. Combined pharmacotherapy and behavioural interventions for smoking cessation. Cochrane Database Syst Rev 2012;(10):CD008286.
31. Kanazawa H, Tochino Y, Asai K, et al. Validity of HMGB1 measurement in epithelial lining fluid in patients with COPD. Eur J Clin Invest 2012; 42(4):419–26.
32. Williams JM, Steinberg MB, Steinberg ML, et al. Varenicline for tobacco dependence: panacea or plight? Expert Opin Pharmacother 2011;12(11): 1799–812.
33. West R, Zatonski W, Cedzynska M, et al. Placebo-controlled trial of cytisine for smoking cessation. N Engl J Med 2011;365(13):1193–200.
34. Hartmann-Boyce J, Cahill K, Hatsukami D, et al. Nicotine vaccines for smoking cessation. Cochrane Database Syst Rev 2012;(8):CD007072.
35. Hickey AJ. Back to the future: inhaled drug products. J Pharm Sci 2013;102(4):1165–72.
36. Yasuda H, Soejima K, Nakayama S, et al. Bronchoscopic microsampling is a useful complementary diagnostic tool for detecting lung cancer. Lung Cancer 2011;72(1):32–8.
37. D'Souza MS, Markou A. Neuronal mechanisms underlying development of nicotine dependence: implications for novel smoking-cessation treatments. Addict Sci Clin Pract 2011;6(1):4–16.
38. Cazzola M, Page CP, Calzetta L, et al. Emerging anti-inflammatory strategies for COPD. Eur Respir J 2012;40(3):724–41.
39. Cazzola M, Page CP, Calzetta L, et al. Pharmacology and therapeutics of bronchodilators. Pharmacol Rev 2012;64(3):450–504.
40. Cazzola M, Page CP, Rogliani P, et al. Beta2-agonist therapy in lung disease. Am J Respir Crit Care Med 2013;187(7):690–6.
41. Cazzola M, Page C, Matera MG. Long-acting muscarinic receptor antagonists for the treatment of respiratory disease. Pulm Pharmacol Ther 2013;26(3):307–17.
42. Vogelmeier C, Ramos-Barbon D, Jack D, et al. Indacaterol provides 24-hour bronchodilation in COPD: a placebo-controlled blinded comparison with tiotropium. Respir Res 2010;11:135.
43. Barnes PJ, Pocock SJ, Magnussen H, et al. Integrating indacaterol dose selection in a clinical study in COPD using an adaptive seamless design. Pulm Pharmacol Ther 2010;23(3):165–71.
44. Korn S, Kerwin E, Atis S, et al. Indacaterol once-daily provides superior efficacy to salmeterol twice-daily in COPD: a 12-week study. Respir Med 2011;105(5):719–26.
45. Cazzola M. Aclidinium bromide, a novel long-acting muscarinic M3 antagonist for the treatment

of COPD. Curr Opin Investig Drugs 2009;10(5): 482–90.

46. Cazzola M, Rogliani P, Matera MG. Aclidinium bromide/formoterol fumarate fixed-dose combination for the treatment of chronic obstructive pulmonary disease. Expert Opin Pharmacother 2013;14(6): 775–81.

47. Buhl R, Banerji D. Profile of glycopyrronium for once-daily treatment of moderate-to-severe COPD. Int J Chron Obstruct Pulmon Dis 2012;7:729–41.

48. Kerwin E, Hebert J, Gallagher N, et al. Efficacy and safety of NVA237 versus placebo and tiotropium in patients with COPD: the GLOW2 study. Eur Respir J 2012;40(5):1106–14.

49. Beeh KM, Singh D, Di SL, et al. Once-daily NVA237 improves exercise tolerance from the first dose in patients with COPD: the GLOW3 trial. Int J Chron Obstruct Pulmon Dis 2012;7:503–13.

50. van Noord JA, Aumann JL, Janssens E, et al. Combining tiotropium and salmeterol in COPD: effects on airflow obstruction and symptoms. Respir Med 2010;104(7):995–1004.

51. van Noord JA, Aumann JL, Janssens E, et al. Effects of tiotropium with and without formoterol on airflow obstruction and resting hyperinflation in patients with COPD. Chest 2006;129(3):509–17.

52. Tashkin DP, Pearle J, Iezzoni D, et al. Formoterol and tiotropium compared with tiotropium alone for treatment of COPD. COPD 2009;6(1):17–25.

53. van Noord JA, Buhl R, LaForce C, et al. QVA149 demonstrates superior bronchodilation compared with indacaterol or placebo in patients with chronic obstructive pulmonary disease. Thorax 2010; 65(12):1086–91.

54. Dougall IG, Young A, Ince F, et al. Dual dopamine D2 receptor and beta2-adrenoceptor agonists for the treatment of chronic obstructive pulmonary disease: the pre-clinical rationale. Respir Med 2003; 97(Suppl A):S3–7.

55. Hiller FC, Alderfer V, Goldman M. Long-term use of Viozan (sibenadet HCl) in patients with chronic obstructive pulmonary disease: results of a 1-year study. Respir Med 2003;97(Suppl A):S45–52.

56. Vestbo J, Hurd SS, Agusti AG, et al. Global strategy for the diagnosis, management, and prevention of chronic obstructive pulmonary disease: GOLD executive summary. Am J Respir Crit Care Med 2013;187(4):347–65.

57. de Miguel-Diez J, Carrasco-Garrido P, Rejas-Gutierrez J, et al. Inappropriate overuse of inhaled corticosteroids for COPD patients: impact on health costs and health status. Lung 2011;189(3): 199–206.

58. Yang IA, Clarke MS, Sim EH, et al. Inhaled corticosteroids for stable chronic obstructive pulmonary disease. Cochrane Database Syst Rev 2012;(7):CD002991.

59. Wedzicha JA, Calverley PM, Seemungal TA, et al. The prevention of COPD exacerbations by salmeterol/fluticasone propionate or tiotropium bromide. Am J Respir Crit Care Med 2007;177:19–26.

60. Ehrchen J, Steinmuller L, Barczyk K, et al. Glucocorticoids induce differentiation of a specifically activated, anti-inflammatory subtype of human monocytes. Blood 2007;109(3):1265–74.

61. Barnes PJ. Glucocorticosteroids: current and future directions. Br J Pharmacol 2011;163(1): 29–43.

62. Cazzola M, Ando F, Santus P, et al. A pilot study to assess the effects of combining fluticasone propionate/salmeterol and tiotropium on the airflow obstruction of patients with severe-to-very severe COPD. Pulm Pharmacol Ther 2007;20(5):556–61.

63. Singh D, Brooks J, Hagan G, et al. Superiority of "triple" therapy with salmeterol/fluticasone propionate and tiotropium bromide versus individual components in moderate to severe COPD. Thorax 2008;63:592–8.

64. Renard D, Looby M, Kramer B, et al. Characterization of the bronchodilatory dose response to indacaterol in patients with chronic obstructive pulmonary disease using model-based approaches. Respir Res 2011;12:54.

65. Ito K, Ito M, Elliott WM, et al. Decreased histone deacetylase activity in chronic obstructive pulmonary disease. N Engl J Med 2005;352(19):1967–76.

66. Marwick JA, Caramori G, Stevenson CS, et al. Inhibition of PI3Kdelta restores glucocorticoid function in smoking-induced airway inflammation in mice. Am J Respir Crit Care Med 2009;179(7):542–8.

67. Ito K, Caramori G, Adcock IM. Therapeutic potential of phosphatidylinositol 3-kinase inhibitors in inflammatory respiratory disease. J Pharmacol Exp Ther 2007;321(1):1–8.

68. Lo Tam Loi AT, Hoonhorst SJ, Franciosi L, et al. Acute and chronic inflammatory responses induced by smoking in individuals susceptible and non-susceptible to development of COPD: from specific disease phenotyping towards novel therapy. Protocol of a cross-sectional study. BMJ Open 2013;3(2).

69. Cosio BG, Iglesias A, Rios A, et al. Low-dose theophylline enhances the anti-inflammatory effects of steroids during exacerbations of COPD. Thorax 2009;64(5):424–9.

70. Cosio BG, Tsaprouni L, Ito K, et al. Theophylline restores histone deacetylase activity and steroid responses in COPD macrophages. J Exp Med 2004;200(5):689–95.

71. Warnier MJ, van Riet EE, Rutten FH, et al. Smoking cessation strategies in patients with COPD. Eur Respir J 2013;41(3):727–34.

72. Kanner RE, Anthonisen NR, Connett JE. Lower respiratory illnesses promote FEV_1 decline in current

smokers but not ex-smokers with chronic obstructive pulmonary disease: results from Lung Health Study. Am J Respir Crit Care Med 2001;164: 358–64.

73. Donaldson GC, Seemungal TA, Bhowmik A, et al. Relationship between exacerbation frequency and lung function decline in chronic obstructive pulmonary disease. Thorax 2002;57(10):847–52.

74. Murphy TF. The role of bacteria in airway inflammation in exacerbations of chronic obstructive pulmonary disease. Curr Opin Infect Dis 2006; 19(3):225–30.

75. Sethi S, Maloney J, Grove L, et al. Airway inflammation and bronchial bacterial colonization in chronic obstructive pulmonary disease. Am J Respir Crit Care Med 2006;173(9):991–8.

76. Patel IS, Seemungal TA, Wilks M, et al. Relationship between bacterial colonisation and the frequency, character, and severity of COPD exacerbations. Thorax 2002;57(9):759–64.

77. Barnes PJ. The cytokine network in asthma and chronic obstructive pulmonary disease. J Clin Invest 2008;118(11):3546–56.

78. Nseir S, Ader F. Prevalence and outcome of severe chronic obstructive pulmonary disease exacerbations caused by multidrug-resistant bacteria. Curr Opin Pulm Med 2008;14(2):95–100.

79. Hanlon GW. Bacteriophages: an appraisal of their role in the treatment of bacterial infections. Int J Antimicrob Agents 2007;30(2):118–28.

80. Serhan CN, Chiang N, Van Dyke TE. Resolving inflammation: dual anti-inflammatory and pro-resolution lipid mediators. Nat Rev Immunol 2008; 8(5):349–61.

81. Tamaoki J, Kadota J, Takizawa H. Clinical implications of the immunomodulatory effects of macrolides. Am J Med 2004;117(Suppl 9A):5S–11S.

82. Kanoh S, Rubin BK. Mechanisms of action and clinical application of macrolides as immunomodulatory medications. Clin Microbiol Rev 2010;23(3): 590–615.

83. Albert RK, Connett J, Bailey WC, et al. Azithromycin for prevention of exacerbations of COPD. N Engl J Med 2011;365(8):689–98.

84. Seemungal TA, Wilkinson TM, Hurst JR, et al. Long-term erythromycin therapy is associated with decreased chronic obstructive pulmonary disease exacerbations. Am J Respir Crit Care Med 2008; 178(11):1139–47.

85. Li YJ, Azuma A, Usuki J, et al. EM703 improves bleomycin-induced pulmonary fibrosis in mice by the inhibition of TGF-beta signaling in lung fibroblasts. Respir Res 2006;7:16.

86. Sethi S, Jones PW, Theron MS, et al. Pulsed moxifloxacin for the prevention of exacerbations of chronic obstructive pulmonary disease: a randomized controlled trial. Respir Res 2010;11:10.

87. Varkey JB, Varkey B. Viral infections in patients with chronic obstructive pulmonary disease. Curr Opin Pulm Med 2008;14(2):89–94.

88. Brownlee JW, Turner RB. New developments in the epidemiology and clinical spectrum of rhinovirus infections. Curr Opin Pediatr 2008;20(1):67–71.

89. Patel IS, Roberts NJ, Lloyd-Owen SJ, et al. Airway epithelial inflammatory responses and clinical parameters in COPD. Eur Respir J 2003;22(1):94–9.

90. Baines KJ, Hsu AC, Tooze M, et al. Novel immune genes associated with excessive inflammatory and antiviral responses to rhinovirus in COPD. Respir Res 2013;14:15.

91. Klune JR, Dhupar R, Cardinal J, et al. HMGB1: endogenous danger signaling. Mol Med 2008; 14(7–8):476–84.

92. Ramaswamy M, Groskreutz DJ, Look DC. Recognizing the importance of respiratory syncytial virus in chronic obstructive pulmonary disease. COPD 2009;6(1):64–75.

93. Sikkel MB, Quint JK, Mallia P, et al. Respiratory syncytial virus persistence in chronic obstructive pulmonary disease. Pediatr Infect Dis J 2008; 27(Suppl 10):S63–70.

94. Olszewska W, Openshaw P. Emerging drugs for respiratory syncytial virus infection. Expert Opin Emerg Drugs 2009;14(2):207–17.

95. Novel Swine-Origin Influenza A (H1N1) Virus Investigation Team, Dawood FS, Jain S, et al. Emergence of a novel swine-origin influenza A (H1N1) virus in humans. N Engl J Med 2009; 360:2605–15.

96. Glezen WP. Clinical practice. Prevention and treatment of seasonal influenza. N Engl J Med 2008; 359(24):2579–85.

97. Hayden F. Developing new antiviral agents for influenza treatment: what does the future hold? Clin Infect Dis 2009;48(Suppl 1):S3–13.

98. Sarir H, Henricks PA, van Houwelingen AH, et al. Cells, mediators and Toll-like receptors in COPD. Eur J Pharmacol 2008;585(2–3):346–53.

99. Raymond T, Schaller M, Hogaboam CM, et al. Toll-like receptors, Notch ligands, and cytokines drive the chronicity of lung inflammation. Proc Am Thorac Soc 2007;4(8):635–41.

100. O'Neill LA. The interleukin-1 receptor/Toll-like receptor superfamily: 10 years of progress. Immunol Rev 2008;226:10–8.

101. Kumar H, Kawai T, Akira S. Pathogen recognition in the innate immune response. Biochem J 2009; 420(1):1–16.

102. Paul-Clark MJ, McMaster SK, Sorrentino R, et al. Toll-like receptor 2 is essential for the sensing of oxidants during inflammation. Am J Respir Crit Care Med 2009;179(4):299–306.

103. Williams AS, Leung SY, Nath P, et al. Role of TLR2, TLR4, and MyD88 in murine ozone-induced airway

hyperresponsiveness and neutrophilia. J Appl Physiol 2007;103(4):1189–95.

104. Doz E, Noulin N, Boichot E, et al. Cigarette smoke-induced pulmonary inflammation is TLR4/MyD88 and IL-1R1/MyD88 signaling dependent. J Immunol 2008;180(2):1169–78.

105. Foell D, Wittkowski H, Roth J. Mechanisms of disease: a 'DAMP' view of inflammatory arthritis. Nat Clin Pract Rheumatol 2007;3(7):382–90.

106. Bianchi ME. DAMPs, PAMPs and alarmins: all we need to know about danger. J Leukoc Biol 2007; 81(1):1–5.

107. Areschoug T, Gordon S. Scavenger receptors: role in innate immunity and microbial pathogenesis. Cell Microbiol 2009;11(8):1160–9.

108. Ramasamy R, Yan SF, Schmidt AM. RAGE: therapeutic target and biomarker of the inflammatory response–the evidence mounts. J Leukoc Biol 2009;86(3):505–12.

109. Sukkar MB, Xie S, Khorasani NM, et al. Toll-like receptor 2, 3, and 4 expression and function in human airway smooth muscle. J Allergy Clin Immunol 2006;118(3):641–8.

110. O'Neill LA, Bryant CE, Doyle SL. Therapeutic targeting of toll-like receptors for infectious and inflammatory diseases and cancer. Pharmacol Rev 2009;61(2):177–97.

111. Shirey KA, Lai W, Scott AJ, et al. The TLR4 antagonist Eritoran protects mice from lethal influenza infection. Nature 2013;497(7450):498–502.

112. Chaudhuri N, Whyte MK, Sabroe I. Reducing the toll of inflammatory lung disease. Chest 2007; 131(5):1550–6.

113. Kenny EF, O'Neill LA. Signalling adaptors used by Toll-like receptors: an update. Cytokine 2008; 43(3):342–9.

114. O'Connor BJ, Leaker BR, Barnes PJ, et al. Inhibition of LPS-induced neutrophilic inflammation in healthy volunteers. Eur Respir J 2007;30(Suppl 51):1294.

115. Holz O, Khalilieh S, Ludwig-Sengpiel A, et al. SCH527123, a novel CXCR2 antagonist, inhibits ozone-induced neutrophilia in healthy subjects. Eur Respir J 2010;35(3):564–70.

116. Kerstjens HA, Bjermer L, Eriksson L, et al. Tolerability and efficacy of inhaled AZD4818, a CCR1 antagonist, in moderate to severe COPD patients. Respir Med 2010;104(9):1297–303.

117. Norman P. DP(2) receptor antagonists in development. Expert Opin Investig Drugs 2010;19(8): 947–61.

118. Seggev JS, Thornton WH Jr, Edes TE. Serum leukotriene B4 levels in patients with obstructive pulmonary disease. Chest 1991;99(2):289–91.

119. Beeh KM, Kornmann O, Buhl R, et al. Neutrophil chemotactic activity of sputum from patients with COPD: role of interleukin 8 and leukotriene B4. Chest 2003;123(4):1240–7.

120. Snelgrove RJ, Jackson PL, Hardison MT, et al. A critical role for LTA4H in limiting chronic pulmonary neutrophilic inflammation. Science 2010; 330(6000):90–4.

121. Watz H, Bock D, Meyer M, et al. Inhaled pan-selectin antagonist Bimosiamose attenuates airway inflammation in COPD. Pulm Pharmacol Ther 2012; 26(2):265–70.

122. Bedard PW, Kaila N. Selectin inhibitors: a patent review. Expert Opin Ther Pat 2010;20(6):781–93.

123. Currie GP, Butler CA, Anderson WJ, et al. Phosphodiesterase 4 inhibitors in chronic obstructive pulmonary disease: a new approach to oral treatment. Br J Clin Pharmacol 2008;65(6):803–10.

124. Giembycz MA. Can the anti-inflammatory potential of PDE4 inhibitors be realized: guarded optimism or wishful thinking? Br J Pharmacol 2008;155(3):288–90.

125. Sriskantharajah S, Hamblin N, Worsley S, et al. Targeting phosphoinositide 3-kinase delta for the treatment of respiratory diseases. Ann N Y Acad Sci 2013;1280(1):35–9.

126. Rennard S, Knobil K, Rabe KF, et al. The efficacy and safety of cilomilast in COPD. Drugs 2008; 68(Suppl 2):3–57.

127. Compton CH, Gubb J, Nieman R, et al. Cilomilast, a selective phosphodiesterase-4 inhibitor for treatment of patients with chronic obstructive pulmonary disease: a randomised, dose-ranging study. Lancet 2001;358(9278):265–70.

128. Rennard SI, Schachter N, Strek M, et al. Cilomilast for COPD: results of a 6-month, placebo-controlled study of a potent, selective inhibitor of phosphodiesterase 4. Chest 2006;129(1):56–66.

129. Rabe KF, Bateman ED, O'Donnell D, et al. Roflumilast–an oral anti-inflammatory treatment for chronic obstructive pulmonary disease: a randomised controlled trial. Lancet 2005;366(9485):563–71.

130. Calverley PM, Sanchez-Toril F, McIvor A, et al. Effect of 1-year treatment with roflumilast in severe chronic obstructive pulmonary disease. Am J Respir Crit Care Med 2007;176(2):154–61.

131. Fabbri LM, Calverley PM, Izquierdo-Alonso JL, et al. Roflumilast in moderate-to-severe chronic obstructive pulmonary disease treated with long-acting bronchodilators: two randomised clinical trials. Lancet 2009;374(9691):695–703.

132. Calverley PM, Rabe KF, Goehring UM, et al. Roflumilast in symptomatic chronic obstructive pulmonary disease: two randomised clinical trials. Lancet 2009;374(9691):685–94.

133. Giembycz MA, Field SK. Roflumilast: first phosphodiesterase 4 inhibitor approved for treatment of COPD. Drug Des Devel Ther 2010;4:147–58.

134. Chong J, Poole P, Leung B, et al. Phosphodiesterase 4 inhibitors for chronic obstructive pulmonary disease. Cochrane Database Syst Rev 2011;(5):CD002309.

135. Calverley PM, Martinez FJ, Fabbri LM, et al. Does roflumilast decrease exacerbations in severe COPD patients not controlled by inhaled combination therapy? the REACT study protocol. Int J Chron Obstruct Pulmon Dis 2012;7:375–82.

136. Robichaud A, Stamatiou PB, Jin SL, et al. Deletion of phosphodiesterase 4D in mice shortens alpha(2)-adrenoceptor-mediated anesthesia, a behavioral correlate of emesis. J Clin Invest 2002; 110(7):1045–52.

137. Seguin RM, Ferrari N. Emerging oligonucleotide therapies for asthma and chronic obstructive pulmonary disease. Expert Opin Investig Drugs 2009;18(10):1505–17.

138. Barnes PJ. Corticosteroid resistance in patients with asthma and chronic obstructive pulmonary disease. J Allergy Clin Immunol 2013;131(3): 636–45.

139. Simmons DL. Targeting kinases: a new approach to treating inflammatory rheumatic diseases. Curr Opin Pharmacol 2013;13(3):426–34.

140. Gaestel M, Kotlyarov A, Kracht M. Targeting innate immunity protein kinase signalling in inflammation. Nat Rev Drug Discov 2009;8(6):480–99.

141. Chung KF. p38 mitogen-activated protein kinase pathways in asthma and COPD. Chest 2011; 139(6):1470–9.

142. Lomas DA, Lipson DA, Miller BE, et al. An oral inhibitor of p38 MAP kinase reduces plasma fibrinogen in patients with chronic obstructive pulmonary disease. J Clin Pharmacol 2012;52(3): 416–24.

143. Langereis JD, Raaijmakers HA, Ulfman LH, et al. Abrogation of NF-kappaB signaling in human neutrophils induces neutrophil survival through sustained p38-MAPK activation. J Leukoc Biol 2010; 88(4):655–64.

144. Caramori G, Casolari P, Adcock I. Role of transcription factors in the pathogenesis of asthma and COPD. Cell Commun Adhes 2013;20(1–2):21–40.

145. Patel S. Exploring novel therapeutic targets in gist: focus on the PI3K/Akt/mTOR pathway. Curr Oncol Rep 2013;15(4):386–95.

146. Marwick JA, Caramori G, Casolari P, et al. A role for phosphoinositol 3-kinase delta in the impairment of glucocorticoid responsiveness in patients with chronic obstructive pulmonary disease. J Allergy Clin Immunol 2010;125(5):1146–53.

147. Fung-Leung WP. Phosphoinositide 3-kinase delta (PI3Kdelta) in leukocyte signaling and function. Cell Signal 2011;23(4):603–8.

148. Fung-Leung WP. Phosphoinositide 3-kinase gamma in T cell biology and disease therapy. Ann N Y Acad Sci 2013;1280:40–3.

149. Doukas J, Eide L, Stebbins K, et al. Aerosolized phosphoinositide 3-kinase gamma/delta inhibitor TG100-115 [3-[2,4-diamino-6-(3-hydroxyphenyl) pteridin-7-yl]phenol] as a therapeutic candidate for asthma and chronic obstructive pulmonary disease. J Pharmacol Exp Ther 2009;328(3):758–65.

150. Shen Y, Chen L, Wang T, et al. PPARgamma as a potential target to treat airway mucus hypersecretion in chronic airway inflammatory diseases. PPAR Res 2012;2012:256874.

151. Onoue S, Sato H, Ogawa K, et al. Inhalable dry-emulsion formulation of cyclosporine A with improved anti-inflammatory effects in experimental asthma/COPD-model rats. Eur J Pharm Biopharm 2012;80(1):54–60.

152. Barnes PJ, Celli BR. Systemic manifestations and comorbidities of COPD. Eur Respir J 2009;33(5): 1165–85.

153. Agusti A, Faner R. Systemic inflammation and co-morbidities in chronic obstructive pulmonary disease. Proc Am Thorac Soc 2012;9(2):43–6.

154. Hunninghake DB. Cardiovascular disease in chronic obstructive pulmonary disease. Proc Am Thorac Soc 2005;2(1):44–9.

155. Barnes PJ. Future treatments for chronic obstructive pulmonary disease and its comorbidities. Proc Am Thorac Soc 2008;5(8):857–64.

156. Agusti A, Edwards LD, Rennard SI, et al. Persistent systemic inflammation is associated with poor clinical outcomes in COPD: a novel phenotype. PLoS One 2012;7(5):e37483.

157. Donaldson AV, Maddocks M, Martolini D, et al. Muscle function in COPD: a complex interplay. Int J Chron Obstruct Pulmon Dis 2012;7:523–35.

158. Steiner MC, Roubenoff R, Tal-Singer R, et al. Prospects for the development of effective pharmaco-therapy targeted at the skeletal muscles in chronic obstructive pulmonary disease: a translational review. Thorax 2012;67(12):1102–9.

159. Jain MK, Ridker PM. Anti-inflammatory effects of statins: clinical evidence and basic mechanisms. Nat Rev Drug Discov 2005;4(12):977–87.

160. van Gestel YR, Hoeks SE, Sin DD, et al. Effect of statin therapy on mortality in patients with peripheral arterial disease and comparison of those with versus without associated chronic obstructive pulmonary disease. Am J Cardiol 2008;102(2):192–6.

161. Blamoun AI, Batty GN, DeBari VA, et al. Statins may reduce episodes of exacerbation and the requirement for intubation in patients with COPD: evidence from a retrospective cohort study. Int J Clin Pract 2008;62(9):1373–8.

162. Frost FJ, Petersen H, Tollestrup K, et al. Influenza and COPD mortality protection as pleiotropic, dose-dependent effects of statins. Chest 2007; 131(4):1006–12.

163. Mancini GB, Etminan M, Zhang B, et al. Reduction of morbidity and mortality by statins, angiotensin-converting enzyme inhibitors, and angiotensin receptor blockers in patients with chronic obstructive

pulmonary disease. J Am Coll Cardiol 2006;47(12): 2554–60.

164. Soyseth V, Brekke PH, Smith P, et al. Statin use is associated with reduced mortality in COPD. Eur Respir J 2007;29(2):279–83.

165. Lahousse L, Loth DW, Joos GF, et al. Statins, systemic inflammation and risk of death in COPD: the Rotterdam study. Pulm Pharmacol Ther 2012; 26(2):212–7.

166. van Gestel YR, Hoeks SE, Sin DD, et al. COPD and cancer mortality: the influence of statins. Thorax 2009;64(11):963–7.

167. Mak JC. Pathogenesis of COPD. Part II. Oxidative-antioxidative imbalance. Int J Tuberc Lung Dis 2008;12(4):368–74.

168. Kovacic P, Somanathan R. Pulmonary toxicity and environmental contamination: radicals, electron transfer, and protection by antioxidants. Rev Environ Contam Toxicol 2009;201:41–69.

169. Kirkham P, Rahman I. Antioxidant therapeutic strategies. In: Hansel TT, Barnes PJ, editors. New drugs and targets for respiratory diseases. London: Thomson-Reuters; 2009.

170. Rahman I, MacNee W. Antioxidant pharmacological therapies for COPD. Curr Opin Pharmacol 2012;12(3):256–65.

171. Wood JG, Rogina B, Lavu S, et al. Sirtuin activators mimic caloric restriction and delay ageing in metazoans. Nature 2004;430(7000):686–9.

172. Sharma G, Hanania NA, Shim YM. The aging immune system and its relationship to the development of chronic obstructive pulmonary disease. Proc Am Thorac Soc 2009;6(7):573–80.

173. Ito K, Barnes PJ. COPD as a disease of accelerated lung aging. Chest 2009;135(1):173–80.

174. Harman D. Free radical theory of aging: an update: increasing the functional life span. Ann N Y Acad Sci 2006;1067:10–21.

175. Kumar V, Kumar S, Hassan M, et al. Novel chalcone derivatives as potent Nrf2 activators in mice and human lung epithelial cells. J Med Chem 2011;54(12):4147–59.

176. Rubio ML, Martin-Mosquero MC, Ortega M, et al. Oral N-acetylcysteine attenuates elastase-induced pulmonary emphysema in rats. Chest 2004;125(4):1500–6.

177. Stey C, Steurer J, Bachmann S, et al. The effect of oral N-acetylcysteine in chronic bronchitis: a quantitative systematic review. Eur Respir J 2000;16(2): 253–62.

178. Decramer M, Rutten-van Molken M, Dekhuijzen PN, et al. Effects of N-acetylcysteine on outcomes in chronic obstructive pulmonary disease (Bronchitis Randomized on NAC Cost-Utility Study, BRONCUS): a randomised placebo-controlled trial. Lancet 2005;365(9470): 1552–60.

179. Zheng JP, Kang J, Huang SG, et al. Effect of carbocisteine on acute exacerbation of chronic obstructive pulmonary disease (PEACE Study): a randomised placebo-controlled study. Lancet 2008;371(9629):2013–8.

180. Li L, Salto-Tellez M, Tan CH, et al. GYY4137, a novel hydrogen sulfide-releasing molecule, protects against endotoxic shock in the rat. Free Radic Biol Med 2009;47(1):103–13.

181. Rogers DF. Mucoactive agents for airway mucus hypersecretory diseases. Respir Care 2007;52(9): 1176–93.

182. Foreman MG, DeMeo DL, Hersh CP, et al. Polymorphic variation in surfactant protein B is associated with COPD exacerbations. Eur Respir J 2008; 32(4):938–44.

183. Hudson TJ. Dornase in treatment of chronic bronchitis. Ann Pharmacother 1996;30:674–5.

184. Kueppers F. The role of augmentation therapy in alpha-1 antitrypsin deficiency. Curr Med Res Opin 2011;27(3):579–88.

185. Hunninghake GM, Cho MH, Tesfaigzi Y, et al. MMP12, lung function, and COPD in high-risk populations. N Engl J Med 2009;361(27):2599–608.

186. Korkmaz B, Horwitz MS, Jenne DE, et al. Neutrophil elastase, proteinase 3, and cathepsin G as therapeutic targets in human diseases. Pharmacol Rev 2010;62(4):726–59.

187. Stevens T, Ekholm K, Granse M, et al. AZD9668: pharmacological characterization of a novel oral inhibitor of neutrophil elastase. J Pharmacol Exp Ther 2011;339(1):313–20.

188. Vogelmeier C, Aquino TO, O'Brien CD, et al. A randomised, placebo-controlled, dose-finding study of AZD9668, an oral inhibitor of neutrophil elastase, in patients with chronic obstructive pulmonary disease treated with tiotropium. COPD 2012;9(2):111–20.

189. Brown RA, Lever R, Jones NA, et al. Effects of heparin and related molecules upon neutrophil aggregation and elastase release in vitro. Br J Pharmacol 2003;139(4):845–53.

190. Churg A, Zhou S, Wright JL. Series "matrix metalloproteinases in lung health and disease": matrix metalloproteinases in COPD. Eur Respir J 2012; 39(1):197–209.

191. Bramhall SR, Hallissey MT, Whiting J, et al. Marimastat as maintenance therapy for patients with advanced gastric cancer: a randomised trial. Br J Cancer 2002;86(12):1864–70.

192. Magnussen H, Watz H, Kirsten A, et al. Safety and tolerability of an oral MMP-9 and -12 inhibitor, AZD1236, in patients with moderate-to-severe COPD: a randomised controlled 6-week trial. Pulm Pharmacol Ther 2011;24(5):563–70.

193. Dahl R, Titlestad I, Lindqvist A, et al. Effects of an oral MMP-9 and -12 inhibitor, AZD1236, on

biomarkers in moderate/severe COPD: a randomised controlled trial. Pulm Pharmacol Ther 2012; 25(2):169–77.

194. du Bois RM. Strategies for treating idiopathic pulmonary fibrosis. Nat Rev Drug Discov 2010;9(2): 129–40.

195. Fernandez IE, Eickelberg O. New cellular and molecular mechanisms of lung injury and fibrosis in idiopathic pulmonary fibrosis. Lancet 2012; 380(9842):680–8.

196. Sivakumar P, Ntolios P, Jenkins G, et al. Into the matrix: targeting fibroblasts in pulmonary fibrosis. Curr Opin Pulm Med 2012;18(5):462–9.

197. Datta A, Scotton CJ, Chambers RC. Novel therapeutic approaches for pulmonary fibrosis. Br J Pharmacol 2011;163(1):141–72.

198. Wuyts WA, Agostini C, Antoniou KM, et al. The pathogenesis of pulmonary fibrosis: a moving target. Eur Respir J 2013;41(5):1207–18.

199. Lee SB, Kalluri R. Mechanistic connection between inflammation and fibrosis. Kidney Int Suppl 2010;(119):S22–6.

200. Chilosi M, Poletti V, Rossi A. The pathogenesis of COPD and IPF: distinct horns of the same devil? Respir Res 2012;13:3.

201. Wilson MS, Wynn TA. Pulmonary fibrosis: pathogenesis, etiology and regulation. Mucosal Immunol 2009;2(2):103–21.

202. Laurent GJ, McAnulty RJ, Hill M, et al. Escape from the matrix: multiple mechanisms for fibroblast activation in pulmonary fibrosis. Proc Am Thorac Soc 2008;5(3):311–5.

203. Scotton CJ, Chambers RC. Molecular targets in pulmonary fibrosis: the myofibroblast in focus. Chest 2007;132(4):1311–21.

204. Krueger GG, Langley RG, Leonardi C, et al. A human interleukin-12/23 monoclonal antibody for the treatment of psoriasis. N Engl J Med 2007; 356(6):580–92.

205. Milara J, Peiro T, Serrano A, et al. Epithelial to mesenchymal transition is increased in patients with COPD and induced by cigarette smoke. Thorax 2013;68(5):410–20.

206. Leung SY, Niimi A, Noble A, et al. Effect of transforming growth factor-beta receptor I kinase inhibitor 2,4-disubstituted pteridine (SD-208) in chronic allergic airway inflammation and remodeling. J Pharmacol Exp Ther 2006;319(2):586–94.

207. Suissa S, Ernst P, Hudson M. TNF-alpha antagonists and the prevention of hospitalisation for chronic obstructive pulmonary disease. Pulm Pharmacol Ther 2008;21(1):234–8.

208. Rennard SI, Fogarty C, Kelsen S, et al. The safety and efficacy of infliximab in moderate to severe chronic obstructive pulmonary disease. Am J Respir Crit Care Med 2007;175(9):926–34.

209. Barnes PJ. Unexpected failure of anti-tumor necrosis factor therapy in chronic obstructive pulmonary disease. Am J Respir Crit Care Med 2007;175(9): 866–7.

210. Loza MJ, Watt R, Baribaud F, et al. Systemic inflammatory profile and response to anti-tumor necrosis factor therapy in chronic obstructive pulmonary disease. Respir Res 2012;13:12.

211. Wenzel SE, Barnes PJ, Bleecker ER, et al. A randomized, double-blind, placebo-controlled study of TNF-alpha blockade in severe persistent asthma. Am J Respir Crit Care Med 2009;179: 549–58.

212. Paul-Pletzer K. Tocilizumab: blockade of interleukin-6 signaling pathway as a therapeutic strategy for inflammatory disorders. Drugs Today (Barc) 2006;42(9):559–76.

213. Dhimolea E. Canakinumab. MAbs 2010;2(1):3–13.

214. Ivanov S, Linden A. Targeting interleukin-17 in the lungs. In: Hansel TT, Barnes PJ, editors. New drugs and targets for respiratory diseases. London: Thomson-Reuters; 2009.

215. Prause O, Bossios A, Silverpil E, et al. IL-17-producing T lymphocytes in lung tissue and in the bronchoalveolar space after exposure to endotoxin from Escherichia coli in vivo–effects of anti-inflammatory pharmacotherapy. Pulm Pharmacol Ther 2009;22(3):199–207.

216. Zijlstra GJ, ten Hacken NH, Hoffmann RF, et al. Interleukin-17A induces glucocorticoid insensitivity in human bronchial epithelial cells. Eur Respir J 2012;39(2):439–45.

217. Leonardi C, Matheson R, Zachariae C, et al. Anti-interleukin-17 monoclonal antibody ixekizumab in chronic plaque psoriasis. N Engl J Med 2012;366(13):1190–9.

218. Papp KA, Leonardi C, Menter A, et al. Brodalumab, an anti-interleukin-17-receptor antibody for psoriasis. N Engl J Med 2012;366(13):1181–9.

219. Ito K, Colley T, Mercado N. Geroprotectors as a novel therapeutic strategy for COPD, an accelerating aging disease. Int J Chron Obstruct Pulmon Dis 2012;7:641–52.

220. Yao H, Rahman I. Perspectives on translational and therapeutic aspects of SIRT1 in inflammaging and senescence. Biochem Pharmacol 2012;84(10): 1332–9.

221. Beauharnois JM, Bolivar BE, Welch JT. Sirtuin 6: a review of biological effects and potential therapeutic properties. Mol Biosyst 2013;9(7):1789–806.

222. Agusti A, MacNee W, Donaldson K, et al. Hypothesis: does COPD have an autoimmune component? Thorax 2003;58(10):832–4.

223. Lee SH, Goswami S, Grudo A, et al. Antielastin autoimmunity in tobacco smoking-induced emphysema. Nat Med 2007;13(5):567–9.

224. Feghali-Bostwick CA, Gadgil AS, Otterbein LE, et al. Autoantibodies in patients with chronic obstructive pulmonary disease. Am J Respir Crit Care Med 2008;177(2):156–63.

225. Checkley W, West KP Jr, Wise RA, et al. Maternal vitamin A supplementation and lung function in offspring. N Engl J Med 2010;362(19):1784–94.

226. Butler JP, Loring SH, Patz S, et al. Evidence for adult lung growth in humans. N Engl J Med 2012; 367(3):244–7.

227. Rennard SI, Wachenfeldt K. Rationale and emerging approaches for targeting lung repair and regeneration in the treatment of chronic obstructive pulmonary disease. Proc Am Thorac Soc 2011;8(4):368–75.

228. Hind M, Maden M. Is a regenerative approach viable for the treatment of COPD? Br J Pharmacol 2011;163(1):106–15.

229. Kubo H. Concise review: clinical prospects for treating chronic obstructive pulmonary disease with regenerative approaches. Stem Cells Transl Med 2012;1(8):627–31.

230. Massaro GD, Massaro D. Retinoic acid treatment abrogates elastase-induced pulmonary emphysema in rats. Nat Med 1997;3(6):675–7.

231. Roth MD, Connett JE, D'Armiento JM, et al. Feasibility of retinoids for the treatment of emphysema study. Chest 2006;130(5):1334–45.

232. Stolk J, Stockley RA, Stoel BC, et al. Randomised controlled trial for emphysema with a selective agonist of the gamma-type retinoic acid receptor. Eur Respir J 2012;40(2):306–12.

233. Rankin S. Mesenchymal stem cells. Thorax 2012; 67(6):565–6.

234. Weiss DJ, Casaburi R, Flannery R, et al. A placebo-controlled, randomized trial of mesenchymal stem cells in COPD. Chest 2013;143(6):1590–8.

235. Badylak SF, Weiss DJ, Caplan A, et al. Engineered whole organs and complex tissues. Lancet 2012; 379(9819):943–52.

Pulmonary Rehabilitation

Thierry Troosters, PT, PhD[a,b,*], Heleen Demeyer, PT, MSc[a,b],
Miek Hornikx, PT, MSc[a,b],
Carlos Augusto Camillo, PT, MSc[a,b],
Wim Janssens, MD, PhD[a,b]

KEYWORDS

- Pulmonary rehabilitation • COPD • Screening • Physical activity • Exercise
- Long term management

KEY POINTS

- Pulmonary rehabilitation is an evidence-based therapy for patients with COPD that remain symptomatic despite optimal pharmacological management.
- Pulmonary rehabilitation improves exercise tolerance, symptoms and health related quality of life. It reduces health care cost, particularly in patients with exacerbations.
- Further research should focus on the strategies to ensure the long-term benefits for patients with COPD, particularly in improvements of physical activity.

OUTLINE
Definition

Pulmonary rehabilitation is now an accepted therapy for patients with respiratory diseases. Its effectiveness is supported by countless randomized controlled trials. Over the past 30 to 40 years, pulmonary rehabilitation has evolved from an "art of medicine" to evidence-based therapy. Despite the availability of an updated definition and the increased emphasis on the evidence base, the essence of definitions of pulmonary rehabilitation as an individualized and multidisciplinary treatment has existed since the very first statement on pulmonary rehabilitation of the American Thoracic Society (ATS). **Table 1** provides the history of definitions of pulmonary rehabilitation by ATS and European Respiratory Society (ERS). The most recent definition identifies the core components of a rehabilitation program.[1]

When patients remain symptomatic despite optimized pharmacotherapy, prescription of a rehabilitation program must be considered. In an initial assessment phase, a rehabilitation program aims at mapping out the modifiable nonrespiratory consequences of respiratory diseases (see below, ie, muscle weakness, depressive symptoms, poor coping with the disease, impaired engagement in physical activities, nutritional deficits). Subsequently (or in parallel) the rehabilitation program calls on the self-management of patients to engage in a healthy lifestyle in terms of physical activity, nutrition, smoking, and coping. The rehabilitation team becomes the coach of the patient. Exercise training is considered a crucial element of the rehabilitation program. More recently, the focus of research has gradually shifted toward more lifelong behavioral change. Although the science base of exercise training has reached a very high standard, the evidence base for achieving a true behavior change is less solid. Significant and important progress must be made, particularly to help maintain the benefits of an exercise training

Supported by grant Flemish Research Foundation FWO G.0871.13N.
[a] Respiratory Rehabilitation and Respiratory Division, University Hospital Gasthuisberg, Herestraat 49, 3000 Leuven, Leuven, Belgium; [b] Faculty of Kinesiology and Rehabilitation Sciences, Department of Rehabilitation Sciences, Katholieke Universiteit Leuven, Tervuursevest 101, 3000 Leuven, Belgium
* Corresponding author. Respiratory Rehabilitation and Respiratory Division, University Hospital Gasthuisberg, Herestraat 49, 3000 Leuven, Leuven, Belgium.
E-mail address: thierry.troosters@med.kuleuven.be

Clin Chest Med 35 (2014) 241–249
http://dx.doi.org/10.1016/j.ccm.2013.10.006
0272-5231/14/$ – see front matter © 2014 Elsevier Inc. All rights reserved.

Table 1
Evolution of definitions of pulmonary rehabilitation by the ATS or jointly by the ATS and ERS

Date	Definition
1981 (1974)	Pulmonary rehabilitation is an art of medical practice wherein an *individually* tailored, *multidisciplinary* program is formulated, which through accurate diagnosis, therapy, emotional support, and education stabilizes or reverses both the physiology and psychology of pulmonary diseases and attempts to return the patient to the highest possible functional capacity allowed by his pulmonary handicap and overall life situation. Goals are (1) control and alleviate symptoms and complications of respiratory impairment, and (2) teach patients optimal capability to carry out activities of daily life.
1999	(No definition) The principal goals of pulmonary rehabilitation are to reduce symptoms, decrease disability, increase participation in physical and social activities, and improve the overall quality of life for individuals with chronic respiratory disease.
2006	Pulmonary rehabilitation is an evidence-based, *multidisciplinary*, and *comprehensive intervention* for patients with chronic respiratory diseases who are symptomatic and often have decreased daily life activities. Integrated into the individualized treatment of the patients, it is designed to reduce symptoms, optimize functional status, increase participation, and reduce health care costs through stabilizing or reversing systemic manifestations of the disease.
2013	Pulmonary rehabilitation is a *comprehensive intervention* based on a thorough patient assessment followed by *patient-tailored* therapies, which include, but are not limited to, exercise training, education, and behavior change, designed to improve the physical and psychological condition of people with chronic respiratory disease and to promote the long-term adherence to health-enhancing behaviors.

Definition of pulmonary rehabilitation over the past 40 years. A clear difference is the evolution from art to science. The evidence base has increased[2] over the years but in essence pulmonary rehabilitation has always been defined as an individualized multidisciplinary treatment.

program in the long term and perhaps to have an impact on truly modifying the long-term nonrespiratory consequences of chronic obstructive pulmonary disease (COPD). In this article the different components and the setup of a rehabilitation program are reviewed. Importantly, pulmonary rehabilitation programs are often integrated in other care plans for patients with COPD, such as self-management programs, lung transplantation programs, noninvasive ventilation, or smoking cessation programs. Interaction between the different teams and experts running these care programs across lines of health care and pathologic abnormaltiy (to adequately handle comorbidity) is crucial for the overall success of the management of these patients with complex chronic diseases.

THE EVIDENCE BASE FOR PULMONARY REHABILITATION

Several reviews have summarized the evidence for pulmonary rehabilitation[2–4] and practice guidelines are available.[5,6] Therefore, a comprehensive review of all the evidence on the effectiveness of pulmonary rehabilitation is beyond the scope of this article.

Pulmonary rehabilitation, including exercise training, enhances exercise tolerance mainly through enhanced skeletal muscle function and reduced ventilatory requirements during exercise. Functional performance is increased through physiologic improvements, enhanced movement efficiency, and perhaps increased self-efficacy. Rehabilitation also improves patient-reported outcomes, such as symptoms and health-related quality of life. These improvements are of clear clinical significance in patients with COPD.[4]

Beyond these benefits, rehabilitation also leads to psychological improvements.[7] In patients referred to the authors' rehabilitation program, depressive symptoms were present in 42% of patients and symptoms compatible with anxiety were present in 38% of patients. Improvements of depressive symptoms and anxiety are only to be expected if patients do have these symptoms. Hence the relatively small effect size reported in the meta-analysis[7] may be induced by the dilution of the depressed patients in the larger patient pool.

As per definition, rehabilitation attempts to increase the amount of physical activity patients engage in. The systemic consequences of COPD, such as cardiovascular morbidity, muscle weakness, and osteoporosis, originate to a large extent directly or indirectly from living an inactive lifestyle. When pulmonary rehabilitation aims at achieving a sustained effect, an inactive lifestyle after rehabilitation should be avoided. The effect of pulmonary rehabilitation programs on physical activity levels has only been studied in the past 10 years. It was commonly taken for granted that a comprehensive rehabilitation program would increase physical activity levels, but studies have reported conflicting results. Few randomized controlled trials have addressed the topic[8,9] and no long-term follow-up studies are available. Changing physical activity behavior is challenging and in general results are somewhat disappointing. Although endurance capacity virtually doubles, physical activity levels increase less than 20% across studies.[10] Changing physical activity may not simply follow the increased exercise capacity or improved skeletal muscle function. Probst and colleagues[11] showed that more increased exercise tolerance (by providing higher intense exercise programs) did not lead to further enhanced physical activity levels. Physical activity is a complex behavior that depends on physiologic capacity, but also on psychological processes. In addition, environmental, societal, and cultural factors are important and there is even a genetic component in physical activity behavior.[12] To have a major impact on physical activity, an even more comprehensive approach may be needed that reaches out to the family and social network of the patient and to the community.

In recent years, appealing new strategies have been developed that may potentially help to increase the effects of classical rehabilitation on physical activities. First, providing patients real-time feedback with pedometers on their physical activity levels may, along with setting achievable goals, enhance daily activity levels inside or outside the context of pulmonary rehabilitation.[13] Second, walking at home has been stimulated effectively using group activities such as Nordic Walking or using modern interfaces such as mobile phone technology, which included paced walking on the rhythm of music adapted to the possibilities of the patient. Even more recently, "gaming"-based or Internet-based programs have become available that may support rehabilitation programs, but must be further validated in this context.[14] Future research should focus on further strategies that may help to lead to a sustainable behavior change.

A last benefit of pulmonary rehabilitation is a decrease in the use of health care recourses. Hospital admissions are an important driver of direct costs of COPD. These health care recourses do not occur in all patients, but once they occur they tend to be repetitive[15] and are expensive. In one of the first large randomized controlled trials on pulmonary rehabilitation there was a trend for a lower number of hospital days[16]; a more recent trial showed a significant reduction in the number of hospital days.[17] Comparable findings were obtained in relatively long open studies comparing use of health care recourses before and after taking part in pulmonary rehabilitation. When trials focus on more fragile patients, such as those recently admitted to hospital and at risk for readmission, a meta-analysis showed that the risk for readmission was substantially reduced.[18]

WHERE CAN PULMONARY REHABILITATION BE ORGANIZED

Pulmonary rehabilitation programs have traditionally been developed as outpatient programs. In the early 1990s, however, it was suggested that home-based programs could also be applied. Community-based settings were later proposed as an alternative. Inpatient programs are effective but very expensive and should perhaps be reserved for the most complex patients. Ideally, a center should be able to offer rehabilitation programs that are also individually tailored in terms of setting and supervision, complexity, and duration (**Fig. 1**). If not, the available program format may not be the desired program from a patient perspective or may simply be impossible to cope with. As a consequence many patients decline the invitation to take part in rehabilitation or drop out from programs. Because different forms of programs were shown to be effective, perhaps a way to increase uptake would be to offer different options to patients. Challenges obviously will remain in the funding and management of different programs at once. **Fig. 1** represents the different organizational options for pulmonary rehabilitation. For most of these evidence of efficacy is available if patients are well selected and supervision is provided. Perhaps all these options may not be offered by one rehabilitation team, but ideally links between different teams exist across lines of health care to allow that patients can be offered a program that is in line with their needs and their desires. **Fig. 1** also provides a few examples of clinical scenarios, but obviously these are not exhaustive.

A COMPREHENSIVE INTERVENTION: PROGRAM CONTENT

Exercise training is an essential component in the rehabilitation program of patients with COPD that

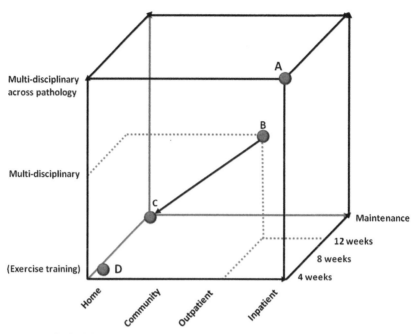

Fig. 1. Different types of rehabilitation. All of the combinations in the 3 dimensions are theoretically possible. A few examples are given. In patient A, a patient on noninvasive mechanical ventilation and with severe COPD, heart failure, and type 2 diabetes, an in-patient complex rehabilitation program is offered. Patient B is a patient with severe COPD, symptoms of depression, and a body mass index of 29 kg m^{-2}, who still drives his own car. He is enrolled in an outpatient program after which he will follow a maintenance program in primary care (a fitness facility (C)). Patient D is a patient with mild COPD who is deconditioned due to a prolonged inactive lifestyle. The patient has mild symptoms and further uncomplicated COPD. He is referred to a simple exercise training program in primary care.

suffer from deconditioning. The program must be individualized in terms of exercise modalities, specificity of the training, the training intensity, and specific inspiratory muscle training. To obtain significant physiologic improvements in skeletal muscle function, it is important to train patients at a training intensity that is "high" relative to the maximum capacity of the patients.[19] Recently, programs eliciting more significant skeletal muscle fatigue were related to better training effects in terms of functional exercise tolerance and reduction of symptoms.[20] To combine an effective training program with patient comfort, clinicians have the choice of several exercise training modalities. These exercise training modalities include endurance training, interval training, and resistance training. Further individualization of the training program can be achieved through more complex training regimens, including the use of oxygen supplements, noninvasive mechanical ventilation, single leg training, or inspiratory muscle training. More fine-tuned modulation of the training intensity and close follow-up of patients during training may also result in better training outcomes.[21] Across the world, programs of different program length have been adopted.

Six-week to 6-month programs have been described. In the latest consensus statement of ATS and ERS the program length is stated as "Optimal duration for the individual can be considered the longest duration that is possible and practical, since programs longer than 12 weeks have been shown to produce greater sustainable benefits than shorter programs." In the real world, the duration often depends on funding schemes, patient's willingness to continue, waiting lists, and so on. To result in physiologic benefits, the duration of an exercise training program is generally thought to be at least 8 weeks with a minimum frequency of 3 training sessions a week. One of these sessions can be conducted outside the formally supervised setting by the patients, provided that the session is comparable in terms of duration and intensity to the supervised sessions.[22] Although the evidence for exercise training is well accepted, less evidence is available on the involvement of other disciplines. Nevertheless, there is, for almost 40 years already (see **Table 1**), consensus that other disciplines may add value to a pulmonary rehabilitation program in specific patients. Other disciplines that can be considered to intervene in selected patients are occupational therapists, psychologists, nutritional experts, physiotherapists, nurses, and social workers. Tasks of these health care providers should be discussed in a specific rehabilitation team. Indications and possible tasks are provided in **Table 2**. It is clear that not all patients will benefit to the same extent of the involvement of a particular health care provider. For example, a patient with a normal body mass index and body composition and healthy nutritional habits will likely not benefit from seeing a nutritional specialist. Conversely, patients with symptoms of depression may benefit from seeing a psychologist to establish the potential diagnosis of depression and if so suggest appropriate treatment.

Proper screening of patients at the moment of the intake will orient patients toward the different health care providers in a rehabilitation program.

Because many patients with COPD can be considered "frail elderly" patients, aspects of rehabilitation for this patient group can be included in the rehabilitation process. For example, because of poor proprioceptive balance control and skeletal muscle weakness, the balance of patients with COPD may be disturbed,[29] leading to increased risk of falling. Combined with osteoporosis, it is clear that falls are an important precursor of fractures. Recently the added value of a balance training program was shown in patients with COPD.[27]

PATIENT SCREENING AND SELECTION

The 2006 definition of pulmonary rehabilitation included the goals of rehabilitation: pulmonary rehabilitation is "designed to reduce symptoms,

Table 2
Health care providers and their suggested task in a rehabilitation team

Health Care Provider	Suggested Tasks
Chest physician (preferably with pulmonary rehabilitation specialty)	Medical treatment and patient referral Diagnosis and follow-up of comorbidities Setup and supervision of multidisciplinary team Referral for comorbidities
Exercise specialist (physiotherapist)	Setup and supervision of the exercise program Home exercise program (follow-up) Arrangement of maintenance training strategies
Psychologist	Management of uncertainty[23] Management of depression in depressed patients[24,a] Smoking cessation
Occupational therapist	Home energy efficiency[25] Specific training of home activities[26] Use of walking aids Pacing techniques
Nutritional experts	Management of overweight Management of cachexia Nutrient intake in line with exercise training program Nutritional supplements
Nurse specialist	Medication adherence Smoking cessation Self-management program for exacerbation management
Physiotherapist	Mucous clearance in patients with mucous hypersecretion and difficulties to clear spontaneously[5] Balance/proprioceptive training in frail patients at risk for falling[27]
Social worker	Solve transportation issues in outpatient programs Map out the social support network around a patient to anticipate on dropout[28] Implementation of social support measures provided by the health care system to alleviate financial burden

An overview of different health care providers and their tasks in a rehabilitation team. This list is not exhaustive and may be complemented by speech therapists, specific disciplines involved in the management of comorbidity, and so on. Family members as well as general practitioners are also members of the rehabilitation team around a patient.

[a] Intervention implemented by trained nurse.

optimize functional status, increase participation, and reduce health care costs through stabilizing or reversing systemic manifestations of the disease."[22] From this it followed that the ideal candidate for rehabilitation is symptomatic, has impaired functional status, participation, and high utilization of health care resources, and should suffer from the "systemic consequences of COPD" or perhaps better "the nonrespiratory consequences" of COPD. Hence the selection of patients should not be done based on lung function, but rather on the proper assessment of the extrapulmonary consequences of COPD found to be reversible with rehabilitation, symptoms, functional status, the levels of participation in daily life, and health-related quality of life. Other factors, such as age, gender, and smoking status, are not important to predict the outcome of rehabilitation. It is important that patients are screened for pulmonary rehabilitation after establishing optimal pharmacotherapy. Although being screened for rehabilitation, patients can also be considered for other programs, such as a lung transplantation or lung volume reduction program, a program of noninvasive ventilatory support, or oxygen therapy. Such programs have no exclusion criteria for pulmonary rehabilitation. On the contrary, oftentimes pulmonary rehabilitation is strongly recommended in these patients.

Screening for the Extrapulmonary Consequences of COPD

In the context of exercise training the most important "systemic consequence" of COPD is skeletal muscle dysfunction. In clinical practice this can be assessed by skeletal muscle force or local skeletal muscle endurance, which is often even more affected. Roughly 70% of patients referred to an outpatient COPD clinic suffer from skeletal muscle weakness and skeletal muscle force is acutely further reduced during acute exacerbations. In patients with less severe, newly detected Global Initiative for Chronic Obstructive Lung Disease 2, COPD, about 30% of patients may suffer from muscle weakness. In these patients quadriceps force was related to exercise capacity as was shown previously in more severe patients. In milder patients (forced expiratory volume in 1 second >80% of the predicted normal value) muscle weakness was a predictor of physical inactivity levels.[30] Reversal of skeletal muscle dysfunction is an important goal of the exercise training component of a rehabilitation program and hence patients suffering from skeletal muscle weakness are particularly good candidates for exercise training.[31] Improving skeletal muscle strength

can be done particularly effectively by including resistance training exercises in the exercise training sessions. When successful muscle force does increase, muscle oxidative capacity is enhanced.

Pharmacologic support with anabolic drugs can be considered in combination with exercise training to increase the effectiveness, but altogether research has focused on the average patient referred for rehabilitation rather than on targeted patient populations (for review, see ref.[32]). One study that did specifically target hypogonadal men and provided them with testosterone supplements in combination with resistance training did show benefits of the pharmacologic intervention to increase muscle strength.[33]

Impaired exercise tolerance and functional exercise capacity are the result of the pulmonary and systemic consequences of COPD. In the context of pulmonary rehabilitation the exercise tolerance is best formally assessed before the program using an incremental exercise test, which will help guide the exercise training program in terms of its intensity, the training modalities, and safety. The functional exercise capacity is best assessed using field tests such as the 6-minute walking test. For this test reference values exist and benchmark improvements for program quality[3] and clinical and statistical importance have been reported. When a patient's exercise tolerance is normal, the indication for exercise training is questionable.

Another important extrapulmonary consequence of COPD is the derangement of the body composition. Both obesity, as a consequence of an inactive lifestyle and poor nutritional hygiene, and cachexia, as observed in other chronic inflammatory disorders are important to pickup and treat in pulmonary rehabilitation programs. Obesity (defined as an increased body mass index greater than 30 kg m^{-2}) will limit the functional abilities of patients with limited ventilatory capacity as it increases the ventilatory needs for exercises against gravity. Cachexia, an involuntary loss of fat free mass, leads inevitably to skeletal muscle weakness. It is a complex problem and its origin is not yet fully understood. Energy imbalance, disuse atrophy, hormonal imbalance, chronic hypoxia, accelerated aging, and systemic inflammation have been discussed as potential factors contributing to cachexia. When present, the treatment of cachexia is an important goal of rehabilitation in patients with COPD and requires individualized interventions by nutritional specialists. To appropriately assess this aspect, body composition should be assessed using Dual-energy X-ray Absorptiometry (DXA)-scan or bio-electrical impedance measures.

Symptoms

The most disabling symptom in COPD is clearly shortness of breath. Patients report dyspnea, particularly during exercise or activity, as a significant burden. Another important symptom is fatigue.[34] Symptoms can be assessed during exercise using Borg symptom scores or during activities of daily living using specific questionnaires.[35] Dyspnea with activity (or exercise) is substantially improved with exercise training. The mechanism through which such large effects are observed is not entirely clear. Certainly there is less required pulmonary ventilation at iso-work and at iso-VO_2, leading to improved (ie, less) dynamic hyperinflation. In addition, the way the dyspnea experience is processed by the patient may improve, due to the repetitive exposure to this threatening stimulus under well-controlled circumstances (ie, in the exercise training setting). Whether genetic factors also play a role is an attractive hypothesis, but this surely requires further study.

Physical Activity

The methodology to assess physical activity was reviewed elsewhere and is beyond the scope of the present review. Several questionnaires have been used, but increasingly activity monitors find their way to the clinical arena and validation studies of several monitors are available.[36] Validation studies, conducted under the umbrella of the PROactive (www.PROactivecopd.com) IMI-JU project, have identified 3 monitors that are valid for use in COPD. In the future it is likely that benchmark values for physical activity will become available for patients with COPD. Patients not meeting current guidelines on physical healthy physical activity (30 minutes of moderate intense exercise on 5 days of the week) can be considered candidates for pulmonary rehabilitation whereby the focus lies on improving the physical activity lifestyle of the patient.

Severe Exacerbations

Patients with COPD who have been hospitalized with an acute exacerbation are particularly good candidates to be enrolled in pulmonary rehabilitation programs. Recent systematic[37] reviews exist on the topic. Patients suffering from exacerbations have lost muscle force, functional exercise tolerance, and health-related quality of life acutely as the result of an exacerbation. Physical activity levels are also dramatically low during the hospital admission and at least up to a month afterward. That observation prompted investigators to look at the effects of muscle activation during the hospitalization phase by means of resistance training or neuromuscular electrical stimulation, which proved to be effective to maintain muscle function during this acute phase. In addition, it is well known that patients who had a hospital admission for COPD are very likely to face new hospital admissions in the year following the previous admission, imposing a high burden on health care cost.

In these frail patients, the rehabilitation program may need significant modification. The emphasis should be on acquiring appropriate self-management skills to prevent subsequent admissions[38] and the exercise training program may need to be adapted to the more severe ventilatory and/or skeletal muscle limitation, using resistance training or interval training at high intensities. A recent meta-analysis of a handful of studies, however, showed that patients who suffered from exacerbations are very good candidates for pulmonary rehabilitation.[39] Clearly these patients may impose a higher burden on the rehabilitation team and recruitment in programs and dropout from the program is a particularly important problem.[40] Although in a recent European audit 42% of eligible patients were reported to have received rehabilitation,[41] a prospective survey in the United Kingdom of close to 500 subsequent admissions found that 31% of eligible patients (63% of the population was found to be eligible) were referred to rehabilitation but only 15% of the eligible patients completed the rehabilitation program.[42] There is clearly margin for improvement by providing more tailored rehabilitation solutions (see **Fig. 1**) to these patients by integrating community- or home-based approaches with appropriate involvement of experts. Future avenues involving tele-health solutions may offer attractive novel ways of interacting across lines of care, to the benefit of these frail patients.

MAINTAINING THE EFFECTS OF PULMONARY REHABILITATION

Our current understanding of the development of systemic consequences of COPD may help to design successful longer-term strategies to maintain the effects of pulmonary rehabilitation. First, all efforts should be made to change the physical activity behavior in patients. Physical inactivity is likely to be the most important modifiable contributor to the development of systemic consequences in COPD. Providing patients direct feedback on their physical activity levels or using structured behavioral interventions may prove to yield results more rapidly. Second, exercise at home should be facilitated and can be done using feedback on home exercises, or incentives. Such exercises must be individually tailored to achieve effective intensity to provide a continued training stimulus. Ideally the exercises are regularly supervised. In patients with moderate COPD there is no evidence that continued outpatient rehabilitation (once per week) has better outcomes than a well-prescribed home-based training program. Tele-coaching interventions, where a coaching interface is available in the home of the patients, may be a promising future direction. Last, specific attention should go to patients who suffer from exacerbations. Prevention of such events can be done in patients at risk by implementing self-management strategies and the implementation of a case manager.[38] Although it seems intuitively useful, there is currently little evidence for a short "booster" program after a hospital admission to maintain the benefits of rehabilitation. If these repeated programs are preplanned, they seem to contribute little to the overall long-term success of programs.[43]

SUMMARY

Nowadays, pulmonary rehabilitation is an evidence-based intervention for patients with COPD. Programs are individually tailored to the needs of patients in terms of the program structure and its components. According to the definition of pulmonary rehabilitation, the aim of the rehabilitation program is to lead to long-term change in physical activity and self-management behavior. Although the short-term effects of rehabilitation are well known, the long-term effects are not always guaranteed. Further research should focus on the strategies to ensure the long-term benefits for patients with COPD. Further knowledge of the processes underlying an endurable shift in lifestyle, as well as better understanding of the pathophysiologic mechanisms leading to the systemic consequences of COPD and its treatments, may lead to major advances in the future.

REFERENCES

1. Spruit MA, Singh S, Garvey C, et al. An official American Thoracic Society/European Respiratory Society Statement: key concepts and advances in pulmonary rehabilitation - an Executive Summary. Am J Respir Crit Care Med 2013;188(8):e13–64.
2. Clini EM, Ambrosino N. Nonpharmacological treatment and relief of symptoms in COPD. Eur Respir J 2008;32:218–28.
3. Lacasse Y, Goldstein R, Lasserson TJ, et al. Pulmonary rehabilitation for chronic obstructive pulmonary disease. Cochrane Database Syst Rev 2006;(4):CD003793.
4. Troosters T, Casaburi R, Gosselink R, et al. Pulmonary rehabilitation in chronic obstructive pulmonary disease. Am J Respir Crit Care Med 2005; 172:19–38.
5. Langer D, Hendriks E, Burtin C, et al. A clinical practice guideline for physiotherapists treating patients with chronic obstructive pulmonary disease based on a systematic review of available evidence. Clin Rehabil 2009;23:445–62.
6. Ries AL, Bauldoff GS, Carlin BW, et al. Pulmonary rehabilitation: joint ACCP/AACVPR evidence-based clinical practice guidelines. Chest 2007;131: 4S–42S.
7. Coventry PA, Hind D. Comprehensive pulmonary rehabilitation for anxiety and depression in adults with chronic obstructive pulmonary disease: systematic review and meta-analysis. J Psychosom Res 2007;63:551–65.
8. Effing T, Zielhuis G, Kerstjens H, et al. Community based physiotherapeutic exercise in COPD self-management: a randomised controlled trial. Respir Med 2011;105:418–26.
9. Breyer MK, Breyer-Kohansal R, Funk GC, et al. Nordic walking improves daily physical activities in COPD: a randomised controlled trial. Respir Res 2010;11:112.
10. Troosters T, Gosselink R, Janssens W, et al. Exercise training and pulmonary rehabilitation: new insights and remaining challenges. Eur Respir Rev 2010; 19:24–9.
11. Probst VS, Kovelis D, Hernandes NA, et al. Effects of 2 exercise training programs on physical activity in daily life in patients with COPD. Respir Care 2011; 56:1799–807.
12. Hoed Md, Brage S, Zhao JH, et al. Heritability of objectively assessed daily physical activity and sedentary behavior. Am J Clin Nutr 2013;98(5): 1317–25.
13. Vaes AW, Cheung A, Atakhorrami M, et al. Effect of 'activity monitor-based' counseling on physical activity and health-related outcomes in patients with chronic diseases: a systematic review and meta-analysis. Ann Med 2013;45:397–412.
14. Moy ML, Janney AW, Nguyen HQ, et al. Use of pedometer and Internet-mediated walking program in patients with chronic obstructive pulmonary disease. J Rehabil Res Dev 2010;47:485–96.
15. Hurst JR, Vestbo J, Anzueto A, et al. Susceptibility to exacerbation in chronic obstructive pulmonary disease. N Engl J Med 2010;363:1128–38.
16. Ries AL, Kaplan RM, Limberg TM, et al. Effects of pulmonary rehabilitation on physiologic and psychosocial outcomes in patients with chronic obstructive pulmonary disease. Ann Intern Med 1995;122: 823–32.

17. Griffiths TL, Burr ML, Campbell IA, et al. Results at 1 year of outpatient multidisciplinary pulmonary rehabilitation: a randomised controlled trial. Lancet 2000;355:362–8.

18. Puhan M, Scharplatz M, Troosters T, et al. Pulmonary rehabilitation following exacerbations of chronic obstructive pulmonary disease. Cochrane Database Syst Rev 2009;(1):CD005305.

19. Garber CE, Blissmer B, Deschenes MR, et al. American College of Sports Medicine position stand. Quantity and quality of exercise for developing and maintaining cardiorespiratory, musculoskeletal, and neuromotor fitness in apparently healthy adults: guidance for prescribing exercise. Med Sci Sports Exerc 2011;43:1334–59.

20. Burtin C, Saey D, Saglam M, et al. Effectiveness of exercise training in patients with COPD: the role of muscle fatigue. Eur Respir J 2012;40:338–44.

21. Klijn P, van Keimpema A, Legemaat M, et al. Nonlinear exercise training in advanced chronic obstructive pulmonary disease is superior to traditional exercise training. A randomized trial. Am J Respir Crit Care Med 2013;188:193–200.

22. Nici L, Donner C, Wouters E, et al. American Thoracic Society/European Respiratory Society statement on pulmonary rehabilitation. Am J Respir Crit Care Med 2006;173:1390–413.

23. Jiang X, He G. Effects of an uncertainty management intervention on uncertainty, anxiety, depression, and quality of life of chronic obstructive pulmonary disease outpatients. Res Nurs Health 2012;35:409–18.

24. Lamers F, Jonkers CC, Bosma H, et al. Improving quality of life in depressed COPD patients: effectiveness of a minimal psychological intervention. COPD 2010;7:315–22.

25. Osman LM, Ayres JG, Garden C, et al. A randomised trial of home energy efficiency improvement in the homes of elderly COPD patients. Eur Respir J 2010;35:303–9.

26. Norweg AM, Whiteson J, Malgady R, et al. The effectiveness of different combinations of pulmonary rehabilitation program components: a randomized controlled trial. Chest 2005;128:663–72.

27. Beauchamp MK, Janaudis-Ferreira T, Parreira V, et al. A randomized controlled trial of balance training during pulmonary rehabilitation for individuals with COPD. Chest 2013. [Epub ahead of print]. http://dx.doi.org/10.1378/chest.13-1093.

28. Young P, Dewse M, Fergusson W, et al. Respiratory rehabilitation in chronic obstructive pulmonary disease: predictors of nonadherence. Eur Respir J 1999;13:855–9.

29. Janssens L, Brumagne S, McConnell AK, et al. Proprioceptive changes impair balance control in individuals with chronic obstructive pulmonary disease. PLoS One 2013;8:e57949.

30. Shrikrishna D, Patel M, Tanner RJ, et al. Quadriceps wasting and physical inactivity in patients with COPD. Eur Respir J 2012;40:1115–22.

31. Troosters T, Gosselink R, Decramer M. Exercise training in COPD: how to distinguish responders from nonresponders. J Cardiopulm Rehabil 2001;21:10–7.

32. Troosters T, Janssens W, Decramer M. Managing skeletal muscle dysfunction in COPD. Eur Respir Monogr 2013;59:164–73.

33. Casaburi R, Bhasin S, Cosentino L, et al. Anabolic effects of testosterone replacement and strength training in men with COPD. Am J Respir Crit Care Med 2004;170:870–8.

34. Theander K, Jakobsson P, Torstensson O, et al. Severity of fatigue is related to functional limitation and health in patients with chronic obstructive pulmonary disease. Int J Nurs Pract 2008;14:455–62.

35. Lareau SC, Meek PM, Roos PJ. Development and testing of the modified version of the pulmonary functional status and dyspnea questionnaire (PFSDQ-M). Heart Lung 1998;27:159–68.

36. Van RH, Giavedoni S, Raste Y, et al. Validity of activity monitors in health and chronic disease: a systematic review. Int J Behav Nutr Phys Act 2012;9:84.

37. Reid WD, Yamabayashi C, Goodridge D, et al. Exercise prescription for hospitalized people with chronic obstructive pulmonary disease and comorbidities: a synthesis of systematic reviews. Int J Chron Obstruct Pulmon Dis 2012;7:297–320.

38. Bourbeau J, Julien M, Maltais F, et al. Reduction of hospital utilization in patients with chronic obstructive pulmonary disease: a disease-specific self-management intervention. Arch Intern Med 2003;163:585–91.

39. Puhan MA, Gimeno-Santos E, Scharplatz M, et al. Pulmonary rehabilitation following exacerbations of chronic obstructive pulmonary disease. Cochrane Database Syst Rev 2011;(10):CD005305.

40. Eaton T, Young P, Fergusson W, et al. Does early pulmonary rehabilitation reduce acute health-care utilization in COPD patients admitted with an exacerbation? A randomized controlled study. Respirology 2009;14:230–8.

41. Lopez-Campos JL, Hartl S, Pozo-Rodriguez F, et al. Variability of hospital resources for acute care of COPD patients: European COPD Audit. Eur Respir J 2013. [Epub ahead of print]. http://dx.doi.org/10.1183/09031936.00074413.

42. Jones SE, Green SA, Clark AL, et al. Pulmonary rehabilitation following hospitalisation for acute exacerbation of COPD: referrals, uptake and adherence. Thorax 2013. [Epub ahead of print]. http://dx.doi.org/10.1136/thoraxjnl-2013-204227.

43. Foglio K, Bianchi L, Ambrosino N. Is it really useful to repeat outpatient pulmonary rehabilitation programs in patients with chronic airway obstruction? A 2-year controlled study. Chest 2001;119:1696–704.

Noninvasive Ventilation and Lung Volume Reduction

Patrick Brian Murphy, MRCP, PhD[a,1],
Zaid Zoumot, MBBS, MRCP, MSc[b,1],
Michael Iain Polkey, PhD, FRCP[b,*]

KEYWORDS

- Lung volume reduction surgery • Noninvasive ventilation • Emphysema • Collateral ventilation

KEY POINTS

- Noninvasive ventilation given to patients with acute hypercapnic exacerbation of chronic obstructive pulmonary disease reduces mortality and morbidity.
- Lung volume reduction surgery is effective in patients with heterogeneous upper zone emphysema and reduced exercise tolerance, and is probably underused.
- Rapid progress is being made in nonsurgical approaches to lung volume reduction, but use outside specialized centers cannot be recommended presently.

INTRODUCTION

As parenchymal lung disease in chronic obstructive pulmonary disease (COPD) becomes increasingly severe there is a diminishing prospect of drug therapies conferring clinically useful benefit. As a result, when the load on the respiratory muscle pump exceeds the capacity, respiratory failure and/or breathlessness ensue.[1] Noninvasive ventilation (NIV) and lung volume reduction (LVR) surgery (LVRS) both address this in different ways; NIV is intended to offload the work of breathing by augmenting airflow into the lung and offsetting intrinsic positive end-expiratory pressure (PEEP), whereas LVR is intended to restore elastic recoil and improve VQ matching.

NIV

NIV provides ventilatory support without the need for endotracheal intubation and thus supports the respiratory muscle pump both by reducing the work of breathing and by improving tidal volume.[2] The ability to provide ventilatory support without the need for invasive mechanical ventilation has been one of the major advances in the management of acute respiratory failure complicating exacerbations of COPD. The use of NIV during decompensated hypercapnic respiratory failure secondary to acute exacerbations of COPD has become standard practice and forms part of national[3] and international[4] guidelines, whereas the use of NIV in patients with stable chronic

This work was supported in part by the NIHR Respiratory Biomedical Research Unit, which part funds the salary of M.I. Polkey and wholly funds the salary of Z. Zoumot. Z. Zoumot's institution has received reimbursement for trial expenses from PneumRx, Spiration, and Broncus. P. Murphy was previously supported by a grant for a study cofounded by ResMed and Respironics. M.I. Polkey receives fees for consulting from Respironics, Broncus, and PortAero, and his institution held on his behalf an award from PortAero for clinical research.

[a] Lane Fox Clinical Respiratory Physiology Group, Guy's & St Thomas' NHS Foundation Trust, London, UK;
[b] NIHR Respiratory Biomedical Research Unit, Royal Brompton and Harefield NHS Foundation Trust, Imperial College London, London, UK
[1] Drs P. Murphy and Z. Zoumot contributed equally to this article.
* Corresponding author. NIHR Respiratory Biomedical Research Unit, Royal Brompton Hospital, Fulham Road, London, UK.
E-mail address: m.polkey@rbht.nhs.uk

hypercapnic respiratory failure remains controversial and its use lacks a clear consensus.[5]

NIV DURING ACUTE HYPERCAPNIC RESPIRATORY FAILURE
Indications

Acute exacerbations of COPD represent a dynamic shift in the load-capacity-drive relationship of the respiratory system caused by an increased load exerted on it.[6] The increased load is mediated principally via changes in both inspiratory resistance and dynamic chest wall elastance, as well as a threshold load exerted by intrinsic PEEP.[7] This acute increase in load on the respiratory system causes a significant increase in the work of breathing, with transdiaphragmatic pressure changes in patients with acute exacerbations of COPD being double those of stable counterparts.[8,9] These effects can be further exacerbated by dynamic hyperinflation resulting from severe airflow limitation impairing expiratory flow time and causing an increase in operating lung volumes to a less advantageous part of the compliance curve.[10] In severe cases this load overcomes the ability of the respiratory muscle pumps to maintain carbon dioxide homeostasis. Increasing arterial partial pressure of carbon dioxide ($PaCO_2$) results in a decrease in arterial pH (<7.35); it is this respiratory acidosis that is the hallmark of acute decompensated respiratory failure.

Acute exacerbations of COPD complicated by respiratory failure are associated with high rates of inpatient mortality[11] and so offer the opportunity for therapeutic intervention. It is in this patient group that NIV was initially used as a means of preventing intubation. Initial promising data from small studies indicated a physiologic response with improvements in arterial pH, $PaCO_2$, and subjective dyspnea and a trend toward improvement in 30-day mortality in comparisons of the addition of NIV with standard care.[12] These encouraging results led to larger trials confirming the physiologic improvement that could be obtained with the application of NIV for acute hypercapnic respiratory failure during acute exacerbations of COPD, as well as indicating reduction in rates of intubation and mortality.[13,14] These initial intensive care–based studies have been supplemented by those conducted in respiratory specialist units confirming the reduction in length of hospital stay and mortality that is attributable to the use of NIV in this patient group.[15] These studies all enrolled patients with acute decompensated respiratory failure secondary to acute exacerbations of COPD and defined respiratory acidosis as a pH less than 7.35. The studies all excluded those

deemed to need immediate intubation on either specific (pH<7.30) or general (clinician discretion) criteria. None of the studies used sham ventilation as a control but used standard care comparisons. Notwithstanding these limitations, the consensus from these studies is that NIV should be initiated in those patients with mild to moderate respiratory acidosis during exacerbations.

Predictors of Treatment Success and Treatment Failure

The use of NIV is now considered gold standard for the management of respiratory failure during COPD exacerbations but the exact characteristics of the patients who benefit remain debated (**Box 1**). The factors that predict treatment failure can be divided into patient-associated and therapy-associated factors.

Patients who, at the onset of therapy, have a poor nutritional state as indicated by lower body weight and lower percentage of ideal body weight, but not by lower serum albumin levels, are more likely to fail a trial of NIV and require invasive mechanical ventilation than patients with better nutritional status.[16] The presence of pneumonic consolidation indicates a higher mortality during unselected admissions caused by acute exacerbations of COPD.[17] In the subgroup of patients requiring NIV, those patients with pneumonic consolidation on chest radiograph are similarly

---

Box 1
Predictors of NIV success in acute hypercapnic exacerbation of COPD

Factors present at initiation:

- Poor nutritional status
- Lower Glasgow Coma Score
- More severe physiologic derangement
  - Higher APACHE II score
  - Lower pH
  - Higher $PaCO_2$
- Excessive secretions

Factors following initial trial of NIV:

- Failure to improve in the first hour
  - Respiratory rate
  - pH
  - $PaCO_2$
  - Glasgow Coma Score
- Poor patient-ventilator interaction
- Excessive mask leak

more likely to fail a trial of NIV.[16,18] As expected, patients who exhibit more severe physiologic derangement, indicated by lower arterial blood pH, higher $PaCO_2$, or higher APACHE II score at presentation of their exacerbation have higher mortality, higher rates of NIV failure, and longer hospital stays.[16,18] However, the severity of initial respiratory failure or the presence of coma at initiation of NIV has not always been unequivocally linked with treatment failure.[19] Other indicators of treatment failure are the ability to apply NIV successfully to patients with high levels of mask leak, poor patient-ventilator synchrony, poor patient comfort, or poor tolerance.[12,16,18]

The best predictor of treatment success during NIV for acute hypercapnic COPD is the patient's response to the initial trial of NIV. Patients in whom the physiologic derangement improves with an increase in Glasgow Coma Score (GCS), improvement in arterial pH and $PaCO_2$, and reduction in respiratory rate have reduced intubation rates and shorter hospital stays.[13,16,20]

Although these small datasets indicate various groups with higher failure rates, none either in isolation or combined provides sufficient accuracy to allow them to dictate clinical decision making. The clinical gestalt is therefore often used, although its limitation in prognostication for patients requiring admission to intensive care because of exacerbations of their airways disease has been shown by Wildman and colleagues.[21] In this observational cohort study the admitting intensive care physician's mortality estimate was compared with the 6-month outcome and showed substantial prognostic pessimism among clinicians.

Ventilator Mode and Setup

The initial trials of NIV in acute hypercapnic COPD used the spontaneous timed or assisted-cycled modes with ventilator-delivered breaths occurring in the absence of patient triggering (ie, during apnea). There are few data available on the exact value of the set backup rate and what, if any, effect this has on patient tolerance or outcomes. Most clinical trials used a bilevel approach,[12,14] although single-level pressure support NIV was used in the study by Brochard and colleagues[13] with no direct comparison of the 2 modes available. Most available ventilators now offer multiple modes and generally the use of bilevel rather than simple pressure support mode is used with the applied expiratory positive air pressure (EPAP), allowing offset of auto-PEEP and thus reducing the work of breathing.[22] Levels of inspiratory positive airway pressure (IPAP) vary between studies, with initial values ranging between 10

and 20 cm H_2O.[13,15] Although higher levels of pressure support aid carbon dioxide clearance they are accompanied by increased leak, with subsequent effects on the patient and ventilator. Concerns regarding the tolerability of high levels of IPAP by patients during NIV for acute exacerbations have been addressed in the European Predictors of Ventilation (EPOV) study. This prospective pan-European study recruited 190 patients and evaluated the duration of NIV usage in patients who had high (IPAP≥20 cm H_2O) or low (IPAP<20 cm H_2O) inspiratory pressures.[23] The data showed that patients with higher IPAP used NIV for longer in the first 24 hours of therapy (13.9 vs 10.9 hours; $P = .003$) and used NIV for longer during admission (51.7 vs 31.6 hours; $P = .008$). Although both groups in the study had similar outcomes in terms of physiologic improvement in the first hour and mortality, the EPOV investigators have also shown that shorter duration of NIV is associated with higher in-hospital and 3-month mortalities.[24]

Newer ventilatory modes exist, for example proportional assist and neurally adjusted modes, but most lack any clear demonstration of superior efficacy in the management of acute hypercapnic exacerbations secondary to COPD. In the same way, modifying the ventilator to provide more information to the clinician is intuitively attractive but thus far has failed to translate to clinical benefit.[25]

DOMICILIARY NIV FOR CHRONIC HYPERCAPNIC RESPIRATORY FAILURE
Physiologic Basis

The development of hypercapnic respiratory failure in COPD occurs because of an imbalance in the load-capacity-drive relationship of the respiratory system and confers a poor prognosis, with significant morbidity and mortality.[26,27] The use of ventilatory support to correct respiratory failure in this context has empirical appeal and is suggested to work via 3 main hypotheses:

1. Resetting central respiratory drive
2. Improving pulmonary mechanics
3. Resting chronically fatigued respiratory muscles

The relative merits of each hypothesis are discussed later.

Respiratory Drive

Because of the heightened load on the respiratory system, patients with COPD have an increased level of neural respiratory drive (NRD) as measured by diaphragm electromyogram (EMG_{di}), hypercapnic ventilatory response (HCVR), or pressure change during the first 100 milliseconds of inspiration ($P_{0.1}$).[28–30] Patients with COPD with chronic hypercapnia fail to increase levels of drive in response to further CO_2 stimulus.[29] This reduction in central chemosensitivity is thought to be a significant mediator of persistent hypercapnia and can be improved by even short periods of NIV.[31] Chemosensitivity is inversely correlated with changes in daytime $PaCO_2$ following domiciliary NIV use, supporting the hypothesis of an mechanistic role in mediating the change.[32] The measurement of central respiratory drive can be challenging and 2 main methods have been used: the HCVR[33] and $P_{0.1}$.[34] Both tests have been shown to improve following domiciliary NIV in hypercapnic COPD.[31,32,35,36]

Respiratory load

COPD is characterized by significant increases in the load on the respiratory system. A major contributor to this is hyperinflation, which places patients on an inefficient portion of the pressure-volume curve. The airflow limitation that is the hallmark of COPD can further exacerbate this problem by leading to dynamic hyperinflation.[10] The degree of hyperinflation as measured by the ratio of inspiratory capacity total lung capcity (IC/TLC) provides a global indication of respiratory load and has prognostic value in stable COPD.[37] Improvements in the degree of hyperinflation following treatment with NIV have been shown, with the degree of improvement correlating with improvements in gas exchange.[31,32] Long-term use of NIV has also been shown to reduce load by improving C_{dyn},[36] $PEEP_{dyn}$,[36] airflow obstruction,[38] and resting respiratory pattern.[35,36] However, the changes have not been consistently found across all of the studies. The mechanical constraints imposed by both static and exercise-induced dynamic hyperinflation seem to be the most significant limiting factor in endurance exercise capacity in COPD.[39] Thus improvements in this area offer the opportunity to release this critical constraint, allowing improved exercise performance.

Respiratory muscle capacity

Initial theories regarding the mechanism of action of NIV in COPD were based on the idea of resting the fatigued respiratory muscles. More recent work has indicated that the respiratory muscles in COPD are more efficient at a cellular level than healthy controls[40] and this is thought to be caused by a fiber shift within the muscle.[41] There has been a failure to show diaphragm fatigue in vivo in patients with COPD,[42] even in those patients requiring mechanical ventilation.[43] Studies to date have not shown any clinically meaningful changes in respiratory muscle function following treatment with NIV in severe hypercapnic COPD, making fatigue an implausible mechanism.[31,44–47]

Early Trials

The first trial of (negative-pressure) ventilation in COPD was compromised by poor adherence to therapy and, perhaps unsurprisingly, it failed to show a treatment benefit.[46]

With the advent of positive-pressure NIV there was renewed interest in ventilation in chronic type 2 respiratory failure, and small studies suggested that positive-pressure ventilation could be effective in carefully selected patients treated in specialist centers.[48,49]

Current Data and Practice

The largest trial to date investigating the role of domiciliary ventilation in COPD was conducted by the Australia Trial of Noninvasive Ventilation in Chronic Airflow Limitation (AVCAL) group and recruited stable patients with hypercapnic respiratory failure secondary to severe COPD without concomitant obstructive sleep apnea (OSA; defined as an apnea-hypopnea index >20/h). One-hundred and forty-four patients were randomized to NIV and LTOT or LTOT alone.[50] NIV setup was performed during full polysomnography and was judged adequate if the patient slept for more than 3 hours with a pressure support of greater than 5 cm H_2O. Primary outcome was 2-year survival and the study was initially powered for 200 patients, but slow recruitment rates led to a prolongation of trial follow-up. The raw data showed no survival benefit of the addition of NIV to standard care (hazard ratio [HR], 0.82; 95% confidence interval [CI], 0.53–1.25; P = nonsignificant) but, when the data were adjusted for baseline confounders (PaO_2, $PaCO_2$, and St George's Respiratory Questionnaire (SGRQ) total score), there was a small but statistically significant survival advantage in the NIV group at 2 years, although the confidence intervals were wide (HR, 0.63; 95% CI, 0.40–0.99; P = .045). The secondary data analysis showed no differences in gas exchange or spirometry between groups but a reduction in measures of health-related quality of life, specifically the domains of general health and vigor in the NIV group compared with the control group. It is perhaps unsurprising that NIV did not change resting gas exchange given the modest pressure support used (mean IPAP, 12.9 cm H_2O; mean EPAP, 5.1 cm H_2O) and that ventilatory settings were titrated to sleep rather than a marker of hypoventilation such as $PaCO_2$.

Could Technical Factors Explain the Failure to Show a Benefit with NIV?

Of critical importance when analyzing failed trials is the assessment of ventilatory support on daytime resting gas exchange; in this regard many prior trials have used inspiratory pressures that are now considered subtherapeutic. There is increasing support for the use of high-intensity NIV in chronic hypercapnic COPD, with longitudinal cohort data suggesting good long-term outcomes.[51,52] It remains unclear whether there is a requirement of both high inspiratory pressures and high backup rates to achieve the improved clinical outcomes associated with high-intensity NIV. A small crossover randomized controlled trial has investigated this area by comparing a high pressure and low backup rate with a high pressure and high backup rate ventilatory approach in chronic hypercapnic COPD.[53] Although the study had a higher-than-expected dropout rate, there were no significant differences in terms of ventilator usage, the primary outcome, or any of the clinically assessed secondary outcomes in terms of overnight oximetry-capnography, gas exchange, health-related quality-of-life scores, subjective sleep quality, or objective actigraphy-assessed sleep quality between the two ventilatory strategies. If control of nocturnal hypoventilation is the important therapeutic goal of domiciliary NIV, then a high-intensity approach may not be required, but an effective ventilatory strategy can be adopted that is tailored to an individual patient to optimize patient comfort and compliance while controlling sleep-disordered breathing.

A second issue is patient selection; most early trials enrolled patients with both chronic respiratory failure and a stable clinical phenotype, with inclusion criteria usually stipulating a minimum 6-week exacerbation-free period. The requirement for the patient to be stable removes the patients most likely to benefit from NIV because previous uncontrolled data suggested that patients with frequent acidotic exacerbations may derive the most therapeutic benefit from domiciliary NIV.[54] To test this hypothesis, Cheung and colleagues[55] randomized 24 patients to domiciliary NIV and 23 to sham continuous positive airway pressure (CPAP) following acute exacerbations of COPD requiring acute NIV. The study population consisted of patients with GOLD stage IV COPD and moderately severe hypercapnia (NIV group $PaCO_2$, 7.3 $\pm$ 1.0 kPa; CPAP group, 7.7 $\pm$ 1.0 kPa) without OSA (excluded via polysomnography). Patients were followed up for 12 months and the primary outcome of recurrent acute hypercapnic exacerbation was analyzed on an intention-to-treat basis. Patients allocated to the NIV arm received moderate inspiratory pressure support (IPAP, 14.8 $\pm$ 1.1 cm H_2O) with sham CPAP set at 5 cm H_2O. Seven patients in the NIV arm and 14 patients in the sham arm reached the primary outcome with a significant reduction in risk of recurrent acute hypercapnic exacerbation in the NIV treatment arm (HR, 0.39; 95% CI, 0.16–0.98; P = .047). As with earlier studies, the use of modest inspiratory pressures produced no significant improvement in gas exchange in the NIV group compared with sham CPAP. Furthermore, if a more generic end point was used, such as time to any readmission rather than the stipulation of an acute hypercapnic readmission, then there was no treatment effect (NIV arm 71 days vs sham CPAP arm 56 days; P = .48). Other similar studies have provided similar results with an improvement in specific outcomes that do not translate to benefit in important generic outcomes such as exacerbation frequency or mortality.[56]

Summaries

In the context of acute acidotic hypercapnic exacerbation of COPD there is good evidence that the use of NIV improves prognosis and reduces the need for endotracheal intubation. In the case of chronic domiciliary use, the case for the addition of NIV to standard therapy remains equivocal. Several clinical trials are in progress addressing the deficiencies in the published literature; the results of these pending studies should guide future management in this area.

LVR FOR THE TREATMENT OF EMPHYSEMA
Physiologic Basis

Emphysema is characterized by damage and destruction of the alveoli and airspaces distal to the terminal bronchioles diminishing the alveolar surface area available for gas exchange. This loss of the alveolar wall, structural elements, and pulmonary vasculature leads to reduced elastic recoil, as well as narrowing of the airways caused by the loss of the outward tension that maintains their patency. Airways are thus compressed and can collapse under the positive intrathoracic pressure of expiration, leading to gas trapping and hyperinflation. To compensate, patients with COPD breathe at higher lung volumes because this improves airway opening and lung recoil, but at the expense of a reduced vital capacity (VC) and a much higher work of breathing. During exercise, shorter expiratory times preclude expiration of the complete inspired volume from each breath, leading to progressive worsening of gas trapping, termed dynamic hyperinflation. In patients with emphysema-predominant COPD, dynamic hyperinflation arguably plays a more important role in the development of exertional dyspnea than airways obstruction.[57,58] Reducing the volume of the hyperinflated lung to make it a better fit for its thoracic cavity is sensible, especially if this is achieved by removing or shrinking the most diseased portions of the lung contributing the least to gas exchange. Surgical and nonsurgical approaches to achieve this have been attempted. LVR surgery (LVRS) and surgical bullectomy involve resection of the worst affected area of emphysematous lung or giant bullae, respectively. The precise mechanisms by which these translate to clinical improvement are not known with certainty, but is likely to be a combination of factors:

First, LVR improves matching between the size of the lungs and the capacity of the thoracic cavity that holds them. The resultant improvement in the outward circumferential pull on small airways and terminal bronchioles improves expiratory airflow by maintaining airway patency, or a retensioning effect. Also, the remaining healthier lung has more preserved parenchymal structural integrity, further increasing elastic recoil, and provides increased structural stability. Hence, expiratory airway collapse is reduced, allowing the lung to empty more effectively[59] and reducing gas trapping, which increases VC and hence the forced expiratory volume in 1 second (FEV_1)[59] and reduces dynamic hyperinflation. Using the coefficient of retraction, an indicator of elastic recoil of the lung calculated as the ratio of maximal static recoil pressure to total lung capacity, Sciurba and colleagues[60] showed a significantly greater increase in exercise capacity in 16 patients who showed increases in elastic recoil following LVRS compared with 4 patients who did not have increased elastic recoil. Reduction in dynamic hyperinflation is probably the most significant factor in terms of the improvement in exertional dyspnea in patients undergoing LVRS.[61]

Second, a return of the diaphragm to the usual curved shape and length caused by the reduction of the functional residual capacity (FRC) leads to improvement in the mechanical function of the diaphragm and intercostal muscles.[62,63] Furthermore, increases in the abdominal contribution to tidal volume and improved synchrony of the diaphragm with other inspiratory muscles have been reported.[64]

Third, reinflation of previously compressed healthier lung parenchyma reduces physiologic dead space, improving matching of ventilation and perfusion, and in addition the reduction of intrathoracic pressure improves left ventricular (LV) end-diastolic dimension and LV filling after LVRS, resulting in improved LV function.[65]

Surgical LVR

A variety of surgical approaches to correct hyperexpansion of emphysematous lungs have been attempted and been unsuccessful in the past: costochondrectomy, phrenic crush, pneumoperitoneum, pleural abrasion, lung denervation, and thoracoplasty. However, two surgical procedures have shown significant success: bullectomy and reduction pneumoplasty (or LVRS).

Bullectomy Bullae can be large enough that they occupy more than 30% of the hemithorax (termed giant bullae). These giant bullae may compress adjacent lung tissue, reducing perfusion and ventilation to healthier lung parenchyma. Surgical removal of giant bullae has been a standard treatment in selected patients for many years,[66] and this has been achieved via standard lateral thoracotomy, bilateral resections via midline sternotomy, and video-assisted thoracoscopy. Patients who are symptomatic and have an FEV_1 of less than 50% of the predicted value have a better outcome after bullectomy.[66] Benefits result from expansion of compressed lung tissue and improved ventilatory mechanics, with short-term benefits in hypoxemia, hypercapnia, gas trapping, and dyspnea reported in the published literature (predominantly uncontrolled retrospective studies).[67] A recent series of 43 patients treated with giant bullectomy reported significant improvements in spirometry, residual volume (RV), and exercise capacity as measured by the 6-minute walk test (6MWT), with benefits persisting for at least 3 years.[68] Randomized controlled trials of giant bullectomy have not been performed. An alternative approach for frail patients with large single bullae is the Monaldi procedure (**Table 1**).[69]

LVRS Brantigan[70] described unilateral thoracotomy and resection of the most diseased-appearing portion of emphysematous lungs coupled with lung denervation in 33 patients in 1957. However, surgical mortalities of more than 18% meant that the procedure never gained widespread acceptance. Cooper and colleagues[71] revived LVRS in the early 1990s by refining the procedure with the use of staple sutures and pericardial strips to buttress the suture line, thereby reducing the incidence of postoperative air leaks and simplifying the procedure. The group showed that LVRS improved symptoms, lung function, and gas trapping with an acceptable operative risk (4.8% perioperative mortality), and several small randomized controlled trials followed that showed the superiority of LVRS compared with best medical care.[72–74]

The National Emphysema Treatment Trial (NETT),[75] a Medicare-funded and well-designed

Table 1
Considerations when selecting patients for bullectomy

Parameter	Favorable	Unfavorable
Clinical	Rapid progressive dyspnea despite maximal medical therapy Ex-smoker	Advanced age (>60 y) Comorbid illness Cardiac disease Pulmonary hypertension >10% weight loss Frequent respiratory infections
Physiologic	FEV_1 >40% predicted Minimal airway reversibility High trapped lung volume Preserved DL_{CO} Normal PaO_2 and $PaCO_2$	FEV_1 <35% predicted Low gas trapping Low DL_{CO}
CT	Large and localized bulla Vascular crowding and normal pulmonary parenchyma around bulla	Poorly defined bullae Homogeneous emphysema in remaining lung parenchyma

Abbreviations: CT, computed tomography; DL_{CO}, carbon monoxide diffusion in the lung.

Data from American Thoracic Society/European Respiratory Society Task Force. Standards for the Diagnosis and Management of Patients with COPD [Internet]. Version 1.2. New York: American Thoracic Society; 2004 [updated 2005 September 8]. Available from: http://www.thoracic.org/go/copd.

controlled trial that randomized more than 1200 patients to bilateral LVRS or best medical care, provides the best evidence for the indications for LVRS. An early result was the identification of a high-risk group with a high mortality (FEV_1< 20% predicted with either a homogeneous pattern of disease or transfer factor of the lung for carbon monoxide [TL_{CO}] <20% predicted). Subsequent enrollment from this patient group was stopped.

At 24 months, patients undergoing LVRS were more likely to have a significant increase in exercise capacity of greater than 10 W (16% vs 3%; P<.001) and greater than an 8-point improvement in health-related quality of life as measured by the SGRQ (37% vs 10%; P<.001). Although there was no overall survival benefit to LVRS, post hoc analysis based on a priori categories of exercise capacity and pattern of emphysema identified the subgroup of patients with heterogeneous emphysema and low baseline exercise capacity as having a reduced risk of death (relative risk [RR], 0.47; P<.005), as well as clinically significant improvements in exercise capacity and quality of life, compared with best medical care. Excluding the high-risk group, 90-day mortality was 5.5% in the NETT trial, with serious morbidity after LVRS observed in 59% of patients (persistent air leak, 33%; respiratory failure, 22%; pneumonia, 18%; cardiac arrhythmias, 24%). However, 33% of patients who had LVRS had not returned home 30 days after randomization.[75]

A subsequent report from this trial showed that the beneficial effects of LVRS were sustained[76]

(as was the case in the Brompton series[77]), with increased survival in the LVRS group at a median 4.3 years of follow-up (0.11 deaths per person year in the LVRS group vs 0.13 in the medical group; RR, 0.85; P<.02). The cost of LVRS was $140,000 per quality-adjusted life year (QALY) gained at 5 years, and was projected to be $54,000 per QALY gained at 10 years.[78]

Some groups have suggested that performing staged unilateral LVRS separated by a period of 2 to 5 years reduces operative risks and extends overall symptomatic benefit compared with bilateral LVRS at a single operation.[79] However, other reported case series showed larger benefits in some outcome measures with no increase in perioperative mortality.[61,80]

National and international guidelines now recommend that LVRS be considered in patients with upper lobe–predominant disease and low exercise capacity.[81,82] However, LVRS remains greatly underutilized with only 90 LVRS operations performed in the United Kingdom in 2010 according to the Society of Cardiothoracic Surgery register, and 119 performed in 2008 under Medicare in the United States. This underutilization of LVRS is likely multifactorial and caused by a combination of lack of expertise, a complicated and expensive certification system for Medicare, lack of knowledge by patients and physicians alike, and a misinterpretation of the NETT trial as showing no mortality benefit and high morbidity. Nevertheless, safer, faster, and less invasive approaches to achieving LVR are needed; **Table 2** summarizes

Table 2
Nonsurgical LVR techniques

Approach	Technique	Mechanism of Action	Pattern of Disease Most Likely to Benefit	Likely Influence of Collateral Ventilation?	Possible Limitations and Complications	Available Evidence	Active Trials
Devices occluding airways	Endobronchial valves	One-way valves allow air and secretions to escape the target segments of lung while preventing air from reentering and causing atelectasis	Heterogeneous disease without collateral ventilation	Collateral ventilation prevents atelectasis and limits success	Effect limited in the presence of collateral ventilation	Zephyr: single arm open label n = 98[99]; RCT n = 321, 171[86,100]	Pivotal trial recruiting
					Risk of pneumothorax likely in the range of ~25% in the responder population	Spiration: observational n = 91[88]	Pivotal trial soon
Agents inducing an inflammatory response	Polymeric LVR	Air within the hydrogel foam located in the alveoli is absorbed, leading to collapse of the alveoli with selective inflammation, shrinkage, and scarring	Heterogeneous disease	No effect	High risk of postprocedural severe pneumonia and COPD exacerbation	Phase 2 dose-ranging study n = 25,[90] unblinded n = 20[101]	Pivotal trial recruiting
	Bronchoscopic thermal vapor ablation (steam)	The steam causes acute tissue injury, which is followed by scarring, fibrosis, and shrinkage of the targeted lung parenchyma	Heterogeneous disease	No effect	High risk of postprocedural pneumonia and COPD exacerbation	Single arm unblinded n = 44[92]	Pivotal trial in planning
	Bronchoscopic intrabullous blood instillation	Instilled blood induces an inflammatory response leading to scarring and contraction of giant bulla	Giant bulla	No effect	Blood in the airways after a procedure may increase the risk of infection	Single arm unblinded n = 5[102]	Safety and feasibility trial recruiting

Airway bypass techniques	Exhale airway bypass drug-eluting stents	Airway stents between emphysematous lung parenchyma and large airways offer a low-resistance path for trapped air to escape	Homogeneous disease	Enhances effect: pathologic connections between lobes allow trapped gas to escape and form a wider area of emphysematous lung	Maintaining stent patency is a major difficulty	Single arm unblinded n = 36[96] RCT n = 315[97]	Nil
	Percutaneous transpleural airway bypass (spiracles)	The pneumonostomy tube provides an alternate route for gas trapped in the emphysematous lung to escape	Homogeneous disease	Enhances effect: pathologic connections between lobes allow trapped gas to escape from a wider area of emphysematous lung	A permanent pneumostoma and the need to change the pneumonostomy tube daily may deter patients Spontaneous closure of pneumostoma	Single arm unblinded n = 6[98]	Nil
Devices leading to mechanical compression	RePneu Coil LVR	The coils may internally compress treated segments of lung and may increase lung recoil, reducing gas trapping and preventing dynamic hyperinflation	Heterogeneous and homogeneous, RV >200% predicted, no bullous destruction	No effect	Many coils are no longer visible in the airways once released, making the procedure irreversible. May preclude future LVRS	Single arm unblinded n = 11,16[93,94] RCT n = 45[95]	Pivotal trial recruiting

Abbreviation: RCT, randomized controlled trial.

the approaches that have been trialled as well as the current evidence and future trials.

Bronchoscopic LVR

Endobronchial airway valves

This approach, the most widely studied nonsurgical approach at LVR, involves placing unidirectional valves into segmental airways, allowing gas to escape but not reenter the worst affected lobe of the lung, with the aim of causing lobar collapse and atelectasis. The mechanisms of benefit resemble those of LVRS: improved ventilation and perfusion of previously crowded healthier lung parenchyma, retensioning of the small airways, and a return to the functional residual capacity (FRC) reducing the work of breathing with improved respiratory mechanics. Early clinical experience showed that, in a proportion of patients, significant LVR occurred following valve placement[83] associated with increased exercise capacity and a reduced dynamic hyperinflation.[84]

For this approach to be successful, complete occlusion and isolation of the target lobe is required. Damage to the interlobar fissures allows air to bypass the valves and enter via the adjacent lobe, preventing atelectasis. In a similar way, imprecise placement of the valves or unusual airway anatomy can disrupt the valve-airway wall seal. Although small improvements in lung function may occur in the absence of radiological volume reduction, perhaps by the diversion of airflow to healthier lung, benefits are greatest where atelectasis occurs. Follow-up of patients from our early case series suggests that successful LVR with radiological atelectasis is associated with a survival advantage with 0 of 5 deaths at 6 years, compared with 8 of 14 deaths in which atelectasis had not occurred ($P<.02$).[85] Atelectasis is associated with a risk of pneumothorax, which may be caused by air leak or may occur ex vacuo as the target area of lung collapses. These pneumothoraces may resolve spontaneously or require intercostal drainage.

There are two CE (Conformité Européenne)-marked valves commercially available in Europe: the Zephyr valve (Pulmonx, Redwood City, CA) (**Fig. 1**) and the Intrabronchial Valve (IBV; Spiration Inc, Redmond, WA), but neither are currently licensed for use in the United States. In the Endobronchial Valves for Emphysema Palliation Trial (VENT),[86] 321 patients with heterogeneous emphysema were randomly assigned to receive either endobronchial valves or best medical care in a 2:1 distribution. At 6 months there was a statistically significant, but not clinically meaningful, benefit in FEV_1 and the 6MWT. This benefit occurred at the expense of a small increase in COPD exacerbations (7.9%) and minor hemoptysis (5.2%). There were 9 pneumothoraces (only 3

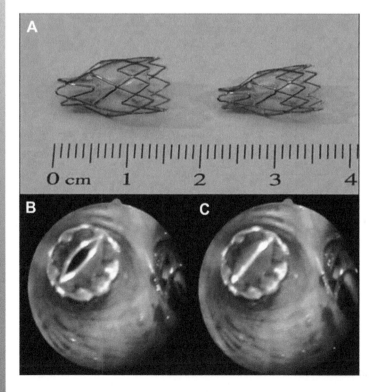

Fig. 1. (*A*) Zephyr valves in both commercially available sizes: 5.5 (*left*) and 4.0 (*right*). Endobronchial appearance (*B*) in inspiration with duckbill closed and (*C*) in expiration with duckbill open.

unresolved after 7 days), but this should be considered as a proportion of the responders with atelectasis (9 of 37, or 24%) rather than the quoted rate of 4.5% in the combined treated population. The response was heterogeneous with higher heterogeneity patients in whom lobar exclusion was accomplished (intact interlobar fissures and correct valve placement confirmed on computed tomography [CT]) having much larger improvements in lung function (ΔFEV_1, 23%; ΔRV, -57%). However, this was the case in only 37 of the 214 patients in the endobronchial valve treatment arm. Prospective trials are needed to establish whether this subgroup of responders (heterogeneous disease with intact fissures) can be accurately identified prospectively, and a pivotal randomized controlled trial will commence recruitment soon.

In addition to CT assessment of fissure intactness (currently arbitrarily defined as fissures >90% complete in at least one axis), an endobronchial catheter-based device (Chartis System, Pulmonx Inc, Palo Alto, CA) has been developed for measuring collateral ventilation (**Fig. 2**). One group showed positive and negative predictive values of 71% and 83% respectively for treatment response. The overall accuracy of the test was 75%.[87] This finding may prove useful for target lobe selection; however, the additional benefit compared with accurate fissure analysis on cross-sectional imaging is unclear, and may not justify the high additional expense.

The IBV (**Fig. 3**) was evaluated in a randomized multicenter trial of 91 patients with severe heterogeneous emphysema, and the investigators elected to leave 1 segment of the right upper lobe and 1 segment of the lingua unoccluded in order to minimize the risk of pneumothorax. Although quality of life and CT-measured lobar volumes improved in this unblinded study, lung function did not.[88] Eberhardt and colleagues[89] later directly compared a unilateral occlusive strategy with a bilateral nonocclusive strategy, which was judged by the change in FEV_1 after 3 months. Greater improvement was seen in the unilateral complete occlusion group, confirming the understanding regarding complete lobar isolation as a predictor of success for endobronchial valves. A pivotal randomized controlled trial of the IBV is in the advanced stages of planning.

Biologic LVR Biologic LVR is intended to reduce lung volume through tissue remodelling, by inducing an inflammatory reaction that leads to scar formation and hence contraction of the treated lung segments, and at the same time reducing collateral ventilation and rendering fissure integrity less important.

Polymeric LVR (PLVR) with Aeriseal (Aeris Therapeutics, Inc; Woburn, MA) involves bronchoscopic deployment of a biodegradable gel into subsegmental bronchi. The solution, which contains aminated polyvinyl alcohol and buffered cross-linker, creates a hydrogel foam when

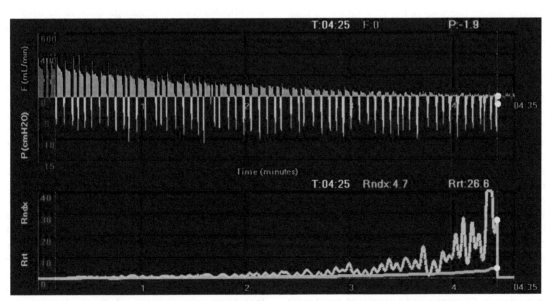

Fig. 2. Chartis assessment of a lobe with no collateral ventilation. Expiratory flow (*orange bars*) decreases as air is aspirated out of the lobe, and inspiratory pressures (*blue bars*) are maintained with each breath. This process is coupled with an increase in resistance (*bottom chart*).

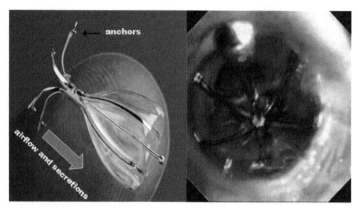

Fig. 3. Spiration valve.

delivered to the distal airways. As gas within the foam (which fills damaged alveoli) is absorbed, the foam, which is now adherent to the alveolar tissue, collapses and as it does so it reduces lung volume and hyperinflation. An open-label, multicenter, exploratory phase 2 clinical study with PLVR hydrogel administered to 8 subsegmental sites in 25 patients with upper lobe emphysema showed improvements in lung function and functional parameters that persisted at 6 months (ΔFEV$_1$, +10%; ΔRV/TLC ratio, -7.4%; ΔmMRC (modified Medical Research Council), -1.0 points; Δ6MWT, +28.7 m; ΔSGRQ, 9.9 points).[90] The procedures were well tolerated but almost all patients experienced an intense flu-like inflammatory reaction, leading to COPD exacerbations in the sickest of this population. Benefits are not achieved for several weeks because of the time taken for scar formation, and the mechanism of action is independent of the presence of collateral ventilation.[91]

A large pivotal randomized controlled trial is currently underway.

Bronchoscopic thermal vapor ablation (steam) The bronchoscopic thermal vapor ablation (BTVA) system (Uptake Medical, Seattle, WA) delivers heated water vapor bronchoscopically via a dedicated catheter into the targeted emphysematous lung segments and, like the Aeris system (vide supra), is designed to reduce lung volume and seal channels of collateral ventilation. The dose of thermal energy to achieve 41.9 J (10 calories)/g lung tissue is calculated from a preprocedure CT assessment of lung density, with procedures to treat a single lobe lasting approximately 30 minutes. The pooled results of 2 single-arm open-label studies[92] comprising 44 patients showed a 716 mL (48%) reduction in CT-measured volume of the target lobe. Significant improvements were also reported in FEV$_1$ (Δ, +17%), SGRQ (Δ, -14 points), mMRC

(Δ, -0.9), and 6MWT (Δ, +46.5 m). Twenty-nine serious adverse events were recorded, of which most were COPD exacerbations or infections attributed to the inflammatory reaction. One death occurred 67 days after the procedure, caused by end-stage COPD. As with PLVR, exacerbations of COPD secondary to the induced inflammatory reaction seem to be the major complication of BTVA.

RePneu LVR coils The RePneu LVR coil (PneumRx Inc, Mountain View, CA) is an implantable coil-like device composed of the biocompatible superelastic memory shape alloy, nitinol. The self-actuating implant is delivered bronchoscopically under fluoroscopic guidance into the targeted airways and, when its sheath is removed, the implant recoils or springs back to its original predetermined shape (**Fig. 4**), so reducing lung volume.

Two small pilot studies predominantly of heterogeneous disease showed the safety of coil insertion procedures with substantial improvements in physiologic and clinical outcomes.[93,94] A recent randomized controlled trial of 46 patients showed a significant difference in ΔSGRQ 90 days following treatment favoring the treatment rather than the control group (-10.54 points; $P = .004$), as well as secondary end points of 6MWT (Δ, +70 m; $P<.001$), FEV$_1$ (Δ, +11.6%; $P = .017$), and RV (Δ, -0.35 L; $P = .026$).[95]

Although the early data are promising, more work is needed to determine the optimal patient selection criteria. There is particular potential for patients with homogeneous emphysema, because this cohort currently has no effective nonmedical therapies available to it. Little is known about long-term complications of these devices and the effect they may have on future thoracic surgery or lung resections. A pivotal multicenter

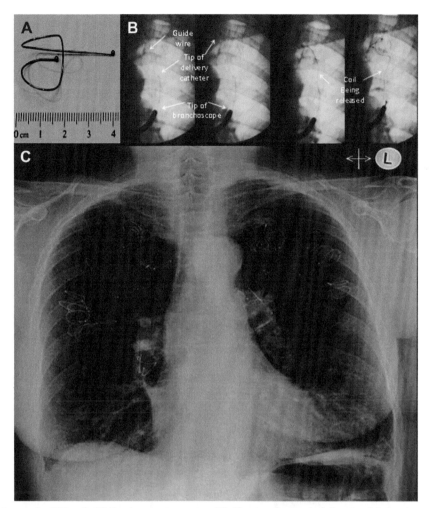

Fig. 4. (*A*): PneumRx LVR coil. (*B*) Deployment process. (*C*) Chest radiograph following bilateral upper lobe coil treatment.

randomized controlled trial intending to recruit 315 subjects with 6MWT at 12 months as the primary outcome is currently recruiting in centers in Europe and North America.

Airways bypass stents Exhale airway bypass paclitaxel-eluting stents (Broncus Inc; Mountain View, CA) are placed bronchoscopically through cartilaginous airways, creating artificial tracts that connect central airways with the emphysematous lung parenchyma and serve as conduits that allow trapped gas to escape, reducing both static and dynamic hyperinflation. Initial pilot data in patients with homogeneous emphysema showed encouraging persistent benefits in physiologic and functional parameters at 6 months.[96] However, a multicenter, double-blind, randomized, sham-controlled pivotal trial was disappointing.[97] Three-hundred and fifteen patients with severe homogeneous emphysema were randomized to have

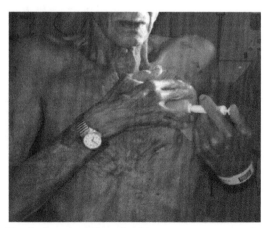

Fig. 5. A patient changing his pneumonostomy tube (spiracles).

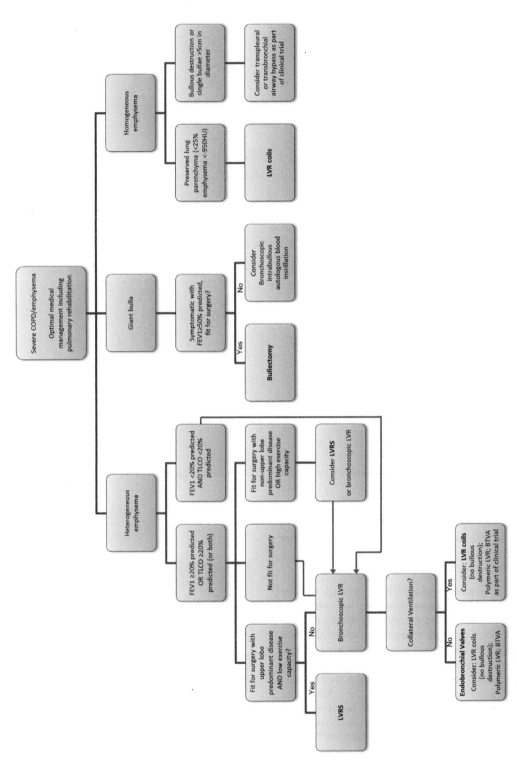

Fig. 6. LVR treatment algorithm.

sham bronchoscopy (n = 107) or up to 6 Exhale stents implanted bronchoscopically (n = 212). On day 1 following the procedure, a difference in the reduction of the RV of 26% (P = .017) and an increase in the forced vital capacity of 27% (P<.001) were seen between the groups. Significant differences were also seen in CT-measured lobar volumes and FEV_1. However, these benefits were not maintained, with lung function measures and CT-measured lobar volumes returning to baseline by 3 months following treatment. This finding is primarily caused by airway bypass stent occlusion by mucus, granulation tissue, or stent expectoration. Although the concept of transbronchial airway bypass has been proved, the problem of stent occlusion needs to be addressed before it can be of value for patients. A similar physiologic approach was trialed by creating an airway bypass directly between the lung and the atmosphere through the chest wall through a minimally invasive transthoracic surgical approach in a procedure that takes approximately 1 hour to complete (**Fig. 5**). A proof-of-concept study was undertaken in 6 patients, and, in the 4 patients who retained the bypass tube for 3 months or more, there was a 23% increase in FEV_1.[98]

SUMMARY

At the time of writing, the only established therapy is surgical LVR, which is indicated for hyperinflated patients with heterogeneous upper zone disease who exceed the NETT safety criteria and who experience symptoms despite rehabilitation. Pivotal trials of several nonsurgical techniques are underway and should inform on efficacy, safety, and optimal patient selection within the next 3 to 5 years. Long-term safety and efficacy data for these novel bronchoscopic techniques are lacking but will emerge in the near future as further follow-up data become available. Our current practice follows the treatment algorithm in **Fig. 6**, with all nonsurgical LVR offered as part of clinical trials. In the future, a randomized control trial of LVRS versus endobronchial valves may be necessary to determine the superiority of either technique.

As the success of bronchoscopic LVR increases with improved patient selection, so too will complication rates. It is therefore likely that the best approach will be through specialist centers able to adopt a multidisciplinary approach offering, according to careful selection, a range of techniques to appropriate patients, with the ability to manage the complications.

REFERENCES

1. Polkey MI, Moxham J. Noninvasive ventilation in the management of decompensated COPD. Monaldi Arch Chest Dis 1995;50:378–82.
2. Nava S, Ambrosino N, Rubini F, et al. Effect of nasal pressure support ventilation and external PEEP on diaphragmatic activity in patients with severe stable COPD. Chest 1993;103:143–50.
3. British Thoracic Society Standards of Care Committee. Non-invasive ventilation in acute respiratory failure. Thorax 2002;57:192–211.
4. Organized jointly by the American Thoracic Society, European Respiratory Society, European Society of Intensive Care Medicine. International consensus conferences in intensive care medicine: noninvasive positive pressure ventilation in acute respiratory failure. Am J Respir Crit Care Med 2001;163:283–91.
5. Elliott MW. Domiciliary non-invasive ventilation in stable COPD? Thorax 2009;64:553–6.
6. Purro A, Appendini L, Polillo C, et al. Mechanical determinants of early acute ventilatory failure in COPD patients: a physiologic study. Intensive Care Med 2009;35:639–47.
7. Jubran A, Tobin MJ. Pathophysiologic basis of acute respiratory distress in patients who fail a trial of weaning from mechanical ventilation. Am J Respir Crit Care Med 1997;155:906–15.
8. Brochard L, Isabey D, Piquet J, et al. Reversal of acute exacerbations of chronic obstructive lung disease by inspiratory assistance with a face mask. N Engl J Med 1990;323:1523–30.
9. Laghi F, Jubran A, Topeli A, et al. Effect of lung volume reduction surgery on diaphragmatic neuromechanical coupling at 2 years. Chest 2004;125: 2188–95.
10. Dal Vecchio L, Polese G, Poggi R, et al. "Intrinsic" positive end-expiratory pressure in stable patients with chronic obstructive pulmonary disease. Eur Respir J 1990;3:74–80.
11. Chu CM, Chan VL, Lin AW, et al. Readmission rates and life threatening events in COPD survivors treated with non-invasive ventilation for acute hypercapnic respiratory failure. Thorax 2004;59:1020–5.
12. Bott J, Carroll MP, Conway JH, et al. Randomised controlled trial of nasal ventilation in acute ventilatory failure due to chronic obstructive airways disease. Lancet 1993;341:1555–7.
13. Brochard L, Mancebo J, Wysocki M, et al. Noninvasive ventilation for acute exacerbations of chronic obstructive pulmonary disease. N Engl J Med 1995;333:817–22.
14. Kramer N, Meyer TJ, Meharg J, et al. Randomized, prospective trial of noninvasive positive pressure ventilation in acute respiratory failure. Am J Respir Crit Care Med 1995;151:1799–806.

15. Plant PK, Owen JL, Elliott MW. Early use of non-invasive ventilation for acute exacerbations of chronic obstructive pulmonary disease on general respiratory wards: a multicentre randomised controlled trial. Lancet 2000;355:1931–5.

16. Ambrosino N, Foglio K, Rubini F, et al. Non-invasive mechanical ventilation in acute respiratory failure due to chronic obstructive pulmonary disease: correlates for success. Thorax 1995;50:755–7.

17. Myint PK, Lowe D, Stone RA, et al. National COPD resources and outcomes project 2008: patients with chronic obstructive pulmonary disease exacerbations who present with radiological pneumonia have worse outcome compared to those with non-pneumonic chronic obstructive pulmonary disease exacerbations. Respiration 2011;82:320–7.

18. Soo Hoo GW, Santiago S, Williams AJ. Nasal mechanical ventilation for hypercapnic respiratory failure in chronic obstructive pulmonary disease: determinants of success and failure. Crit Care Med 1994;22:1253–61.

19. Diaz GG, Alcaraz AC, Talavera JC, et al. Noninvasive positive-pressure ventilation to treat hypercapnic coma secondary to respiratory failure. Chest 2005;127:952–60.

20. Meduri GU, Turner RE, Abou-Shala N, et al. Noninvasive positive pressure ventilation via face mask. First-line intervention in patients with acute hypercapnic and hypoxemic respiratory failure. Chest 1996;109:179–93.

21. Wildman MJ, Sanderson C, Groves J, et al. Implications of prognostic pessimism in patients with chronic obstructive pulmonary disease (COPD) or asthma admitted to intensive care in the UK within the COPD and Asthma Outcome Study (CAOS): multicentre observational cohort study. BMJ 2007; 335:1132.

22. Fanfulla F, Delmastro M, Berardinelli A, et al. Effects of different ventilator settings on sleep and inspiratory effort in patients with neuromuscular disease. Am J Respir Crit Care Med 2005;172:619–24.

23. Miller SD, Elliott MW. High inspiratory pressures are tolerated by patients with acute COPD requiring noninvasive ventilation. Eur Respir J 2009;34:39s.

24. Miller SD, Elliott MW. The duration of non-invasive ventilation is associated with outcome in acute COPD. Eur Respir J 2009;34:39s.

25. Di Marco F, Centanni S, Bellone A, et al. Optimization of ventilator setting by flow and pressure waveforms analysis during noninvasive ventilation for acute exacerbations of COPD: a multicentric randomized controlled trial. Crit Care 2011;15: R283.

26. Connors AF Jr, Dawson NV, Thomas C, et al. Outcomes following acute exacerbation of severe chronic obstructive lung disease. The SUPPORT investigators (Study to Understand Prognoses and Preferences for Outcomes and Risks of Treatments). Am J Respir Crit Care Med 1996;154: 959–67.

27. Murray I, Paterson E, Thain G, et al. Outcomes following non-invasive ventilation for hypercapnic exacerbations of chronic obstructive pulmonary disease. Thorax 2011;66:825–6.

28. Hamnegard CH, Polkey MI, Kyroussis D, et al. Maximum rate of change in oesophageal pressure assessed from unoccluded breaths: an option where mouth occlusion pressure is impractical. Eur Respir J 1998;12:693–7.

29. Montes de Oca M, Celli BR. Mouth occlusion pressure, CO_2 response and hypercapnia in severe chronic obstructive pulmonary disease. Eur Respir J 1998;12:666–71.

30. Jolley CJ, Luo YM, Steier J, et al. Neural respiratory drive in healthy subjects and in COPD. Eur Respir J 2009;33:289–97.

31. Nickol AH, Hart N, Hopkinson NS, et al. Mechanisms of improvement of respiratory failure in patients with COPD treated with NIV. Int J Chron Obstruct Pulmon Dis 2008;3:453–62.

32. Elliott MW, Mulvey DA, Moxham J, et al. Domiciliary nocturnal nasal intermittent positive pressure ventilation in COPD: mechanisms underlying changes in arterial blood gas tensions. Eur Respir J 1991; 4:1044–52.

33. Read DJ. A clinical method for assessing the ventilatory response to carbon dioxide. Australas Ann Med 1967;16:20–32.

34. Whitelaw WA, Derenne JP, Milic-Emili J. Occlusion pressure as a measure of respiratory center output in conscious man. Respir Physiol 1975;23:181–99.

35. Nava S, Fanfulla F, Frigerio P, et al. Physiologic evaluation of 4 weeks of nocturnal nasal positive pressure ventilation in stable hypercapnic patients with chronic obstructive pulmonary disease. Respiration 2001;68:573–83.

36. Diaz O, Begin P, Torrealba B, et al. Effects of noninvasive ventilation on lung hyperinflation in stable hypercapnic COPD. Eur Respir J 2002;20:1490–8.

37. Moore AJ, Soler RS, Cetti EJ, et al. Sniff nasal inspiratory pressure versus IC/TLC ratio as predictors of mortality in COPD. Respir Med 2010;104: 1319–25.

38. Diaz O, Begin P, Andresen M, et al. Physiological and clinical effects of diurnal noninvasive ventilation in hypercapnic COPD. Eur Respir J 2005;26: 1016–23.

39. Laveneziana P, Webb KA, Ora J, et al. Evolution of dyspnea during exercise in chronic obstructive pulmonary disease: impact of critical volume constraints. Am J Respir Crit Care Med 2011;184: 1367–73.

40. Stubbings AK, Moore AJ, Dusmet M, et al. Physiological properties of human diaphragm muscle

fibres and the effect of chronic obstructive pulmonary disease. J Physiol 2008;586:2637–50.

41. Levine S, Kaiser L, Leferovich J, et al. Cellular adaptations in the diaphragm in chronic obstructive pulmonary disease. N Engl J Med 1997;337:1799–806.

42. Polkey MI, Kyroussis D, Hamnegard CH, et al. Diaphragm performance during maximal voluntary ventilation in chronic obstructive pulmonary disease. Am J Respir Crit Care Med 1997;155:642–8.

43. Laghi F, Cattapan SE, Jubran A, et al. Is weaning failure caused by low-frequency fatigue of the diaphragm? Am J Respir Crit Care Med 2003;167:120–7.

44. Clini E, Sturani C, Rossi A, et al. The Italian multicentre study on noninvasive ventilation in chronic obstructive pulmonary disease patients. Eur Respir J 2002;20:529–38.

45. Casanova C, Celli BR, Tost L, et al. Long-term controlled trial of nocturnal nasal positive pressure ventilation in patients with severe COPD. Chest 2000;118:1582–90.

46. Shapiro SH, Ernst P, Gray-Donald K, et al. Effect of negative pressure ventilation in severe chronic obstructive pulmonary disease. Lancet 1992;340:1425–9.

47. Wijkstra PJ, Lacasse Y, Guyatt GH, et al. Nocturnal non-invasive positive pressure ventilation for stable chronic obstructive pulmonary disease. Cochrane Database Syst Rev 2002;(3):CD002878.

48. Strumpf DA, Millman RP, Carlisle CC, et al. Nocturnal positive-pressure ventilation via nasal mask in patients with severe chronic obstructive pulmonary disease. Am Rev Respir Dis 1991;144:1234–9.

49. Fleetham JA, Forkert L, Clarke H, et al. Regional lung function in the presence of pleural symphysis. Am Rev Respir Dis 1980;122:33–8.

50. McEvoy RD, Pierce RJ, Hillman D, et al. Nocturnal non-invasive nasal ventilation in stable hypercapnic COPD: a randomised controlled trial. Thorax 2009;64:561–6.

51. De Angelis G, Sposato B, Mazzei L, et al. Predictive indexes of nocturnal desaturation in COPD patients not treated with long term oxygen therapy. Eur Rev Med Pharmacol Sci 2001;5:173–9.

52. Budweiser S, Jorres RA, Riedl T, et al. Predictors of survival in COPD patients with chronic hypercapnic respiratory failure receiving noninvasive home ventilation. Chest 2007;131:1650–8.

53. Murphy PB, Brignall K, Moxham J, et al. High pressure versus high intensity noninvasive ventilation in stable hypercapnic chronic obstructive pulmonary disease: a randomized crossover trial. Int J Chron Obstruct Pulmon Dis 2012;7:811–8.

54. Tuggey JM, Plant PK, Elliott MW. Domiciliary non-invasive ventilation for recurrent acidotic exacerbations of COPD: an economic analysis. Thorax 2003;58:867–71.

55. Cheung AP, Chan VL, Liong JT, et al. A pilot trial of non-invasive home ventilation after acidotic respiratory failure in chronic obstructive pulmonary disease. Int J Tuberc Lung Dis 2010;14:642–9.

56. Funk GC, Breyer MK, Burghuber OC, et al. Long-term non-invasive ventilation in COPD after acute-on-chronic respiratory failure. Respir Med 2011;105:427–34.

57. Ofir D, Laveneziana P, Webb KA, et al. Mechanisms of dyspnea during cycle exercise in symptomatic patients with gold stage I chronic obstructive pulmonary disease. Am J Respir Crit Care Med 2008;177:622–9.

58. O'Donnell DE, Banzett RB, Carrieri-Kohlman V, et al. Pathophysiology of dyspnea in chronic obstructive pulmonary disease: a roundtable. Proc Am Thorac Soc 2007;4:145–68.

59. Fessler H, Scharf S, Permutt S. Improvement in spirometry following lung volume reduction surgery. Application of a physiologic model. Am J Respir Crit Care Med 2002;165:34–40.

60. Sciurba FC, Rogers RM, Keenan RJ, et al. Improvement in pulmonary function and elastic recoil after lung-reduction surgery for diffuse emphysema. N Engl J Med 1996;334:1095–9.

61. Martinez FJ, de Oca MM, Whyte RI, et al. Lung-volume reduction improves dyspnea, dynamic hyperinflation, and respiratory muscle function. Am J Respir Crit Care Med 1997;155:1984–90.

62. Gorman RB, McKenzie DK, Butler JE, et al. Diaphragm length and neural drive after lung volume reduction surgery. Am J Respir Crit Care Med 2005;172:1259–66.

63. Lando Y, Boiselle PM, Shade D, et al. Effect of lung volume reduction surgery on diaphragm length in severe chronic obstructive pulmonary disease. Am J Respir Crit Care Med 1999;159:796–805.

64. Bloch Konrad E, Li Y, Zhang J, et al. Effect of surgical lung volume reduction on breathing patterns in severe pulmonary emphysema. Am J Respir Crit Care Med 1997;156:553–60.

65. Jorgensen K, Houltz E, Westfelt U, et al. Effects of lung volume reduction surgery on left ventricular diastolic filling and dimensions in patients with severe emphysema. Chest 2003;124:1863–70.

66. Snider GL. Reduction pneumoplasty for giant bullous emphysema. Implications for surgical treatment of nonbullous emphysema. Chest 1996;109:540–8.

67. Martinez FJ, Chang A. Surgical therapy for chronic obstructive pulmonary disease. Semin Respir Crit Care Med 2005;26:167–91.

68. Schipper PH, Meyers BF, Battafarano RJ, et al. Outcomes after resection of giant emphysematous

bullae. Ann Thorac Surg 2004;78:976–82 [discussion: 976–82].

69. Shah SS, Goldstraw P. Surgical treatment of bullous emphysema: experience with the Brompton technique. Ann Thorac Surg 1994;58:1452–6.

70. Brantigan OC. Surgical treatment of pulmonary emphysema. Md State Med J 1957;6:409–14.

71. Cooper JD, Trulock EP, Triantafillou AN, et al. Bilateral pneumectomy (volume reduction) for chronic obstructive pulmonary disease. J Thorac Cardiovasc Surg 1995;109:106–16 [discussion: 116–9].

72. Criner GJ, Cordova FC, Furukawa S, et al. Prospective randomized trial comparing bilateral lung volume reduction surgery to pulmonary rehabilitation in severe chronic obstructive pulmonary disease. Am J Respir Crit Care Med 1999;160:2018–27.

73. Geddes D, Davies M, Koyama H, et al. Effect of lung-volume-reduction surgery in patients with severe emphysema. N Engl J Med 2000;343:239–45.

74. Al-Hadithy N, Zoumot Z, Parida S, et al. Panton-Valentine leukocidin pneumonia: an emerging threat. Clin Respir J 2010;4:61–4.

75. Fishman A, Martinez F, Naunheim K, et al, National Emphysema Treatment Trial Research Group. A randomized trial comparing lung-volume-reduction surgery with medical therapy for severe emphysema. N Engl J Med 2003;348:2059–73.

76. Naunheim KS, Wood DE, Krasna MJ, et al. Predictors of operative mortality and cardiopulmonary morbidity in the national emphysema treatment trial. J Thorac Cardiovasc Surg 2006;131:43–53.

77. Lim E, Ali A, Cartwright N, et al. Effect and duration of lung volume reduction surgery: mid-term results of the Brompton trial. Thorac Cardiovasc Surg 2006;54:188–92.

78. Ramsey SD, Berry K, Etzioni R, et al. Cost effectiveness of lung-volume-reduction surgery for patients with severe emphysema. N Engl J Med 2003;348:2092–102.

79. Oey IF, Morgan MD, Singh SJ, et al. The long-term health status improvements seen after lung volume reduction surgery. Eur J Cardiothorac Surg 2003;24:614–9.

80. Palla A, Desideri M, Rossi G, et al. Elective surgery for giant bullous emphysema: a 5-year clinical and functional follow-up. Chest 2005;128:2043–50.

81. Celli BR, MacNee W, Agusti A, et al. Standards for the diagnosis and treatment of patients with COPD: a summary of the ATS/ERS position paper. Eur Respir J 2004;23:932–46.

82. Management of chronic obstructive pulmonary disease in adults in primary and secondary care (partial update). This guideline partially updates and replaces nice clinical guideline 12. 2010. Available at: http://guidance.nice.org.uk/CG101. Accessed March 2013.

83. Toma TP, Hopkinson NS, Hillier J, et al. Bronchoscopic volume reduction with valve implants in patients with severe emphysema. Lancet 2003;361:931–3.

84. Hopkinson NS, Toma TP, Hansell DM, et al. Effect of bronchoscopic lung volume reduction on dynamic hyperinflation and exercise in emphysema. Am J Respir Crit Care Med 2005;171:453–60.

85. Hopkinson NS, Kemp SV, Toma TP, et al. Atelectasis and survival after bronchoscopic lung volume reduction for COPD. Eur Respir J 2011;37:1346–51.

86. Sciurba FC, Ernst A, Herth FJ, et al. A randomized study of endobronchial valves for advanced emphysema. N Engl J Med 2010;363:1233–44.

87. Gompelmann D, Eberhardt R, Michaud G, et al. Predicting atelectasis by assessment of collateral ventilation prior to endobronchial lung volume reduction: a feasibility study. Respiration 2010;80:419–25.

88. Springmeyer SC, Bolliger CT, Waddell TK, et al. Treatment of heterogeneous emphysema using the Spiration IBV valves. Thorac Surg Clin 2009;19:247–53, ix–x.

89. Eberhardt R, Gompelmann D, Schuhmann M, et al. Complete unilateral vs partial bilateral endoscopic lung volume reduction in patients with bilateral lung emphysema. Chest 2012;142:900–8.

90. Herth FJ, Gompelmann D, Stanzel F, et al. Treatment of advanced emphysema with emphysematous lung sealant (AeriSeal®). Respiration 2011;82:36–45.

91. Magnussen H, Kramer MR, Kirsten AM, et al. Effect of fissure integrity on lung volume reduction using a polymer sealant in advanced emphysema. Thorax 2012;67:302–8.

92. Snell G, Herth FJ, Hopkins P, et al. Bronchoscopic thermal vapour ablation therapy in the management of heterogeneous emphysema. Eur Respir J 2012;39:1326–33.

93. Herth FJ, Eberhard R, Gompelmann D, et al. Bronchoscopic lung volume reduction with a dedicated coil: a clinical pilot study. Ther Adv Respir Dis 2010;4:225–31.

94. Slebos DJ, Klooster K, Ernst A, et al. Bronchoscopic lung volume reduction coil treatment of patients with severe heterogeneous emphysema. Chest 2012;142:574–82.

95. Shah PL, Zoumot Z, Singh S, et al. Endobronchial coils for the treatment of severe emphysema with hyperinflation (RESET): a randomised controlled trial. Lancet 2013;1:233–40.

96. Lausberg HF, Chino K, Patterson GA, et al. Bronchial fenestration improves expiratory flow in emphysematous human lungs. Ann Thorac Surg 2003;75:393–7.

97. Sybrecht GW, Shah P, Slebos DJ, et al. Exhale airway stents for emphysema (ease) trial: safety and procedural outcomes for airway bypass. Eur Respir J 2009;35:A4129.

98. Moore AJ, Cetti E, Haj-Yahia S, et al. Unilateral extrapulmonary airway bypass in advanced emphysema. Ann Thorac Surg 2010;89:899–906, 906.e1–2.

99. Wan IY, Toma TP, Geddes DM, et al. Broncho-scopic lung volume reduction for end-stage emphysema: report on the first 98 patients. Chest 2006;129:518–26.

100. Herth FJ, Noppen M, Valipour A, et al. Efficacy predictors of lung volume reduction with Zephyr valves in a European cohort. Eur Respir J 2012; 39:1334–42.

101. Kramer MR, Refaely Y, Maimon N, et al. Bilateral endoscopic sealant lung volume reduction ther-apy for advanced emphysema. Chest 2012;142: 1111–7.

102. Zoumot Z, Kemp SV, Caneja C, et al. Broncho-scopic intrabullous autologous blood instillation; a novel approach for the treatment of giant bullae. Ann Thorac Surg 2013;96:1488–91.

Index

Note: Page numbers of article titles are in **boldface** type.

A

AATD. See Alpha1-antitrypsin deficiency (AATD)
Acidosis
  hypercapnic
    COPD–cardiovascular disease and, 104–105
Acute hypercapnic respiratory failure
  NIV during, 252–253
Acute phase proteins
  in COPD, 79
Acute phase reactants regulated by IL-6
  as biomarkers in COPD, 135–136
Aging
  accelerated
    in COPD, 80
  as factor in COPD
    management of, 230
Air pollution
  COPD related to, 9
  indoor
    exposure to
      COPD related to, 20–22
  outdoor
    COPD related to, 24
Airway fibrosis
  in COPD, 80
Airway hyperresponsiveness
  in asthma and COPD, 146–147
Airway obstruction and reversibility
  in asthma and COPD, 145–146
Airways bypass stents
  for emphysema, 263–265
Alpha1-antitrypsin deficiency (AATD), **39–50**
  augmentation of, 43–45
  biomarkers of, 46–47
  clinical impact of, 40–41
  introduction, 39
  pathophysiology of, 41–43
  prevalence of, 39–40
  treatment of, 46
Anemia
  COPD and, 113–115
    management of, 115
    pathogenesis of, 113, 115
    prevalence of, 113
Antibiotics. See Antimicrobial agents
Antiinfective agents
  in COPD management, 223–228
Antiinflammatory agents
  in COPD management, 223–228

Antimicrobial agents
  in COPD management, 223–225
    CAP related to, 92
  long-term
    in prevention of acute exacerbations of COPD, 161
Antimicrobial peptides
  chronic infection in COPD related to, 94–95
Antimuscarinic agents
  in COPD management, 192–193
Antioxidants
  in COPD management, 228–229
Antiviral agents
  in COPD management, 225
Asthma
  COPD and, **143–156**
    airway hyperresponsiveness in, 146–147
    airway obstruction and reversibility in, 145–146
    atopy in, 146
    clinical features of, 144–148
    definitions related to, 144
    environment in, 148–150
    genetics in, 148–150
    inflammation in, 150–151
    introduction, 143–144
    overlap phenotype in, 147–148
    pharmacologic responses in, 151–152
    symptoms of, 144–145
  defined, 144
Atopy
  in asthma and COPD, 146
Autoimmunity
  as factor in COPD
    management of, 230
Autonomic dysfunction
  COPD and, 115

B

β_2-agonists
  in COPD management, 192
Bacteria
  exacerbation of acute infection in COPD due to, 89–90
  with virus
    exacerbation of acute infection in COPD due to, 91
Biologic agents
  in COPD management, 230

Clin Chest Med 35 (2014) 271–278
http://dx.doi.org/10.1016/S0272-5231(13)00188-3
0272-5231/14/$ – see front matter © 2014 Elsevier Inc. All rights reserved.

Biomarker(s)
  of AATD, 46–47
  in COPD, **131–141**
    current status, 133–138
      acute phase reactants regulated by IL-6, 135–136
      fibrinogen, 133–135
    defined, 132
    emerging, 136
    future directions in, 138–139
    general concepts, 131–132
    inflammome, 137–138
    introduction, 131
    pneumoproteins, 136–137
    requirements for, 132
    of therapeutic responses, 137
Bronchodilator(s)
  classes of, 192–193
  in COPD management, **191–201**
    antimuscarinic agents, 192–193
    β_2-agonists, 192
    choice of
      determining factors in, 193–195
    future developments in, 195–198
    importance of, 191
    methylxanthines, 193
    new traditional, 196–198
    novel classes in, 195–196
  dual
    in prevention of acute exacerbations of COPD, 160–161
  inhaled
    in COPD management, 222–223
  long-acting
    in prevention of acute exacerbations of COPD, 159–160
Bronchoscopic LVR
  for emphysema, 260–265
Bronchoscopic thermal vapor ablation (BTVA)
  for emphysema, 262
BTVA. See Bronchoscopic thermal vapor ablation (BTVA)
Bupropion
  in smoking cessation, 171

C

Calcification paradox
  COPD–related osteoporosis related to, 111
CAMP-induced, adverse-effect genes, 212
Cancer
  lung
    COPD and, 115–117. See also Lung cancer, COPD and
Candidate antiinflammatory genes
  in COPD of severe, bronchitic, frequent exacerbator phenotype, 209–212

CAP. See Community-acquired pneumonia (CAP)
Cardiovascular disease
  COPD and, 101–107
    complications of, 105–106
      interventions for, 106–107
    pathogenesis of, 102–105
    prevalence of, 102
Chemoattractant receptor-homologous receptor antagonism
  in COPD management, 226
Chemokine(s)
  in mediation of inflammation in COPD, 76
Chemokine receptor antagonists
  in COPD management, 226
Chronic hypercapnic respiratory failure
  domiciliary NIV for, 253–255
Chronic obstructive pulmonary disease (COPD), **1–16**
  AATD and, **39–50**. See also Alpha1-antitrypsin deficiency (AATD)
  acute exacerbations of, **157–163**
    causes of, 158–159
    definition of, 157–158
    frequent phenotype, 159
    impact of, 157
    management of, 161–162, 177–179
    pathogenesis of, 158–159
    prevention of, 159–161
      dual bronchodilators in, 160–161
      home oxygen in, 161
      inhaled corticosteroids in, 159–160
      long-acting bronchodilators in, 159–160
      long-term antibiotics in, 161
      PDE inhibitors in, 161
      pulmonary rehabilitation in, 161
      vaccines in, 159
      ventilatory support in, 161
  airflow limitation and reversibility in
    measures of, 8
  asthma and, **143–156**. See also Asthma, COPD and
  biomarkers in, **131–141**. See also Biomarker(s), in COPD
  burden of, 11–14
  cellular and molecular mechanisms of, **71–86**
    dendritic cells, 74
    eosinophils, 74
    epithelial cells, 72
    inflammatory cells, 72
      mediators of, 75–76
    introduction, 71
    macrophages, 72–74
    management of
      implications for future therapy, 80–82
        disease phenotypes, 81–82
        need for biomarkers, 81
        new antiinflammatory therapies, 81
        new pathways, 81

reversal of corticosteroid resistance,
80–81
treating acute exacerbations, 82
neutrophils, 74
oxidative stress, 77–78
proteases, 76
T lymphocytes, 75
chronic exacerbations of
management of, 179
classification of, 101
clinical features of, 8
clinical integrative physiology of, **51–69**
introduction, 51
mild COPD, 51–56
clinical relevance, 51–52
exercise responses, 54–56
resting physiologic abnormalities, 52–54
small airways dysfunction, 52–53
ventilation-perfusion abnormalities, 53–54
moderate-to-severe COPD, 56–61
exercise responses, 57–61
resting physiologic abnormalities, 56–57
comorbidities of, **101–130**. *See also specific*
types, e.g., Cardiovascular disease, COPD and
anemia, 113–115
autonomic dysfunction, 115
cardiovascular disease, 101–107
diabetes, 117–118
lung cancer, 115–117
metabolic syndrome, 117–118
nutritional abnormalities, 111–112
obesity, 112–113
OSA, 112–113
osteoporosis, 109–111
psychological illnesses, 117
skeletal muscle dysfunction, 107–109
defined, 1–2, 7–8
diagnostic criteria for, 2–3
future
considerations for, 3–4
dyspnea in
physiologic mechanisms of, 61–62
extrapulmonary consequences of
screening for, 246
fibrosis associated with
management of, 229–230
genetics in, 9, **29–38**. *See also* Genetic(s), in
COPD
infections in
role of, **87–100**. *See also* Infection(s), in COPD
inflammation in. *See* Inflammation
as inflammatory disease, 72
introduction, 7, 51, 71, 101, 203–204, 251
management of, **177–189**
for acute exacerbations, 177–179
aging- and autoimmunity-related, 230
alternative therapies in, 183–184

antimicrobial therapy in
CAP related to, 92
bronchodilators in, **191–201**. *See also*
Bronchodilator(s), in COPD management
chemoattractant receptor-homologous
receptor antagonism in, 226
for chronic exacerbations, 179
emerging issues in, 184–185
evidence-based therapy in, 182
initial drug therapy in, 183
introduction, 177
lung regeneration in, 230–231
LVR in, **255–265**. *See also* Left volume
reduction (LVR)
new drugs, **219–239**
agents acting on innate immunity, 225–226
antiinfective agents, 223–228
antiinflammatory agents, 223–228
antioxidants, 228–229
antiviral agents, 225
biologics, 230
chemokine receptor antagonists, 226
ICSs, 222–223
inhaled bronchodilators, 222–223
introduction, 219–220
kinase inhibitors, 227
LAMAs, 222–223
LTB_4 receptor antagonists, 226
mucoactive drugs, 229
PDE4 inhibitors in, 226–227
proteases, 229
selectin antagonism, 226
statins, 227–228
NIV in, **251–255**. *See also* Noninvasive
ventilation (NIV)
patient evaluation in, 182–183
pulmonary rehabilitation in, **241–249**. *See also*
Pulmonary rehabilitation, in COPD
management
smoking cessation in, **165–176**. *See also*
Smoking cessation
steroid resistance in, 223
mortality data, 11–14, 101
occupational, 22–24
overlap syndromes, 8
pathology of, 71–72
phenotypes of, 4–5
physical activity and, 247
prevalence of, **9–11**
criteria for, 9–10
estimates, 10–11
gender differences in, 11
risk factors for, 8–9
air pollution, 9
cigarette smoking, 8–9
environmental, **17–27**
indoor air pollutants, 20–22

Chronic (*continued*)
      indoor biomass fuel smoke, 20–21
      introduction, 17–18
      outdoor air pollution, 24
      second-hand smoke, 19–20
    genetics, 9
    occupational, 9
  of severe, bronchitic, frequent exacerbator
    phenotype
      PDE4 inhibitors in, **203–217**. *See also*
        Phosphodiesterase 4 (PDE4) inhibitors, in
        COPD of severe, bronchitic, frequent
        exacerbator phenotype
    severe exacerbations of, 247
    symptoms of, 247
    systemic effects of, **101–130**
      inflammation, 78–79, 117–121
Cigarette smoking
  cessation of, **165–176**. *See also* Smoking
    cessation
  COPD related to, 8–9
  COPD–related cardiovascular disease and, 104
Cluster of differentiation 200
  in COPD of severe, bronchitic, frequent
    exacerbator phenotype, 210
Community-acquired pneumonia (CAP)
  exacerbation of acute infection in COPD due to,
    91–92
COPD. *See* Chronic obstructive pulmonary disease
  (COPD)
Corticosteroid(s)
  COPD–related osteoporosis related to, 110
  inhaled. *See* Inhaled corticosteroids (ICSs)
CRISPLD2
  in COPD of severe, bronchitic, frequent
    exacerbator phenotype, 210
Cylindromatosis, 211
Cytokines
  in COPD, 79
  in mediation of inflammation in COPD, 75–76

D

Dendritic cells
  in COPD, 74
Depression
  COPD and, 117
Diabetes
  COPD and, 117–118
Dyspnea
  in COPD
    physiologic mechanisms of, 61–62

E

ECM. *See* Extracellular matrix (ECM)
Emphysema

  management of
    LVR in, **255–265**. *See also* Left volume
      reduction (LVR)
Environment
  as factor in asthma, 148–150
  as factor in COPD, **17–27,** 148–150
Environmental tobacco smoke
  COPD related to, 19–20
Eosinophils
  in COPD, 74
Epithelial cells
  in COPD, 72
Exercise
  in mild COPD
    responses to, 54–56
      cardiocirculatory impairment, 54–56
      dynamic respiratory mechanics
        impairment, 54
      high ventilatory requirements, 54
      skeletal muscle dysfunction, 56
  in moderate-to-severe COPD
    responses to, 57–61
      cardiocirculatory impairment, 59–61
      dynamic respiratory mechanics across
        continuum of COPD, 58
      increased central respiratory drive, 57–58
      skeletal muscle dysfunction, 61
Extracellular matrix (ECM)
  in genetic susceptibility in COPD, 30–31

F

Farming
  COPD related to, 22–23
Fibrinogen
  as biomarker in COPD, 133–135
Fibrosis
  airway
    in COPD, 80
  COPD and
    management of, 229–230

G

Gender
  as factor in COPD, 11
Gene therapies
  for AATD, 46
Gene transactivation
  in COPD of severe, bronchitic, frequent
    exacerbator phenotype
      glucocorticoid resistance and, 205–207, 212
Generalized anxiety disorder
  COPD and, 117
Genetic(s)
  in asthma, 148–150
  cAMP-induced, adverse-effect genes, 212

in COPD, 9, **29–38,** 148–150
 candidate gene approaches, 30–34
  ECM, 30–31
  inflammation, 33–34
  protease-antiprotease balance, 31–32
  reactive oxygen species, 32–33
 introduction, 29–30
 unbiased approaches, 30
GILZ. *See* Glucocorticoid-induced leucine zipper
 (GILZ)
Glucocorticoid-induced leucine zipper (GILZ)
 in COPD of severe, bronchitic, frequent
  exacerbator phenotype, 209–210
Glucocorticoid resistance
 gene transactivation and
  in COPD of severe, bronchitic, frequent
   exacerbator phenotype, 212
Growth factors
 in mediation of inflammation in COPD, 76

H

Home oxygen
 in prevention of acute exacerbations of COPD,
  161
Hypercapnic acidosis
 COPD–related cardiovascular disease and,
  104–105
Hypoxia
 COPD–related cardiovascular disease and, 104

I

ICSs. *See* Inhaled corticosteroids (ICSs)
IL-6. *See* Interleukin-6 (IL-6)
Immunoglobulin A
 chronic infection in COPD related to, 94
Indoor air pollutants
 exposure to
  COPD related to, 20–22
Indoor biomass fuel smoke
 exposure to
  COPD related to, 20–21
Infection(s)
 in COPD, **87–100**
  acute infection, 88–92
   CAP, 91–92
   causes of exacerbations, 88–91
  chronic infection, 92–96
   antimicrobial peptides and, 94–95
   evidence for, 93–94
   host defects, 94–96
   immunoglobulin A and, 94
   macrophage function and, 95–96
   mechanism of increased susceptibility to,
    94
   mucociliary clearance and, 94

   pathogen mechanisms in, 96
   vicious-cycle hypothesis, 92
  future directions in, 96
  introduction, 87–88
Inflammation
 in asthma, 150–151
 in COPD, 72, 117–121, 150–151
  defective resolution of, 79–80
  mediators of, 75–76
  network approach to, 137–138
  systemic, 78–79
 COPD–related cardiovascular disease and,
  102–104
 COPD–related osteoporosis related to, 110
 in genetic susceptibility in COPD, 33–34
Inflammatory cells
 in COPD, 72
Inflammome
 as biomarker in COPD, 137–138
Inhaled bronchodilators
 in COPD management, 222–223
Inhaled corticosteroids (ICSs)
 CAP in COPD related to, 91–92
 in COPD management, 179–182, 222–223
 in prevention of acute exacerbations of COPD,
  159–160
Innate immunity
 agents acting on
  in COPD management, 225–226
Interleukin-6 (IL-6)
 acute phase reactants regulated by
  as biomarkers in COPD, 135–136

K

Kinase inhibitors
 in COPD management, 227

L

Left volume reduction (LVR)
 bronchoscopic
  for emphysema, 260–265
   airways bypass stents, 263–265
   biologic LVR, 261–262
   BTVA, 262
   endobronchial airway valves, 260–265
   RePneu LVR coils, 262–263
 in COPD management, **255–265**
  for emphysema, **255–265**
   physiologic basis of, 255–260
Lipid mediators
 in COPD, 75
 proresolving
  in COPD, 80
LTB$_4$ receptor antagonists
 in COPD management, 226

Lung cancer
   COPD and, 115–117
      clinical implications of, 116–117
      pathogenesis of, 116–117
      prevalence of, 115–116
Lung regeneration
   in COPD management, 230–231
LVR. See Left volume reduction (LVR)
Lymphocyte(s)
   T
      in COPD, 75

M

Macrophage(s)
   in COPD, 72–74
   function of
      chronic infection in COPD related to, 95–96
Metabolic syndrome
   COPD and, 117–118
Methylxanthines
   in COPD management, 193
Mining
   COPD related to, 23
Mitogen-activated protein kinase phosphatase 1
   in COPD of severe, bronchitic, frequent
      exacerbator phenotype, 209
Mucoactive drugs
   in COPD management, 229
Mucociliary clearance
   chronic infection in COPD related to, 94

N

Neutrophils
   in COPD, 74
Nicotine inhaler
   in smoking cessation, 170–171
Nicotine nasal spray
   in smoking cessation, 171
Nicotine polacrilex gum
   in smoking cessation, 170
Nicotine polacrilex lozenge
   in smoking cessation, 170
Nicotine replacement therapy (NRT)
   in smoking cessation, 169–172
      bupropion, 171
      combinations, 171
      nicotine inhaler, 170–171
      nicotine nasal spray, 171
      nicotine polacrilex gum, 170
      nicotine polacrilex lozenge, 170
      off-label agents, 172
      transdermal nicotine, 170
      varenicline, 171–172
NIV. See Noninvasive ventilation (NIV)
Noninvasive ventilation (NIV)

in COPD management, **251–255**
   during acute hypercapnic respiratory failure,
      252–253
   described, 251–252
   domiciliary
      in COPD management
         for chronic hypercapnic respiratory failure,
         253–255
NRT. See Nicotine replacement therapy (NRT)
Nutritional abnormalities
   COPD and, 111–112

O

Obesity
   COPD and, 112–113
Obstructive sleep apnea (OSA)
   COPD and, 112–113
Occupational COPD, 22–24
OSA. See Obstructive sleep apnea (OSA)
Osteoporosis
   COPD and, 109–111
      contributors to, 110–111
      interventions for, 111
      prevalence of, 110
Outdoor air pollution
   COPD related to, 24
Overlap phenotype
   in asthma and COPD, 147–148
Oxidative stress
   in COPD, 77–78
Oxygen
   home
      in prevention of acute exacerbations of COPD,
      161

P

PDE4 inhibitors. See Phosphodiesterase 4 (PDE4)
   inhibitors
Phosphodiesterase 4 (PDE4) inhibitors
   in COPD management, 226–227
   in COPD of severe, bronchitic, frequent
      exacerbator phenotype, **203–217**
      cAMP-induced, adverse-effect genes, 212
      candidate antiinflammatory genes, 209–212
      cluster of differentiation 200, 210
      CRISPLD2, 210
      cylindromatosis, 211
      GILZ, 209–210
      mitogen-activated protein kinase
         phosphatase 1, 209
      p57^{kip2}, 211
      RGS 2, 210
      SOCS 3, 211
      tristetraprolin, 211–212
      described, 204–205

future directions in, 212–213
gene transactivation in, 205–207
glucocorticoid resistance and, 212
triple combination therapy for, 205
why ICS/LABA combination therapies are not
enough, 207–209
in prevention of acute exacerbations of COPD,
161
Physical activity
COPD effects on, 247
p57^{kip2}
in COPD of severe, bronchitic, frequent
exacerbator phenotype, 211
Pneumonia(s)
community-acquired
exacerbation of acute infection in COPD due
to, 91–92
Pneumoproteins
as biomarkers in COPD, 136–137
Polycythemia
COPD–related cardiovascular disease and, 104
Protease(s)
in COPD, 76
in COPD management, 229
Protease-antiprotease balance
in genetic susceptibility in COPD, 31–32
Psychological illnesses
COPD and, 117
Pulmonary rehabilitation
in COPD management, **241–249**
evidence base for, 242–243
introduction, 241–242
maintaining effects of, 247–248
organization of, 243
patient screening and selection for, 245–247
program content, 243–245
defined, 241–242
in prevention of acute exacerbations of COPD,
161

Q

Quarrying
COPD related to, 23

R

Reactive oxygen species
in genetic susceptibility in COPD, 32–33
Regulators of G-protein signaling (RGS) 2
in COPD of severe, bronchitic, frequent
exacerbator phenotype, 210
Rehabilitation
pulmonary. See Pulmonary rehabilitation
RePneu LVR coils
for emphysema, 262–263

S

Secretion strategies
for AATD, 46
Selectin antagonism
in COPD management, 226
Skeletal muscle
COPD effects on, 107–109
Smoke
indoor biomass fuel
exposure to
COPD related to, 20–21
second-hand
COPD related to, 19–20
Smoking
cessation of, **165–176**. See also Smoking
cessation
COPD related to, 8–9, **17–27**
COPD–related cardiovascular disease and, 104
physiology of, 165–167
Smoking cessation, **165–176**
approach to, 167–168
in COPD management
drugs to aid, 221–222
in harm reduction, 172–173
introduction, 165
pharmacotherapy in, 169–172
NRT, 169–172
strategy for, 168–169
SOCS 3. See Suppressor of cytokine signaling
(SOCS) 3
Statins
in COPD management, 227–228
Steel industries
COPD related to, 23
Stress
oxidative
in COPD, 77–78
Suppressor of cytokine signaling (SOCS) 3
in COPD of severe, bronchitic, frequent
exacerbator phenotype, 211
Systemic inflammation
in COPD, 78–79

T

T lymphocytes
in COPD, 75
Tobacco smoke
environmental
COPD related to, 19–20
Tobacco smoking. See also Smoking; Smoking
cessation
COPD related to, **17–27**
Transdermal nicotine
in smoking cessation, 170

Tristetraprolin
    in COPD of severe, bronchitic, frequent
        exacerbator phenotype, 211–212

V

Vaccine(s)
    in prevention of acute exacerbations of COPD, 159
Varenicline
    in smoking cessation, 171–172
Vascular endothelial function/vessel wall
    abnormalities in
        COPD–related cardiovascular disease and, 105

Ventilation
    noninvasive
        in COPD management, **251–255**. *See also*
            Noninvasive ventilation (NIV)
Ventilatory support
    in prevention of acute exacerbations of COPD,
        161
Virus(es)
    with bacteria
        exacerbation of acute infection in COPD due
            to, 91
        exacerbation of acute infection in COPD due to,
            88–89

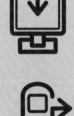

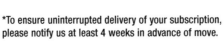

Printed and bound by CPI Group (UK) Ltd, Croydon, CR0 4YY

03/10/2024

01040309-0007